Basic and Clinical Neurocardiology

Basic and Clinical Neurocardiology

Edited by
J. Andrew Armour
Jeffrey L. Ardell

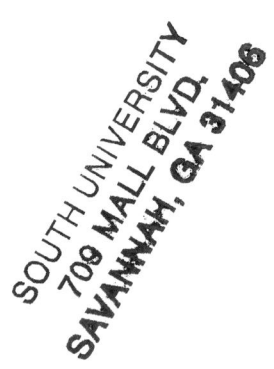

OXFORD
UNIVERSITY PRESS
2004

OXFORD
UNIVERSITY PRESS

Oxford   New York
Auckland   Bangkok   Buenos Aires   Cape Town   Chennai
Dar es Salaam   Delhi   Hong Kong   Istanbul   Karachi   Kolkata
Kuala Lumpar   Madrid   Melbourne   Mexico City   Mumbai   Nairobi
São Paulo   Shanghai   Taipei   Tokyo   Toronto

Copyright © 2004 by Oxford University Press, Inc.

Published by Oxford University Press, Inc.
198 Madison Avenue, New York, New York 10016
http://www.oup.com

Oxford is a registered trademark of Oxford University Press

All rights reserved. No part of this publication may be reproduced,
stored in a retrieval system, or transmitted, in any form or by any means,
electronic, mechanical, photocopying, recording, or otherwise,
without the prior permission of Oxford University Press.

Library of Congress Cataloging-in-Publication Data
Basic and clinical neurocardiology /
edited by J. Andrew Armour, Jeffrey L. Ardell.
p. ; cm.   Includes bibliographical references and index.
ISBN 0-19-514129-6
1. Cardiovascular system—Diseases—Complications.
2. Cardiological manifestations of general diseases.
3. Neurological manifestations of general diseases.
4. Heart—Innervation.   5. Heart—Pathophysiology.
I. Armour, J. Andrew. II. Ardell, Jeffrey L.
[DNLM: 1. Cardiovascular System—innervation.
2. Autonomic Nervous System—physiology.
3. Cardiovascular System—physiopathology. 4. Neurotransmitters—physiology.
WG 102 B311 2004]   RC682.B286 2004   616.1—dc22   2003062220

9 8 7 6 5 4 3 2 1
Printed in the United States of America
on acid-free paper

Preface

Understanding the neurohumoral basis of reflex control of the diseased heart is critical to determining why some patients experience sudden death while others sustain life when cardiac function is severely compromised. Ischemic heart disease represents competing processes characterized by the activation of multiple systems, including the autonomic nervous system, which coordinate regional cardiac function. Neurohumoral derangement produced by cardiac stressors can initiate heart damage, and we now know that therapy with β-adrenoceptor blockers or ACE inhibitors significantly reduces the incidence of death from myocardial infarction. Accordingly, the hypothesis has been put forward that remodeling of the cardiac nervous system plays a critical role in the development of overt signs and symptoms associated with specific cardiac diseases instead of merely being a response to the disease process. Indeed, it is now recognized that neurohumoral remodeling of the cardiac neuronal axis occurs before overt signs of cardiac disease become manifest, thereby affecting prognosis and clinical management. The American Heart Association and the American College of Cardiology have issued a consensus statement about the staging of congestive heart failure that is based on the clinical observation that among patients with risk factors for heart failure are those characterized by excessive activation of the cardiac sympathetic efferent neurons and the renin-angiotensin system.

Recently, evidence for the relevance of the autonomic nervous system in cardiac disease has given neurocardiology a more therapeutic perspective.[4] This has been driven in large part by the recognition that complex, synergistic interactions among neurons located throughout the cardiac neuronal axis help to maintain cardiac output over a lifetime. During the last decade the complexity of the reflex arcs involved in the ongoing coordination of regional cardiac function has begun to emerge. Building on data presented in our 1994 book,[1] we have focused this volume on changes over the last decade in our understanding of cardiac control in health and disease. Central to this changing view is the realization that transduction of the cardiac milieu to cardiac efferent neurons occurs not only within the central nervous system but also within the intrathoracic autonomic nervous system. Indeed, the way in which its target organ component interacts with the rest of the cardiac neuronal hierarchy to maintain autonomic efferent neuronal tone to cardiomyocytes may well determine adequate cardiac function.

To match cardiac output to the demands of various bodily functions, neurons in the intrinsic cardiac nervous system are in constant communication with those in intrathoracic extracardiac ganglia as well as those in the spinal cord and medulla that in turn are under the influence of higher center neurons. The interactions occurring throughout this hierarchy to effect stable cardiac control are now commanding attention. If any component within this neuronal hierarchy becomes deranged, including its cortical one, cardiac pathology can arise. It is the whole cardiac nervous system that must be considered if one is to manage cardiac disease from a neurological perspective. That the processing of centrifugal and centripetal information occurs on an ongoing basis among the varied populations of neurons intrinsic to the heart necessitates a reappraisal of our understanding of cardiac control, from a clinical as well as basic scientific perspective.

In the past, there has been a tendency to assume that neurons in the brain stem (parasympathetic efferent preganglionic neurons) and spinal cord (sympathetic efferent preganglionic neurons) are the sole source of cardiac neuronal control. Cardiac control has been considered to reside solely among neurons within the central nervous system. In such a scenario, intrathoracic paravertebral ganglia (containing sympathetic efferent postganglionic neurons) and intrinsic cardiac ganglia (containing parasympathetic efferent postganglionic neurons) have been assumed to function solely as efferent neuronal relay stations for the cardiac sympathetic and parasympathetic efferent nervous systems, respectively. For decades it has also been assumed that the two efferent limbs of the autonomic nervous system act in a reciprocal fashion to regulate cardiodynamics so that as one becomes activated the other is suppressed.[3,6] In light of the fact that the processing of cardiovascular sensory information occurs not only within the central nervous system but also within the intrathoracic nervous system, including its intrinsic cardiac component, those assumptions no longer stand.

That the heart possesses its own little brain has major implications for understanding how the entire cardiac neuroaxis processes cardiovascular sensory information to maintain adequate efferent neuronal output to cardiomyocytes.[1,5] The finding that complex interdependent communication occurs among neurons in the heart and brain, as well as those located in between, is in accord with data that gastroenterologists have obtained from the enteric nervous system.[2]

The first seven chapters of this volume show how intrinsic cardiac neurons, acting in concert with neurons in intrathoracic extracardiac ganglia and the central nervous system, transduce alterations in the cardiovascular milieu on an ongoing basis to the cardiac efferent postganglionic neurons that regulate cardiac output and thus help to meet the demands of body function over a lifetime. The first two chapters describe the structure and function of neurons located in various strata of the cardiac neuronal hierarchy. This is followed by a discussion of the transduction properties of cardiovascular sensory neurons located throughout the cardiac neuroaxis (Chapter 3) that directly or indirectly influence autonomic efferent neurons controlling regional cardiac function (Chapter 4). With respect to the central components of the cardiac hierarchy, reflexes involving neurons in the spinal cord (Chapter 5) and medulla (Chapter 6) are presented next, followed by a discussion of the integration of cardiovascular sensory information by higher center neurons (Chapter 7). Thus, the first seven chapters present an overview of our current knowledge about the processing of cardiovascular sensory information by neurons located throughout the cardiac neuronal hierarchy that modulates cardiac motor neurons.

Recent data indicate that key components of the intrathoracic cardiac neuronal hierarchy remodel themselves during the evolution of specific cardiac pathologies. Inherent to this remodeling concept is the finding that this hierarchy can become deranged even following relatively minor insults to the myocardium. In the presence of pathology, remodeling involves both short- and long-term alterations in its capacity to coordinate regional cardiac function. To address the complexities of this remodeling, the anatomical and physiological bases for understanding active information processing within the cardiac neuronal hierarchy during ontogeny and aging are described in Chapters 8 and 9, respectively. Then remodeling of the cardiac neuroaxis during the evolution of myocardial ischemia (Chapter 10), cardiac arrhythmias (Chapter 11), and heart failure (Chapter 12) and the neurogenic underpinnings for the genesis of hypertension (Chapter 13) are discussed. Chapter 14 presents recent data concerning the relevance of the psychological aspects of cardiac disease (Chapter 14), a topic of increasing importance given current awareness of psychological stressors in the genesis of heart disease. Thus, these seven chapters provide an overview of how the cardiac neuronal hierarchy responds to important cardiac pathologies as it remodels in an attempt to stabilize cardiac output.

Given the recent explosion of basic science and clinical information about how the cardiac nervous system stabilizes cardiac output, the ultimate goals of this volume are to *(1)* present a consensus concerning the complex interactions that occur within the cardiac neuronal hierarchy that maintain homeostatic cardiac function, and *(2)* present a rationale for developing novel therapeutic strategies that target specific components of the cardiac neuroaxis as it adapts or maladapts to altered cardiac status during the evolution of specific cardiac pathologies.

Montreal, Quebec   J.A.A.
Johnson City, Tennessee   J.L.A.

REFERENCES

1. Armour JA and Ardell JL, eds. *Neurocardiology.* New York: Oxford University Press, 1994.
2. Furness, JB. Intestinofugal neurons and sympathetic reflexes that bypass the central nervous system. *J Comp Neurol* 455:281–284, 2003.
3. Hillarp N-A. Peripheral autonomic mechanisms. In: Field J, ed. *Handbook of Physiology, Section I: Neurophysiology.* Washington, DC: American Physiological Society, 1960, pp 979–1006.
4. Lathrop DA and Spooner PM. On the neural connection. *J Cardiovasc Electrophysiol* 12:841–844, 2001.
5. Shepherd JT and Vatner SF, eds. *Nervous Control of the Heart.* Amsterdam: Harwood Academic Publishers, 1996.
6. Skok VI. *Physiology of Autonomic Ganglia.* Tokyo: Igaku Shoin, 1973.

Contents

Contributors, xi

1. Electrophysiological Properties of Intrinsic Cardiac Neurons, 1
   David J. Adams and Javier Cuevas

2. Colocalization of Multiple Neurochemicals in Mammalian Intrathoracic Neurons, 61
   Magda Horackova

3. Cardiac Sensory Neurons, 79
   J. Andrew Armour and Guy C. Kember

4. Intrathoracic Neuronal Regulation of Cardiac Function, 118
   Jeffrey L. Ardell

5. Integrative Control of Cardiac Function by Cervical and Thoracic Spinal Neurons, 153
   Robert D. Foreman, Mike J.L. DeJongste, and Bengt Linderoth

6. Central Nervous System Regulation of the Heart, 187
   Michael C. Andresen, Diana L. Kunze, and David Mendelowitz

7. Forebrain Control of Healthy and Diseased Hearts, 220
   David F. Cechetto

8. Ontogeny of the Cardiac Nervous System, 252
   Phyllis M. Gootman

9. Aging and Neural Responses in the Heart, 272
   James G. Dobson, Jr. and Richard A. Fenton

10. The Genesis of Pain during Myocardial Ischemia and Infarction, 298
    Christer Sylvén

11. Neuronal Modulation of Atrial and Ventricular
    Electrical Properties, 315
    René Cardinal and Pierre L. Pagé

12. Sympathetic Nervous System in the Evolution of Heart Failure, 340
    Louis J. Dell'Italia and Jeffrey L. Ardell

13. The Pathogenesis of Hypertension, 368
    J. Michael Wyss, Scott H. Carlson, and Suzanne Oparil

14. Psychological Aspects of Heart Disease, 393
    Christine Gagnon, Srikanth Ramachandruni, Edith E. Bragdon, and David S. Sheps

15. Epilogue: Relevance of the Cardiac Neuronal Hierarchy in
    Heart Disease, 419
    Jeffrey L. Ardell, Louis J. Dell'Italia, and J. Andrew Armour

    Index, 425

Contributors

DAVID J. ADAMS, PH.D.
Department of Physiology and
 Pharmacology
School of Biomedical Sciences
University of Queensland
Brisbane, Australia

MICHAEL C. ANDRESEN, PH.D.
Department of Physiology and
 Pharmacology
Oregon Health & Science University
Portland, Oregon

JEFFREY L. ARDELL, PH.D.
Department of Pharmacology
James H. Quillen College of Medicine
East Tennessee State University
Johnson City, Tennessee

J. ANDREW ARMOUR, M.D.,
 PH.D.
Department of Pharmacology
University of Montréal
Montréal, Québec, Canada

EDITH E. BRAGDON, PH.D.
School of Dentistry
University of North Carolina
Chapel Hill, North Carolina

RENÉ CARDINAL, PH.D.
Department of Pharmacology
University of Montréal
Montréal, Québec, Canada

SCOTT H. CARLSON, PH.D.
Department of Biology
Luther College
Decorah, Iowa

DAVID F. CECHETTO, PH.D.
Department of Anatomy and Cell
 Biology
University of Western Ontario
London, Ontario, Canada

JAVIER CUEVAS, PH.D.
Department of Pharmacology and
 Therapeutics
University of South Florida
College of Medicine
Tampa, Florida

MIKE J.L. DEJONGSTE, M.D.,
 PH.D.
Department of Cardiology
Thorax Center
University Hospital of Groningen
Groninger, The Netherlands

LOUIS J. DELL'ITALIA, M.D.
Division of Cardiology
Department of Medicine
University of Alabama at Birmingham
Birmingham, Alabama

JAMES G. DOBSON, JR., PH.D.
Department of Physiology
University of Massachusetts Medical
 School
Worcester, Massachusetts

RICHARD A. FENTON, PH.D.
Department of Physiology
University of Massachusetts Medical
  School
Worcester, Massachusetts

ROBERT D. FOREMAN, PH.D.
Department of Physiology
College of Medicine
University of Oklahoma Health
  Sciences Center
Oklahoma City, Oklahoma

CHRISTINE GAGNON, PH.D.
Department of Allied Health
  Psychology
Saint Margaret Mercy Healthcare
  Center
Hammond, Indiana

PHYLLIS M. GOOTMAN, PH.D.
Department of Physiology and
  Pharmacology
State University of New York
Downstate Medical Center
Brooklyn, New York

MAGDA HORACKOVA, PH.D.
Department of Physiology &
  Biophysics
Dalhousie University
Halifax, Nova Scotia, Canada

GUY C. KEMBER, PH.D.
Department of Physics
Dalhousie University
Halifax, Nova Scotia, Canada

DIANA L. KUNZE, PH.D.
Rammelkamp Center
MetroHealth System
Case Western Reserve University
Cleveland, Ohio

BENGT LINDEROTH, M.D., PH.D.
Department of Neurosurgery
Karolinska Institutet
Stockholm, Sweden

DAVID MENDELOWITZ, PH.D.
Department of Pharmacology
George Washington University
Washington, District of Columbia

SUZANNE OPARIL, M.D.
Hypertension Training Program of the
  Department of Medicine
University of Alabama at Birmingham
Birmingham, Alabama

PIERRE L. PAGÉ, M.D.
Centre de Recherche
Hôpital du Sacré-coeur de Montréal
Montréal, Québec, Canada

SRIKANTH RAMACHANDRUNI, M.D.
Division of Internal Medicine
Department of Medicine
University of Florida
Gainesville, Florida

DAVID S. SHEPS, M.D.
Department of Cardiovascular
  Medicine
University of Florida,
Gainesville, Florida

CHRISTER SYLVÉN, M.D., PH.D.
Department of Cardiology
Karolinska Institute
Huddinge University Hospital
Stockholm, Sweden

J. MICHAEL WYSS, PH.D.
Department of Cell Biology
University of Alabama at Birmingham
Birmingham, Alabama

Basic and Clinical Neurocardiology

1
Electrophysiological Properties of Intrinsic Cardiac Neurons

DAVID J. ADAMS AND JAVIER CUEVAS

Cardiac performance is determined by the rate and strength of contraction of the heart. There is increasing evidence indicating that intrinsic cardiac neurons interact with extracardiac intrathoracic ganglia and the central nervous system to control the heart and are capable of independently monitoring and influencing cardiac function. Aspects of cardiac function that are subject to control by intracardiac neurons include chronotropic actions (changes in heart rate), dromotropic actions (changes in conduction of excitation) mediated by pacemaker and conducting cells, and inotropic actions (changes in contractile force) mediated by atrial and ventricular myocytes. In addition, the coronary circulation and aspects of cardiac valve function are likely to be influenced. Evidence obtained from histochemical, electrophysiological, and pharmacological studies both in vivo and in vitro strongly suggest that neurons form functional afferent, efferent, and local circuits within the cardiac nerve plexus. This plexus acts as a complex site for the integration and modification of sensory input and cardiac output. Indeed, rather than being a simple relay station, the cardiac nerve plexus seems to share many similarities with the complex neural network of the enteric nervous system.

Neural control of the heart is under the influence of the two major divisions of the autonomic system, the sympathetic and the parasympathetic nervous systems. The sympathetic nervous system projects to the heart through the intrathoracic ganglia. Preganglionic neurons in the spinal cord project to postganglionic neurons in the stellate, middle cervical, and mediastinal ganglia, which in turn project to the heart. Activation of the sympathetic nervous system causes an increase in heart rate, an increase in conduction velocity, and an increase in ventricular contractile force. In contrast, activation of the parasympathetic division of the nervous system, which arises from the neurons in the medulla region of the brain stem, causes a decrease in heart rate, a decrease in conduction velocity through the atrioventricular (AV) node, and a decrease in the force of atrial and ventricular contraction.

This review focuses on the role and electrophysiological properties of neurons of the mammalian intrinsic cardiac nervous system. Several earlier reviews have considered primarily the anatomy, neurochemistry, and function of intrinsic cardiac ganglia.[8,10,128,129,132]

Anatomical Organization

Innervation of the Heart

Parasympathetic innervation of the heart is carried by the Xth cranial (vagus) nerve. Nuclei in the ventral lateral medulla project via the vagus nerve to postganglionic neurons in the cardiac nerve plexus. Neurons of the dorsal motor nucleus of the vagus (DVM) and of the nucleus ambiguus (NA) innervate the heart as shown by physiological, viral-tracing, and degeneration studies.[149] Furthermore, it has been shown that the ganglion cluster located at the left atrium adjacent to the inferior vena cava ("AV ganglion") receives input from both the DVM and NA,[104,148] whereas, the ganglion cluster located at the right pulmonary vein–left atrial junction ("SA ganglion") receives fibers from the NA only.[105] There is a degree of asymmetry in the distribution of preganglionic neurons in the medulla. Injection of a retrograde tracer into the AV ganglion of the cat results in the labeling of twice as many cells on the left side of the medulla as on the right side,[104] whereas injection of a retrograde tracer into the SA ganglion and subsequent histological examination of the ventral lateral medulla reveals asymmetrical distribution of labeled preganglionic neurons.[105] The precise distribution of neurons innervating the specific intracardiac ganglion exhibits substantial interindividual variation.

Preganglionic neurons synapse on postganglionic neurons in autonomic ganglia, and it has been assumed that there is a substantial degree of "convergence" in the parasympathetic nervous system. However, there is considerable diversity in the degree of convergence and divergence among species, as well as among different autonomic ganglia and individuals of a single species.[164] With regard to cardiac ganglia, there appears to be a degree of *divergence* rather than convergence in the cardiac ganglion of the cat whereby one preganglionic neuron projects on average to 13 or 32 postganglionic neurons.[164] Similarly, studies by Massari et al.[104]

indicate that a small number of neurons in the medulla are capable of controlling significant numbers of postganglionic cardiac neurons.

Cardiac Ganglion Nerve Plexus

The extensive network of neuronal cell bodies receiving parasympathetic vagal input and comprising the intrinsic cardiac ganglia of the mammalian heart has long been known,[109,171] yet the precise function of the network and the way in which it mediates vagal input are largely unknown. A detailed description of the location, distribution, and projections of the intracardiac ganglia has been provided for the heart in numerous mammalian species.[40,89,112,120] These ganglia could well represent the final common pathway through which the diverse, extrinsic neural signals to the heart are modified before being transmitted to the effector tissues. Cardiac ganglia are located on epicardial fat pads adjacent to the myocardium and within the myocardium itself. The exact anatomical distribution of the intracardiac ganglia varies among species. For example, four ganglia in the atria and three in the ventricles have been described in the dog,[11,15,16] whereas in the rat, four major ganglion clusters have been found and are only located in the atria.[120] Whereas some of the ganglia are extracardial, the septal ganglia are located on the inner surface of the atria. Cardiac ganglion neurons located in the right atrium are associated with control of the sinoatrial node and neurons in the region of the inferior vena cava modulate AV conduction.[10] A schematic diagram to illustrate the distribution of intracardiac ganglia in rat atria is shown in Figure 1–1A.

A photomicrograph of neurons of the neonatal rat cardiac ganglion in the living preparation is shown in Figure 1–1B. Figure 1–1C shows the morphology of the neurons following enzymatic dissociation and after being maintained in tissue culture for 48 hours.

There appear to be at least three different types of neurons in the mammalian cardiac plexus on the basis of morphology[39,136,174] (see Table 1–2). A morphological study of neurons in the nerve plexus that lies beneath the pulmonary arteries on the myocardium of the left atrium of rats and guinea pigs revealed at least two major types of neuron: unipolar (61.2%) and multipolar (38.8%). The neuron somata exhibit no significant difference in their length or width.[122] Classification of nerve cells in the terminal plexus of the rat AV junction according to their three-dimensional (3-D) morphology confirmed that they could be divided into three categories: *(1)* large unipolar neurons with axonal projections directed toward the interventricular junction, *(2)* large unipolar or bipolar neurons, and *(3)* small multipolar interneurons.[114]

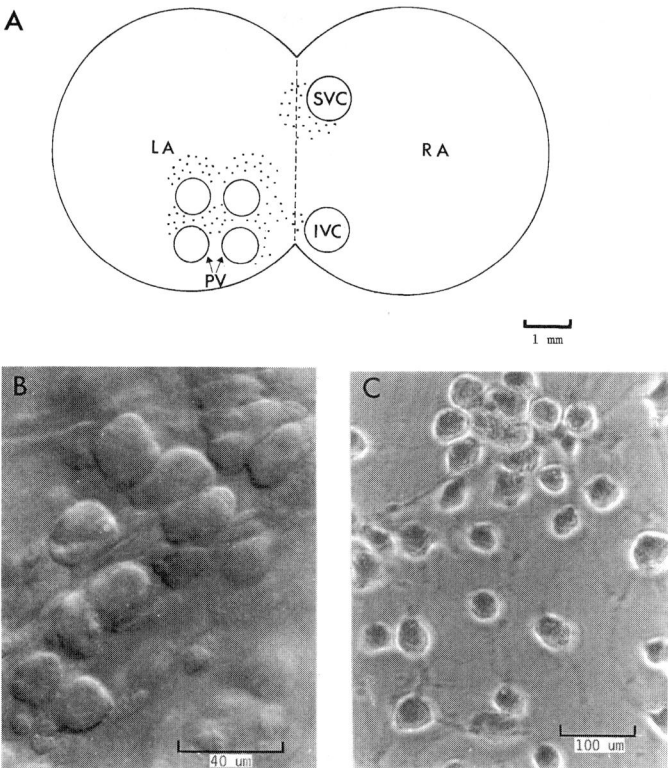

FIGURE 1–1 Rat intracardiac ganglia in situ and dissociated intracardiac neurons in tissue culture. **A.** Distribution of intracardiac ganglia (stippled regions) on the epicardial surface of neonatal rat atria. IVC, inferior vena cava; LA, left atria; PV, pulmonary veins; RA, right atria; SVC, superior vena cava. Scale bar, 1 mm. **B.** Intrinsic cardiac neurons in a living preparation viewed with Hoffman modulation contrast optics. Scale bar, 40 μm. **C.** Phase-contrast photomicrograph of neurons dissociated from explants of rat cardiac ganglia and placed in tissue culture for 48 hours. Neuronal soma (25–35 μm diameter) and axonal processes are visualized at 400× magnification. Scale bar, 100 μm. (From Xu and Adams.[178])

It has been shown that neurons with distinct electrophysiological behavior differ in their number of dendritic processes and patterns of synaptic inputs.[39,90] Many cardiac neurons are synaptically coupled to each other and/or excited by stimulation of extrinsic nerves. However, approximately 10% of intrinsic cardiac neurons appear to lack a synaptic input as determined by staining whole-mount preparations of guinea pig cardiac plexus with antibodies to synaptophysin.[90] The important questions that have not been answered relate to the function of the discrete neuron types and how they connect together to form the reflex circuits that appear to exist in cardiac ganglia.

Histological studies have shown that a complex network of neurons exists within the mammalian cardiac ganglion. Postganglionic parasympathetic neurons are not the only neurons present and there is evidence suggesting that sensory neurons, interneurons, and efferent neurons are found in intracardiac ganglia. Furthermore, the presence of sympathetic fibers[145] and afferent nerve fibers[56] suggests that there is potential for interaction between these elements. Sympathetic nerve terminals are often found in close proximity to parasympathetic nerve terminals.[27] This anatomical arrangement of sympathetic and parasympathetic nerve terminals makes it possible for transmitters released from the nerve terminals of one division to diffuse readily to terminals of the other division, as well as to cardiac muscle cells. Small intensely fluorescent (SIF) cells, which contain catecholamines, have also been shown to be present within mammalian intracardiac ganglia.[59,83,134] Therefore, both the soma and axon terminal of parasympathetic neurons may be under the physiological influence of catecholamines.

Sympathetic and parasympathetic (vagal) nervous systems exert antagonistic effects on the heart and interaction between the two systems is well established.[92] For example, stimulation of muscarinic receptors on sympathetic nerve terminals in the heart reduces the release of norepinephrine (NE).[45,98,101,162] However, reports of the existence of the reciprocal effect, that is, NE-mediated antagonism of acetylcholine (ACh) release from parasympathetic nerve terminals via α-adrenergic receptors, have been conflicting.[4,93,99,170]

In addition to parasympathetic efferent and sensory afferent neurons, there also exists a population of interneurons within the cardiac ganglia. These interneurons may be *intra*ganglionic or *inter*ganglionic,[173] that is, the axons of these cells may reside within its particular ganglion or travel out into another ganglion cluster. This arrangement has been found in most species, including the dog,[173] guinea pig,[151] and rabbit.[118] Electrical stimulation of an interganglionic nerve is sufficient to produce excitatory postsynaptic potentials (EPSPs) and action potentials in ganglion neurons innervated.[174,175] The function of the interneurons within cardiac ganglia is unknown, though presumably these neurons mediate lateral interactions between various ganglion neurons and allow a convergence of different inputs. Electrical stimulation of the stellate ganglion or the vagosympathetic trunk produces responses in ganglion cells, with variable latencies indicating polysynaptic connections.[50]

Analogous to the enteric division of the autonomic nervous system, sensory neurons innervate the heart. Visceral cardiac afferent neurons also exist in cardiac ganglia, which are identified by the presence of the neuropeptides substance P (SP) and calcitonin gene–related peptide (CGRP).[48] The presence of these afferents in close association with parasympathetic neurons has led to postulation of the existence of a local reflex circuit within the heart. Spontaneous activity has been demonstrated in canine cardiac neurons.[50] The spontaneous firing is entrained to events in the cardiac and respiratory cycles even with disconnection from the central nervous system, although the amount of activity is substantially less. These observations strongly suggest that cardiac afferent fibers transmit cardiopulmonary information to ganglion cells in a local reflex arc as well as through higher centers. A schematic representation for the organization and possible integration within the mammalian intracardiac ganglia is presented in Figure 1–2. There is considerable potential for complex integration of activity regulating cardiac function within the intracardiac ganglia. The term *heart brain* has been proposed to describe the integrative role of this intrinsic nervous system within the heart.[129]

Neurochemical Coding in Mammalian Intracardiac Ganglia

Acetylcholine is the primary chemical transmitter in the extrinsic (parasympathetic) innervation of the mammalian cardiac nerve plexus; however, there is considerable evidence to suggest that noncholinergic mechanisms also operate in intrinsic cardiac ganglia. There are numerous studies demonstrating that a variety of neurotransmitters and neuropeptides are localized and operate within mammalian intrinsic cardiac ganglia. The existence of several transmitters and, in particular, the colocalization of more than one neurotransmitter/neuropeptide in a neuron are highly suggestive of complex control of the heart.

Acetylcholine is released from parasympathetic preganglionic nerve terminals and acts as the principal excitatory neurotransmitter at the intracardiac ganglionic synapse.[136,175] Choline acetyltransferase (ChAT) immunoreactivity has been shown to be expressed in all postganglionic neurons in guinea pig cardiac ganglia.[106] Furthermore, varicose nerve fibers that were immunoreactive for ChAT were abundant in ganglia, with every intracardiac neuron lying in close apposition to one or more varicosities. This observation indicates that each neuron is likely to receive cholinergic input.

Acetylcholine is not the only neurotransmitter released at the pre- to postganglionic synapse. Stimulation of the preganglionic neuron in the presence of nicotinic ACh receptor antagonists in vivo fails to abolish the response in the postganglionic intracardiac neuron in many species, suggesting that other neurotransmitters may be involved in synaptic transmission. Other transmitters implicated in neurotransmission within the mammalian cardiac ganglion include a variety of catecholamines and neuropeptides, as well as serotonin (5-hydroxytryptamine), histamine, adenosine 5'-triphosphate (ATP), and nitric oxide (NO).

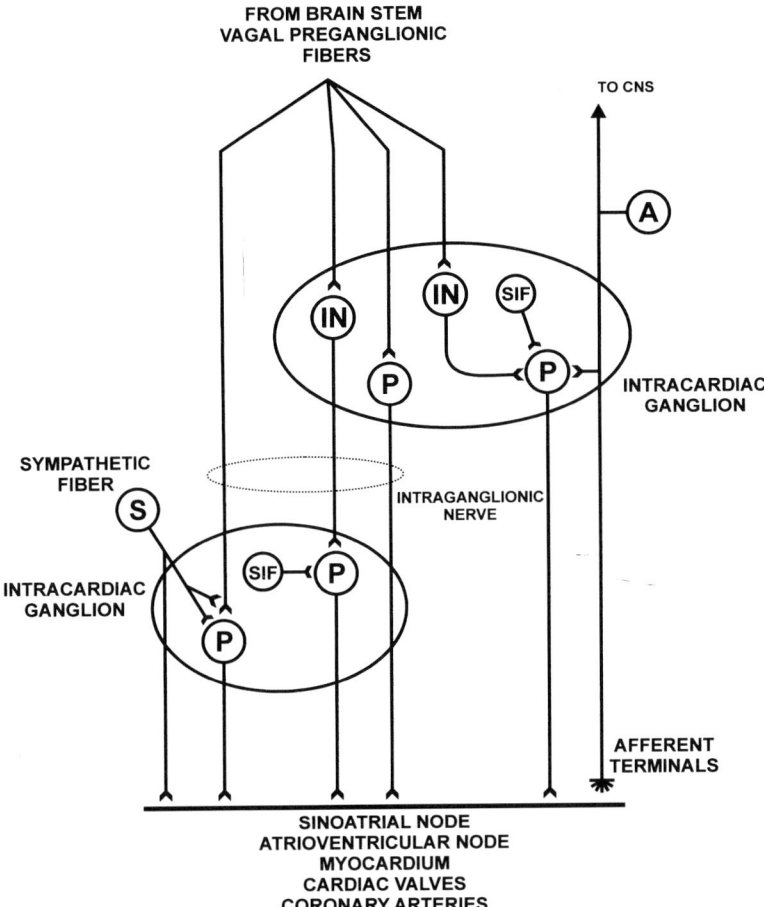

FIGURE 1–2 Schematic diagram of the possible integration within the mammalian intracardiac ganglia. Vagal preganglionic nerve fibers from the brain stem terminate on principal ganglion cells (P) or interneurons (IN) which may send connection to P cells. Some preganglionic nerve fibers course between ganglia as well as postganglionic fibers and axons of IN cells via an intraganglionic nerve. P cells may also receive inputs from small, intensely fluorescent (SIF) cells and cardiac afferent fibers (A). Postganglionic sympathetic nerve fibers (S) may influence P cells via presynaptic or postsynaptic contacts. CNS, central nervous system. (Modified from Randall and Wurster.[128])

Catecholamines

The presence of catecholamines in the cardiac nerve plexus has been demonstrated previously in SIF cells[59,91,134,142] and in sympathetic nerve fibers that course through the ganglion (see review[128]). While catecholamines have not been found in the principal ganglion cells, many neurons do display immunoreactivity for dopamine β-hydroxylase (DBH).[20,59,60,83] However, DBH immunoreactivity appears to be lost from guinea pig intracardiac neurons maintained in tissue culture[61] and is not detected in intracardiac neurons cultured from fetal human heart.[62] Baluk and Gabella[20] have found that 70%–80% of the neurons taken from the posterior atrial wall of the guinea pig contained special mechanisms for the uptake of L-dopa. Curiously, the neurons also contained the enzymes L-amino acid decarboxylase and DBH, two enzymes involved in the synthesis of catecholamines. Administration of α_1-, α_2-, β_1-, and β_2-agonists and antagonists to a population of spontaneously active intrinsic cardiac neurons via either local epicardial application or local arterial blood supply in anesthetized dogs indicated that intracardiac neurons involved in cardiac regulation possess α- and β-adrenoceptors.[13,156] Alpha-adrenoceptor agonists either increased or decreased neuronal activity whereas activity was augmented by β-adrenoceptor agonists. Spontaneous neuronal activity was suppressed by β-adrenoceptor, but not α-adrenoceptor, blockade, indicating that intrinsic cardiac adrenergic neurons receive tonic inputs via β-adrenoreceptors, but not α-adrenoceptors.[13]

Neuropeptides

The guinea pig has been the most common model for the study of neuropeptides in the intrinsic cardiac ganglion. A variety of potential neurotransmitters and neuromodulators have been identified, including somatostatin,[36,121,152] neuropeptide Y (NPY),[58,59,61,152] vasoactive intestinal polypeptide (VIP),[59,134,168] substance P,[19] and opioid peptides (dynorphin A, dynorphin B, leu-enkephalin).[150,152] Steele et al.[152] demonstrated immunoreactivity for somatostatin, NPY, VIP, dynorphin B, and substance P within the intracardiac neurons of the guinea pig. Most of the neurons examined contained at least one of these peptides and indeed some neurons displayed immunoreactivity for all five of these neuropeptides. A large percentage of the neurons (45%) demonstrated immunoreactivity for somatostatin and eight distinct populations of neurons were identified on the basis of neuropeptide content (see Figure 1–3).

Neuropeptides have been detected in somata, processes, and synaptic termini within intracardiac ganglia. Whereas the presence of neuropeptide-like immunoreactivity in the soma of cardiac neurons is well established, there has been considerable debate concerning the origin of neuropeptides in cardiac ganglia and in the myocardium. The presence of peptides and enzymes in intrinsic cardiac ganglia has been studied using immunocytochemical and histochemical techniques, often in conjunction with the axoplasmic transport inhibitor, colchicine, to raise the levels of peptides in the somata.[100,152] Neuropeptide Y expression was in-

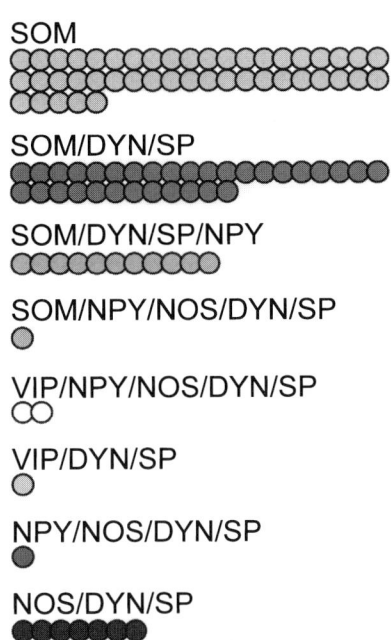

FIGURE 1–3 Combinations and relative populations of neuropeptides in guinea pig cardiac ganglion neurons. Guinea pig intracardiac neurons exhibit immunoreactivity for the neuropeptides somatostatin (SOM), dynorphin (DYN), substance P (SP), neuropeptide Y (NPY), vasoactive intestinal polypeptide (VIP), and the enzyme nitric oxide synthase (NOS). (Data taken from Steele et al.[152])

creased in 36- to 72-hour explanted guinea pig cardiac ganglia preparations compared to that in control preparations and colchicine treatment further increased the percentage of NPY-immunoreactive neurons.[100] Neuropeptide Y constitutes the main peptide containing subpopulation of nerve fibers in the conduction system in a wide variety of species. Its distribution mirrors that of tyrosine hydroxylase, VIP, and somatostatin. The presence of SP and CGRP is thought to be characteristic of local afferent nerves.

While the vagus nerve is a major source of efferent neural input into the mammalian cardiac ganglia, sympathetic efferent and afferent sympathetic and sensory neurons also project onto the cardiac nerve plexus.[10,112] Whereas the efferent nerves primarily release NE to the heart from nerve terminals found in close proximity to parasympathetic nerve terminals,[83] afferent neurons of spinal and vagal origin also form a moderately dense network of SP-immunoreactive fibers in the myocardium and around blood vessels in the atria.[34,46] These SP-containing nerve fibers have been found closely associated with the parasympathetic intracardiac ganglia, often surrounding ganglion cells.[34,56,74,152] Further evidence suggesting that SP may play a major role in the cardiac ganglia is the fact that this neuropeptide is also found in neurons of vagal sensory origin. Treatment of the vagus nerve with capsaicin, which depletes nerves of SP content, significantly reduced SP immunoreactivity in the right atrium of guinea pigs.[34,119] Substance P may be acting as a neurotransmitter or neuromodulator in the intracardiac ganglia, thus influencing neuronal transmission and ultimately cardiac function.

These findings demonstrate the considerable neurochemical diversity within the heart of the guinea pig and among different species. Neuropeptides serve a useful purpose as markers for neural pathways, given that neurons containing different combinations of peptides project to discrete areas of the heart. However, what function do these neuropeptides serve? Some neuropeptides may be actively involved in neurotransmission within the cardiac ganglion, while other peptides such as NPY are known to have vasoconstrictor effects on blood vessels. It is likely that the axons of intracardiac neurons containing neuropeptides may innervate and modulate the function of not only the myocardium but also the coronary vasculature and cardiac valves.[3,151,168]

Monamines and histamine
Although the existence of serotonergic neurons in the cardiac nerve plexus remains controversial, however, immunoreactivity to 5-hydroxytryptamine (5-HT) has been reported in the heart of the guinea pig.[61] In addition, there is evidence that these neurons were able to synthesize 5-HT from its precursor, 5-hydroxytryptophan. It was concluded, however, that the reason the neurons displayed 5-HT immunoreactivity was that there was neuronal uptake of serotonin from the culture medium. A more recent study in adult human heart tissue convincingly demonstrated that neurons within the cardiac ganglia contain enzymes involved in the synthesis of monamines and histamine and that they contain dopamine, NE, serotonin, and histamine immunoreactivity.[141] In guinea pig cardiac ganglia, the only apparent source of histamine is mast cells. However, mast cell degranulation or exogenous histamine application evoked membrane depolarization and an increase in neuronal excitability via the activation of H_1 receptors.[125] Although histamine has been shown to modify the spontaneous activity of canine right atrial neurons in situ,[12] additional functional evidence will be necessary to evaluate the physiological role of monamines and histamine in neural control of the heart.

Adenosine 5'-triphosphate
A population of intrinsic neurons in atria isolated from guinea pig and rabbit hearts has been shown to exhibit a positive histochemical reaction with quinacrine, indicating a high ATP content.[28] In the mammalian heart, ATP stimulates cardiac vagal afferent fibers, producing a negative chronotropic effect,[123] and has been reported to inhibit NE release from efferent nerve fibers.[163] Local administration of ATP to canine intrinsic

cardiac ganglia in situ either enhanced or attenuated spontaneous neuronal activity concomitant with either bradycardia or tachycardia.[78] The release of ATP in the heart from nerve terminals, activated platelets, endothelium, and cardiomyocytes may mediate ischemia-induced cardiovascular reflexes and cardiac arrhythmias via modulation of neuronal activity of the intrinsic cardiac nervous system (see Armour[14]).

Nitric oxide
The role of NO as an endogenous neurotransmitter/neuromodulator in the heart has been studied extensively over the past decade. Immunoreactivity for nitric oxide synthase (NOS) has been found in neurons and nerve fibers of rat and guinea pig cardiac ganglia.[26,63,152,154,155] Thirty to forty percent of neurons in canine intrinsic cardiac ganglia were histochemically labeled for NADPH diaphorase (a specific marker of NO production) and, in a subpopulation of neurons studied in vitro, the application of NO donors such as nitroprusside and nitroglycerine evoked membrane depolarization.[18] Nitric oxide donors induced concentration-dependent increases in neuronal activity of intracardiac neurons in situ frequently associated with augmentation in ventricular systolic pressure and heart rate, which was attenuated by the NOS inhibitor N-nitro-L-arginine methyl ester (L-NAME).[18] Following acute decentralization, NO donors continued to augment neuronal activity in intracardiac ganglia, but the cardiovascular responses were suppressed or eliminated.[18] Although it has been demonstrated that NO can modulate neuronal activity of canine cardiac ganglia, the precise sites and mechanisms of action remain to be determined. For example, it is difficult to differentiate between the effects of NO on the preganglionic terminals and those on the postganglionic neurons or their terminals, or both, as the ganglia are located in close proximity to the neuroeffector junction. Nevertheless, NO has been shown to act presynaptically to enhance cardiac vagal neurotransmission and facilitate vagal slowing of heart rate.[65,66,135] Furthermore, inhibition of neuronally released NOS by injection of 1-(2-trifluoromethylphenyl) imidazole (TRIM) into the sinus node artery reduced bradycardia evoked by vagal stimulation, indicating that the facilitatory role of NO is likely to occur at vagal pre- and postganglionic synaptic mechanisms in the intrinsic cardiac ganglia.[103]

Amino acids
Amino acids have also been shown to modulate neuroexcitability in parasympathetic intracardiac neurons. Local application of the excitatory amino acids glutamate and aspartate onto spontaneously active canine intracardiac neurons in situ increased neuronal activity in most neurons

tested and decreased the activity in a smaller subpopulation.[18,77] Conversely, gamma aminobutyric acid (GABA) decreased the activity of most spontaneously active neurons but increased the activity in some neurons.[77] The presence of ionotropic and metabotropic glutamate receptors in the rat heart has been demonstrated immunohistochemically and they have been preferentially localized to cardiac nerve terminals, ganglion cells, and components of the conducting system.[52,53] A significant component of amino acid modulation of intracardiac neurons appears to be dependent on connections to the central nervous system, since acute decentralization resulted in loss of responsiveness of neurons to amino acid application.[77]

Passive Membrane Properties

Electrophysiological studies allow the characterization of passive and active electrical properties and analysis of the types of ion channels expressed in excitable cells. Most of the electrophysiological studies of mammalian intracardiac neurons over the last two decades have been carried out using intracellular microelectrode and patch clamp recording techniques. Voltage clamp methods allow direct measurement of ionic currents associated with the activation of ligand-gated and voltage-gated ion channels in excitable cells and have provided considerable insight into the function and modulation of electrical activity in intrinsic cardiac ganglion neurons. Electrophysiological recording methods used in the investigation of the electrical properties and ion currents in autonomic neurons have been described previously.[1] Specific details of whole-cell patch clamp recording techniques and the analysis of macroscopic and single channel currents can be obtained from other sources.[67,116,133]

Passive electrical properties of somata of mammalian intrinsic cardiac neurons are listed in Table 1–1. The resting membrane potential measured in different mammalian intracardiac neurons ranges from -45 mV to -76 mV with a mean value of -54 mV. There appear to be no significant differences in resting membrane potential for different populations of intracardiac neurons within individual species.[39,145,174] The variation in values is likely to reflect the difference in recording conditions and techniques as much as genuine diversity among species. The bath solutions used had varying K^+ concentrations and temperatures ranged from 22°C to 37°C. The intracellular voltage-recording electrode was usually filled with 0.5–3 M KCl solution, and often the process of cell impalement in high-resistance neurons produced significant "shunt" conductance with variable recovery.

TABLE 1-1 Passive Electrical Properties of Mammalian Intracardiac Neurons

Species	Preparation	Recording Method (electrode [Ksalt])	Soma Diameter (μm) (length × width)	E_m (mV)	Input Resistance (MΩ)	Time Constant (ms)	Reference
Pig	In vitro	M (3 M KCl)	20–50	-52 ± 4.9	37 ± 23.5	5.1 ± 3.8	146
Pig	In vitro	M (3 M KCl)	Phasic	-49 ± 4	72 ± 8	5.8 ± 0.7	145
			Accommodating	-47 ± 5	33 ± 7	7.2 ± 1.1	
			Tonic	-49 ± 5	39 ± 7	6.1 ± 1.2	
Canine	In vitro	M (3 M KCl)	40 × 62	-61.5 ± 17.8	70.3 ± 51.1	3.3 – 5.4	173, 175
Canine	In situ	M (3 M KCl)	Tonic (R-cell) 35 × 61	-52.5 ± 1.8	84.4 ± 5.1		174
			Phasic (S-cell) 44 × 62	-58 ± 1.5	65.6 ± 4.1	2.2–7.5	
Guinea pig	Cultured	M (2 M K citrate)	8–40	-45 to -76	123.4 ± 66.7	—	7
Guinea pig	In vitro	M (3 M KCl/2 M K acetate)	30–50 × 20–40	-50– to -70	20–50	2–10	110
Guinea pig	In situ	M (2 M KCl)	S	-55.3 ± 1.0	107 ± 7.4	—	56
Guinea pig	In situ	M (0.5 M KCl)	25 × 17	-49.8 ± 1.1	129 ± 14	5.8 ± 0.6	39
			SAH 43 × 32	-52.6 ± 1.3	167 ± 21	10.8 ± 1.2	
			P 51 × 34	-49.2 ± 1.2	171 ± 18	13.2 ± 1.5	
Rat (neonatal)	In situ	M (4 M K acetate)	25–40	-58.9 ± 3.5	107.5 ± 2.6	—	134
Rat (adult)	In vitro	M (3 M KCl)	63 ± 25 (pF)	-52.6 ± 6.3	85.6 ± 0.3	4.6 ± 1.2	136
Rat (neonatal)	Cultured	P (dialyzed)	25–35	-52 ± 11	850 ± 34		178
Rat	Cultured	P (perforated)	19 ± 10 (pF)	-51.3 ± 3.5	854 ± 252	53.1 ± 8.4	33, 69
Rat (adult)	Cultured	P (perforated)	54 ± 22 (pF)	-52.5 ± 4.13	321 ± 115	—	69

*Cell capacitance (pF) is approximately equivalent to soma diameter (μm). Values are mean ± standard deviation.

The cell input resistance (R_{in}) is determined from the current–voltage (I-V) relation, which can be measured experimentally. A survey of the values for R_{in} (MΩ) in mammalian intracardiac neurons varies by an order of magnitude and may therefore reflect to a large extent the method of recording rather than real differences (see Table 1–I). Values obtained with microelectrodes vary with the resistance of the recording electrode and are substantially lower than those found in the same preparation with whole-cell patch recording techniques. The electrical characteristics of dissociated neurons from neonatal and adult rat intracardiac ganglia have been examined at 22°C and 37°C using the perforated patch whole-cell recording technique. The mean resting membrane potential was −52.0 mV at 37°C and exhibited no temperature dependence. However, lowering the temperature from 37°C to 22°C decreased the mean input resistance from 854 MΩ to 345 MΩ, respectively.[33]

The I-V relationship in many autonomic neurons has been found to be linear for membrane potentials negative to the resting potential, consistent with a voltage-independent leakage conductance (see Fig. 1–4). Rectification is frequently observed with depolarization, resistance typically being less than half that for hyperpolarizing currents. Hyperpolarizing current pulses induced time-dependent rectification of the voltage response in all neurons at both temperatures. This behavior was observed in perforated patch whole-cell recording but not in dialyzed neurons,[33] and was reversibly blocked by external Cs^+ (2 mM) but not Ba^{2+} (1 mM).

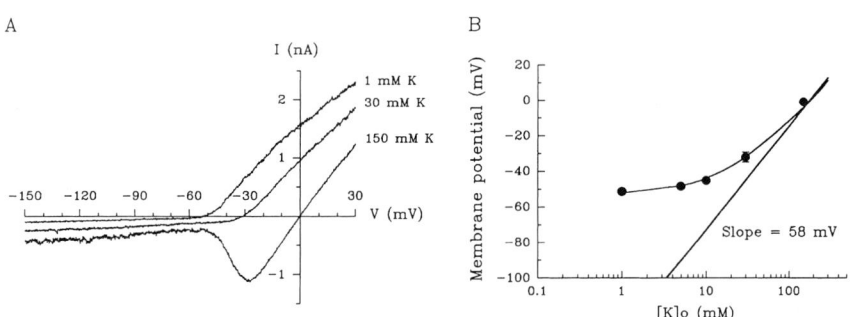

FIGURE 1–4 Dependence of the resting membrane potential of neonatal rat intracardiac neurons on the extracellular K^+ concentration. **A.** Current–voltage (I-V) relations obtained by applying a voltage ramp from −150 to +30 mV in the presence of 1, 30, or 150 mM extracellular K^+ in the same neuron. **B.** Resting membrane potential plotted as a function of the extracellular K^+ concentration. Data points represent mean ± SEM ($n = 4$). The data were fitted with the Goldman-Hodgkin-Katz voltage equation with $P_{Na}/P_K = 0.12$. The straight line was drawn according to the Nernst equation for a K^+-selective electrode with a slope of 58 mV. (From Xu and Adams.[178])

Subsequent experiments demonstrated that this time-dependent rectification was mediated by activation of the hyperpolarization-activated nonselective cation current, I_h.[69]

Discharge Charactersitics

Mammalian intracardiac neurons display a range of action potential and afterpotential characteristics. Somatic action potentials can be evoked by depolarizing current pulses or electrical stimulation of the preganglionic nerves. The functional classification of intracardiac neurons, based on their firing properties, was originally made on cultured intracardiac neurons of guinea pig.[7] The most common neurons (65%–70% of cells studied), termed AH_s-type neurons, were highly refractory and exhibited a pronounced Ca^{2+}-dependent spike afterhyperpolarization (AHP). A second population of neurons (10%–15% of neurons) also exhibited a pronounced AHP but was capable of multiple firing, discharging a short high-frequency burst of action potentials at the onset of current stimulation. These phasic firing neurons are termed AH_m-type neurons. The third type of neuron, termed M cells, which constituted 10%–15% of the neurons studied, did not exhibit a prolonged AHP and discharged tonically in response to prolonged stimulation. To date, at least three different types of neurons have been characterized in the *intact* mammalian cardiac ganglion with regard to their response to depolarizing and hyperpolarizing current pulses. These are phasic, accommodating, and tonic in pig,[145] S, R, and N cells in canine,[174,175] type I (I_b and I_m) and type II neurons in rat,[136] and S, SAH, and P cell in guinea pig[39] intracardiac ganglia. The discharge characteristics and action potential parameters of each of these types of neuron in different species are summarized in Table 1–2. Examination of the distribution of synaptic boutons on the cell body of identified cardiac ganglion cells in guinea pig showed that ~67% of the somata of S cells, 58% of SAH cells, but only 12% of the somata of P cells were covered with synaptophysin-positive varicosities.[90]

In >90% of dissociated neurons from neonatal rat intracardiac ganglia, depolarizing currents evoked firing of multiple, adapting, action potentials at 22°C[33]. The number of action potentials increased, with current strength producing a mean discharge of 5.1 (+100 pA, 1 second pulse), which was attenuated at 37°C to a mean of 1.4. The discharge activity of these neurons exhibits a high temperature dependence and is induced by external Ba^{2+}, which is consistent with the regulation of discharge activity, by the muscarine-sensitive K^+ current (I_M).[33]

TABLE 1–2 Discharge Activity in Neuronal Subtypes of Mammalian Intracardiac Ganglia

Preparation	Discharge Activity of Neuronal Types					AHP (ms)	AP Amplitude (mV)	Reference
	None	Phasic	Adapting	Tonic	Spontaneous			
In situ								
Pig		I (40%)	II (33%)			48 ± 4	73 ± 5	
						39 ± 5	75 ± 4	145
				III (27%)		130 ± 11	72 ± 5	
Canine	N (21%)	S (52%)		R (27%)		—	84 ± 2	174
Rat		Type I (11%)		Type II (8%)		68 ± 6.7		
						400 ± 21	61 ± 2	136
Guinea pig	I (11%)		Type I$_b$ (34%)	Type I$_m$ (39%)	Type I$_m$ (8%)	132 ± 7		39
						—		
		S (37%)		SAH (26%)		30 ± 11		
				P (16%)	P (10%)	144 ± 13		
						166 ± 22		
In Vitro								
Guinea pig		AH$_s$ (70%)	AH$_m$ (15%)	AH$_m$		928 ± 65		7
				M (15%)	M	<100		

AHP, after hyperpolarization; AP, action potential.

Spontaneous discharge activity has been recorded in neurons of canine[172] adult rat[136] and guinea pig intracardiac ganglia in vitro[39] but not in dissociated neurons from neonatal rat or guinea pig heart maintained in tissue culture.[7,178] The firing characteristics of the different types of neuron in adult rat intracardiac ganglia in situ are shown in Figure 1–5. The occurrence of spontaneous activity may be associated with injury produced by electrode impalement and activation of sensory afferent fibers, as pacemaker activity has not been recorded in isolated or dissociated intracardiac neurons.

VOLTAGE-GATED ION CHANNELS

Voltage clamp studies indicate that many kinds of ion channels underlie the electrical behavior of intracardiac neurons. Table 1–3 summarizes the current knowledge of the voltage-sensitive ion channels found in the soma membrane of mammalian intracardiac neurons.

Sodium Channels

All mammalian intracardiac neurons are capable of generating action potentials in response to electrical stimulation. Action potentials are abolished upon the removal of external Na^+ or in the presence of the specific Na^+ channel blocker, tetrodotoxin (TTX; 0.3 μM), indicating the presence of TTX-sensitive voltage-dependent Na^+ channels in rat,[179] canine,[175] and guinea pig (multiple-firing M cells only[7]) intracardiac neurons. In contrast, TTX (0.3 μM) slowed the rate of rise and diminished spike amplitude but failed to abolish action potentials in cultured AH_s- and AH_m-type cells of guinea pig,[7] and phasic (S cells) and tonic (R cells) cells of canine cardiac ganglia.[174] Lowering external Ca^{2+} or addition of $CdCl_2$ together with TTX blocked the action potential, which suggests that both voltage-sensitive Na^+ and Ca^{2+} channels contribute to action potentials in these neurons.

Studies of the voltage-gated Na^+ conductance in intracardiac neurons have been carried out on isolated neurons to achieve spatial and temporal voltage control during the rapid depolarization-activated Na^+ current (I_{Na}). The Na^+ conductance in rat intracardiac neurons was isolated by replacing intracellular K^+ with Cs^+ and adding Cd^{2+} and tetraethylammonium (TEA) to the external solution. The depolarization-activated Na^+ current (I_{Na}) was reversibly blocked by TTX (0.3 μM) and the peak amplitude was dependent on the external Na^+ concentration.[179] The Na^+ conductance activates positive to -40 mV and increases with a sigmoidal

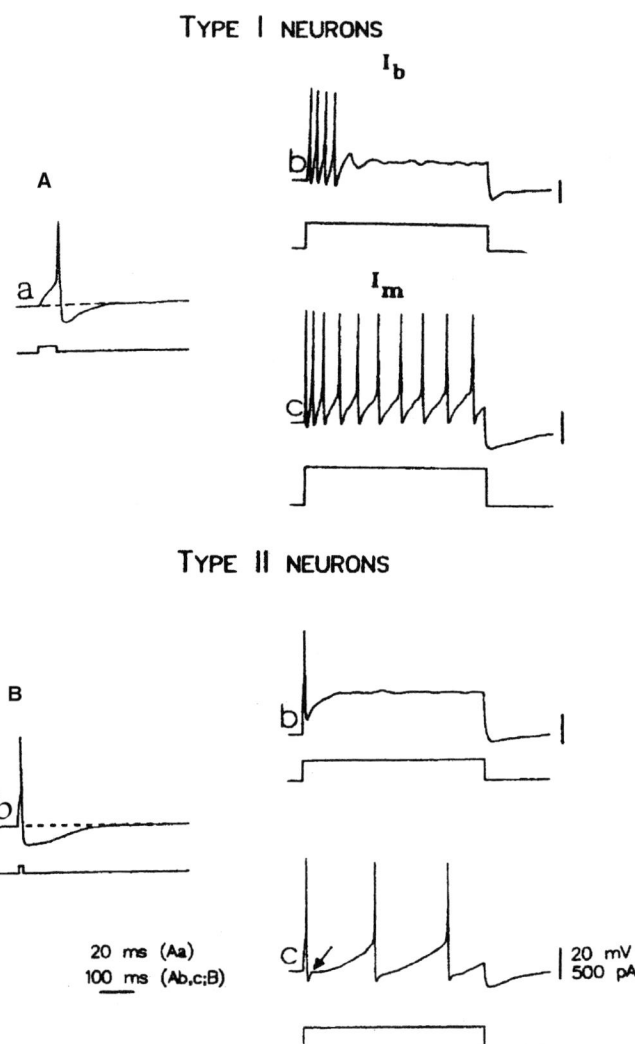

FIGURE 1–5 Firing characteristics of adult rat intracardiac neurons in situ. **A.** Firing of cardiac type I neurons. Type I_b neurons discharged a single spike followed by a short afterhyperpolarization (AHP) in response to a 10 ms depolarizing current pulse (*a*) and a burst of spikes at the onset of a prolonged pulse (500 ms) of depolarizing current of increased strength (*b*). Multiple firing in I_m neuron to 500 ms depolarizing current pulse (*c*). **B.** Firing of cardiac type II neurons. A type II neuron discharged a single spike followed by a long AHP in response to a 10 ms depolarizing current pulse (*a*) and a single spike at the onset of a prolonged pulse (500 ms) of depolarizing current of increased strength (*b*). Multiple firing in type II neuron to 500 ms depolarizing current pulse (*c*). Records in **A**(*a,b*), **A**(*c*), **B**(*a,b*), and **B**(*c*) were obtained from four different neurons—resting membrane potentials −51 mV, −45 mV, −47 mV, and −57 mV respectively. The upper record shows voltage, the lower record shows current. (From Selyanko.[136])

TABLE 1–3 Voltage-sensitive Ion Channels Identified in Mammalian Intracardiac Neurons

Ion Channel Family (major permeant ion)	Common Name	Molecular Identity	Antagonist	Reference
Sodium (Na^+)	TTX-sensitive	$Na_v1.1$–3, $Na_v1.7$	TTX, STX	179
Calcium (Ca^{2+})	L	$Ca_v1.2$ (α_{1C})	Dihydropyridines	85, 179
	N	$Ca_v2.1$ (α_{1B})	ω-conotoxin GVIA	85, 179
	P/Q	$Ca_v2.2$ (α_{1A})	ω-conotoxin MVIIC ω-agatoxin IVA	85
	R	$Ca_v2.3$ (α_{1E})	Ni^{2+}, SNX-482	85
Potassium (K^+)	K_V	Kv1.x	TEA	176, 178
	A	Kv3.x, Kv4.x	4-aminopyridine	176
	BK_{Ca}	Slo	TEA, charybdotoxin	47, 176, 178
	AHP	?	Ryanodine	7
	K_{IR}*	Kir2.x, Kir3.x	Ba^{2+}	39, 69
	K_{ATP}*	Kir6.x/SUR1–2	Glibenclamide, tolbutamide	68
	M	KCNQ1–5	Linopirdine (XE991)	33, 176
Nonselective cation (Na^+/K^+)	H	HCN1–4	Cs^+, ZD 7288	33, 39, 176

*K_{IR} and K_{ATP} are only expressed in mature intracardiac neurons.

relationship relative to voltage, reaching half-maximal activation at −25 mV. The number of Na^+ channels available for activation is steeply dependent on the membrane potential (steady-state inactivation) and, under the experimental conditions, half of the channels are inactivated at about −60 mV, which is close to the resting membrane potential of mammalian intracardiac neurons. During maintained depolarization, I_{Na} turns on and then inactivates with an exponential time course. The onset of inactivation determined from the time constant of I_{Na} decay is about 1 ms (at −20 mV) and decreased upon further depolarization. At the resting membrane potential (−60 mV), I_{Na} recovered slowly (τ = 20 ms) but was accelerated with membrane hyperpolarization. The stimulus-dependent decrease of nerve-evoked excitatory postsynaptic potentials observed in rat intracardiac ganglion neurons[134] may be attributed to the slow recovery from Na^+ channel inactivation.

Voltage-gated Na^+ channels are also a potential target for neurotoxins and drugs, including local anesthetics, antidepressants, and NO. The Na^+ channel activator, veratridine, has been shown to increase neuronal activity in canine intrinsic cardiac neurons in situ.[156,158] Similarly, ciguatoxin increases neuronal excitability and causes spontaneous opening of single Na^+ channels by shifting the voltage of activation of TTX-sensitive

Na$^+$ channels to more negative potentials.[70] Assessment of the actions of cardioactive drugs on Na$^+$ channel activity in intracardiac neurons needs to be considered in determining the site and mechanism of action of drugs that have been reported to modulate cardiac function.

Calcium Channels

Calcium channels contribute to neuronal excitability and convert electric activity into changes in intracellular free Ca^{2+} concentration, which regulates an array of cellular events including transmitter release, synaptic plasticity, gene expression, or modulation of excitability via Ca^{2+}-activated ion channels. The presence of voltage-gated Ca^{2+} channels was originally detected as a TTX-resistant, Ca^{2+}-dependent action potential in a population of guinea pig and canine intracardiac neurons.[7,175] Voltage-dependent Ca^{2+} currents are isolated by inhibiting Na$^+$ currents with TTX or replacing external Na$^+$ with an impermeant cation and suppressing K$^+$ currents with intracellular Cs$^+$ and/or extracellular TEA ions. Depolarization-activated ionic currents carried by Ca^{2+}, Ba^{2+}, or Na$^+$ through open Ca^{2+} channels have been characterized in rat intracardiac neurons.[85,179] The peak Ca^{2+} current density was ~45 pA/pF (2.5 mM Ca^{2+}), which increased ~1.5-fold with Ba^{2+} as the charge carrier. Peak Ca^{2+} current increased with increasing extracellular Ca^{2+} concentration and above 10 mM approached saturation (K_d of 2–4 mM), indicating the existence of saturable binding sites for Ca^{2+} within the calcium channel pore.

Voltage clamp studies of mammalian intracardiac neurons reveal only high-threshold Ca^{2+} channels, that is, no Ca^{2+} currents are activated at membrane potentials more negative than −40 mV. Rat intracardiac neurons exhibit Ca^{2+} currents that activate upon step depolarization positive to −30 mV, and the Ca^{2+} conductance increases sigmoidally with increasing depolarization reaching half-maximal activation at ~−5 mV with a slope of 4 mV per e-fold change.[179] The Ca^{2+} channel activation curve obtained with Ba^{2+} as the charge carrier was shifted approximately 10 mV to more negative potentials.[85] The steady-state inactivation of the Ca^{2+} current was also voltage-dependent, with half-inactivation occurring at −37 mV and complete inactivation at 0 mV. The kinetics and pharmacological properties of the whole-cell Ca^{2+} currents in mammalian intracardiac neurons suggest the existence of more than one type of Ca^{2+} channel. The kinetics of activation and inactivation of the Ca current were voltage-dependent and the time course of inactivation was fitted by the sum of two exponentials. The rate of recovery from inactivation increased with hyperpolarization with both time constants reduced e-fold by a 60 mV hyperpolarization.

At least three distinct pharmacological types of high-threshold Ca^{2+} channels have been identified to date in rat intracardiac neurons: *(1)* dihydropyridine (DHP)-sensitive L-type ($Ca_v1.2$) Ca^{2+} channels, *(2)* ω-conotoxin GVIA-sensitive N-type ($Ca_v2.1$) Ca^{2+} channels, and *(3)* DHP- and ω-conotoxin GVIA-resistant Ca^{2+} channels, all of which are blocked by 100 μM Cd^{2+} externally.[85,179] Amiloride, a potassium-sparing diuretic and antagonist of T-type ($Ca_v3.x$) Ca^{2+} channels, had no effect on Ca^{2+} current amplitude, consistent with the absence of a low-threshold T-type Ca^{2+} current in rat intracardiac neurons.[179] In neonatal rat intracardiac neurons, the DHP antagonist, nifedipine, and ω-conotoxin GVIA blocked ~50% and ~70%, respectively, of the total Ca^{2+} current at saturating concentrations, indicating that considerable overlap exists with regard to the inhibition of Ca^{2+} channels by DHPs and ω-conotoxin GVIA in these neurons.[179] In contrast, in adult rat intracardiac neurons, a saturating concentration of nifedipine (10 μM) blocked 11% of the control Ba^{2+} current whereas 63% of the total Ba^{2+} current was blocked by saturating concentration (1 μM) of ω-conotoxin GVIA with no significant overlap.[85] The resistant Ca^{2+} channel current (26%) in adult intracardiac neurons was largely inhibited by the P/Q-type ($Ca_v2.2$) Ca^{2+} channel antagonist, ω-conotoxin MVIIC (5 μM), but was insensitive to low concentrations (<100 nM) of ω-agatoxin IVA. The current that was insensitive to nifedipine and ω-conotoxins GVIA and MVIIC (7% of the total current) was sensitive to 100 μM Ni^{2+} and purported to represent the R-type ($Ca_v2.3$) Ca^{2+} channel current (see Fig. 1–6). Taken together, intracardiac neurons from adult rats express functional L-, N-, P/Q-, and R-type Ca^{2+} channels; however, the relative contribution(s) of other Ca^{2+} channel subtypes to the remaining DHP- and ω-conotoxin-resistant Ca^{2+} current (15% of the total current) in neonatal rats remains to be determined. The clearest distinction between functionally distinct Ca^{2+} channel types in intracardiac neurons may be achieved by direct measurement of the single channel properties correlated with analysis of mRNA expression and protein levels to determine the specific Ca^{2+} channel subunits expressed in individual neurons.

The physiological roles of multiple subtypes of Ca^{2+} channels are as yet unclear in mammalian intracardiac neurons. Extracellular recordings from canine right atrial cardiac neurons in situ show that local arterial infusion of the nonselective Ca^{2+} channel antagonist, Cd^{2+} (200 μM), increased neuronal activity, whereas, the L-type Ca channel antagonist, nifedipine (5 μM), reduced neuronal activity.[158] These data suggest that Ca^{2+} channel subtypes differentially contribute to electrical activity in intracardiac neurons and cardiac responses. Voltage-gated Ca^{2+} channel currents have also been shown to be modulated by various neurotransmitters and neuromodulators localized in intracardiac ganglia, indicating

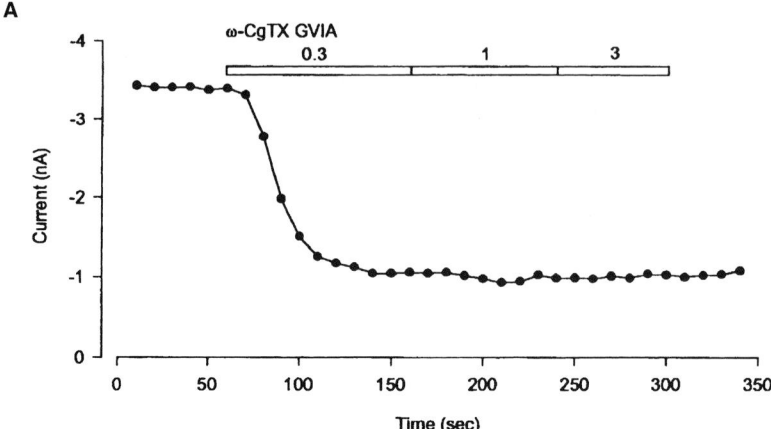
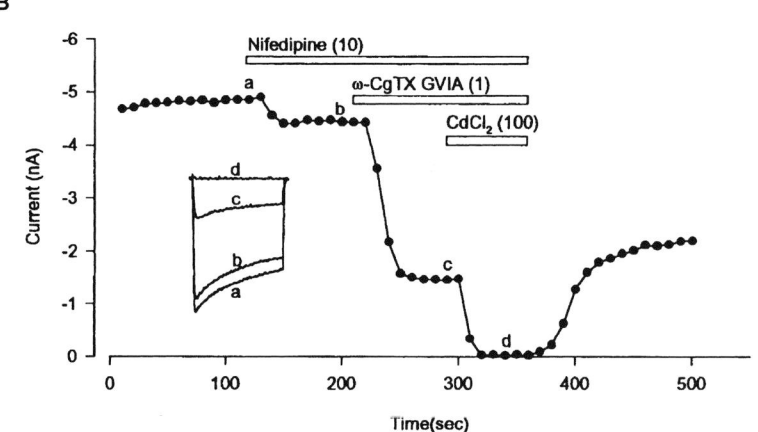
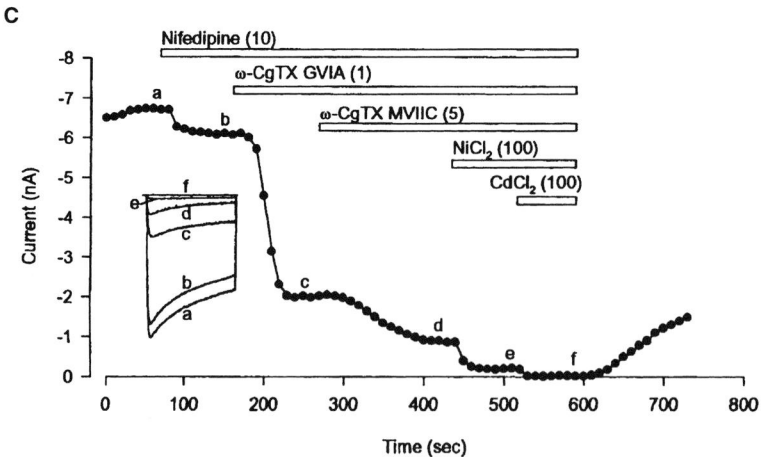

that regulation of Ca^{2+} channels is likely to influence neuronal excitability and ganglionic transmission in vivo. The major target of the different neurotransmitters appears to be the ω-conotoxin GVIA-sensitive N-type Ca^{2+} channel in both neonatal and adult rat intracardiac neurons. In most peripheral neurons, pertussis toxin-sensitive G proteins transduce the voltage-dependent and membrane-delimited inhibition of N-type Ca^{2+} channels.[67,81]

Potassium Channels

At least five distinct voltage-dependent K^+ currents have been identified in mammalian intrinsic cardiac neurons: *(1)* a delayed outward rectifying K^+ current (I_{Kv}), *(2)* a transient outward K^+ current, *(3)* a Ca^{2+}-dependent K^+ current(s) ($I_{K,Ca}$), *(4)* an inwardly rectifying K current (I_{Kir}), and *(5)* a muscarine-sensitive K^+ current (I_M).

Delayed outward rectifying K^+ current (I_{Kv})

The delayed rectifier (non-inactivating K^+ current) functions primarily to terminate the action potential rapidly. Membrane depolarization from a holding potential of -60 mV, which is close E_m, activates a slowly developing outward current that persists while the depolarization is maintained and deactivates with an outward tail current upon repolarization. Outward rectification is primarily a manifestation of this time-dependent gating process, but is enhanced by a time-independent rectification inherent to the open channel. The delayed rectifier has been described in mammalian intracardiac neurons, where it was isolated from Ca^{2+}-dependent K^+ currents using Ca^{2+}-free and/or Cd^{2+}-containing external solutions.[178] Elevation of bath K^+ concentration reduced the steady-state

FIGURE 1–6 Effect of ω-conotoxin GVIA (ω-CgTX GVIA) and ω-conotoxin MVIIC (ω-CgTX MVIIC) on Ca^{2+} channel currents. **A.** Determination of a saturating concentration of ω-CgTX GVIA. The saturation of blocking current was assessed by successive application of increasing concentrations of ω-CgTX GVIA (0.3, 1, and 3 μM). **B.** Blockade of N-type currents by a saturating concentration of ω-CgTX GVIA. ω-CgTX GVIA (1 μM) was applied after nifedipine (10 μM), which blocked a small portion (L type) of currents. **Inset:** Current traces obtained at different time points (labeled *a–d*). In both A and B, the peak Ba^{2+} current was evoked every 10 seconds by a depolarizing step to 0 mV for 100 ms. **C.** Blockade of the total Ba^{2+} current by ω-CgTX MVIIC (5 μM). Nifedipine (10 μM), ω-CgTX GVIA (1 μM), ω-CgTX MVIIC (5 μM), and $NiCl_2$ (100 μM) were successively applied. The peak Ba^{2+} current was evoked every 10 seconds by a depolarizing step to 0 mV for 100 ms. **Inset:** Current traces obtained at different time points (labeled *a–f*). (From Jeong and Wurster.[85])

outward current and shifted the reversal potential for tail currents to more positive potentials, as expected for a K^+-selective electrode. The delayed rectifier K^+ conductance activates at membrane potentials positive to -40 mV and increases in amplitude with increasing depolarization until saturation occurs beyond $+20$ mV.[178] Single-cell reverse transcription–polymerase chain reaction (RT-PCR) experiments indicate that rat intrinsic cardiac neurons express a heterogenous population of Kv channel subtypes, including Kv1.5 and Kv1.6. However, these cells do not appear to express Kv1.2, Kv1.3, or Kv1.7 (unpublished observation, H. Zhang and J. Cuevas).

The delayed outward current was inhibited by replacement of internal K^+ with Cs^+ and/or the addition of external TEA. Externally applied TEA produced a dose-dependent inhibition of the Ca^{2+}-insensitive, delayed outward current with 50% inhibition of I_{Kv} obtained with $\sim$3 mM TEA.[178] The delayed outwardly rectifying K^+ current in rat intracardiac neurons is also inhibited reversibly by verapamil and the related phenylalkylamine, D600.[72] Verapamil inhibited I_{Kv} in a concentration-dependent manner with an IC_{50} of 11 μM, which is about sevenfold more potent than its inhibition of high voltage–activated Ca^{2+} channel currents in these neurons.[72] The verapamil binding site on the delayed rectifier K^+ channel has been identified as part of the inner mouth of the K^+ channel pore.[127]

Transient outward K^+ current (I_A)
The fast, transient outward current is a membrane conductance that is activated in the subthreshold range of neuronal excitation and functions to reduce the excitatory effects of depolarizing stimuli in a time-dependent manner.

A transient outward K^+ current activated by membrane depolarization from potentials more negative than the resting membrane potential was described in a majority of adult rat intracardiac neurons.[176] The transient outward K^+ current was small in amplitude ($<$1 nA) and increased as it was evoked from more negative potentials. I_A exhibited both voltage- and time-dependent inactivation; the inactivation time course was fitted by a single exponential and usually complete within 100 ms, and inactivation of I_A was removed at hyperpolarized potentials with a time constant for removal of inactivation of 20 ms. Steady-state activation and inactivation overlapped between -70 and -40 mV. I_A amplitude was reversibly reduced by $\geq$80% by 1 mM 4-aminopyridine (4-AP) but was not affected by external TEA or Cs^+.

In addition to inhibiting I_A, 4-AP increased the frequency of repetitive firing, which suggests that in adult rat intracardiac neurons, I_A acts to slow repetitive discharge by reducing the rate of decay of the AHP.[176] I_A was not observed in neonatal rat intracardiac neurons.[178] This finding suggests that developmental changes in the expression ion channels in these neurons may contribute to the changes in autonomic control of the rat heart observed during the first few weeks of postnatal life.[126]

Ca^{2+}-dependent K^+ current ($I_{K,Ca}$)
Ca^{2+}-dependent K^+ currents are activated by an elevated cytoplasmic $[Ca^{2+}]$ and have an intrinsic voltage sensitivity. Their function is to hyperpolarize the cell following a burst of action potentials or single action potentials sufficient to raise intracellular Ca^{2+} levels. Action potentials in mammalian intracardiac neurons are followed by AHPs lasting from tens of milliseconds to several seconds.[7,39,136,146,174] These have been shown to be due to prolonged K^+ conductance activation by Ca^{2+} influx via depolarization-activated Ca^{2+} channels. In neonatal and adult rat intracardiac neurons, $I_{K,Ca}$ accounts for approximately one-third of the total outward K^+ current.[178] The action potential repolarization was not affected by the Ca^{2+} channel blocker Cd^{2+}, but the magnitude and duration of the AHP were reduced in the presence of either Cd^{2+} or Ca^{2+}-free external solutions.[39,178] Superfusion of Ca^{2+}-free solutions has been reported to cause a small membrane depolarization in guinea pig[7] and rat intracardiac neurons[136] and it has been suggested that $I_{K,Ca}$ may contribute to the resting membrane potential. Bath application of either TEA (1 mM) or Ba^{2+} (1 mM) depolarized neonatal rat intracardiac neurons by $\geq$10 mV, but Ca^{2+}-free external solutions or intracellular BAPTA, a Ca^{2+} chelator, did not change the resting potential, in dialyzed neurons.[178]

Single Ca^{2+}-activated K^+ (BK) channels have been characterized in excised membrane patches from neonatal rat intracardiac neurons and exhibited a single channel conductance of 207 pS in symmetrical 140 mM K^+.[47] Channel activity increased with the cytoplasmic $[Ca^{2+}]$ with a half-saturating $[Ca^{2+}]$ of 1.35 μM and was inhibited reversibly by external TEA ions and charybdotoxin. The resting BK channel activity in the cell-attached recording configuration was consistent with an intracellular $[Ca^{2+}]$ <100 nM, and the Ca^{2+} ionophore, ionomycin, increased channel activity consistent with a rise in intracellular $[Ca^{2+}]$ to $\geq$0.3 μM. TEA (1 mM) increased the action potential duration ~1.5-fold and reduced the amplitude and duration of the AHP by 26%. In contrast, charybdotoxin (100 nM) did not significantly alter the action potential duration or AHP amplitude but reduced the AHP duration by ~40%. These findings indicate that BK channel activation contributes to the action potential and AHP duration in rat intracardiac neurons.

Inwardly rectifying K$^+$ current (I$_{Kir}$)
A hyperpolarization-activated conductance producing a region of inward rectification in the steady-state I-V relationship and reversing at E$_K$ has been described in mammalian autonomic neurons.[1] This rectification is due to a time-dependent gating process and to a time-independent or instantaneous rectification either inherent to the permeability of the open channel or to block of outward current by intracellular Mg^{2+}. An inwardly rectifying K$^+$ current was found in intracardiac neurons from adult but not neonatal rats.[69] I$_{Kir}$ was present in approximately one-third of the adult intracardiac neurons studied, with a current density of 0.6 pA/pF at -130 mV, and was blocked by extracellular Ba^{2+} (10 μM). I$_{Kir}$ displayed rapid activation kinetics and no time-dependent rectification consistent with the rapidly activating, inward K$^+$ rectifier described in other mammalian autonomic neurons. A time-independent, Ba^{2+}-sensitive inward current that rectified at membrane potentials negative to -80 mV was also described in a population of guinea pig intracardiac neurons (SAH cells[39]). I$_{Kir}$ was sensitive to changes in external K$^+$, whereby raising the external K$^+$ concentration from 3 mM to 15 mM shifted the reversal potential by $\sim +36$ mV.[69] Substitution of external Na$^+$ had no effect on the reversal potential or amplitude of I$_{Kir}$. I$_{Kir}$ density increases as a function of postnatal development in a population of rat intracardiac neurons, which together with a concomitant decrease in I$_h$ (see below) may contribute to changes in the modulation of neuronal excitability in adult but not neonatal rat intracardiac ganglia.

ATP-sensitive K$^+$ current (I$_{K,ATP}$)
ATP-sensitive K$^+$ (K$_{ATP}$) channels serve to transduce changes in cell metabolism into changes in membrane potential; they are closed in the presence of micromolar concentrations of cytoplasmic ATP and are open when the ATP concentration decreases below a threshold. K$_{ATP}$ channels can be identified pharmacologically by their sensitivity to K$^+$ channel openers, including cromakalim, pinacidil, and diazoxide, and to the sulphonylurea drugs glibenclamide and tolbutamide.[49] Inhibition of sulphonylurea-sensitive K$^+$ channels has been shown to increase the heart rate response to vagal nerve stimulation in rat and guinea pig isolated atria by a presynaptic mechanism.[9,42] Furthermore, recordings from canine intracardiac ganglia in situ using extracellular microelectrodes demonstrated that transient coronary occlusion or administration of cromakalim in the local blood supply has been shown to alter the neuronal firing.[76,159] A K$_{ATP}$ conductance was identified in a population ($\sim$50%) of dissociated neurons from adult but not neonatal rat intracardiac ganglia,[68] based on the following evidence: (1) the K$^+$ channel opener, levcromakalim, evoked

a hyperpolarization that was inhibited by glibenclamide and tolbutamide, and (2) the presence of the sulphonylurea receptor in approximately half of the intracardiac neurons was confirmed by labeling with fluorescent glibenclamide-BODIPY. Bath application of either glibenclamide or tolbutamide depolarized (~5 mV) adult intracardiac neurons, a finding suggesting that a K_{ATP} conductance is activated under resting conditions and contributes to the resting membrane potential. Under voltage clamp conditions in symmetrical (140 mM) K^+ solutions, bath application of levcromakalim evoked an inward current of ~8 pA/pF at −50 mV that reversed close to E_K. Cell dialysis with an ATP-free intracellular solution also evoked an inward current, which was inhibited by tolbutamide. Metabolic inhibition or hypoxic solutions (PO_2 <30 mmHg) also activated a membrane current, which exhibited I-V characteristics that were similar to those of the levcromakalim-induced current and were inhibited by glibenclamide. These results suggest that K_{ATP} channel activation in intracardiac neurons may contribute to changes in neural regulation of the mature heart and cardiac function during ischemia-reperfusion.[14] Furthermore, the presence of K_{ATP} channels in adult intracardiac neurons only may contribute to the differential effects of hypoxia on heart rate in neonates and adults.[54]

Muscarine-sensitive K^+ current (I_M)
The muscarine-sensitive, non-inactivating K^+ current (M current) has been described in neonatal and adult rat intracardiac neurons.[33,176] In most mammalian intracardiac neurons, application of either muscarine or ACh evokes a slow depolarization associated with an increase in membrane resistance resulting from inhibition of an M-current that is partially activated at rest.[5,33,137] This muscarinic ACh-evoked depolarization corresponds to a decrease in outward K^+ current. M current is a small voltage-dependent K^+ current that is activated at more hyperpolarized membrane potentials than the delayed rectifier (I_{Kv}), Ca^{2+}-dependent K^+ ($I_{K,ca}$), or transient K^+ (I_A) currents, and is inhibited by ACh and other muscarinic receptor agonists.[24] I_M is activated in the voltage range between the resting potential and threshold (from −70 mV to −30 mV) and therefore may contribute as a background K^+ current to the resting membrane current and affects the general level of excitability. Step hyperpolarization from depolarized potentials, i.e., −30 mV, reveals a slow inward relaxation associated with the deactivation of the time- and voltage-dependent current. The inward relaxation became faster at more hyperpolarized potentials whereby the time constant for deactivation of I_M changed e-fold for a 19 mV change in membrane potential at 37°C.[33] The amplitude and kinetics of I_M in rat intracardiac neurons were highly tem-

perature-dependent; lowering the temperature from 37° to 22°C reduced the steady-state current amplitude by one-third and the rate of deactivation by six- to ninefold (Q_{10} of 3.7).

Nonselective cation channels: hyperpolarization-activated current
In the population of neurons (P cells) in the guinea pig cardiac plexus that displayed inward rectification at potentials near rest, rectification resulted from the activation of an inward current that was blocked by external Cs^+ but not Ba^{2+}.[39] Hyperpolarizing current pulses induced time-dependent rectification of the voltage response in all neonatal rat intracardiac neurons, which was not observed in dialyzed neurons.[33] Voltage clamp studies of isolated rat intracardiac neurons revealed a hyperpolarization-activated inward current that was isolated from other membrane currents using external Cs^+.[33,69,176] The time- and voltage-

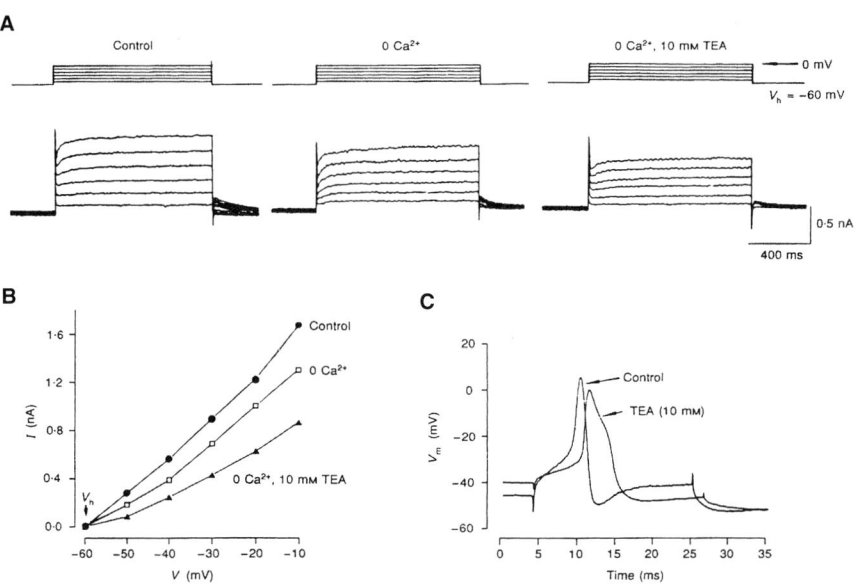

FIGURE 1-7 Detection of I_K and $I_{K,Ca}$ in an adult rat intracardiac neuron. A. The depolarization-activated outward relaxation and tail current were first decreased by removing Ca^{2+} from the media and then further depressed by addition of TEA (10 mM) in a single neuron. $V_h = -60$ mV; $V_c = -50$ to -10 mV in 10 mV increments. B. Current–voltage (I-V) relationship from a different neuron shows the presence of Ca^{2+}-sensitive and Ca^{2+}-insensitive outward K^+ currents. Voltage protocol shown in A. C. Effects of TEA (10 mM) on the resting potential, action potential, and afterhyperpolarization from a single intracardiac neuron. Experiments A and B were carried out in the presence of TTX (3 μM), Ba^{2+} (1 mM), and 4-AP (1 mM). (From Xi-Moy and Dun.[176])

dependence of this current is consistent with the hyperpolarization-activated nonselective cation current, I_h, and contributes to the electrical properties of intracardiac neurons. I_h was observed in both neonatal and adult rat intracardiac neurons and displayed slow time-dependent rectification with a time constant of activation of ~500 ms at -100 mV (22°C), which was voltage-sensitive with the rate of activation of I_h increasing with membrane hyperpolarization.[33,39,176] The time constant of activation of I_h was about threefold faster in intracardiac neurons from adult than in those from neonatal rats and decreased e-fold change for 27 mV hyperpolarization.[69] Raising the temperature from 22°C to 37°C increased I_h amplitude and the rate of activation fivefold with a corresponding Q_{10} of 3.[33] I_h was isolated by blockade with external Cs^+ (2 mM) and was inhibited irreversibly by the bradycardic agent ZD 7288. Current density of I_h was approximately twofold greater in neurons from neonatal rats (4.1 pA/pF at -130 mV) than that in adult rats (2.3 pA/pF), however, the reversal potential and activation parameters were unchanged. The reversal potential and amplitude of I_h were sensitive to changes in external Na^+ and K^+ concentrations with P_{Na}/P_K ratio of 0.42.[69,176] The effects of Cs^+ on the resting membrane potential and action potential discharge at 37°C suggest that I_h may play a role in regulating action potential firing in mammalian intracardiac neurons.[39,69] I_h is also subject to modulation by neurotransmitters and neuropeptides that converge to act via adenyl cyclase[117] and the membrane-permeable analogue of cAMP, 8-bromo-cAMP, has been shown to increase the amplitude of I_h in rat intracardiac neurons.[69] Transmitter-induced modulation of I_h can potentially allow prolonged alterations of the sensitivity of intracardiac neurons to synaptic and nonsynaptic stimuli.

MODULATION OF VOLTAGE-GATED ION CHANNELS

One of the fundamental requirements of the hypothesis that mammalian intracardiac ganglia serve as integration centers for sympathetic, parasympathetic, and afferent innervation of the heart is that intracardiac neurons be able to convert signals from these discrete inputs into a code that may be relayed to the effector tissue. Furthermore, there must be sufficient plasticity in this code to adequately reflect the summation of these converging signals and to produce a concomitant response in the target tissue. Recent advances in our understanding of neurotransmitters and neuromodulators in mammalian intracardiac ganglia have given insight into putative mechanisms involved in the integration process. The ability of various neurotransmitters and neuromodulators to alter the electrical properties of neurons, and thus this code, forms the basis for the neural network integrator. As discussed previously, immunohistochemical studies have revealed the presence of a wide array of neurochemicals in neurons and nerve fibers within intracardiac ganglia. In this section, we focus on the changes in electrical properties of intracardiac neurons that are evoked by the different neurotransmitters and neuromodulators identified in cardiac ganglia. Table 1–4 summarizes the effects of these agents on ion channels in mammalian intracardiac neurons.

Cholinergic Modulation of Ion Channels

Acetylcholine is the primary neurotransmitter mediating intrinsic and extrinsic (vagal) innervation of the intracardiac ganglia. One of the mechanisms by which ACh modulates neurotransmission to these neurons is by activating muscarinic receptors, which in turn produce a variety of changes in membrane conductances. Transcripts encoding four of the five known muscarinic receptor (M_1–M_4) genes have been detected in intracardiac neurons in vitro and in situ,[64,73] and muscarinic receptor expression in the ganglia has been demonstrated by autoradiography.[55] Early experiments using muscarinic receptor agonists and antagonists that did not effectively discriminate between muscarinic ACh receptor (mAChR) subtypes demonstrated that mAChRs mediated several membrane responses in guinea pig, canine, and rat intracardiac neurons.[5,137,177] Recent studies using mAChR subtype selective antagonists have used pharmacological blockade to characterize the cellular effects due to each receptor subtype.[30,33,86]

Muscarinic ACh-evoked responses are observed in the majority (>75%) of isolated intracardiac neurons from neonatal rats[30,33] and adult guinea pigs.[5] In most neurons, both muscarine and ACh evoke a slow depolarization associated with an increase in membrane resistance.[5,33,137] This muscarinic ACh–evoked depolarization corresponds to a decrease in outward K^+ current. The voltage- and time-dependent properties of the K^+ current suggest that it is the muscarinic-sensitive M current (I_M) originally described in amphibian sympathetic neurons.[25] Inhibition of I_M in rat intracardiac neurons was shown to be mediated by activation of M_1 muscarinic receptors[33] and was blocked by low concentrations of the M_1 receptor antagonists pirenzepine or m1-toxin (MT1), a specific peptide toxin from *Dendroaspis angusticeps*.[107]

Muscarinic receptor activation was also associated with an increase in the number of action potentials evoked by a depolarizing current pulse, causing a phasic to tonic shift in the firing pattern of rat intracardiac neurons that could be blocked by pirenzepine (Fig. 1–8). A similar phenom-

TABLE 1-4 Neurotransmitter-evoked Responses in Mammalian Intracardiac Neurons

Neurotransmitter	Receptor	Species	Target	Effect	References
ACh	nAChR	Rat		Rapid depolarization	43, 115
		Guinea pig		Rapid depolarization	7
	M_1	Rat	I_M	Inhibition of I_M, phasic to tonic shift	33
		Guinea pig			5
	M_2		$I_{K?}$	Decreased excitability	110, J. Cuevas and D.J. Adams, unpublished observation
	M_4		I_{Ca}	Inhibition	30, 86
ATP	P2X	Rat		Rapid depolarization	44, 95
		Guinea pig		Rapid depolarization	6
	P2Y	Rat	I_M	Slow hyperpolarization	97
GABA/glycine		Canine		Increased neuronal activity	77
Glutamate		Canine		Increased neuronal activity	156
Histamine	H_1	Canine		Increased excitability	12
		Guinea pig		Depolarization; increased excitability	125
NE	α_1		I_{Ca}	Inhibition	82
	α_2				180
	β_1	Canine		Increased neuronal activity	13, 156
	β_2				
NO		Canine		Increased neuronal activity	18, 156

ACh, acetylcholine; ATP, adenosine 5′-triphosphate; GABA, γ-amino butyric acid; nAChR, nicotinic acetylcholine receptor; NE, norepinephrine; NO, nitric oxide.

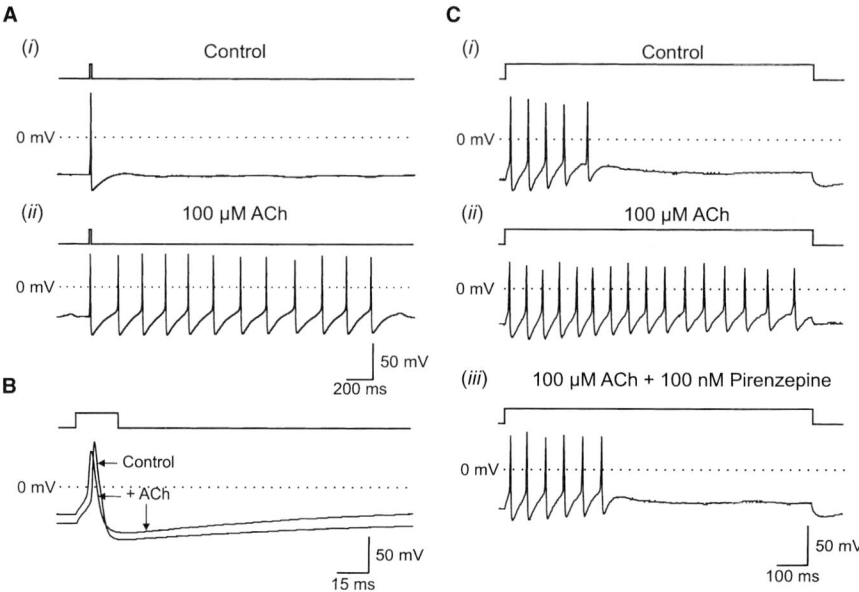

FIGURE 1–8 Acetylcholine (ACh) modulation of discharge activity by muscarinic receptor activation. **A.** Action potentials recorded in response to brief current pulses (+140 pA, 10 ms) in control, physiological saline solution *(i)* and in the presence of focally applied 100 μM ACh co-applied with 3 μM mecamylamine *(ii)*. **B.** Superimposed traces of action potentials, shown on expanded time scale, obtained in the absence (control) and presence of ACh (ACh⁺). In the absence (control) and presence of ACh (+ACh), the resting membrane potentials were −54 mV and −42 mV, respectively. **C.** Discharge activity recorded in response to a depolarizing current pulse (+50 pA, 1 second) in the absence *(i)* and presence of 100 μM ACh *(ii)* and following co-application of ACh with muscarinic receptor antagonist, pirenzepine (100 nM) *(iii)*. Temperature 22°C. (From Cuevas et al.[33])

enon has also been observed in guinea pig intracardiac neurons.[5] However, in guinea pig intracardiac neurons, muscarine was suggested to promote multiple firing predominantly by inhibiting a Ca^{2+}-activated K^+ conductance (I_{KCa}). External application of Cd^{2+}, which inhibits Ca^{2+} influx and depresses I_{KCa} activation, mimicked the actions of muscarine in promoting repetitive firing.[5] In rat intracardiac neurons, however, it is the inhibition of I_M by M_1 muscarinic receptor activation, rather than the modulation of I_{KCa} that appears to mediate muscarinic-induced repetitive firing. Although the I_M inhibitors UTP and Ba^{2+} facilitate multiple firing, neither charybdotoxin (an inhibitor of I_{KCa}) nor Cd^{2+} increases the number of action potentials evoked by depolarizing current pulses in these cells.[33,178]

Guinea pig, canine, and rat intracardiac ganglia contain a population of neurons in which muscarinic agonists evoke a transient hyperpolarization that is followed by the I_M-mediated sustained depolarization[5,177] (J. Cuevas and D.J. Adams, unpublished observation). The transient hyperpolarization corresponds to an inwardly rectifying outward current with the dependence of the current amplitude on $[K^+]$, which suggests that K^+ is the charge carrier (J. Cuevas and D.J. Adams, unpublished observation). Muscarinic ACh activation of the outward K^+ conductance appears to be mediated by an M_2 muscarinic receptor, since the tricyclic antimuscarinic AF-DX 116, which is specific for the M_2 receptor subtype,[80] inhibits muscarinic agonist activation of the transient K^+ current. Furthermore, this ACh-induced K^+ current was not significantly affected by pirenzepine at concentrations that inhibit M_1 or M_4 receptors, or by the specific M_4 receptor antagonist, m4-toxin.

Muscarine also evokes a slow depolarization associated with an increase in membrane conductance in guinea pig intracardiac neurons.[5,110] This third muscarine-evoked current was also observed in ~12% of rat intracardiac neurons (J. Cuevas and D.J. Adams, unpublished observation) and reversed near the Cl^- equilibrium potential, suggesting that it is due to activation of a Cl^- conductance. The muscarine-evoked conductance was not inhibited by either pirenzepine or AF-DX 116 (J. Cuevas and D.J. Adams, unpublished observation).[5] Therefore, it appears that M_3 receptors couple to Cl^- channels in a subpopulation of intracardiac neurons.

Muscarinic agonists also produce a rapid, reversible inhibition of depolarization-activated Ca^{2+} channel currents in rat intracardiac neurons. Acetylcholine and oxotremorine methiodide (oxo-M) inhibit peak Ca^{2+} channel current amplitude by ~75% via voltage-dependent and -independent mechanisms, with inhibition of multiple Ca^{2+} channel subtypes, including N-type, L-type, and non-L, non-N-type Ca^{2+} channels being involved.[29] Experiments using selective muscarinic receptor antagonists, including pirenzepine and m-4 toxin (MT3), suggest that the M_4 muscarinic receptor subtype inhibits Ca^{2+} channel currents in neonatal rat intracardiac neurons.[30] In contrast, in adult rat intracardiac neurons, mAChR activation by oxo-M has been shown to selectively and reversibly inhibit N-, Q-, and R- but not L-type Ca^{2+} channel currents.[86] The selective antagonists to M_2 (methoctramine), but not M_1/M_4 (pirenzepine) or M_3 (hexahydro-sila-difenidol) receptors, antagonized the inhibitory effect of oxo-M to inhibit Ba^{2+} currents. This suggests that M_2 receptors mediate the inhibition of Ca^{2+} channel currents in adult rat intracardiac neurons.[86]

Muscarinic agonist attenuation of Ca^{2+} channel currents via either the M_2 or M_4 receptor activation is mediated by a pertussis toxin (PTX)-sensitive G protein, and differs from the BAPTA-sensitive pathway for

I_{Ca} inhibition of rat sympathetic neurons.[21] Pretreatment of rat intracardiac neurons with PTX or the heterologous expression of transducin, a known chelator of G-protein $\beta\gamma$ subunits, significantly attenuated the mAChR-mediated current inhibition.[84] Furthermore, experiments using relatively specific activators and inhibitors of diacylglycerol, protein kinase C, and adenylate cyclase fail to mimic or occlude the inhibitory effects of muscarinic agonists on Ca^{2+} channel currents in rat intracardiac neurons.[86,180] Therefore, mAChR-mediated inhibition of Ca^{2+} channels in neonatal and adult rat intracardiac neurons is likely mediated by direct interaction of a PTX-sensitive G protein(s) and the Ca^{2+} channels, as suggested in other systems.[67]

Adrenergic Modulation of Ion Channels

Norepinephrine is released in the heart from sympathetic nerve terminals located in close proximity to intracardiac neurons. Numerous studies suggest direct interaction between the sympathetic and parasympathetic nervous systems at the level of the intracardiac ganglia.[50,108] Although presynaptic adrenoceptor-mediated inhibition of ACh release from postganglionic intracardiac neurons is likely to occur (see Anatomical Organization, above), other mechanisms of integration between the two systems are likely to involve changes in the electrical properties of intracardiac neurons in response to catecholamine release.

Direct application of NE to the soma of isolated rat intracardiac neurons decreased the amplitude and duration of Ca^{2+}-dependent action potentials.[180] This effect was shown to be the result of attenuation of depolarization-activated Ca^{2+} currents. In contrast to M_4 muscarinic inhibition of Ca^{2+} channels in these neurons, adrenergic receptor activation inhibited primarily a high-threshold, ω-conotoxin GVIA-sensitive current. Maximum inhibition of peak I_{Ca} amplitude was ~60% and was the result of voltage-dependent and -independent changes in the activation kinetics of these channels.[84,180] Pharmacological studies suggest that the effect of NE on these neurons is mediated by an α-adrenoreceptor with properties that may differ from those of classical α_1- and α_2-receptor subtypes. The signal transduction cascade mediating the effects of NE indicates that the α-adrenoceptor, like the M_4 muscarinic receptor, is coupled to Ca^{2+} channels via a PTX-sensitive G protein.[180]

In addition to the inhibition of Ca^{2+} channels, in a subpopulation of rat intracardiac neurons, NE activates a time-independent, cation-selective background current.[180] Activation of an outward nonselective cation current at voltages that open Ca^{2+} channels would repolarize the cell and further inhibit Ca^{2+} influx. This effect, together with the direct inhibition of I_{Ca} by NE, may account for the reduction in action potential amplitude and duration produced by NE in rat intracardiac neurons. More recently, NE has been shown to activate a cation channel that is inhibited by extracellular Ca^{2+} or Mg^{2+} via α_1-adrenoceptors in intracardiac neurons.[82] This channel produced an inward current in neurons held at -60 mV. In cells studied under current-clamp mode, activation of this conductance depolarized the neurons and elicited repetitive firing of action potentials.[82]

Peptidergic Modulation of Ion Channels

A considerable number of neuropeptides have been identified in cell bodies and neuron fibers within the mammalian intracardiac ganglia. The origin of these peptides varies considerably as discussed above and the function of these neuropeptides is likely to reflect the type of influence that the particular source of these neuromodulators has on the intracardiac ganglia. For example, neuropeptide Y is primarily released from sympathetic nerve terminals that are adjacent to intracardiac neurons and thus this peptide is likely to shift the balance toward increased sympathetic tone in the heart. The mechanisms by which NPY and other peptides may achieve their effect on the intracardiac ganglia is discussed here. A summary of the effects of neuropeptides studied to date is presented in Table 1–5.

Angiotensin II

Angiotensin II (ANG II) has been reported to induce positive chronotropic and inotropic effects.[130] Many of these effects appear to be related to direct interaction with cardiac myocytes and with increased sympathetic tone due to changes in central nervous system (CNS) sympathetic outflow.[38] However, some of the cardiovascular effects of ANG II appear to be related to its ability to directly modulate the function of peripheral neurons. Angiotensin II has been shown to activate postganglionic sympathetic neurons[130] and to facilitate the release of NE from sympathetic nerve terminals.[94] Recently, ANG II has been shown to modulate the activity of intracardiac neurons in situ.[75] Administration of ANG II onto active neurons from the canine right atrial ganglionated plexus increased the activity of most of the neurons (83%) tested, but in some neurons (17%) ANG II depressed the firing rate. Antagonism of the effects of ANG II by a selective AT_1 receptor antagonist (losartan) but not a selective AT_2 receptor antagonist (PD-123319) suggests that the effects of ANG II on intracardiac neurons are mediated by AT_1 receptors. However, the cellular mechanisms mediating the changes in neuroexcitability remain to be determined.

TABLE 1-5 Neuropeptide Regulation of Mammalian Intracardiac Neurons

Neuropeptide	Species	Receptor	Target	Effect	Reference
Angiotensin II	Canine	AT_1	I_{Ca}?	Increased neuronal activity	75, 156
Bradykinin	Canine			Increased neuronal activity	156
Met-enkephalin	Rat	μ-opioid	$I_{Ca(L-, N-Type)}$	Inhibition	2, 84
NPY	Guinea pig		I_{Ca}	Membrane hyperpolarization; decreased AHP amplitude and duration	88
	Rat		I_{Ca}	Inhibition of I_{Ca}	84
Somatostatin	Rat		I_{Ca}	Inhibition	84
Substance P	Rat		nAChR	Inhibition	31
	Guinea pig				182
VIP	Rat	VPAC1 and VPAC2	nAChR	Potentiation	29, 96
PACAP	Rat	PAC1	nAChR	Potentiation	96
	Guinea pig	PAC1	I_A?	Depolarization	121

Voltage-gated Ca^{2+} channel currents were recorded at 22°C with Ba^{2+} as the charge carrier. AHP, afterhyperpolarization; NPY, neuropeptide Y; PACAP, pituitary adenylate cyclase-activating peptide; VIP, vasoactive intestinal polypeptide.

Met-enkephalin

Endogenous opioid peptides have been found in the extrinsic and intrinsic innervation of rat and guinea pig heart as well as cardiac muscle.[79,147,167] One such peptide, met-enkephalin, has been shown to reduce bradycardia associated with vagus nerve stimulation,[169] while application of an enkephalin derivative, [d-Ala^2, d-Leu^5] enkephalin, increased neuronal activity in the epicardial ganglia and produced concomitant changes in heart rate.[17] These data suggest that endogenous opioid peptides may exert some of their cardiovascular effects at the level of the intracardiac ganglia.

Modulation of depolarization-activated ionic conductances by opioid receptor agonists has been investigated in isolated neurons from neonatal and adult rat intracardiac ganglia using whole-cell perforated patch clamp recording techniques. Met-enkephalin (10 μM) was shown to alter the action potential waveform, reducing the maximum amplitude, slowing the rate of rise, and increasing the action potential duration.[2] The effects of met-enkephalin on the action potential appear to be mediated by a selective and reversible reduction of the peak amplitude of high voltage–activated Ca^{2+} channel currents and a change in Ca^{2+} channel gating.[2,84] Peak Ca^{2+} channel current evoked by step depolarizations to 0 mV from -90 mV was decreased by 50%–60% and the time to peak was increased nearly fourfold. Analogous to muscarinic and α-adrenergic receptor–mediated inhibition of I_{Ca}, met-enkephalin had no effect on the voltage dependence of steady-state inactivation but shifted the voltage dependence of activation to more positive membrane potentials, whereby stronger depolarization was required to open Ca^{2+} channels.[2,84] Furthermore, addition of met-enkephalin after exposure to ω-conotoxin GVIA failed to cause a further decrease of the residual current. Thus, met-enkephalin, like NE, inhibits primarily ω–conotoxin GVIA–sensitive Ca^{2+} channels in rat intracardiac neurons. Pharmacological studies further demonstrated that these effects are mediated by μ-opioid receptors via activation of a PTX-sensitive G protein.[2,84] Heterologous expression of transducin in rat intracardiac neurons almost completely abolished met-enkephalin–induced inhibition of I_{Ca}, an effect similar to that observed for ACh-, NE-, and NPY-induced current inhibition.[84] Taken together, these data suggest that four different neurotransmitters (met-enkephalin, ACh, NE, and NPY) inhibit Ca^{2+} channel currents in rat intracardiac neurons via a common pathway that is voltage-dependent and membrane delimited, and utilizes $\beta\gamma$ subunits released from PTX-sensitive G proteins.

A second mechanism by which met-enkephalin may modulate neuronal excitability in intracardiac neurons was recently identified. In isolated intracardiac neurons of neonatal rats, met-enkephalin activation of μ-opioid receptors evoked a transient increase in intracellular [Ca^{2+}].[143]

This increase in $[Ca^{2+}]_i$ was dependent on extracellular Ca^{2+} and inhibited by ryanodine, which suggests that it was due to Ca^{2+} release from ryanodine-sensitive intracellular Ca^{2+} stores. This mobilization of intracellular Ca^{2+} activated an outward current mediated by large-conductance Ca^{2+}-dependent K^+ (BK_{Ca}) channels that were voltage-sensitive and blocked by charybdotoxin.[143] Activation of these channels therefore represents a second mechanism by which endogenous enkephalins may depress neuronal excitability and alter firing behavior in mammalian intracardiac neurons.

Neuropeptide Y

Neuropeptide Y has been implicated as one of the major neurotransmitters facilitating parasympathetic–sympathetic interaction in the cardiovascular system. Investigation of cardiac autonomic responses has shown that the sequence of sympathetic and vagal stimulation determines the predominant tone in the heart. Longer antecedent sympathetic stimulation progressively diminished parasympathetic output, a phenomenon that was attributed to NPY-mediated inhibition of vagal transmission.[181] Furthermore, studies on the effects of NPY on basal contractile force and nerve-mediated atrial inotropic responses in guinea pigs suggested that NPY is a prejunctional inhibitor of vagus-mediated negative inotropic responses.[139]

What are the cellular mechanisms mediating this effect of NPY? As in the case of NE, a component of the inhibition is likely the ability of NPY to modulate ACh release through activation of presynaptic receptors on parasympathetic nerve terminals. For example, NPY has been shown to depress ACh release from parasympathetic nerve terminals in the rat urinary bladder[160] and the guinea pig myenteric plexus.[153] However, NPY also exerts direct effects on parasympathetic intracardiac neurons and these effects may result in depression of parasympathetic tone. Intracellular recordings of guinea pig intracardiac neurons in situ showed that NPY (100 μM) hyperpolarized 60% of the cells tested by an average of 9 mV.[88] Both phasic and tonic neurons exhibited this hyperpolarizing membrane response to NPY, and this effect was coupled with a decrease in membrane resistance. No changes in action potential amplitude or duration were noted, but the spike AHP was decreased.

The attenuation of the action potential AHP is likely due to NPY-mediated decreases in depolarization-activated Ca^{2+} currents. Bath application of NPY (1 μM) inhibits reversibly 65% of the peak Ca^{2+} current in rat intracardiac neurons.[84] Neuropeptide Y receptors have been shown to couple to a PTX-sensitive G protein that modulates Ca^{2+} channel currents in guinea pig and rat intracardiac neurons.[84,88] This signal transduction cascade for Ca^{2+} channel inhibition appears to represent a convergence of adrenergic, cholinergic (muscarinic), and peptidergic (NPY and μ-opioid) receptor–mediated pathways. The major target of these receptors appears to be N-type or ω-conotoxin GVIA-sensitive Ca^{2+} channels, which accounts for 60%–70% of the total whole-cell Ca^{2+} current.

Pituitary adenylate cyclase-activating polypeptide
Messenger RNA encoding pituitary adenylate cyclase-activating polypeptide (PACAP)-selective PAC1 receptor isoforms has been reported in adult guinea pig and neonatal rat intracardiac neurons.[23,37] Immunohistochemical studies have also detected PAC_1 receptor immunoreactivity localized to cardiac ganglia neuronal plasma membranes in adult guinea pig hearts, with almost all of the parasympathetic neurons expressing membrane-associated PAC_1 receptor proteins.[23] The immunocytochemical localization of these cells correlated with the population of cells that responded physiologically to PACAP.[23] In these cells, pituitary adenylate cyclase-activating polypeptide was shown to depolarize both tonic and phasic neurons. Furthermore, PACAP directly modulates neuronal excitability, inducing a phasic to tonic shift in the neurons. The rank order of peptide potency on membrane excitability in response to depolarizing currents was consistent with PAC_1 receptor activation. The changes in neuroexcitability did not appear to be a direct result of the peptide-induced membrane depolarization or alterations in action potential configuration, but may be due to an inhibition in I_A, as has been reported in rat sacral preganglionic neurons.[111]

In contrast to the effects of PACAP on neuroexcitability in adult guinea pig intracardiac neurons, this neuropeptide does not appear to have any direct effects on neonatal rat intracardiac neurons.[96] There are two possible explanations for this discrepancy. First, the predominant PAC_1 isoform expressed in neonatal rat intracardiac neurons is the PAC_1-HOP_1,[37] whereas in guinea pig intracardiac neurons, the PAC_1-*very-short* is most abundant.[23] This difference in receptor subtype may result in distinct cellular effects, particularly in light of the fact that the sequence variations between these isoforms occur in the region known to determine G-protein coupling. Second, neonatal rat intracardiac neurons do not express some membrane currents present in adult intracardiac neurons[68] and may therefore not be expressing the channel modulated by PAC_1 receptor activation in cells from adult animals.

Substance P
Primary afferent fibers that innervate the mammalian intracardiac ganglia contain substance P immunoreactivity[51,161] and are likely to provide direct

sensory input to cardiac neurons, forming the first segment of local reflex arcs that serve to modulate cardiac function. In canine hearts, SP modulates autonomic nerve activity, increasing cardiac contractility during vagal stimulation and decreasing contractility during stellate ganglion stimulation.[146] Application of capsaicin, which releases SP and CGRP from afferent nerve terminals, evokes noncholinergic, nonadrenergic depolarizations in mammalian intrinsic cardiac neurons. In guinea pig intracardiac neurons, the capsaicin-induced, Ca^{2+}-dependent slow depolarization could be mimicked by tachykinins.[56] In addition to increasing membrane excitability by depolarizing the neuron, SP also increased the number of action potentials in response to depolarizing current pulses, converting phasic neurons to adapting or tonic neurons.[56] Pharmacological investigation of the mechanism(s) mediating SP-induced depolarization of intracardiac neurons in guinea pigs showed that SP activated a nonselective cation conductance via an NK_3 receptor,[57] to induce bradycardia in guinea pig hearts.[159]

Purinergic Modulation of Ion Channels

There is substantial evidence that ATP is stored and co-released with NE from sympathetic nerves in the cardiovascular system and is likely to be involved in neural control of cardiac function. In the mammalian heart, ATP stimulates vagal efferent fibers producing a negative chronotropic effect[123] and has been reported to inhibit NE release from efferent nerve fibers.[163] Local administration of ATP to canine intrinsic cardiac ganglia in situ either enhanced or attenuated spontaneous neuronal activity, resulting in bradycardia or tachycardia, respectively.[78] Although ATP may have direct effects on cardiac myocytes, intrinsic cardiac neurons may mediate some of the actions of ATP on the heart.

Mammalian intracardiac neurons exhibit multicomponent responses to exogenous ATP, analogous to mAChR activation of a compound response in these neurons. In guinea pig intracardiac neurons, up to three membrane responses to ATP have been observed, consisting of a transient depolarization followed by a brief hyperpolarization and a slow, sustained depolarization.[6] This complexity of response is the result of multiple ATP receptor types being expressed differentially amongst subpopulations of intracardiac neurons. Recent studies using RT-PCR demonstrated that rat intracardiac neurons express transcripts for $P2Y_2$ and $P2Y_4$ purinergic receptors.[97] Microfluorimetric measurements in fura-2–loaded intracardiac neurons showed that the activation of $P2Y_2$ purinoceptors by either ATP or UTP elevates the intracellular $[Ca^{2+}]$ in all neurons tested. This increase in cytoplasmic $[Ca^{2+}]$ is due to the activation of a PTX-insensitive G protein coupled to phospholipase C (PLC) generation of inositol trisphosphate (IP$_3$), which triggers the release of Ca^{2+} from ryanodine-insensitive Ca^{2+} stores.[97]

The increase in intracellular [Ca^{2+}] in response to P2Y$_2$ receptor activation in voltage-clamped rat intracardiac neurons evokes a slow outward current at -60 mV.[97] The correlation between the membrane current and increase in [Ca^{2+}]$_i$ suggests that it is mediated by activation of I$_{KCa}$. This current (I$_{KCa}$) likely underlies the ATP-evoked slow, sustained inhibitory response in these neurons under current-clamp conditions and the hyperpolarization also observed in the guinea pig.[6] The initial transient depolarization is mediated by activation of P2X receptors and will be discussed in the next section; the mechanism mediating the slow ATP-induced depolarization in guinea pig intracardiac neurons is yet to be determined.

LIGAND-GATED ION CHANNELS

Nicotinic Acetylcholine Receptors

In mammalian intracardiac neurons, cholinergic agonists evoke a rapid excitatory response mediated by nicotinic acetylcholine receptor (nAChR) activation similar to that described in other autonomic ganglion neurons. However, the structure, function, and cellular and subcellular distribution of nAChRs in intracardiac ganglion neurons remain to be fully elucidated. The rapid inward current evoked by ACh in isolated neurons of neonatal rat intracardiac ganglia was insensitive to atropine and mimicked by nicotine.[43] The activation of nAChR-mediated currents exhibited a short latency (<10 ms) consistent with a direct ligand-gated ion channel and was reversibly inhibited in a concentration-dependent manner by the ganglionic nAChR antagonists mecamylamine and hexamethonium. Acetylcholine-evoked membrane currents recorded from an isolated rat intracardiac ganglion neuron and the corresponding current-voltage (I-V) relationship are shown in Figure 1–9. Whole-cell ACh-evoked currents exhibited strong inward rectification and a reversal (zero-current) potential close to 0 mV. The dependence of ACh-evoked current amplitude on the extracellular Na$^+$ concentration, and the direction and magnitude of the shift in reversal potential upon replacement of NaCl by mannitol, indicated that nAChRs in intracardiac neurons are cation-selective.[43] Anion substitution experiments showed the relative anion permeability (P$_{Cl}$/P$_{Na}$) to be <0.05. The cation permeability (P$_X$/P$_{Na}$) followed the ionic selectivity sequence Cs$^+$ (1.06) > Na$^+$ (1.0) > Ca^{2+} (0.93). The relative Ca^{2+} permeability is substantially higher than that obtained for muscle nAChRs at the neuromuscular junction, where P$_{Ca}$/P$_{Na}$ is 0.02.[35]

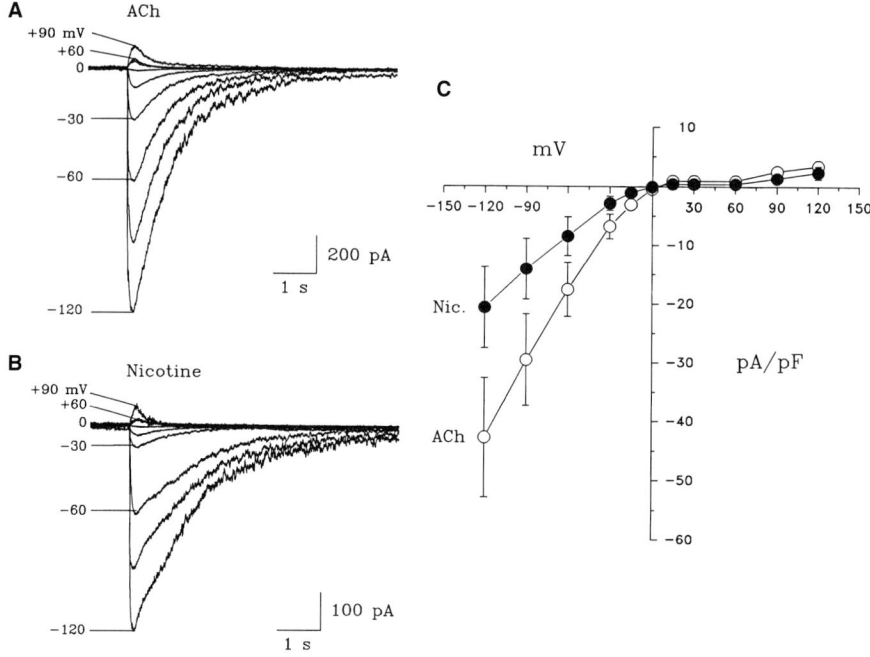

FIGURE 1–9 Excitatory acetylcholine (ACh)-evoked currents in dissociated neurons from rat intracardiac ganglia. **A.** Whole-cell currents evoked in response to a brief (10 ms) pulse of 100 μM ACh focally applied from an extracellular pipette, at the membrane potentials indicated. **B.** Whole-cell currents elicited in response to a 10 ms pulse of 100 μM nicotine. Same cell as in A. **C.** Current–voltage relationship for peak current amplitude evoked by ACh and nicotine in external Na$^+$ solution. Each point represents the mean current density (pA/pF) ± SEM from six cells. (From Nutter and Adams.[115])

Recent studies of nAChRs in rat intracardiac neurons have revealed considerable complexity in the nAChR subtypes expressed. Single-channel analysis of unitary conductances indicates that at least five nAChR subtypes are present in rat intracardiac neurons.[31,124] The nAChR subtypes varied from patch to patch, suggesting cell-to-cell differences in nAChR subtype composition. Figure 1–10A shows unitary AChR-mediated currents recorded from an excised membrane patch (outside-out). An amplitude histogram of single-channel events demonstrates the presence of at least three channel types in this patch (Fig. 1–10C). The heterogeneity of nAChR subtypes expressed is also indicated by pharmacological studies showing cell-to-cell differences in the responses to the cholinergic agonists, which is consistent with heterogeneous nAChR subtype expression by individual neurons.[124] Results from studies using single-cell RT-PCR to examine AChR subunit mRNA expression by indi-

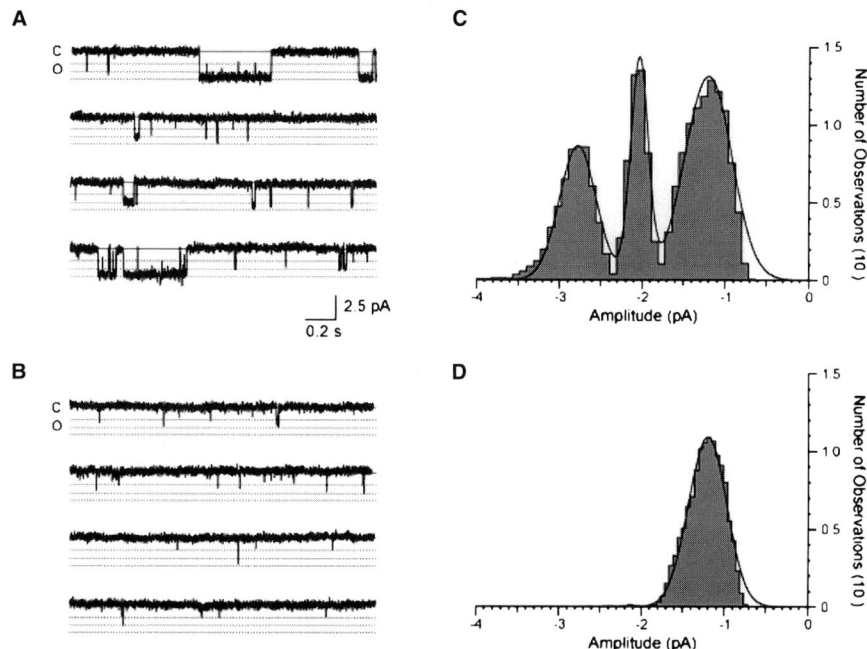

FIGURE 1–10 Acetylcholine (ACh)-evoked single-channel currents obtained in the absence and presence of substance P (SP). **A,B.** Unitary currents recorded from an excised outside-out membrane patch held at −60 mV and perfused with physiological saline solution containing either 3 μM ACh (**A**) or 3 μM ACh + 3 μM SP (**B**). Continuous line represents closed state (C) and dashed lines represent open states (O). **C,D.** Amplitude histograms of unitary currents obtained from the same patch. Histograms are fitted with Gaussian distributions with amplitudes of −1.25 ± 0.28 pA (51% total fit area), −2.09 ± 0.11 pA (22%), and −2.83 ± 0.22 pA (27%) for ACh (**C**); and −1.21 ± 0.23 pA (99%), −2.14 ± 0.09 pA (<1%), and −2.80 ± 0.33 pA (<1%) for ACh + SP (**D**). (From Cuevas and Adams.[31])

vidual neurons was consistent with this AChR heterogeneity.[124] Multicellular cultures were shown to contain mRNAs encoding all eight neuronal nAChR subunits (α_2, α_3, α_4, α_5, α_7, β_2, β_3, and β_4), a complexity greater than that reported for superior cervical ganglion neurons, which express transcripts only encoding the α_3, α_5, α_7, β_2, and β_4 subunits.[102] Furthermore, individual epicardial neurons express distinct subsets of these nAChR subunit mRNAs.[124] While α_3/β_2 containing receptors have been shown to mediate synaptic transmission in canine intracardiac neurons,[22] receptors containing other subunits appear to be important for ganglionic throughput. Most if not all of these subunits are likely to contribute to the nerve-evoked postsynaptic response in intracardiac ganglia. For example, mice deficient in either the α_5 or the β_4 subunit were more resistant to bradycardia induced by high-frequency vagal stimulation than wild-type animals.[165,166]

Nicotinic receptors containing the α_7 subunit also appear to be important contributors to ganglionic transmission, since they have been implicated in the initial decrease in heart rate produced by nicotine administration.[87] Rat intracardiac neurons have recently been shown to express a novel nAChR subtype containing the α_7 subunit (α_7-nAChRs). These α_7-nAChRs have kinetic and pharmacological properties that differ from those of conventional α_7-nAChRs.[32] The α_7-nAChRs in intracardiac neurons exhibit a slow rate of desensitization and bind α-bungarotoxin reversibly, in contrast to recombinant α_7-nAChRs and α_7-nAChRs in mammalian hippocampal neurons that desensitize rapidly and bind α-bungarotoxin in an irreversible manner.[32] Pharmacological experiments using antagonists specific for α_7-nAChRs suggest that these receptors account for ~50% of the ACh-evoked response in isolated intracardiac neurons from neonatal rats, and thus appear to be the predominant α_7-nAChR subtype in these cells.[32,71] More recent studies have suggested that this novel α_7-nAChRs incorporates a splice variant of the α_7-gene product.[140]

Neuropeptide Modulation of Nicotinic Acetylcholine Receptors

Whereas the modulation of voltage-sensitive ion channels often results in alteration of intracardiac neuronal firing patterns or a form of frequency modulation, a second form of modulation of membrane electrical activity also exists—amplitude modulation. The rapid synaptic transmission mediated by ligand-gated ion channels, in particular nAChR channels, is subject to amplitude modulation by neuropeptides. Attenuation or augmentation of nicotinic responses is a mechanism by which neuromodulators may inhibit or facilitate the reaching of threshold by excitatory postsynaptic potentials and thus regulate neuronal firing.

Vasoactive intestinal polypeptide and pituitary adenylate cyclase–activating polypeptide potentiation of nicotinic acetylcholine receptor-mediated currents

The effects of VIP and pituitary adenylate cyclase-activating polypeptide (PACAP27 and PACAP38) on ACh-evoked currents has been studied in isolated parasympathetic neurons of neonatal and adult rat intracardiac ganglia. Vasoactive intestinal polypeptide and PACAP ($\leq$10 nM) selectively and reversibly increased agonist affinity nAChRs resulting in a potentiation of ACh-evoked whole-cell currents at low agonist concentrations.[29,96] The signal transduction pathway mediating VIP- and PACAP-induced potentiation of nicotinic ACh-evoked currents has been shown to be membrane delimited and to involve the PTX-sensitive G protein, G_o.[29,96] Recent experiments using single-cell RT-PCR demonstrate that neonatal rat intracardiac neurons express transcripts encoding PAC_1, $VPAC_1$, and $VPAC_2$ receptors[37] and suggest that VIP and PACAP exert their effects by acting on different receptors.

Substance P inhibition of nicotinic acetylcholine
receptor-mediated currents

The neuropeptide substance P is commonly found within the mammalian intracardiac ganglia as described above. In canine hearts, SP modulates autonomic nerve activity, increasing cardiac contractility during vagal stimulation and decreasing contractility during stellate ganglion stimulation.[146] Furthermore, in guinea pig hearts, SP has been shown to activate a nonselective cation conductance via an NK_3 receptor in intracardiac neurons[57] and to induce bradycardia.[159] A recent study in intracardiac neurons of guinea pig has shown that bath application of SP (0.5–100 μM) caused a dose-dependent depolarization but rarely evoked action potentials. However, SP enhanced nicotinic responses evoked by local pressure ejection of ACh in 77% of neurons studied and attenuated responses to ACh in 15% of intracardiac neurons studied primarily during exposure to higher concentrations (10–100 μM) of SP.[182] In contrast, in rat intracardiac neurons, SP (1–300 μM) has been shown to inhibit nicotinic AChR-evoked currents in a concentration-dependent manner in all neurons examined.[31] Focal application of SP onto the soma of isolated intracardiac neurons reversibly decreased ACh-evoked current amplitude and increased the rate of decay of ACh-evoked currents fourfold, a result suggesting that SP increased the rate of desensitization of the nAChR channel.[31] The inhibition of ACh-evoked currents by SP is voltage-independent and does not involve a diffusible cytosolic second messenger, unlike SP inhibition of nAChRs in chick sympathetic and ciliary ganglion neurons.[131] The effects of SP on ACh-evoked single-channel currents recorded from an excised (outside-out) membrane patch from a rat intracardiac neuron is shown in Figure 1–10B. Substance P reduced the open channel probability of nAChRs in the patch and preferentially inhibited the large-conductance nAChR channel present in these neurons (Fig. 1–10D).[31]

Recent studies have demonstrated that the subunit composition of nAChRs influences the targeting of the receptor, raising the possibility that even within an individual neuron the nAChR subunit composition may vary from synapse to synapse. Thus, substance P may modulate nAChRs targeted to specific synapses, influencing particular pathways in intracardiac ganglia rather than having global effects on cholinergic transmission. The attenuation of nicotinic responses by SP may prevent nAChRs from depolarizing the neuron sufficiently to reach the threshold for action potential firing. If this effect is restricted to particular inputs to a cell, specific pathways in the circuit may be influenced and could therefore explain the observed variability in responses elicited by application of SP onto intracardiac ganglia in situ, where the neuropeptide could increase or decrease neuronal activity, depending on the locus tested.[17] Direct application of SP to spontaneously active canine intrinsic cardiac neurons in situ can both increase and decrease neuronal activity, resulting in concomitant changes in heart rate.[17] Some of the effects of SP may be attributed to modulation of membrane conductances and increased excitability,[57,159] however, the effects of SP may also be mediated by modulation of nicotinic ACh ganglionic transmission. Given that ACh is the primary neurotransmitter mediating vagal innervation of the mammalian heart, SP inhibition of neuronal nAChR channels is likely to alter neuronal activity within intrinsic cardiac ganglia and ultimately affect cardiac performance.

ATP-activated (P2X) Purinoceptors

In addition to its effects on voltage-sensitive ion channels and mobilization of Ca^{2+} from intracellular stores, extracellular ATP also activates direct ligand-gated ion channels in dissociated neurons from mammalian intracardiac ganglia. Direct application of ATP evoked rapid membrane depolarization in ~40% and 75% of isolated intracardiac neurons from adult guinea pigs and neonatal rats, respectively.[6,44] The ATP-evoked depolarization was due to a conductance increase and was of sufficient magnitude to evoke an action potential. The ATP-evoked inward current and depolarization were mediated by activation of P2X purinoceptor channels and inhibited by P2 receptor antagonists, suramin and PPADS. The I-V relationship for whole-cell ATP-evoked currents exhibited marked inward rectification in the presence and absence of external divalent cations and a reversal potential of +10 mV.[44] The cation permeability relative to Na^+ (P_X/P_{Na}) followed the ionic selectivity sequence Ca^{2+} (1.48) > Na^+ (1.0) > Cs^+ (0.67). A recent detailed study of the relative permeability of the P2X receptor channel to monovalent and divalent inorganic and organic cations in dissociated neurons from rat parasympathetic ganglia[95] has shown that the P2X receptor-channel exhibits weak selectivity among the alkali metals ($Na^+ > Li^+ > Cs^+ > Rb^+ > K^+$) and the divalent alkaline earth cations ($Ca^{2+} > Sr^{2+} > Ba^{2+} > Mn^{2+} > Mg^{2+}$). Furthermore, the permeability sequence obtained for the saturated organic cations is inversely correlated with the size of the cation. The relative permeability of the monovalent inorganic and organic cations tested are similar to those reported previously for cloned rat P2X$_2$ receptors expressed in mammalian cells.[41] The pH sensitivity and inhibition of ATP-evoked current amplitude upon cell dialysis with either anti-P2X$_2$ and/or anti-P2X$_4$ but not anti-P2X$_1$ antibodies is consistent with homomeric and/or heteromeric P2X$_2$ and P2X$_4$ receptor subtypes expressed in rat intracardiac neurons.[95]

The function of P2X receptor channels in situ has not been characterized and their role remains controversial. Recent experiments suggest that P2X receptor channels may not be expressed in postganglionic neurons in vivo and their presence in dissociated neurons may be due to an up-regulation of P2X receptor expression.[144] Disruption of ganglionic transmission in vivo by either nerve damage or synaptic blockade may cause an increase in expression or availability of a different class of receptor and mediate a membrane response. For example, ischemic injury and release of ATP may up-regulate P2X receptor expression or availability and alter neuronal excitability in the heart and vasculature.[14]

Synaptic Transmission

The summation of the numerous signaling mechanisms discussed above may be studied by recording synaptic transmission in intracardiac ganglion. Several studies have focused on cell-to-cell signaling in the ganglia and have provided insight into how these mechanisms relate to vagal control of the heart. Intracellular recordings from rat intracardiac ganglion neurons in situ showed that stimulation of the vagus nerve evoked fast excitatory postsynaptic potentials (EPSPs).[134,137] Similar fast EPSPs have also been recorded from pig, canine, and guinea pig intracardiac neurons.[88,146,177] Figure 1–11A shows a representative depolarizing postsynaptic potential recorded intracellularly from a neonatal rat intracardiac neuron in response to electrical stimulation of the vagus nerve. The amplitude of EPSPs evoked by orthodromic stimulation was directly proportional to the intensity of nerve stimulation, and EPSPs decreased in amplitude at higher stimulation frequencies (Fig. 1–11B). Single stimulation of fibers innervating the ganglia often resulted in multiple EPSPs, consistent with polyneural innervation.[134,177] Fast EPSPs were inhibited by low concentrations of mecamylamine, which suggests that these responses are mediated by activation of nAChRs. Nicotinic fast EPSPs were also observed in canine and pig intracardiac neurons in situ, and were enhanced by the cholinesterase inhibitor, physostigmine, and blocked by the ganglionic nAChR antagonist, hexamethonium.[146,177] In these studies, fast EPSPs were evoked by stimulation of intraganglionic nerve fibers,

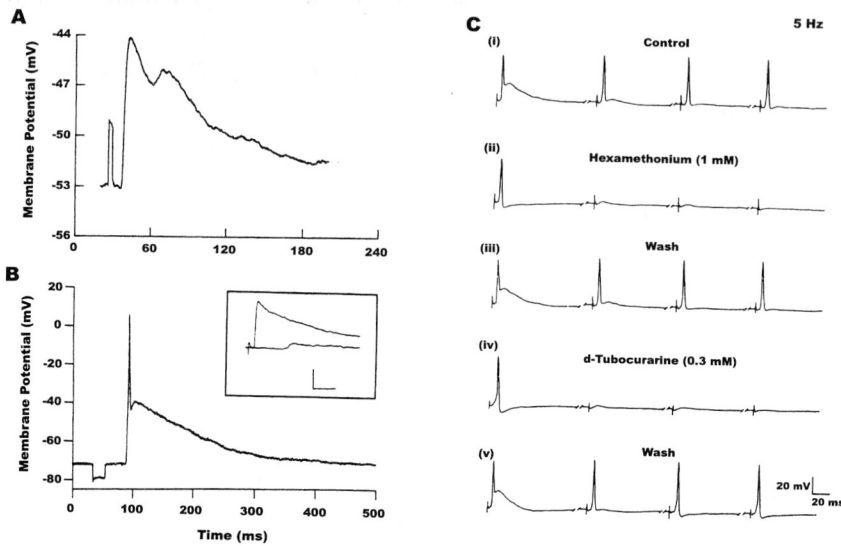

FIGURE 1–11 Nerve-evoked excitatory postsynaptic potentials (EPSPs) from intracardiac neurons in situ in response to vagal stimulation. A. Multiple EPSPs with differing delays evoked in response to a single stimulus applied to the left vagus nerve. B. An action potential elicited by a neurally evoked EPSP. *Inset:* Relative amplitudes and durations of neurally evoked EPSP and a spontaneous miniature EPSP recorded from an intracardiac neuron. Scale: 10 mV, 50 ms. Temperature: 23°C. (From Seabrook et al.[134]) C. Effects of hexamethomium and d-tubocurarine on responses of the same cell to high-frequency fiber tract stimulation. Four responses were evoked at 5 Hz before *(i)* and after *(ii)* adding 1 mM hexamthonium, after washing out hexamethonium *(iii)* and after adding *(iv)* and washing out of 0.3 mM d-tubocurarine *(v)*. Resting membrane potential, −54 mV. Temperature: 36°C. (From Selyanko and Skok.[138])

a result suggesting that intrinsic innervation of the intracardiac nerve plexus is also cholinergic and neurotransmission is mediated by nAChRs. Spontaneous fast EPSPs have also been reported in adult and neonatal rat intracardiac neurons, although the frequency of these events is low (>2 min^{-1}). Given the magnitude of spontaneous events, it was estimated that the quantal content of neurally evoked responses was between 10 and 30 quanta.[134]

Single nerve stimulus can evoke fast EPSPs of sufficient magnitude to generate orthodromic action potentials (Fig. 1–11C). These action potentials exhibit characteristics identical to those of antidromically elicited action potentials, but their duration has been shown to be greater.[146]

In addition to fast EPSPs, slow EPSPs have also been observed in response to stimulation of presynaptic nerve fibers.[134,177] Unlike fast EPSPs, which could be evoked by a single stimulus, slow excitatory potentials were observed only following repetitive presynaptic stimulation. Slow EPSPs, with latencies of <1 second, were observed in 60% of canine intracardiac neurons following orthodromic stimulation. These slow EPSPs were associated with an increase in input resistance and increased neuronal excitability, often resulting in the genesis of a single action potential or trains of action potentials. Muscarinic receptor antagonists, atropine and pirenzepine, blocked the slow EPSPs, which suggests that they are mediated by the activation of muscarinic ACh receptor.[138,177] These neurally evoked responses are likely mediated by M_1 muscarinic receptor inhibition of the M current described previously in this chapter.

In a subpopulation of canine intracardiac neurons, high-frequency stimulation of intraganglionic fibers has been shown to evoke a slow inhibitory postsynaptic potential (IPSP). The slow IPSP, which was associated with a decrease in input resistance, was mimicked by bethanechol and blocked by atropine, but was insensitive to low concentrations of pirenzepine or 4-DAMP.[177] Thus, this response is likely mediated by activation of either M_2 or M_3 receptors coupled to the opening of K^+ or Cl^- channels, respectively,

FUTURE DIRECTIONS

While our understanding of the function of mammalian intracardiac ganglia has grown significantly over the last few years, much remains to be learned about these neurons. Numerous mechanisms for neurotransmission and neuromodulation have been identified in intrinsic cardiac neurons, yet little is known about the contribution of these mechanisms to synaptic transmission in the ganglia. Multiple neuron types have been identified, yet the means by which these components of the circuit contribute to the overall signal processing in the ganglia and through the ganglia remain to be elucidated. Furthermore, there is little information on the effects of aging on intracardiac neurons. It is now clear that the electrical properties of cardiac ganglion neurons dissociated from neonatal or immature animals are different from those of mature animals, thus these neurons will likely function differently during development, maturation, and aging. Finally, the role of these ganglia in the response of the heart to cardiovascular disease or the etiology of cardiovascular pathophysiology remains to be elucidated. A considerable amount of research effort is being focused on the role of the ganglia during ischemia and cardiac hypertrophy. Some of our advances in this area, which will remain of significant interest in years to come, will be discussed in later chapters of this book.

ACKNOWLEDGMENTS

This work was supported by National Health and Medical Research Council of Australia Grant to D.J.A. and National Institute of Health (USA) grant R01-HL63247 to J.C.

REFERENCES

1. Adams DJ and Harper AA. Electrophysiological properties of autonomic ganglion neurons. In: McLachlan EM, ed. *The Autonomic Nervous System* (Series Editor G. Burnstock. Vol. 6, *Autonomic Ganglia*) Luxembourg: Harwood Academic Publishers 1995, pp 153–212.
2. Adams DJ and Trequattrini C. Opioid receptor-mediated inhibition of omega-conotoxin GVIA-sensitive calcium channel currents in rat intracardiac neurons. *J Neurophysiol* 79:753–762, 1998.
3. Ahmed A, Johansson O, and Folan-Curran J. Distribution of PGP 9.5, TH, NPY, SP and CGRP immunoreactive nerves in the rat and guinea pig atrioventricular valves and chordae tendineae. *J Anat* 191(Pt 4):547–560, 1997.
4. Akiyama T and Yamazaki T. Adrenergic inhibition of endogenous acetylcholine release on postganglionic cardiac vagal nerve terminals. *Cardiovasc Res* 46:531–538, 2000.
5. Allen TG and Burnstock G. M_1 and M_2 muscarinic receptors mediate excitation and inhibition of guinea-pig intracardiac neurones in culture. *J Physiol* 422:463–480, 1990.
6. Allen TG and Burnstock G. The actions of adenosine 5'-triphosphate on guinea-pig intracardiac neurones in culture. *Br J Pharmacol* 100:269–276, 1990.
7. Allen TGJ and Burnstock G. Intracellular studies of the electrophysiological properties of cultured intracardiac neurones of the guinea-pig. *J Physiol* 388:349–366, 1987.
8. Allen TGJ, Hassall CJS, and Burnstock G. Mammalian intrinsic cardiac neurons in cell culture. In: Armour JA and Ardell JL, eds. *Neurocardiology*. New York: Oxford University Press, 1994, pp. 115–138.
9. Almond SC and Paterson DJ. Sulphonylurea-sensitive channels and NO-cGMP pathway modulate the heart rate response to vagal nerve stimulation in vitro. *J Mol Cell Cardiol* 32:2065–2073, 2000.
10. Ardell JL. Structure and function of mammalian intrinsic cardiac neurons in neurocardiology. In: Armour JA and Ardell JL, eds. *Neurocardiology*. New York: Oxford University Press, 1994, pp. 95–114.
11. Ardell JL and Randall WC. Selective vagal innervation of sinoatrial and atrioventricular nodes in canine heart. *Am J Physiol* 251:H764–H773, 1986.
12. Armour JA. Histamine-sensitive intrinsic cardiac and intrathoracic extracardiac neurons influence cardiodynamics. *Am J Physiol* 270:R906–R913, 1996.
13. Armour JA. Intrinsic cardiac neurons involved in cardiac regulation possess alpha 1-, alpha 2-, beta 1- and beta 2-adrenoceptors. *Can J Cardiol* 13:277–284, 1997.
14. Armour JA. Myocardial ischaemia and the cardiac nervous system. *Cardiovasc Res* 41:41–54, 1999.
15. Armour JA and Hopkins DA. Activity of canine in situ left atrial ganglion neurons. *Am J Physiol* 259:H1207–H1215, 1990.

16. Armour JA and Hopkins DA. Activity of in vivo canine ventricular neurons. *Am J Physiol* 258:H326–H336, 1990.
17. Armour JA, Huang MH, and Smith FM. Peptidergic modulation of in situ canine intrinsic cardiac neurons. *Peptides* 14:191–202, 1993.
18. Armour JA, Smith FM, Losier AM, Ellenberger HH, and Hopkins DA. Modulation of intrinsic cardiac neuronal activity by nitric oxide donors induces cardiodynamic changes. *Am J Physiol* 268:R403–R413, 1995.
19. Baluk P and Gabella G. Some intrinsic neurons of the guinea-pig heart contain substance P. *Neurosci Lett* 104:269–273, 1989.
20. Baluk P and Gabella G. Some parasympathetic neurons in the guinea-pig heart express aspects of the catecholaminergic phenotype in vivo. *Cell Tissue Res* 261:275–285, 1990.
21. Bernheim L, Mathie A, and Hille B. Characterization of muscarinic receptor subtypes inhibiting Ca^{2+} current and M current in rat sympathetic neurons. *Proc Natl Acad Sci USA* 89:9544–9548, 1992.
22. Bibevski S, Zhou Y, McIntosh JM, Zigmond RE, and Dunlap ME. Functional nicotinic acetylcholine receptors that mediate ganglionic transmission in cardiac parasympathetic neurons. *J Neurosci* 20:5076–5082, 2000.
23. Braas KM, May V, Harakall SA, Hardwick JC, and Parsons RL. Pituitary adenylate cyclase–activating polypeptide expression and modulation of neuronal excitability in guinea pig cardiac ganglia. *J Neurosci* 18:9766–9779, 1998.
24. Brown DA. M-currents. In: Narahashi T, ed. *Ion Channels*. New York: Plenum Press, 1988, pp. 55–94.
25. Brown DA and Adams PR. Muscarinic suppression of a novel voltage-sensitive K+ current in a vertebrate neurone. *Nature* 283:673–676, 1980.
26. Calupca MA, Vizzard MA, and Parsons RL. Origin of neuronal nitric oxide synthase (NOS)-immunoreactive fibers in guinea pig parasympathetic cardiac ganglia. *J Comp Neurol* 426:493–504, 2000.
27. Cooper T. Terminal innervation of the heart. In: Randall WC, ed. *Nervous Control of the Heart*. Baltimore: Williams and Wilkins, 1965, pp. 130–153.
28. Crowe R and Burnstock G. Fluorescent histochemical localisation of quinacrine-positive neurones in the guinea-pig and rabbit atrium. *Cardiovasc Res* 16:384–390, 1982.
29. Cuevas J and Adams DJ. Vasoactive intestinal polypeptide modulation of nicotinic ACh receptor channels in rat intracardiac neurones. *J Physiol* 493(Pt 2):503–515, 1996.
30. Cuevas J and Adams DJ. M4 muscarinic receptor activation modulates calcium channel currents in rat intracardiac neurons. *J Neurophysiol* 78:1903–1912, 1997.
31. Cuevas J and Adams DJ. Substance P preferentially inhibits large conductance nicotinic ACh receptor channels in rat intracardiac ganglion neurons. *J Neurophysiol* 84:1961–1970, 2000.
32. Cuevas J and Berg DK. Mammalian nicotinic receptors with $\alpha 7$ subunits that slowly desensitize and rapidly recover from α-bungarotoxin blockade. *J Neurosci* 18:10335–10344, 1998.
33. Cuevas J, Harper AA, Trequattrini C, and Adams DJ. Passive and active membrane properties of isolated rat intracardiac neurons: regulation by H- and M-currents. *J Neurophysiol* 78:1890–1902, 1997.
34. Dalsgaard CJ, Franco-Cereceda A, Saria A, Lundberg JM, Theodorsson-

Norheim E, and Hokfelt T. Distribution and origin of substance P- and neuropeptide Y–immunoreactive nerves in the guinea-pig heart. *Cell Tissue Res* 243:477–485, 1986.
35. Dani JA. Structure, diversity, and ionic permeability of neuronal and muscle acetylcholine receptors. *EXS* 66:47–59, 1993.
36. Day SM, Gu J, Polak JM, and Bloom SR. Somatostatin in the human heart and comparison with guinea pig and rat heart. *Br Heart J* 53:153–157, 1985.
37. DeHaven WI and Cuevas J. Heterogeneity of pituitary adenylate cyclase-activating polypeptide and vasoactive intestinal polypeptide receptors in rat intrinsic cardiac neurons. *Neurosci Lett* 328:45–49, 2002.
38. DiBona GF. Central sympathoexcitatory actions of angiotensin II: role of type 1 angiotensin II receptors. *J Am Soc Nephrol* 10(Suppl 11):S90–S94, 1999.
39. Edwards FR, Hirst GD, Klemm MF, and Steele PA. Different types of ganglion cell in the cardiac plexus of guinea-pigs. *J Physiol* 486(Pt 2):453–471, 1995.
40. Ellison JP and Hibbs RG. An ultrastructural study of mammalian cardiac ganglia. *J Mol Cell Cardiol* 8:89–101, 1976.
41. Evans RJ, Lewis C, Virginio C, Lundstrom K, Buell G, Surprenant A, and North RA. Ionic permeability of, and divalent cation effects on, two ATP-gated cation channels (P2X receptors) expressed in mammalian cells. *J Physiol* 497(Pt 2): 413–422, 1996.
42. Fabiani ME and Story DF. Effects of cromakalim, pinacidil and glibenclamide on cholinergic transmission in rat isolated atria. *Pharmacol Res* 32:155–163, 1995.
43. Fieber LA and Adams DJ. Acetylcholine-evoked currents in cultured neurones dissociated from rat parasympathetic cardiac ganglia. *J Physiol* 434:215–237, 1991.
44. Fieber LA and Adams DJ. Adenosine triphosphate–evoked currents in cultured neurones dissociated from rat parasympathetic cardiac ganglia. *J Physiol* 434:239–256, 1991.
45. Foldes FF, Kobayashi O, Kinjo M, Harsing LG Jr., Nagashima H, Duncalf D, Goldiner PL, and Vizi ES. Presynaptic effect of muscle relaxants on the release of 3H-norepinephrine controlled by endogenous acetylcholine in guinea pig atrium. *J Neural Transm* 76:169–180, 1989.
46. Forsgren S, Moravec M, and Moravec J. Catecholamine-synthesizing enzymes and neuropeptides in rat heart epicardial ganglia: an immunohistochemical study. *Histochem J* 22:667–676, 1990.
47. Franciolini F, Hogg R, Catacuzzeno L, Petris A, Trequattrini C, and Adams DJ. Large-conductance calcium-activated potassium channels in neonatal rat intracardiac ganglion neurons. *Pflugers Arch* 441:629–638, 2001.
48. Franco-Cereceda A. Calcitonin gene-related peptide and tachykinins in relation to local sensory control of cardiac contractility and coronary vascular tone. *Acta Physiol Scand Suppl* 569:1–63, 1988.
49. Fujita A and Kurachi Y. Molecular aspects of ATP-sensitive K^+ channels in the cardiovascular system and K^+ channel openers. *Pharmacol Ther* 85:39–53, 2000.
50. Gagliardi M, Randall WC, Bieger D, Wurster RD, Hopkins DA, and Armour JA. Activity of in vivo canine cardiac plexus neurons. *Am J Physiol* 255:H789–H800, 1988.

51. Gibbins IL, Furness JB, Costa M, MacIntyre I, Hillyard CJ, and Girgis S. Co-localization of calcitonin gene-related peptide-like immunoreactivity with substance P in cutaneous, vascular and visceral sensory neurons of guinea pigs. *Neurosci Lett* 57:125–130, 1985.
52. Gill SS, Pulido OM, Mueller RW, and McGuire PF. Molecular and immunochemical characterization of the ionotropic glutamate receptors in the rat heart. *Brain Res Bull* 46:429–434, 1998.
53. Gill SS, Pulido OM, Mueller RW, and McGuire PF. Immunochemical localization of the metabotropic glutamate receptors in the rat heart. *Brain Res Bull* 48:143–146, 1999.
54. Gootman PM and Gootman N. Postnatal changes in cardiovascular regulation during hypoxia. *Adv Exp Med Biol* 475:539–548, 2000.
55. Hancock JC, Hoover DB, and Hougland MW. Distribution of muscarinic receptors and acetylcholinesterase in the rat heart. *J Auton Nerv Syst* 19:59–66, 1987.
56. Hardwick JC, Mawe GM, and Parsons RL. Evidence for afferent fiber innervation of parasympathetic neurons of the guinea-pig cardiac ganglion. *J Auton Nerv Syst* 53:166–174, 1995.
57. Hardwick JC, Mawe GM, and Parsons RL. Tachykinin-induced activation of non-specific cation conductance via NK3 neurokinin receptors in guinea-pig intracardiac neurones. *J Physiol* 504(Pt 1):65–74, 1997.
58. Hassall CJ and Burnstock G. Neuropeptide Y-like immunoreactivity in cultured intrinsic neurones of the heart. *Neurosci Lett* 52:111–115, 1984.
59. Hassall CJ and Burnstock G. Intrinsic neurones and associated cells of the guinea-pig heart in culture. *Brain Res* 364:102–113, 1986.
60. Hassall CJ and Burnstock G. Evidence for uptake and synthesis of 5-hydroxytryptamine by a subpopulation of intrinsic neurons in the guinea-pig heart. *Neuroscience* 22:413–423, 1987.
61. Hassall CJ and Burnstock G. Immunocytochemical localisation of neuropeptide Y and 5-hydroxytryptamine in a subpopulation of amine-handling intracardiac neurones that do not contain dopamine beta-hydroxylase in tissue culture. *Brain Res* 422:74–82, 1987.
62. Hassall CJ, Penketh R, Rodeck C, and Burnstock G. The intracardiac neurones of the fetal human heart in culture. *Anat Embryol (Berl)* 182:329–337, 1990.
63. Hassall CJ, Saffrey MJ, Belai A, Hoyle CH, Moules EW, Moss J, Schmidt HH, Murad F, Forstermann U, and Burnstock G. Nitric oxide synthase immunoreactivity and NADPH-diaphorase activity in a subpopulation of intrinsic neurones of the guinea-pig heart. *Neurosci Lett* 143:65–68, 1992.
64. Hassall CJ, Stanford SC, Burnstock G, and Buckley NJ. Co-expression of four muscarinic receptor genes by the intrinsic neurons of the rat and guinea-pig heart. *Neuroscience* 56:1041–1048, 1993.
65. Herring N, Golding S, and Paterson DJ. Pre-synaptic NO-cGMP pathway modulates vagal control of heart rate in isolated adult guinea pig atria. *J Mol Cell Cardiol* 32:1795–1804, 2000.
66. Herring N and Paterson DJ. Nitric oxide-cGMP pathway facilitates acetylcholine release and bradycardia during vagal nerve stimulation in the guinea-pig in vitro. *J Physiol* 535:507–518, 2001.
67. Hille B. *Ionic Channels of Excitable Membranes, 3rd ed.* Sunderland, MA: Sinauer, 2001.

68. Hogg RC and Adams DJ. An ATP-sensitive K($^+$) conductance in dissociated neurones from adult rat intracardiac ganglia. *J Physiol* 534:713–720, 2001.
69. Hogg RC, Harper AA, and Adams DJ. Developmental changes in hyperpolarization-activated currents I_h and $I_{K(IR)}$ in isolated rat intracardiac neurons. *J Neurophysiol* 86:312–320, 2001.
70. Hogg RC, Lewis RJ, and Adams DJ. Ciguatoxin (CTX-1) modulates single tetrodotoxin-sensitive sodium channels in rat parasympathetic neurones. *Neurosci Lett* 252:103–106, 1998.
71. Hogg RC, Miranda LP, Craik DJ, Lewis RJ, Alewood PF, and Adams DJ. Single amino acid substitutions in alpha-conotoxin PnIA shift selectivity for subtypes of the mammalian neuronal nicotinic acetylcholine receptor. *J Biol Chem* 274:36559–36564, 1999.
72. Hogg RC, Trequattrini C, Catacuzzeno L, Petris A, Franciolini F, and Adams DJ. Mechanisms of verapamil inhibition of action potential firing in rat intracardiac ganglion neurons. *J Pharmacol Exp Ther* 289:1502–1508, 1999.
73. Hoover DB, Baisden RH, and Xi-Moy SX. Localization of muscarinic receptor mRNAs in rat heart and intrinsic cardiac ganglia by in situ hybridization. *Circ Res* 75:813–820, 1994.
74. Hoover DB and Hancock JC. Distribution of substance P binding sites in guinea-pig heart and pharmacological effects of substance P. *J Auton Nerv Syst* 23:189–197, 1988.
75. Horackova M and Armour JA. ANG II modifies cardiomyocyte function via extracardiac and intracardiac neurons: in situ and in vitro studies. *Am J Physiol* 272:R766–R775, 1997.
76. Huang MH, Ardell JL, Hanna BD, Wolf SG, and Armour JA. Effects of transient coronary artery occlusion on canine intrinsic cardiac neuronal activity. *Integr Physiol Behav Sci* 28:5–21, 1993.
77. Huang MH, Smith FM, and Armour JA. Amino acids modify activity of canine intrinsic cardiac neurons involved in cardiac regulation. *Am J Physiol* 264:H1275–H1282, 1993.
78. Huang MH, Sylven C, Pelleg A, Smith FM, and Armour JA. Modulation of in situ canine intrinsic cardiac neuronal activity by locally applied adenosine, ATP, or analogues. *Am J Physiol* 265:R914–R922, 1993.
79. Hughes J, Kosterlitz HW, and Smith TW. The distribution of methionine-enkephalin and leucine-enkephalin in the brain and peripheral tissues. 1977. *Br J Pharmacol* 120:428–436; discussion 426–427, 1997.
80. Hulme EC, Birdsall NJ, and Buckley NJ. Muscarinic receptor subtypes. *Annu Rev Pharmacol Toxicol* 30:633–673, 1990.
81. Ikeda SR and Dunlap K. Voltage-dependent modulation of N-type calcium channels: role of G protein subunits. *Adv Second Messenger Phosphoprotein Res* 33:131–151, 1999.
82. Ishibashi H, Umezu M, Jang IS, Ito Y, and Akaike N. Alpha 1-adrenoceptor-activated cation currents in neurones acutely isolated from rat cardiac parasympathetic ganglia. *J Physiol* 548:111–120, 2003.
83. Jacobowitz D, Cooper T, and Barner HB. Histochemical and chemical studies of the localization of adrenergic and cholinergic nerves in normal and denervated cat hearts. *Circ Res* 20:289–298, 1967.
84. Jeong SW, Ikeda SR, and Wurster RD. Activation of various G-protein coupled receptors modulates Ca^{2+} channel currents via PTX-sensitive and volt-

age-dependent pathways in rat intracardiac neurons. *J Auton Nerv Syst* 76:68–74, 1999.
85. Jeong SW and Wurster RD. Calcium channel currents in acutely dissociated intracardiac neurons from adult rats. *J Neurophysiol* 77:1769–1778, 1997.
86. Jeong SW and Wurster RD. Muscarinic receptor activation modulates Ca^{2+} channels in rat intracardiac neurons via a PTX- and voltage-sensitive pathway. *J Neurophysiol* 78:1476–1490, 1997.
87. Ji S, Tosaka T, Whitfield BH, Katchman AN, Kandil A, Knollmann BC, and Ebert SN. Differential rate responses to nicotine in rat heart: evidence for two classes of nicotinic receptors. *J Pharmacol Exp Ther* 301:893–899, 2002.
88. Kennedy AL, Harakall SA, Lynch SW, Braas KM, Hardwick JC, Mawe GM, and Parsons RL. Expression and physiological actions of neuropeptide Y in guinea pig parasympathetic cardiac ganglia. *J Auton Nerv Syst* 71:190–195, 1998.
89. King TS, Coakley JB. The intrinsic nerve cells of the cardiac atria of mammals and man. *J Anat* 92:353–379, 1958.
90. Klemm MF, Wallace DJ, and Hirst GD. Distribution of synaptic boutons around identified neurones lying in the cardiac plexus of the guinea-pig. *J Auton Nerv Syst* 66:201–207, 1997.
91. Leger J, Croll RP, and Smith FM. Regional distribution and extrinsic innervation of intrinsic cardiac neurons in the guinea pig. *J Comp Neurol* 407:303–317, 1999.
92. Levy MN. Sympathetic–parasympathetic interactions in the heart. *Circ Res* 29:437–445, 1971.
93. Lew MJ and Angus JA. Clonidine and noradrenaline fail to inhibit vagal induced bradycardia. Evidence against prejunctional alpha-adrenoceptors on vagal varicosities in guinea pig right atria. *Naunyn Schmiedebergs Arch Pharmacol* 323:228–232, 1983.
94. Lindpaintner K and Ganten D. The cardiac renin–angiotensin system: a synopsis of current experimental and clinical data. *Acta Cardiol* 46:385–397, 1991.
95. Liu DM and Adams DJ. Ionic selectivity of native ATP-activated (P2X) receptor channels in dissociated neurones from rat parasympathetic ganglia. *J Physiol* 534:423–435, 2001.
96. Liu DM, Cuevas J, and Adams DJ. VIP and PACAP potentiation of nicotinic ACh-evoked currents in rat parasympathetic neurons is mediated by G-protein activation. *Eur J Neurosci* 12:2243–2251, 2000.
97. Liu DM, Katnik C, Stafford M, and Adams DJ. P2Y purinoceptor activation mobilizes intracellular Ca^{2+} and induces a membrane current in rat intracardiac neurones. *J Physiol* 526(Pt 2):287–298, 2000.
98. Löffelholz K and Muscholl E. A muscarinic inhibition of the noradrenaline release evoked by postganglionic sympathetic nerve stimulation. *Naunyn Schmiedebergs Arch Pharmacol* 265:1–15, 1969.
99. Loiacono RE and Story DF. Effect of alpha-adrenoceptor agonists and antagonists on cholinergic transmission in guinea-pig isolated atria. *Naunyn Schmiedebergs Arch Pharmacol* 334:40–47, 1986.
100. Lynch SW, Braas KM, Harakall SA, Kennedy AL, Mawe GM, and Parsons RL. Neuropeptide Y (NPY) expression is increased in explanted guinea pig parasympathetic cardiac ganglia neurons. *Brain Res* 827:70–78, 1999.
101. Manabe N, Foldes FF, Torocsik A, Nagashima H, Goldiner PL, and Vizi ES.

Presynaptic interaction between vagal and sympathetic innervation in the heart: modulation of acetylcholine and noradrenaline release. *J Auton Nerv Syst* 32:233–242, 1991.

102. Mandelzys A, Pie B, Deneris ES, and Cooper E. The developmental increase in ACh current densities on rat sympathetic neurons correlates with changes in nicotinic ACh receptor alpha-subunit gene expression and occurs independent of innervation. *J Neurosci* 14:2357–2364, 1994.

103. Markos F, Snow HM, Kidd C, and Conlon K. Nitric oxide facilitates vagal control of heart rate via actions in the cardiac parasympathetic ganglia of the anaesthetised dog. *Exp Physiol* 87:49–52, 2002.

104. Massari VJ, Johnson TA, and Gatti PJ. Cardiotopic organization of the nucleus ambiguus? An anatomical and physiological analysis of neurons regulating atrioventricular conduction. *Brain Res* 679:227–240, 1995.

105. Massari VJ, Johnson TA, Llewellyn-Smith IJ, and Gatti PJ. Substance P nerve terminals synapse upon negative chronotropic vagal motoneurons. *Brain Res* 660:275–287, 1994.

106. Mawe GM, Talmage EK, Lee KP, and Parsons RL. Expression of choline acetyltransferase immunoreactivity in guinea pig cardiac ganglia. *Cell Tissue Res* 285:281–286, 1996.

107. Max SI, Liang JS, and Potter LT. Stable allosteric binding of m1-toxin to m1 muscarinic receptors. *Mol Pharmacol* 44:1171–1175, 1993.

108. McGrattan PA, Brown JH, and Brown OM. Parasympathetic effects on in vivo rat heart can be regulated through an alpha 1-adrenergic receptor. *Circ Res* 60:465–471, 1987.

109. Meiklejohn J. On the topography of the intracardiac ganglia of the rat's heart. *J Anat Physiol* 48:378–381, 1914.

110. Mihara S, Ikeda K, and Nishi S. Muscarinic M_2 receptors on cardiac ganglion neurons of the guinea-pig heart. *Kurume Med J* 35:183–192, 1988.

111. Miura A, Kawatani M, and de Groat WC. Effects of pituitary adenylate cyclase activating polypeptide on lumbosacral preganglionic neurons in the neonatal rat spinal cord. *Brain Res* 895:223–232, 2001.

112. Moravec M and Moravec J. Intrinsic innervation of the atrioventricular junction of the rat heart. *Am J Anat* 171:307–319, 1984.

113. Moravec J and Moravec M. Intrinsic nerve plexus of mammalian heart: morphological basis of cardiac rhythmical activity? *Int Rev Cytol* 106:89–148, 1987.

114. Moravec M and Moravec J. 3-D characterization of ganglion cells of the terminal nerve plexus of rat atrioventricular junction. *J Auton Nerv Syst* 74:1–12, 1998.

115. Nutter TJ and Adams DJ. Monovalent and divalent cation permeability and block of neuronal nicotinic receptor channels in rat parasympathetic ganglia. *J Gen Physiol* 105:701–723, 1995.

116. Ogden D. *Microelectrode Techniques, 2nd ed*. Cambridge: The Company of Biologists Limited, 1994.

117. Pape HC. Queer current and pacemaker: the hyperpolarization-activated cation current in neurons. *Annu Rev Physiol* 58:299–327, 1996.

118. Papka RE. Studies of cardiac ganglia in pre- and postnatal rabbits. *Cell Tissue Res* 175:17–35, 1976.

119. Papka RE, Furness JB, Della NG, and Costa M. Depletion by capsaicin of substance P–immunoreactivity and acetylcholinesterase activity from nerve fibres in the guinea-pig heart. *Neurosci Lett* 27:47–53, 1981.

120. Pardini BJ, Patel KP, Schmid PG, and Lund DD. Location, distribution and projections of intracardiac ganglion cells in the rat. *J Auton Nerv Syst* 20:91–101, 1987.
121. Parsons RL, Rossignol TM, Calupca MA, Hardwick JC, and Brass KM. PACAP peptides modulate guinea pig cardiac neuron membrane excitability and neuropeptide expression. *Ann N Y Acad Sci* 921:202–210, 2000.
122. Pauza DH, Skripkiene G, Skripka V, Pauziene N, and Stropus R. Morphological study of neurons in the nerve plexus on heart base of rats and guinea pigs. *J Auton Nerv Syst* 62:1–12, 1997.
123. Pelleg A, Katchanov G, and Xu J. Autonomic neural control of cardiac function: modulation by adenosine and adenosine 5′-triphosphate. *Am J Cardiol* 79:11–14, 1997.
124. Poth K, Nutter TJ, Cuevas J, Parker MJ, Adams DJ, and Luetje CW. Heterogeneity of nicotinic receptor class and subunit mRNA expression among individual parasympathetic neurons from rat intracardiac ganglia. *J Neurosci* 17:586–596, 1997.
125. Powers MJ, Peterson BA, and Hardwick JC. Regulation of parasympathetic neurons by mast cells and histamine in the guinea pig heart. *Auton Neurosci* 87:37–45, 2001.
126. Quigley KS, Shair HN, and Myers MM. Parasympathetic control of heart period during early postnatal development in the rat. *J Auton Nerv Syst* 59:75–82, 1996.
127. Rampe D, Wible B, Fedida D, Dage RC, and Brown AM. Verapamil blocks a rapidly activating delayed rectifier K^+ channel cloned from human heart. *Mol Pharmacol* 44:642–648, 1993.
128. Randall WC and Wurster RD. Peripheral innervation of the heart. In: Levy MN and Schwartz P, eds. *Vagal Control of the Heart: Experimental Basis and Clinical Implications*. Armonk, NY: Futura Publishing Co. 1994, pp. 21–32.
129. Randall WC, Wurster RD, Randall DC, and Xi-Moy SX. From cardioaccelerator and inhibitory nerves to a "heart brain": an evolution of concepts. In: Shepherd JT and Vatner SF, eds. *Nervous Control of the Heart*. Amsterdam: Harwood Academic Publishers, 1996, pp. 173–199.
130. Reid IA. Interactions between ANG II, sympathetic nervous system, and baroreceptor reflexes in regulation of blood pressure. *Am J Physiol* 262:E763–E778, 1992.
131. Role LW. Substance P modulation of acetylcholine-induced currents in embryonic chicken sympathetic and ciliary ganglion neurons. *Proc Natl Acad Sci USA* 81:2924–2928, 1994.
132. Rubino A, Hassall CJS, and Burnstock G. Autonomic control of the myocardium: non-adrenergic non-cholinergic (NANC) mechanisms. In: Shepherd JT and Vatner SF, eds. *Nervous Control of the Heart*. Amsterdam: Harwood Academic Publishers, 1996, pp. 139–171.
133. Sakmann B and Neher E. *Single-Channel Recording, 2nd ed*. New York: Plenum Press, 1995.
134. Seabrook GR, Fieber LA, and Adams DJ. Neurotransmission in neonatal rat cardiac ganglion in situ. *Am J Physiol* 259:H997–H1005, 1990.
135. Sears CE, Choate JK, and Paterson DJ. NO-cGMP pathway accentuates the decrease in heart rate caused by cardiac vagal nerve stimulation. *J Appl Physiol* 86:510–516, 1999.

136. Selyanko AA. Membrane properties and firing characteristics of rat cardiac neurones in vitro. *J Auton Nerv Syst* 39:181–189, 1992.
137. Selyanko AA and Skok VI. Acetylcholine receptors in rat cardiac neurones. *J Auton Nerv Syst* 40:33–47, 1992.
138. Selyanko AA and Skok VI. Synaptic transmission in rat cardiac neurones. *J Auton Nerv Syst* 39:191–199, 1992.
139. Serone AP and Angus JA. Neuropeptide Y is a prejunctional inhibitor of vagal but not sympathetic inotropic responses in guinea-pig isolated left atria. *Br J Pharmacol* 127:383–390, 1999.
140. Severance EG, Amin JA, Hadley SH, and Cuevas J. Tissue distribution and functional expression of the mammalian α7-2 nicotinic acetylcholine receptor subunit isoform. *Soc Neurosci Abst* 28:617.3, 2002.
141. Singh S, Johnson PI, Javed A, Gray TS, Lonchyna VA, and Wurster RD. Monoamine- and histamine-synthesizing enzymes and neurotransmitters within neurons of adult human cardiac ganglia. *Circulation* 99:411–419, 1999.
142. Slavikova J, Kuncova J, Reischig J, and Dvorakova M. Catecholaminergic neurons in the rat intrinsic cardiac nervous system. *Neurochem Res* 28:593–598, 2003.
143. Smith AB and Adams DJ. Met-enkephalin-induced mobilization of intracellular Ca^{2+} in rat intracardiac ganglion neurones. *Neurosci Lett* 264:105–108, 1999.
144. Smith AB, Hansen MA, Liu DM, and Adams DJ. Pre- and postsynaptic actions of ATP on neurotransmission in rat submandibular ganglia. *Neuroscience* 107:283–291, 2001.
145. Smith FM. Extrinsic inputs to intrinsic neurons in the porcine heart in vitro. *Am J Physiol* 276:R455–R467, 1999.
146. Smith FM, Hopkins DA, and Armour JA. Electrophysiological properties of in vitro intrinsic cardiac neurons in the pig (*Sus scrofa*). *Brain Res Bull* 28:715–725, 1992.
147. Springhorn JP and Claycomb WC. Translation of heart preproenkephalin mRNA and secretion of enkephalin peptides from cultured cardiac myocytes. *Am J Physiol* 263:H1560–H1566, 1992.
148. Standish A, Enquist LW, Escardo JA, and Schwaber JS. Central neuronal circuit innervating the rat heart defined by transneuronal transport of pseudorabies virus. *J Neurosci* 15:1998–2012, 1995.
149. Standish A, Enquist LW, and Schwaber JS. Innervation of the heart and its central medullary origin defined by viral tracing. *Science* 263:232–234, 1994.
150. Steele PA, Aromataris EC, and Riederer BM. Endogenous opioid peptides in parasympathetic, sympathetic and sensory nerves in the guinea-pig heart. *Cell Tissue Res* 284:331–339, 1996.
151. Steele PA, Gibbins IL, and Morris JL. Projections of intrinsic cardiac neurons to different targets in the guinea-pig heart. *J Auton Nerv Syst* 56:191–200, 1996.
152. Steele PA, Gibbins IL, Morris JL, and Mayer B. Multiple populations of neuropeptide-containing intrinsic neurons in the guinea-pig heart. *Neuroscience* 62:241–250, 1994.
153. Takahashi T, Yamamura T, and Utsunomiya J. Human pancreatic polypeptide, neuropeptide Y and peptide YY reduce the contractile motility by depressing the release of acetylcholine from the myenteric plexus of the guinea pig ileum. *Gastroenterol Jpn* 27:327–333, 1992.

154. Tanaka K, Hassall CJ, and Burnstock G. Distribution of intracardiac neurones and nerve terminals that contain a marker for nitric oxide, NADPH-diaphorase, in the guinea-pig heart. *Cell Tissue Res* 273:293–300, 1993.
155. Tanaka K, Takanaga A, Hayakawa T, Maeda S, and Seki M. The intrinsic origin of nitric oxide synthase immunoreactive nerve fibers in the right atrium of the guinea pig. *Neurosci Lett* 305:111–114, 2001.
156. Thompson GW, Collier K, Ardell JL, Kember G, and Armour JA. Functional interdependence of neurons in a single canine intrinsic cardiac ganglionated plexus. *J Physiol* 528:561–571, 2000.
157. Thompson GW, Horackova M, and Armour JA. Sensitivity of canine intrinsic cardiac neurons to H_2O_2 and hydroxyl radical. *Am J Physiol* 275:H1434–H1440, 1998.
158. Thompson GW, Horackova M, and Armour JA. Ion channel modifying agents influence the electrical activity generated by canine intrinsic cardiac neurons in situ. *Can J Physiol Pharmacol* 78:293–300, 2000.
159. Tompkins JD, Hoover, D.B. and Hancock, J.C. Substance P evokes bradycardia by stimulation of postganglionic cholinergic neurons. *Peptides* 20:623–628, 1999.
160. Tran LV, Somogyi GT, and De Groat WC. Inhibitory effect of neuropeptide Y on adrenergic and cholinergic transmission in rat urinary bladder and urethra. *Am J Physiol* 266:R1411–R1417, 1994.
161. Urban L and Papka RE. Origin of small primary afferent substance P–immunoreactive nerve fibers in the guinea-pig heart. *J Auton Nerv Syst* 12: 321–331, 1985.
162. Vizi ES, Kobayashi O, Torocsik A, Kinjo M, Nagashima H, Manabe N, Goldiner PL, Potter PE, and Foldes FF. Heterogeneity of presynaptic muscarinic receptors involved in modulation of transmitter release. *Neuroscience* 31:259–267, 1989.
163. von Kugelgen I, Stoffel D, and Starke K. P_2-purinoceptor-mediated inhibition of noradrenaline release in rat atria. *Br J Pharmacol* 115:247–254, 1995.
164. Wang FB, Holst MC, and Powley TL. The ratio of pre- to postganglionic neurons and related issues in the autonomic nervous system. *Brain Res Brain Res Rev* 21:93–115, 1995.
165. Wang N, Orr-Urtreger A, Chapman J, Rabinowitz R, and Korczyn AD. Deficiency of nicotinic acetylcholine receptor beta 4 subunit causes autonomic cardiac and intestinal dysfunction. *Mol Pharmacol* 63:574–580, 2003.
166. Wang N, Orr-Urtreger A, Chapman J, Rabinowitz R, Nachman R, and Korczyn AD. Autonomic function in mice lacking alpha5 neuronal nicotinic acetylcholine receptor subunit. *J Physiol* 542:347–354, 2002.
167. Weihe E, McKnight AT, Corbett AD, and Kosterlitz HW. Proenkephalin- and prodynorphin-derived opioid peptides in guinea-pig heart. *Neuropeptides* 5:453–456, 1985.
168. Weihe E, Reinecke M, and Forssmann WG. Distribution of vasoactive intestinal polypeptide-like immunoreactivity in the mammalian heart. Interrelation with neurotensin- and substance P–like immunoreactive nerves. *Cell Tissue Res* 236:527–540, 1984.
169. Weitzell R, Illes P, and Starke K. Inhibition via opioid mu- and delta-receptors of vagal transmission in rabbit isolated heart. *Naunyn Schmiedebergs Arch Pharmacol* 328:186–190, 1984.

170. Wetzel GT and Brown JH. Presynaptic modulation of acetylcholine release from cardiac parasympathetic neurons. *Am J Physiol* 248:H33–H39, 1985.
171. Woolard HH. The innervation of the heart. *J Anat* 60:345–373, 1926.
172. Xi X, Randall WC, and Wurster RD. Intracellular recording of spontaneous activity of canine intracardiac ganglion cells. *Neurosci Lett* 128:129–132, 1991.
173. Xi X, Randall WC, and Wurster RD. Morphology of intracellularly labeled canine intracardiac ganglion cells. *J Comp Neurol* 314:396–402, 1991.
174. Xi X, Randall WC, and Wurster RD. Electrophysiological properties of canine cardiac ganglion cell types. *J Auton Nerv Syst* 47:69–74, 1994.
175. Xi XH, Thomas JX Jr, Randall WC, and Wurster RD. Intracellular recordings from canine intracardiac ganglion cells. *J Auton Nerv Syst* 32:177–182, 1991.
176. Xi-Moy SX and Dun NJ. Potassium currents in adult rat intracardiac neurones. *J Physiol* 486(Pt 1):15–31, 1995.
177. Xi-Moy SX, Randall WC, and Wurster RD. Nicotinic and muscarinic synaptic transmission in canine intracardiac ganglion cells innervating the sinoatrial node. *J Auton Nerv Syst* 42:201–213, 1993.
178. Xu ZJ and Adams DJ. Resting membrane potential and potassium currents in cultured parasympathetic neurones from rat intracardiac ganglia. *J Physiol* 456:405–424, 1992.
179. Xu ZJ and Adams DJ. Voltage-dependent sodium and calcium currents in cultured parasympathetic neurones from rat intracardiac ganglia. *J Physiol* 456:425–441, 1992.
180. Xu ZJ and Adams DJ. Alpha-adrenergic modulation of ionic currents in cultured parasympathetic neurons from rat intracardiac ganglia. *J Neurophysiol* 69:1060–1070, 1993.
181. Yang T and Levy MN. Effects of intense antecedent sympathetic stimulation on sympathetic neurotransmission in the heart. *Circ Res* 72:137–144, 1993.
182. Zhang L, Tompkins JD, Hancock JC, and Hoover DB. Substance P modulates nicotinic responses of intracardiac neurons to acetylcholine in the guinea pig. *Am J Physiol Regul Integr Comp Physiol* 281:R1792–R1800, 2001.

2

Colocalization of Multiple Neurochemicals in Mammalian Intrathoracic Neurons

MAGDA HORACKOVA

The electrical and contractile properties of the heart are regulated to a great degree by mechanisms intrinsic to cardiomyocytes themselves. In addition to these intrinsic properties, cardiac myocyte contractile behavior is modulated by neurons within and outside the heart[5] that are constantly transducing sensory inputs from various cardiac regions.[5,42] While many physiological studies have been carried out to determine the role of extrinsic cardiac neurons in the control of the heart, much less is known about the capacity of intrinsic cardiac neurons to regulate regional cardiac function. Recent evidence indicates that intrinsic cardiac neurons receive inputs not only from neurons extrinsic to the heart but also directly or indirectly from local afferent neurons (Chapter 3), so that they may act as integrative centers mediating local reflexes (Chapter 4).

Regional cardiodynamics appear to be constantly modified by inputs from subsets of intrathoracic afferent neurons that are under the influence of a variety of chemicals (Chapter 3). How populations of intrathoracic extracardiac and intrinsic cardiac neurons interact to do so is just beginning to be investigated. One difficulty in trying to study the interactions that occur among such neurons in situ is that when systemic vascular pressure changes cardiomyocytes may be affected and cardiac function is thus compromised. As a result, the direct effects of altered cardiac sensory inputs to the cardiac neuronal hierarchy cannot be separated from indirect effects induced by altering the arterial blood supply of, for instance, intrinsic cardiac neurons. This problem can be avoided when studying adult cardiomyocytes cocultured with peripheral autonomic neurons.[17] In this model, the influence that cardiac neurons exert on cardiomyocytes can be studied without compromising cardiomyocyte function, as occurs when arterial blood pressure is reduced in situ, for instance, by administering hexamethonium or tetrodotoxin (TTX). Furthermore, separating direct effects on cardiomyocytes from those mediated via associated intrinsic cardiac neurons may be difficult in the in situ situation. Employing the in vitro model, one can compare the influence of various pharmacological interventions directly on cardiomyocyte function with those induced indirectly via peripheral autonomic neurons.

Cardiomyocyte–Autonomic Neuronal Interactions

We have provided evidence that adult cardiomyocytes contractile properties can be maintained for more than 2 months (beating frequency of 80–120 per minute) when such myocytes are cocultured with adult intrathoracic autonomic neurons.[22] By comparison, the beating frequency of adult cardiomyocytes cultured alone is low (beating frequency of about 50–80 beats per minute), becoming intermittent after 4 weeks in culture. Thereafter, non-innervated cardiomyocytes fail to contract as they dedifferentiate and lose their pacemaker activity. The morphology of cardiomyocytes cultured in the presence of intrathoracic autonomic neurons remains similar to that found in cardiomyocytes in situ (Fig. 2–1) for up to 2 months, the longest period studied to date. The fact that adult mammalian cardiomyocytes lose their ability to beat spontaneously when cultured in the absence of cardiac neurons, but retain their contractile function when cocultured with cardiac neurons, indicates that peripheral autonomic neurons exert tonic influences on cardiomyocytes in vitro. Furthermore, the electrical properties of cardiomyocytes cocultured with intrinsic neurons retain characteristics similar to those identified in vivo.[22] These data indicate that intrathoracic (extrinsic and intrinsic) autonomic neurons tonically influence cardiomyocytes in vitro, as they do in situ.[31]

The spontaneous contraction rate of cultured cardiomyocytes is, on average, consistently higher when they are cultured in the presence of intrinsic cardiac neurons than when cardiomyocytes are cultured alone (Table 2–1). Furthermore, intrinsic cardiac neurons exert considerably greater influence on cultured cardiac myocytes than do stellate ganglion neurons.[22] The fact that TTX, applied at a concentration that does not affect the generation of action potentials in freshly isolated cardiac myocytes (4×10^{-7} M), decreases the beating rate of cardiomyocytes cocultured with either stellate or intrinsic cardiac neurons more than non-innervated cardiomyocyte cultures (Table 2–1) indicates that intrathoracic autonomic neurons exert tonic influence over cardiac myocytes in vitro. Several pharmacological investigations indicate the importance of functional interac-

Cardiac Neuron-Myocyte Interactions

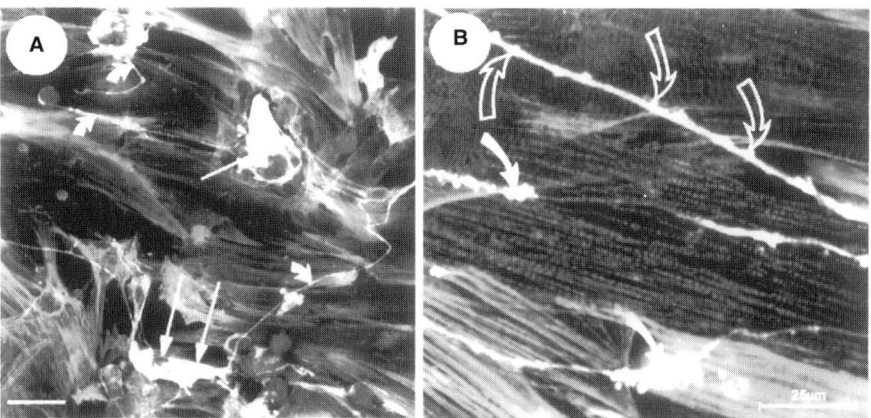

FIGURE 2–1 Confocal scanning micrograph of adult guinea pig cardiomyocytes (stained for F-actin) cocultured with intrinsic cardiac neurons (stained for PGP 9.5 conjugated with FITC) for 28 days. Identified intrinsic neurons (**A**, long arrows) had grown long neurites (small arrows), depicted at larger magnification in panel **B**. These neurites exhibit numerous varicosities along the course of their processes (open curved arrows), with clusters of varicosities present in some (closed curved arrow). Scale bar in A = 50 μM.

tions occurring between cardiac myocytes and cocultured extrinsic (stellate) or intrinsic cardiac neurons (Chapter 4). We have established that the interactions that occur between intrathoracic neurons and cardiomyocytes in response to various neurochemicals in vitro are similar to those that the same neurochemicals induce in situ.[6,9,10,20,23,26,27]

Adrenergic Receptors

The β-adrenergic agonist isoproterenol exerts greater augmentation of the contractile rate of cardiomyocytes cocultured with both types of neurons than that occurring with non-innervated cultured myocytes.[22] Furthermore, the effects elicited by isoproterenol are abolished by TTX in these cocultures but not in non-innervated cardiomyocyte cultures (Fig. 2–2A, Table 2–1). These data indicate that TTX exerts its effects primarily on neurons indirectly controlling cardiomyocyte contractility in such a model (Table 2–1). The β-adrenoceptor blocking agent timolol, when administered in 10^{-6} M doses, also depresses the contractile rate of cardiomyocytes cocultured with intrathoracic neurons (Table 2–1). These data support the contention that adrenergic neurons tonically influence cardiomyocytes in vitro (Fig. 2–2B), as is found in situ.[6,26]

In addition there is anatomical evidence of α- and β-adrenergic receptors associated with neurons within mammalian intrinsic cardiac gan-

TABLE 2-1 Effects of Tetrodotoxin, Isoprenaline, and Timolol on Contractions of Myocytes Alone and in Coculture

Culture Type	Age (weeks)	Myocyte Contraction (beats per minute)												
		BR	C	TTX	Δ%	C	ISO	Δ%	ISO	ISO+TTX	Δ%	C	TIM	Δ%
Myocyte culture	4.1 ± 0.5	67 ± 5 (n = 20)	73 ± 6	62 ± 6** (n = 8)	−15	64 ± 4	93 ± 8** (n = 19)	45	117 ± 31	112 ± 37 (n = 5)	−4	73 ± 6	68 ± 6* (n = 17)	−7
Stellate NM coculture	4.4 ± 0.4	75 ± 6 (n = 20)	62 ± 10	8 ± 3* (n = 12)	−87†	64 ± 5	128 ± 6* (n = 14)	100†	141 ± 4	67 ± 15* (n = 8)	−60†	73 ± 8	38 ± 7* (n = 12)	−48†
Intrinsic NM coculture	4.1 ± 0.4	104 ± 6† (n = 23)	99 ± 10	20 ± 8* (n = 11)	−80†	83 ± 6	151 ± 8* (n = 23)	82†	144 ± 15	77 ± 29* (n = 5)	−47†	102 ± 9	66 ± 8* (n = 23)	−43†

Tonic beating rates of non-innervated cardiomyocyte cultures (myocyte culture) versus cardiomyocytes cultured with stellate (stellate NM [nerve myocyte] coculture) or intrinsic cardiac (intrinsic NM coculture) neurons in vitro changed from basal rates (BR) during different interventions. Tetrodotoxin ([TTX]; 4×10^{-7} M) suppressed the beating frequency of cardiomyocytes cultured with either population of neurons (−80% to 87%) more than cardiomyocytes cultured alone ([C] −15%). The β-adrenergic agonist isoproterenol (ISO) enhanced the beating frequency of cocultured cardiomyocytes more than it did cardiomyocytes alone, indicating the importance of adrenergic inputs to the former cardiomyocytes. That isoproterenol failed to enhance coculture beating rates when administered in the presence of TTX indicates the importance of adrenergic neurons in such tonic input. These data are supported by the fact that β-adrenoceptor blockade (timolol [TIM] 10^{-6} M) suppressed the contractile rates of myocytes in both cocultures (−43% and −48%) much more than cardiomyocytes cultured alone (−7%). Age, number of weeks in culture; Δ% = difference between control and drug-treated cultures in which 100% represents control values. † = difference between each intervention; Δ% = difference between control and drug-treated cultures in which 100% represents control values.

**$P < 0.01$; *$P < 0.05$ comparing data before and during each intervention; † = difference between each intervention; $P < 0.01$, comparing data from non-innervated and innervated cardiomyocyte cultures.

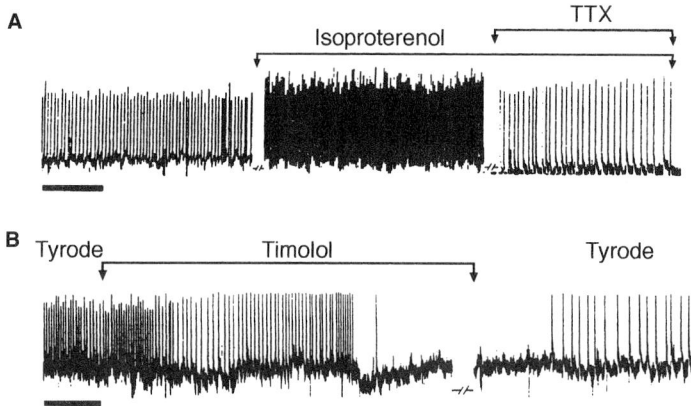

FIGURE 2–2 A. Recordings of contractions (shortening) generated by adult guinea pig cardiac myocytes cocultured with intrinsic cardiac neurons. The beating frequency of cocultured myocytes increased (45–100 beats per minute) when they were exposed to the β-adrenoceptor agonist isoproterenol (10^{-7} M). Their beating frequency was reduced below control values (30 beats per minute) when 4×10^{-7} M tetrodotoxin (TTX) was administered in the presence of isoproterenol. B. Application of the β-adrenoceptor antagonist timolol (10^{-6} M) stopped all beating in these myocytes cocultured with intrinsic cardiac neurons. This effect was reversed upon removal of timolol. Time scales = 20 seconds.

glia.[19,22,24,28,30] Functional evidence indicates the presence of sympathetic efferent postganglionic neurons in not only intrathoracic extracardiac ganglia but also intrinsic cardiac ganglia.[7,10,14] Data derived from coculture studies support the concept that adrenergic neurons are present in mammalian intrathoracic extracardiac ganglia and intrinsic cardiac ganglia,[21] as well as the concept that such neurons tonically influence cardiomyocyte behavior. Three types of catecholaminergic neurons have been identified in whole-mount preparations of guinea pig atria.[19] Presumably these populations have different functional roles in the overall regulation of cardiodynamics.

Nicotinic Receptors

The nicotinic blocking agent hexamethonium (10^{-6} M) also modifies the beating frequency of cardiomyocytes cocultured with stellate or intrinsic cardiac neurons.[22] In contrast, hexamethonium does not change the beating rate of non-innervated cardiac myocytes in vitro (Table 2–2). These data suggest that the cardiac myocyte contractile rate is partially maintained in situ via tonic inputs from neurons that utilize nicotinic synapses. They also support the contention that nicotinic neurons in-

TABLE 2-2 Effects of Hexamethonium, Atropine, Bethanechol, and Nicotine on Contractions of Myocytes Alone and in Culture

Culture Type	Myocyte Contraction (beats per minute)											
	C	HEX	Δ%	C	ATR	Δ%	C	BETH	Δ%	C	NIC	Δ%
Myocyte culture	63 ± 5 (n = 10)	−62 ± 5	—	62 ± 6 (n = 10)	57 ± 5	−8	76 ± 14 (n = 6)	−64 ± 16*	−10	61 ± 5 (n = 19)	60 ± 5	—
Stellate NM coculture	76 ± 2 (n = 7)	62 ± 11*	−18[a]	63 ± 7* (n = 12)	47 ± 4*	−25	94 ± 18 (n = 5)	63 ± 14*	−32	58 ± 3 (n = 5)	80 ± 6	+38
										64 ± 8 (n = 6)	60 ± 8	−6
Intrinsic NM coculture	87 ± 12 (n = 15)	−57 ± 8*	−34[a]	74 ± 9 (n = 9)	59 ± 11	−20	89 ± 9 (n = 6)	59 ± 7*	−35	79 ± 16 (n = 5)	126 ± 17	+59
										80 ± 12 (n = 13)	54 ± 8	−32

Effects of a number of pharmacological agents on the beating frequencies of non-innervated (myocytes) versus innervated (with stellate or intrinsic cardiac neurons) cardiomyocytes. Nicotinic receptor blockage (10^{-6} M hexamethonium [HEX]) affected the beating frequency of cocultures, but not myocytes cultured alone (C). In accord with that, nicotine ([NIC] 10^{-6} M) affected the beating frequency of cocultures, but not cardiomyocytes cultured alone; nicotine induced either increases or decreases in beating frequencies in these cocultures, presumably via adrenergic or cholinergic efferent neurons, respectively. Atropine ([ATR] 10^{-5} M) modified the beating frequency of stellate ganglion cocultures; bethanechol ([BETH] 10^{-6}M) affected cocultures more that cardiomyocytes alone. These data implicate the presence of nicotinic cholinergic and muscarinic cholinergic receptors associated with intrathoracic neurons that regulate cardiomyocyte behavior. Δ%, *$P < 0.01$, significant differences between control and drug-treated cultures. a = $P < 0.01$, comparing data from non-innervated and innervated cardiomyocyte cultures.

volved in cardiac regulation that are located in stellate and intrinsic cardiac ganglia exert tonic influence on the heart in vivo.[6,21] The fact that the rate of spontaneous contractions of cardiomyocytes cocultured with stellate or intrinsic neurons was reduced by TTX, as well as by β-adrenergic or nicotinic receptor blockade (Tables 2–1 and 2–2), indicates that such neurons do exert augmentor effects on cocultured cardiomyocytes (see Fig. 2–7; Tables 2–1 and 2–2). That is not to say that some nicotine-sensitive neurons do not exert depressor effects on cardiac myocytes (Table 2–2). Thus, as is found in intact animals,[26] application of nicotine to intrinsic cardiac neurons can produce either cardiodepressor or cardioaugmentor effects (Fig. 2–3), depending on the neuronal population affected. These findings indicate that there may be two different populations of nicotine-sensitive neurons associated with the heart.[22]

Muscarinic Receptors

Muscarinic receptors have been associated with cultured intrinsic cardiac neurons.[1] The muscarinic receptor agonist bethanechol (10^{-6} M) exerts depressor effects on the contraction rate of innervated cultured cardiomyocytes (Table 2–2). Although the muscarinic blocker atropine (10^{-5} M) does not affect the contractile rate of non-innervated cultured cardiomyocytes, it does result in a decrease in contractile rate of cardiomyocytes cocultured with stellate ganglion neurons or intrinsic cardiac

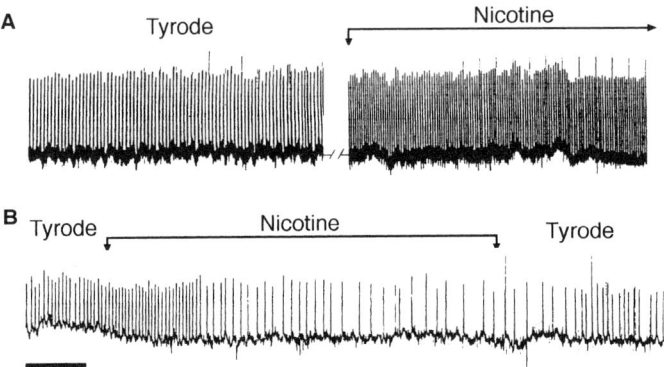

FIGURE 2–3 A. The excitatory effect of nicotine on contractile rate of adult guinea pig cardiomyocytes cocultured with intrinsic cardiac neurons. Exposure to nicotine (10^{-6} M) increased their beating rate from 60 to 90 beats per minute. B. Inhibitory effects of nicotine on beating frequency of this coculture were reversed once nicotine was removed from bathing medium (right side). Time scale = 20 seconds.

neurons (Table 2–2). Furthermore, synaptic transmission within canine stellate and middle cervical ganglia can be modified by muscarinic receptor blockade.[4] Not only are these in vitro data in accord with those obtained in vivo, but they also indicate that some cardiac effects may be mediated in part by intrathoracic neurons possessing muscarinic receptors.[5,6]

Noncholinergic, Nonadrenergic Receptors

As mentioned above, the contractile rate of cardiomyocytes cultured with intrathoracic autonomic neurons is very dependent on tonic input arising from autonomic neurons. Various chemicals are involved in the interneuronal interactions occurring in such a preparation that maintain cardiac myocyte contractile function. Intrathoracic extrinsic and intrinsic cardiac neurons exert differential control over cardiomyocytes, particularly when they are modified by specific chemicals.[5,6,18,28] The fact that cardiac effects mediated by intrinsic cardiac neurons can persist following adrenergic and nicotinic receptor blockade in vivo[8,25,27,44] or in vitro[22] suggests that nonadrenergic and noncholinergic neurons exist in intrathoracic ganglia involved in regulating cardiomyocyte behavior (see Fig. 2–7).

Peptides can also influence intrinsic cardiac neurons.[12,19,39] For instance, angiotensin II (100 nM) induces positive chronotropic effects in cocultures of adult guinea pig cardiomyocytes with adult extrinsic or intrinsic cardiac neurons (Fig. 2–4A). This agent does not influence cardiomyocytes cultured alone.[18] The contractile frequency of innervated cardiomyocytes does not increase when angiotensin II is applied in the presence of the AT_1 receptor blocking agent losartan; the effects of angiotensin II on cardiomyocyte contractile frequency, by contrast, is unaffected by prior application of the AT_2 receptor blocking agent PD-123319.[18] These data indicate that angiotensin II–sensitive neurons exist in intrathoracic extracardiac and intrinsic cardiac ganglia that possess AT_1 receptors. Angiotensin II is known to increase the activity generated by intrinsic cardiac neurons in situ, whether administered to them locally or via their regional arterial blood supply.[18] Since angiotensin II–induced effects in cocultures are significantly attenuated by the β-adrenoceptor blocking agent timolol (Fig. 2–4B), it appears that angiotensin II–sensitive intrinsic cardiac neurons act on cardiomyocytes indirectly by activating efferent adrenergic neurons. Taken together, these data indicate that angiotensin II acts to enhance cardiomyocyte function in vitro in a fashion similar to that observed in situ. Furthermore, angiotensin II–sensitive intrathoracic neurons involved in cardiac regulation have AT_1 receptors.

Among the family of chemicals that modify mammalian intrinsic cardiac neurons and thereby influence cardiac rate and force are nitric ox-

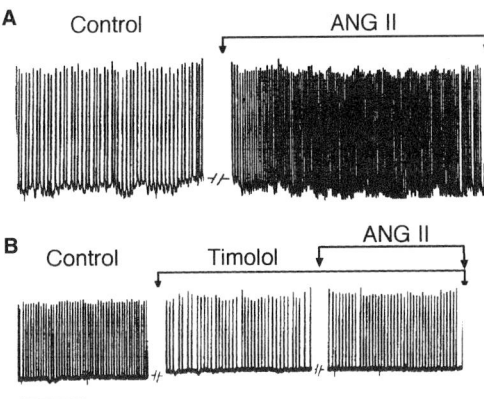

FIGURE 2–4 Angiotensin II (ANG II)–induced responses in adult guinea pig intrinsic cardiac neuronal–ventricular myocytes cocultures. **A.** The beating frequency of cardiomyocytes increased when the coculture was exposed to angiotensin II (100 nM). **B.** Timolol reduced the beating frequency, an effect that was slightly overcome by exposure to angiotensin II. Time scale = 20 seconds.

ide (NO) donors.[9] The mechanisms involved in such cardiac regulation are difficult to resolve using the in situ model. Using our in vitro model we have demonstrated that intrinsic neurons not only are sensitive to NO but can also produce it.[20] L-arginine, a precursor of NO, increases the beating frequency of innervated but not non-innervated cardiomyocytes in vitro. This effect is minimal in the presence of a NO synthase inhibitor (Fig. 2–5A). Thus it appears that NO synthase is present within the intrinsic cardiac nervous system. As the effects elicited by the NO donor SNAP are no longer generated in the presence of the guanylate cyclase inhibitor LY-83583 (Fig. 2–5B), some of the effects that intrinsic cardiac neurons induce are mediated by a NO-sensitive cGMP system. Because some of the augmentor effects that NO donors (i.e., SNAP) exert on mature guinea pig cardiomyocyte–intrinsic cardiac neuronal cocultures occurs also in the presence of the β-adrenoceptor blocking agent timolol, nonadrenergic neuronal mechanisms may be involved in cardiac regulation induced by NO-sensitive intrinsic cardiac neurons.[20]

Purinergic agents also modify autonomic neurons, including cultured intrinsic cardiac neurons.[2,16,23] That is in accord with the fact that the activity generated by intrinsic neurons can be altered in situ by locally applied adenosine or ATP. These effects can be accompanied by altered cardiac function.[27] Using the in vitro experimental model, we found that ATP-sensitive intrathoracic autonomic neurons exert cardioaugmentor effects (Fig. 2–6). This response parallels responses elicited by ATP in situ.[27] The positive chronotropic effects induced by ATP are mediated by P_2 receptors associated with intrinsic cardiac neurons.[14,23] These neurons also possess P_1 receptors, as adenosine produces negative chronotropic effects in cocultures of intrinsic cardiac neurons and cardiomyocytes.[23]

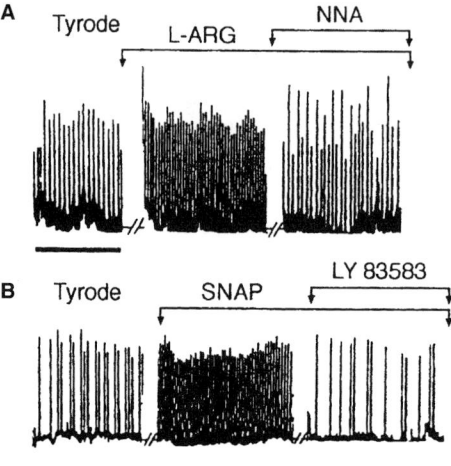

FIGURE 2–5 **A.** The contractile rate of adult guinea pig myocytes cocultured with intrinsic cardiac neurons increased (70–120 beats per minute) following exposure to the nitric oxide donor L-arginine ([L-ARG] 5×10^{-4} M). The subsequent addition to the bathing medium of an inhibitor of nitric oxygen synthase, N^G-nitro-L-arginine ([NNA] 3×10^{-4} M), decreased cardiomyocyte beating frequency (80 beats per minute) despite the presence of L-arginine. **B.** The nitric oxide donor S-nitroso-N-acetylpenicillamine ([SNAP] 5×10^{-4} M) also increased the beating frequency of myocytes cocultured with intrinsic cardiac neurons (40 to 90 beats per minute). SNAP no longer elicited a response in the presence of a guanylate cyclase inhibitor (LY-83583; 10^{-5} M, beating frequency of 36 beats per minute), indicating that NO stimulation of guanylate cyclase leading to increased cGMP is important for the intrinsic cardiac neuronally induced response. Time scale = 20 seconds.

COMPARISONS OF ANATOMICAL AND FUNCTIONAL STUDIES IN VITRO AND IN VIVO

Although we are just beginning to determine how these neuronal subpopulations influence regional cardiomyocyte behavior, it seems likely that many of their effects indeed occur presynaptically, at the level of the neurons. This is because most of the responses depicted above were elicited by pharmacological agents that act primarily on autonomic efferent neurons (TTX, hexamethonium, nicotine) rather than directly on cardiac myocytes. Adult cardiac myocytes cocultured with intrathoracic autonomic neurons exhibit different response characteristics than those reported for neonatal cocultures when the effects are predominantly postsynaptic in nature—that is, they occur at the level of the cardiac myocyte.[13,33,40,45] Although we cannot exclude the possibility of a change in phenotype expression of cultured neurons in adult cocultures, we believe

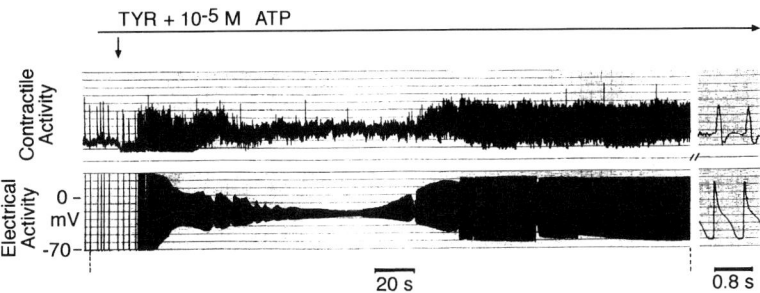

FIGURE 2–6 Representative recording of contractile behavior and intracellular activity displayed by adult guinea pig cardiac myocytes cocultured with intrinsic cardiac neurons. Application of adenosine 5'-triphosphate (ATP) to the tyrodes (TYR) solution in the bath (10^{-5} M ATP; arrow above) altered the spontaneous electrical and contractile activities of the cardiomyocytes (beating frequency increased from 30 to 120 beats per minute) during the early phase of the response. Subsequently, this was followed by depolarization of the cardiomyocyte to about −25 mV, accompanied by an attenuation of peak contraction and an increase in diastolic tension. Cardiomyocyte membrane potentials started to depolarize when the spontaneous beating frequency increased to 150 beats per minute during this phase. The average resting membrane potential of this cardiac myocyte was −72 mV (SEM 5 mV). Note the representative fast speed recordings of contractions (above) and transmembrane action potentials (below) on the right-hand side of the panels. Time scales = 20 and 0.8 seconds.

that changes induced in the neonatal neuronal cocultures represent interactions between the immature neuronal autonomic network and the neonatal myocytes.[34,35] It is unlikely that such interactions represent those that occur among adult neurons that are fully phenotypically developed (Chapter 8). This notion is supported by the fact that the pharmacological effects reported above are not expressed in cultured cells derived from 2- to 10-week-old guinea pigs.[19] On the contrary, phenotypic developmental changes occur in intrinsic cardiac neurons early in the neonatal period.[24] These changes appear to be related to the postnatal development of extrinsic sympathetic and parasympathetic efferent neuronal inputs to the heart during that time.[29,32,38] It is important to note that the various effects induced by adrenergic, muscarinic, and nicotinic agents on cultured adult guinea pig cardiomyocytes via their associated intracardiac neurons are similar to those induced by these agents in vivo.[5,6]

Varied morphological and immunohistochemical properties are associated with intrinsic cardiac neurons identified in different species.[3,11,15,19,21,37,39] Most anatomical studies have employed individual tissue sections, which present difficulties in interpreting the three-dimensional nature of the intrinsic cardiac nervous system as well as its spatial distribution in different regions of the heart. Distinct populations of intrinsic cardiac neurons have been identified in various ganglionated plexuses over the past century.[36] Similar data have arisen from cultures of intrinsic cardiac neurons[15,21] or whole-mount atrial preparations.[17]

In situ and in vitro studies indicate the heterogeneous nature of the anatomy and function of neurons in mammalian intrinsic cardiac ganglia.[5,6,36,43] Intrinsic cardiac neuronal networks are made up of afferent, efferent, and interconnecting local circuit neurons (for a review see Armour[5] and Hogg and Adams[16]) that can process cardiac sensory information independent of central neuronal inputs (Chapter 3). Light and electron microscopic analyses have demonstrated the presence of unipolar, bipolar, and multipolar neurons, as well as small intensely fluorescent (SIF) cells, within the mammalian intrinsic cardiac nervous system.[17,36,43] Cultured intrinsic cardiac neurons are associated with a number of neurochemicals (such as tyrosine hydroxylase, choline acetyltransferase, vasoactive intestinal peptide, neuropeptide Y, etc., see Table 2–3), more than one chemical having been associated with individual intrinsic cardiac neurons.[15,19,39]

We studied whole-mount preparations of guinea pig atrial tissues using confocal scanning microscopy to determine the distribution of neurons of various morphologies within the mammalian intrinsic cardiac nervous system.[19] As in other species, guinea pig atria contain large numbers of intrinsic cardiac neurons. Within their varied distributions we

TABLE 2–3 Staining Positively for General Neuronal Marker PGP 9.5 and for Specific Markers for Nine Neurochemicals

	Intrinsic Cardiac Ganglia		Stellate Ganglia	
Marker	Cultured Alone	Cultured with Myocytes	Cultured with Alone	Myocytes
PGP 9.5	20 ± 5.1 (6)	26 ± 4.3 (24)	60 ± 15.4 (4)	76 ± 12.4 (27)
TH	2.5 ± 1.1 (17)	2 ± 1.2 (7)	60 ± 20.0 (4)	54 ± 18.7 (5)
ChAT	20 ± 2.2 (5)	20 ± 8.1 (5)	10 ± 8.3 (4)	8 ± 7.1 (4)
AChE	18 ± 6.1 (5)	23 ± 7.5 (7)	20 ± 10.2 (4)	20 ± 11.2 (4)
NADPH-d	10 ± 1.56 (19)	12 ± 4.0 (13)	25 ± 10.1 (12)	10 ± 10.8 (11)
NPY	16 ± 11.0 (3)	10 ± 5.1 (4)	12 (1)	10 ± 5.4 (5)
VIP	17 ± 7.8 (6)	—	50 ± 30 (6)	—
Oxytocin	10 ± 2.7 (6)	—	16 ± 11 (5)	—
Bradykinin	16 ± 4.1 (5)	—	38 ± 20.5 (5)	—
CGRP	10 ± 5.1(8)	—	2 ± 1.2 (8)	—

Neurons from intrinsic cardiac ganglia and stellate ganglia, were cultured alone or in the presence of adult guinea pig cardiomyocytes. PGP 9.5, protein gene product 9.5; TH, tyrosine hydroxylase; ChAT, choline acetyltransferase; AChE, acetycholinesterase; NADPH-d, NADPH-diaphorase; NPY, neuropeptide Y; VIP, vasoactive intestinal peptide; CGRP, calcitonin gene–related peptide. Values are the rounded mean (±SEM) number of neurons per culture that stained positively for a marker; the number of culture studies is in parentheses.

TABLE 2–4 Four Populations of Intrinsic Cardiac Neurons: Immunoreactive Subpopulations and Localizations Throughout the Atria (Whole Mount)

Neuronal Distribution	Somata Diameter	Locations	MAP-IR and PGP-IR	TH-IR	ChaT-IR	NPY-IR, SP-IR and VIP-IR
Ganglionic Neurons 85%–90% of all neurons)	Large (15–40 μM) 75% of ganglionic neurons	Clusters of neurons in ganglia located in the interatrial septum and adjacent to origins of the vena cavae	Positive: distributed throughout the somata	Positive: distributed in sarcolemma region	Positive: located throughout somata	Positive: distributed evenly throughout somata
	Small (<15 μM) 20% of ganglionic neurons	Clusters of neurons in ganglia located in the interatrial septum and adjacent to origins	Positive: distributed throughout the somata of the vena cavae	Positive: distributed in sarcolemma region	Positive: located throughout somata	Positive: distributed evenly throughout somata
	Small (<15 μM) 5% of ganglionic neurons	Clusters embedded among PGP-IR ganglionic cells	Negative	Positive: evenly distributed throughout somata	Negative	Negative
Individual Neurons (10%–15% of all neurons)	Small (10–25 μM)	Neurons individually distributed adjacent to origin of the SVC	Negative	Positive: evenly distributed throughout somata	Positive: a. located throughout somata b. located in somata and surrounding neurites c. located in neurites surrounding somata	Positive: located throughout somata, but differing in distribution compared to ganglionic cells

ChAT, choline acetyltransferase; IR, immunoreactive; MAP, microtubule-associated protein; NPY, neuropeptide Y; PGP9.5, protein gene product 9.5; SP, substance P; SVC, superior vena cava; TH, tyrosine hydroxylase; VIP, vasoactive intestinal peptide.

were able to identify the following anatomical features: *(1)* the distribution of neurons with specific morphologies throughout the atria; *(2)* some of the neurochemicals that are expressed by the different populations of these neurons; *(3)* specific neuronal subtypes in specific atrial regions; and *(4)* various transmitter phenotypes associated with individual intrinsic cardiac neurons (Table 2–4). Such varied neuronal subtypes have been identified in cultures of intrinsic cardiac neurons as well.[21] By employing a model of long-term cocultures of cardiomyocytes with intrathoracic neurons, it has been possible to identify varied functional properties of the different populations of intrathoracic cardiac autonomic neurons.[17] This is particularly relevant with respect to determining how intrathoracic afferent, local circuit, and efferent (adrenergic and cholinergic) neurons interact to tonically influence cardiomyocyte behavior in vivo (Fig. 2–7).

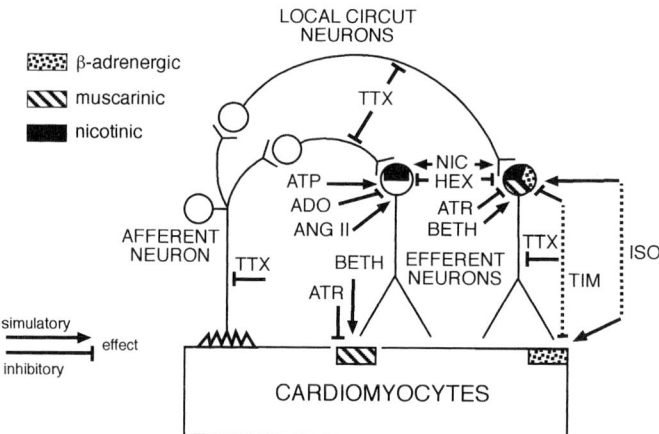

FIGURE 2–7 Schematic representation of some putative interactions that have been identified among intrinsic cardiac neurons and cocultured cardiomyocytes. Neurons influenced by nicotinic (NIC) or muscarinic (bethanechol [BETH]) agonists or the β-adrenergic receptor agonist isoproterenol (ISO) enhance the contractile rate of cocultured cardiomyocytes. Correspondingly, the beating rate of cocultured cardiomyocytes was suppressed following exposure to a nicotinic (hexamethonium [HEX]) or β-adrenergic (timolol [TIM]) receptor–blocking agent. The muscarinic receptor blocking agent atropine (ATR) also modified contractile rate. These and other data indicate that local circuit neurons may be interposed between afferent and efferent neurons within this nervous system, as indicated by the fact that contractile behavior is reduced following tetrodotoxin (TTX) administration, even in the presence of nicotinic agonists. Neuronal input to cardiomyocytes can also be affected by angiotensin II (ANG II) via AT_1 receptors or by purinergic agonists (ATP via P_1 receptors or adenosine [ADO] via P_2 receptors). It should be noted that specific stimulatory or inhibitory effects might involve local circuit or efferent neurons.

CLINICAL RELEVANCE OF MULTIPLE PHENOTYPIC NEURONS

Until recently, intrathoracic ganglia have been considered simple efferent neuronal relay stations, with the intrinsic cardiac nervous system represented by parasympathetic efferent postganglionic neurons that innervate the heart. The in vitro studies employing cocultures of adult cardiomyocytes with extrinsic or intrinsic cardiac neurons depicted in this chapter have provided direct evidence for not only multiple neuronal phenotypes present in intrathoracic extracardiac and intrinsic cardiac ganglia,[21] but also the regulatory role that some neurons in intrathoracic extracardiac and intrinsic cardiac ganglia play in the regulation of regional cardiac function.[4,6] The similarity of their responses to those observed in the in vivo model supports the contention that neurons in intrinsic cardiac and extracardiac intrathoracic ganglia display complex and unique interconnections and chemical sensitivities. While challenging current understanding of cardiac regulation, this view provides novel opportunities to develop pharmacological and even surgical strategies to manipulate the cardiac neuronal hierarchy in the management of cardiac disease.[41]

ACKNOWLEDGMENTS

The author gratefully acknowledges the financial support of the Canadian Institute of Health Research as well as the New Brunswick Heart and Stroke Foundation.

REFERENCES

1. Allen TGJ and Burnstock G. M_1 and M_2 muscarinic receptors mediate excitation and inhibition of guinea-pig intracardiac neurons in culture. *J Physiol (Lond)* 422:463–480, 1990.
2. Allen TGJ and Burnstock G. The actions of adenosine 5-trihosphate on guinea-pig intracardiac neurons in culture. *Br J Pharmacol* 100:269–276, 1990.
3. Allen TGJ, Hassall CJS, and Burnstock G. Mammalian intrinsic cardiac neurons in cell culture. In: Armour JA and Ardell JL, eds. *Neurocardiology.* New York: Oxford University Press, 1994, pp. 115–138.
4. Armour JA. Synaptic transmission in thoracic autonomic ganglia of the dog. *Can J Physiol Pharmacol* 61:793–801, 1983.
5. Armour JA. Intrinsic cardiac neurons. *J Cardiovasc Electrophysiol* 2:331–341, 1991.
6. Armour JA. The role of peripheral autonomic neurons in cardiac regulation. In: Armour JA and Ardell JL, eds. *Neurocardiology.* New York: Oxford University Press, 1994, pp. 219–244.
7. Armour JA and Hopkins DA. Activity of in situ canine left atrial ganglion neurons. *Am J Physiol* 259:H1207–H1215, 1990.
8. Armour JA, Huang MH, and Smith FM. Peptidergic modulation of in situ canine intrinsic cardiac neurons. *Peptides* 14:191–202, 1993.

9. Armour JA, Smith FM, Losier AM, Ellenberger HH, and Hopkins DA. Modulation of intrinsic cardiac neuronal activity by nitric oxide donors induces cardiodynamic changes. *Am J Physiol* 268:R403–R413, 1995.
10. Butler CK, Smith FM, Nicholson J, and Armour JA. Cardiac effects induced by chemical activation of neurons in discrete loci within canine stellate and middle cervical ganglia. *Am J Physiol* 259:H1108–H1117, 1990.
11. Darvesh S, Nance DM, Hopkins DA, and Armour JA. Distribution of neuropeptide immunoreactivity in intact and chronically decentralized middle cervical and stellate ganglia of dogs. *J Auton Nerv Syst* 21:167–180, 1987.
12. DeHaven WI and Cuevas J. Heterogeneity of pituitary adenylate cyclase-activating polypeptide and vasoactive intestinal polypeptide receptors in rat intrinsic cardiac neurons. *Neurosci Lett* 328:45–49, 2002.
13. Drugge ED, Rosen MR, and Robinson RB. Neuronal regulation of the development of the alpha-adrenergic chronotropic response in the rat heart. *Circ Res* 57:415–423, 1985.
14. Gagliardi M, Randall WC, Bieger D, Wurster RD, Hopkins DA, and Armour JA. Activity of in vivo canine cardiac plexus neurons. *Am J Physiol* 255:H789–H800, 1988.
15. Hassall CJS and Burnstock G. Intrinsic neurons and associated cells of the guinea pig heart in culture. *Brain Res* 364:102–113, 1986.
16. Hogg RC and Adams DJ. An ATP-sensitive K^+ conductance in dissociated neurones from adult rat intracardiac ganglia. *J Physiol (Lond)* 534:713–720, 2001.
17. Horackova M, and Armour JA. Role of peripheral autonomic neurons in maintaining adequate cardiac function. *Cardiovasc Res* 30:326–335, 1995.
18. Horackova M and Armour JA. ANG II modifies cardiomyocyte function via extracardiac and intracardiac neurons: in situ and in vitro studies. *Am J Physiol* 41:R766–R775, 1997.
19. Horackova M, Armour JA, and Byczko Z. Distribution of intrinsic cardiac neurons in whole-mount guinea-pig atria identified by multiple neurochemical coding. *Cell Tissue Res* 297:409–421, 1999.
20. Horackova M, Armour JA, Hopkins DA, and Huang MH. Nitric oxide modulates signaling between cultured adult peripheral cardiac neurons and cardiomyocytes. *Am J Physiol* 269:C504–C510, 1995.
21. Horackova M, Croll RP, Hopkins DA, Losier AM, and Armour JA. Morphological and immunohistochemical properties of primary long-term cultures of adult guinea pig ventricular cardiomyocytes with peripheral cardiac neurons. *Tissue Cell* 28:411–425, 1996.
22. Horackova M, Huang MH, Armour JA, Hopkins DA, and Mapplebeck C. Cocultures of adult ventricular myocytes with stellate ganglia or intrinsic cardiac neurons from guinea pig: spontaneous activity and pharmacological properties. *Cardiovasc Res* 27:1101–1108, 1993.
23. Horackova M, Huang MH, and Armour JA. Purinergic modulation of adult guinea pig cardiomyocytes in long-term cultures and cocultures with extracardiac or intracardiac neurons. *Cardiovasc Res* 28:673–679, 1994.
24. Horackova M, Slavikova J, and Byczko Z. Postnatal development of the rat intrinsic cardiac nervous system: a confocal laser scanning microscopy study in whole-mount atria. *Tissue Cell* 32:377–388, 2000.
25. Huang MH, Smith FM, and Armour JA. Amino acids modify the activity of

canine intrinsic cardiac neurons involved in cardiac regulation. *Am J Physiol* 264:H1275–H1282, 1993.
26. Huang MH, Smith FM, and Armour JA. Modulation of in situ canine intrinsic cardiac neuronal activity by nicotinic, muscarinic and β-adrenergic agonists. *Am J Physiol* 265:R659–R669, 1993.
27. Huang MH, Sylvén C, Pelleg A, Smith FM, and Armour JA. Modulation of in situ canine intrinsic cardiac neurons by locally applied adenosine, ATP or their analogs. *Am J Physiol* 165:R914–R922, 1993.
28. Ishibashi H, Umezu M, Jang I-S, Ito Y, and Akaike N. α_1-adrenoceptor-activated cation currents in neurones acutely isolated from rat cardiac parasympathetic ganglia. *J Physiol (Lond)* 548:111–120, 2003.
29. Marvin WJ, Atkins DL, Chittick VL, Lund DD, and Hermsmeyer K. In vitro adrenergic and cholinergic innervation of the developing rat myocyte. *Circ Res* 55:49–58, 1984.
30. Moravec M, and Moravec J. Adrenergic neurons and short proprioceptive feedback loops involved in the integration of cardiac function in the rat. *Cell Tissue Res* 258:381–385, 1989.
31. Murphy DA, O'Blenes S, Hanna BD, and Armour JA. Functional capacity of nicotine sensitive canine intrinsic neurons to modify the heart. *Am J Physiol* 266:R1127–R1135, 1994.
32. Nyquist-Battie C, Cochran PK, Sands SA, and Chronwall BM. Development of neuropeptide Y and tyrosine hydroxylase immunoreactive innervation of postnatal rat heart. *Peptides* 15:1461–1469, 1994.
33. Ogawa S, Barnett JV, Sen L, Galper JB, Smith TW, and March JD. Direct contact between sympathetic neurons and rat cardiac myocytes in vitro increases expression of calcium channels. *J Clin Invest* 89:1085–1093, 1992.
34. Patterson PH and Chun LLY. The induction of acetylcholine synthesis in primary cultures of dissociated rat sympathetic neurons. *Dev Biol* 60:473–481, 1977.
35. Patterson PH, Potter DD, and Furshpan EJ. The chemical differentiation of nerve cells. *Sci Am* 239:50–59, 1978.
36. Robb JS. *Comparative Basic Cardiology*. New York: Grune & Stratton, 1965.
37. Singh S, Johnson PI, Javed A, Gray TS, Lonchyna VA, and Wurster RD. Monamine- and histamine-synthesizing enzymes and neurotransmitters within neurons in adult human cardiac ganglia. *Circulation* 99:411–419, 1999.
38. Slavikova J, Goldstein M, and Dahlström A. The postnatal development of tyrosine hydroxylase immunoreactive nerves in rat atrium, studied with immunofluorescence and confocal laser scanning microscopy. *J Auton Nerv Syst* 43:159–170, 1993.
39. Steele PA, Gibbons IL, Morris JL, and Mayer B. Multiple populations of neuropeptide-containing intrinsic neurons in the guinea pig heart. *Neuroscience* 62:241–250, 1994.
40. Sun LS, Ursell PC, and Robinson RB. Chronic exposure to neuropeptide Y determines cardiac alpha 1-adrenergic responsiveness. *Am J Physiol* 30:H969–H973, 1991.
41. Tallaj J, Wei CC, Hankes GH, Holland M, Rynders P, Dillon AR, L.Ardell JL, Armour JA, Lucchesi PA, and Dell'Italia LJ. β1-adrenergic receptor blockade attenuates angiotensin II–mediated catecholamine release into the cardiac interstitium in mitral regurgitation. *Circulation* 108:225–230, 2003.

42. Thompson GW, Collier J, Ardell JL, Kember G, and Armour JA. Functional interdependence of neurons in a single canine intrinsic cardiac ganglionated plexus. *J Physiol* 528:561–571, 2000.
43. Yuan B-X, Ardell JL, Hopkins DA, Losier AM, and Armour JA. Gross and microscopic anatomy of the canine intrinsic cardiac nervous system. *Anat Rec* 239:75–87, 1994.
44. Yuan B-X, Hopkins DA, Ardell JL, and Armour JA. Differential cardiac responses induced by nicotinic sensitive canine intrinsic atrial and ventricular neurones. *Cardiovasc Res* 27:760–769, 1993.
45. Zhang J, Robinson RB, and Siegelbaum SB. Sympathetic neurons mediate development change in cardiac sodium channel gating through long-term neurotransmitter action. *Neuron* 9:97–103, 1992.

3

Cardiac Sensory Neurons

J. Andrew Armour and Guy C. Kember

The nervous system intrinsic to the heart contains all of the components necessary for information processing. That parasympathetic efferent postganglionic neurons are associated with the intrinsic cardiac nervous system has been known for some time.[22,63] Recently, afferent neurons,[2,10,29,44] sympathetic efferent postganglionic neurons,[25,86] and interconnecting local circuit neurons[13,14,37] have been identified within the intrinsic cardiac nervous system. As a matter of fact, it was the functional identification of the somata of afferent neurons within this system[2] that permitted the development of the thesis that there is a *little brain* on the heart that modulates regional cardiodynamics on a beat-to-beat basis.[10,63]

Cardiac sensory nerve terminals (neurites) are associated with somata in ganglia located relatively distant from the heart, those in nodose and dorsal root ganglia.[64,84] These neurons, plus those associated with sensory neurites in intrathoracic and cervical vessels, transduce the cardiac and intrathoracic vascular milieu to medullary (Chapter 6) and spinal cord (Chapter 5) neurons, respectively. Recent evidence indicates that afferent neuronal somata located in intrathoracic extracardiac ganglia are associated with sensory neurites in cardiac tissues and the adventitia of intrathoracic vessels.[8,23] The latter population of afferent neurons transduces the cardiovascular milieu to cardiac postganglionic motor neurons in intrathoracic ganglia, doing so primarily via intrathoracic local circuit neurons.[10] Each cardiac afferent neuron displays unique transduction capabilities so that the information they provide to second-order processing neurons within different levels of the cardiac neuronal axis varies. These in turn influence cardiac efferent neurons, some of which also receive indirect inputs via central neurons from afferent neurons with sensory neurites in extrathoracic tissues. The latter include the carotid arteries[1,12] and skin of the extremities.[6,7] Ultimately, most efferent neuronal outflow to the heart depends on direct or indirect inputs from cardiac and vascular sensory neurites.[6,7,13,14,37] Thus, the nature of the sensory information transduced by these varied populations of cardiovascular afferent neurons, impinging as it does on intrinsic cardiac, intrathoracic extracardiac, and central interneurons, ultimately determines the capacity of cardiac efferent neurons to coordinate regional cardiac function.[4]

Intrathoracic ganglia have long been thought to act as simple efferent relay stations that involve both "limbs" of the autonomic nervous system—cardiac vagal efferent postganglionic neurons residing in intrinsic cardiac ganglia and sympathetic efferent postganglionic neurons residing in paravertebral ganglia. In this scenario, the two major efferent limbs of the cardiac nervous system act in a purely reciprocal fashion to exert control over cardiac rate and force.[40] This is in accord with the long-held view that visceral afferent fibers have their cells of origin exclusively in cerebrospinal ganglia.[64] Recently this concept has been extended in recognition of the fact that cardiovascular sensory information is also processed within the intrathoracic nervous system, including its component intrinsic to the heart.[10]

Sensory neurites associated with intrinsic cardiac afferent neuronal somata are located in selected regions of the atria and ventricles and in the adventitia of major coronary arteries.[2,13,14,37] Sensory neurites associated with the somata of afferent neurons in intrathoracic extracardiac ganglia are also located in these tissues as well as in the vena cava and thoracic aorta.[3,5] Populations of nodose and dorsal root ganglion afferent neurons also receive inputs from sensory neurites located in these tissues, as well as the carotid arteries, to provide feed-forward information to neurons located primarily in the nucleus tractus solatarius and spinal cord, respectively.

The varied transduction properties displayed by these differing populations of afferent neurons probably reflect not only the location of their sensory neurites but also the anatomical distance between these somata and their associated sensory neurites. Their varied transduction characteristics determine to a large extent the redundancy of function and non-coupled behavior displayed by neurons in differing levels of the cardiac neuronal hierarchy.[10] This minimizes any dependency of regional cardiac control on a single population of afferent neurons.[12] Thus, sensory neurites located in the heart and great thoracic vessels activate short-, intermediate-, and relatively long-latency cardiovascular–cardiac reflexes within this neuronal hierarchy, depending on where their associated somata are located.[4,56] The varied transduction capabilities displayed by these different populations of cardiovascular sensory neurons determine response characteristics displayed by various populations within the cardiac neuronal hierarchy for the integrated control of cardiac efferent neuronal function.

This chapter presents first a brief outline of the anatomy of cardiac sensory neurons, followed by an overview of their differing transduction characteristics. This will permit the development of a model based on their functional anatomy, one that is proposed to gain insight into the content of cardiovascular information that is fed to each level of the cardiac neuronal hierarchy.[52] The chapter's underlying thesis is that differential transduction of cardiovascular sensory information is the primary determinant of the complex interactions that occur within the cardiac neuronal hierarchy which ultimately coordinates cardiac efferent neuronal function. It should be kept in mind that reflexes depending on inputs from cardiac and major intrathoracic vascular sensory neurites act in concert with those initiated by sensory neurons transducing the mechanical milieu of carotid arterial walls or other body regions (see Chapters 5 and 6).

CARDIOVASCULAR AFFERENT NEUROANATOMY

Much is known about the information that is transduced by individual cardiac afferent neurons.[3,5,19–21,30,31,54,56,59,61,71] The extensive arrays of atrial sensory neurites associated with individual neurons lie concentrated in the dorsal aspects of the atria, as well as in the region of the sinoatrial node (Fig. 3–1). Ventricular neurites are located primarily in the outflow tracts of either ventricle, including in the cranial interventricular septum, as well as in the right and left ventricular papillary muscles. The transduction properties of these neurons differ according to whether their associated sensory neurites are located in the ventricular epicardium, myocardium, or endocardium.[3] A large number of mechanosensory neurites are located in the aortic adventitia, concentrated particularly in a band of tissue extending continuously along the inner arch of the thoracic aorta; fewer are located on the vena cava or major pulmonary vessels adjacent to the heart.[3] Not only does the anatomical location of these sensory neurites determine in large part the transduction characteristics of individual cardiac afferent neurons, but their overall response characteristics show a stratification that is related to the distance between sensory neurites and their associated somata (Table 3–1).

When tissues containing physiologically identified cardiac sensory neurites associated with these neurons are examined microscopically, bare nerve endings exist without specialized structures surrounding them.[5] Some cardiac afferent neurons have sensory neurites located in two discrete loci. This includes not only separate loci in one cardiac chamber or two chambers but also the heart and tissues adjacent to the heart, such as a pulmonary artery.[3,34] This anatomical arrangement ensures that source-

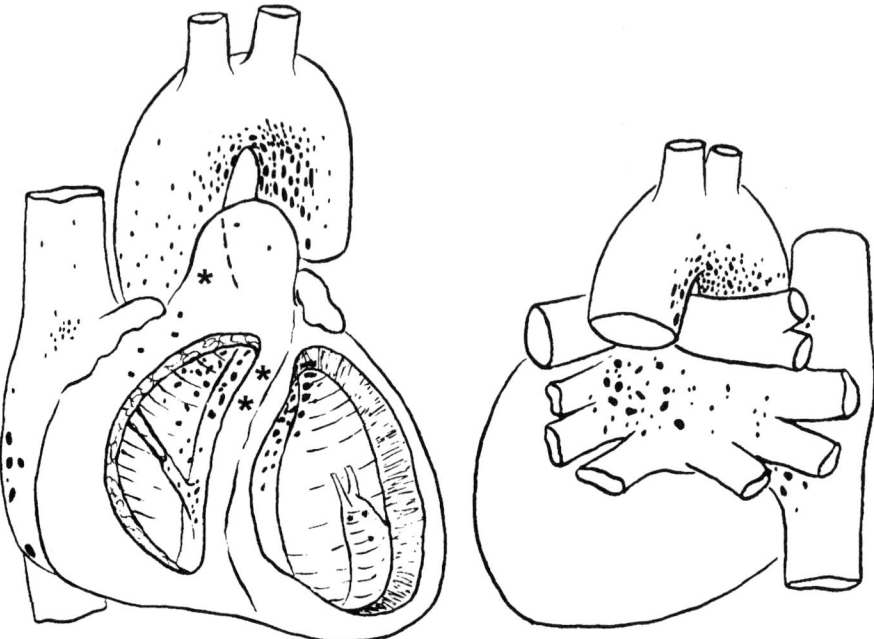

FIGURE 3–1 Schematic representation of the canine heart and major intrathoracic vascular loci where sensory neurites associated with most cardiac afferent neuronal somata are located. Note the predominance of sensory fields in the outflow tracts of the two ventricles. Mechanosensory neurites lie clustered in the region of the sinoatrial node and papillary muscles, as well as along the inner curvature of the aortic arch. The sizes of the dots imply the relative size of identified mechanosensory fields. Chemosensory neurites(*) have been identified in the interventricular septum and aortic root.

based differences can be transduced by cardiac afferent neurons so that spatially derived functional differences are computed at the level of the heart.

As aggregates of cardiac afferent neuronal somata are localized in *(1)* nodose, *(2)* dorsal root, *(3)* intrathoracic extracardiac ganglia, and *(4)* intrinsic cardiac ganglia, the transduction capabilities of these afferent neurons are discussed according to the location of their somata. Individual afferent axons arise from multiple sensory neurites distributed in cardiac or vascular fields of varying size. The degree of their myelination generally varies according to the location of the cardiopulmonary nerve in which they course.[3] For instance, most aortic mechanosensory neurites are associated with Aδ axons that course centrally primarily, but not exclusively, in the intrathoracic dorsal cardiopulmonary nerve.[5] In contrast,

TABLE 3–1 Estimated Cardiac Sensory Neurite Transduction Capabilities Relative to Associated Somata Location

Afferent Neuronal Somata	Mechanosensory (%)	Multimodal (%)	Chemosensory (%)
Nodose ganglia	5	25	70
Dorsal root ganglia	5	90	5
Stellate ganglia	10	15	75
Middle cervical ganglia	10	80	10
Intrinsic cardiac ganglia	10	85	5

Cardiac afferent neurons in various locations are categorized according to whether they transduced the mechanical, mechanical and chemical (multimodal), or solely chemical milieu surrounding their sensory neurites. Dorsal root neurons are primarily multimodal in nature, whereas nodose ganglion ones primarily transduce the chemical milieu of the heart. The populations of cardiac afferent neurons that solely transduce the mechanical milieu surrounding their associated sensory neurites are relatively limited.

carotid artery mechanosensory neurites are associated with afferent axons belonging to the Aδ and c-fiber categories, as defined by Erlanger and Gasser, each displaying unique transduction capabilities.[1]

Nodose Ganglion Afferent Neurons

Using neuroanatomical tracing techniques, about 500 somata associated with cardiac sensory neurites have been identified throughout the right and left nodose ganglia of dogs and pigs.[41,42] Their axons display the functional characteristics of Aδ and C classes of axons.[15,75,76,79] Recent evidence indicates that the somata of nodose ganglion afferent neurons express a variety of receptors. These include adenosine A_1[57] and A_2,[26] bradykinin,[83] and substance P[50] receptors.

Doral Root Ganglion Afferent Neurons

Despite the widely held opinion that most cardiac afferent neurons are located primarily in left-sided dorsal root ganglia, anatomic evidence indicates that the somata of cardiac afferent neurons are distributed relatively equally among right- and left-sided dorsal root ganglia from the C6 to the T6 levels of the spinal cord.[41,81] Afferent neuronal somata are scattered predominantly but not exclusively around the centrally located axons in each ganglion. Over 500 cardiac sensory neurons have been identified anatomically in canine dorsal root ganglia, some ganglia containing over 50 cardiac afferent neuronal somata.[41] The axons connecting cardiac sensory neurites with somata in dorsal root ganglia fall into the Aδ or c classes, axon classes that bear little relationship to their transduction characteristics.[47,48]

Intrathoracic Extracardiac Ganglion Afferent Neurons

Unipolar neurons that display anatomic characteristics similar to those found in nodose and dorsal root ganglia have been identified in intrathoracic extracardiac ganglia.[44] Functional evidence supports the concept that the somata of cardiac sensory neurons are located in stellate, middle cervical, and mediastinal ganglia.[8,23] The axons connecting atrial and ventricular epicardial and myocardial mechanosensory neurites with somata in intrathoracic extracardiac ganglia belong to the Aδ class, as do those connecting major intrathoracic vascular mechanosensory neurites with somata in these ganglia. Cardiac and aortic chemosensory neurites associated with somata in intrathoracic ganglia have Aδ class axons. Ventricular endocardial mechanosensory neurites by contrast are connected to somata in intrathoracic extracardiac ganglia via c-class axons.[3]

Intrinsic Cardiac Ganglion Afferent Neurons

Unipolar neurons are also located in atrial and ventricular intrinsic cardiac ganglionated plexuses.[44,66,85] On the basis of anatomical[29] and functional[10] data, the somata of some intrinsic cardiac afferent neurons project axons centrally; the rest interact only with other intrinsic cardiac neurons.[2] The sensory neurites associated with intrinsic cardiac afferent neurons are located in all four chambers of the heart, particularly in the cranial aspect of the ventricles.[12–14,37] The anatomical characteristics of axons connecting cardiac sensory neurites with intrinsic cardiac afferent neuronal somata remain unknown.

TRANSDUCTION PROPERTIES OF DIFFERENT POPULATIONS OF CARDIAC AFFERENT NEURONS

Depending on the location of their somata, most cardiac sensory neurons transduce the local mechanical and chemical milieu surrounding their sensory neurites (they are multimodal in nature) (Table 3–1). Relatively limited populations of cardiac afferent neurons solely encode the intensity of local mechanical deformation, doing so in a graded fashion. Data accumulated in the canine model indicate that cardiac afferent neurons that transduce only the chemical environment of their sensory neurites are concentrated primarily in nodose and intrathoracic stellate ganglia. However, the estimates provided in Table 3–1 were derived from relatively limited numbers of afferent neurons and thus should be taken as a guide for the fact that different populations of cardiac afferent neurons transduce their cardiac milieu differentially, depending on the anatomic location of their somata and sensory neurites.

We have proposed that common shared mechanosensory inputs to neurons in one intrinsic cardiac ganglionated plexus may account in part for the tight coupling behavior displayed by many of its neurons.[74] Local coordination of neuronal activity is also reflective of sensory inputs impinging on populations of intrathoracic local circuit neurons that disseminate such information to aggregates of cardiac efferent neurons. Short-timescale (>50 ms) coordination does not occur among neurons distributed among intrinsic cardiac and intrathoracic extrinsic ganglia.[12] This reflects the divergent cardiovascular afferent inputs that intracardiac and extracardiac feedback control networks receive, thereby imparting redundancy of function to different populations of cardiac efferent neurons within the cardiac neuronal hierarchy.[12] Thus, the varied transduction characteristics displayed by these different populations of cardiac afferent neurons can initiate short-loop intrinsic cardiac reflexes at the same time as longer-latency reflexes involving central neurons. The transduction properties of each of the principal cardiac afferent neuronal populations presented above will be considered in turn.

Nodose Ganglion Afferent Neurons

Nodose ganglion cardiac afferent neuronal somata project axons centrally to medullary neurons in the nucleus tractus solatarius, as do nodose ganglion afferent neurons associated with aortic and carotid artery sensory neurites (Chapter 6). Most cardiac sensory neurites associated with nodose ganglion somata transduce the chemical milieu of the heart (Table 3–1). Most carotid artery sensory neurites, by contrast, transduce local mechanical deformation related to arterial pressure dynamics.[1] Carotid artery mechanosensory neurites, being located relatively close to somata in nodose ganglia, affect second-order neurons with a minimum of delay to initiate fast-responding reflexes controlling cardiac vagal efferent preganglionic neurons differentially throughout each normal cardiac cycle.[4] They also affect spinal cord sympathetic efferent preganglionic neurons that in turn indirectly affect populations of neurons in intrathoracic sympathetic extracardiac ganglia.[12] These longer-latency reflexes are responsible, in part, for the cardiac-related cyclic activity generated by many of the sympathetic efferent preganglionic neurons that project axons in intrathoracic and abdominal sympathetic nerves.[1,40] With respect to ventricular sensory endings associated with nodose ganglion cardiac afferent neurons, contrary to the generally held opinion that they are confined to the dorsal (inferior) wall of the left ventricle,[77,78] they are located throughout the atria or concentrated in the outflow tracts of either ventricle.[15,75]

Mechanical stimuli

A relatively small population of the nodose ganglion cardiac afferent neurons transduces atrial or ventricular mechanical deformation (Table 3–1). The activity generated by atrial mechanosensory neurites associated with these neurons reflects regional deformation along the major vector parallel to their local muscle fascicles.[19] Presumably, this is why some atrial mechanosensory neurites generate activity that correlates with regional dynamics.[54,59,71] Ventricular mechanosensory neurites associated with a small population of nodose ganglion afferent neurons generate activity that relates to ventricular end diastolic pressure,[20,58] whereas others transduce changes in ventricular systolic pressure.[15] The activity generated by nodose ganglion cardiac mechanosensitive afferent neurons is immediate, proportional to the applied mechanical stimulus, and short lasting upon withdrawal of the stimulus. This relatively small population of afferent neurons can be classified as fast responding with respect to the stimulus transduced (Table 3–2).

Chemical stimuli

Most cardiac afferent neurons in nodose ganglia generate relatively low frequency activity (about 0.1–0.2 Hz) during physiological states that does

TABLE 3–2 Cardiac Afferent Neuron Function

Fast Responding, Mechanotransduction	Slow Responding, Chemotransduction
Sensory-specific (mechanosensory modality)	Frequently multimodal transduction
Transducing constantly varying local mechanics	Transducing multiple, nonuniform events
High-fidelity, relatively uniform signal	"Noisy" (multichemical) signal that limits resolution
Produces phasic activity	Tonic (nonphasic), relatively low frequency activity
Limited memory	Memory capability; affected by past events
Noise-free transduction	Requires noise for transduction
Soma located mostly on or near the heart	Soma located mostly in ganglia distant from the heart
Primarily direct input to cardiac efferent neurons	Inputs to intrathoracic and central interneurons
Primary inputs to short control loops	Inputs to intermediate- and longer-latency control loops

The function of cardiac afferent neurons is categorized according to whether they are (1) fast-responding, mechanotransducing or (2) slow-responding, chemosensory ones. In general, fast-responding, sensory-specific neurons lie closer to the target organ than do slow-responding (tonically active) ones.

not reflect changes in cardiac mechanics.[15,75] Rather, their activity increases many-fold when their sensory neurites are exposed to chemical stimuli.[15] Such responses persist long after (up to 45 minutes) brief exposure of their sensory neurites to an adequate chemical stimulus. This principal subset of nodose afferent neurons can be classified as slow responding.

These nodose ganglion cardiac afferent neurons have been reported to transduce multiple chemicals, including the peptides angiotensin II, bradykinin, calcitonin gene–related peptide (CGRP), substance P, and vasoactive intestinal peptide.[21,36,70,75] They are also sensitive to α- and β-adrenoceptor agonists, acidic solutions (i.e., pH of 6.0), arachidonic acid, histamine, hydrogen peroxide, hydroxyl radicals, and nitric oxide donors.[45,69,72,75,80,81] Thus, this population of cardiac sensory neurons is capable of transducing chemicals known to be liberated by the ischemic myocardium, such as adenosine,[35,67] bradykinin,[39] and oxygen free radicals.[88] Although at the present time we do not understand all the ionic mechanisms underlying their transduction capability, their sensory neurites are known to employ a variety of ion channel mechanisms.[75] These sensory neurites possess membrane Na^+ channels whose permeability is increased in response to chemical stimulation with consequent depolarization and action potential generation.[75] Ca^{2+}-activated K^+ channels associated with their sensory neurites are also involved in this transduction.[75]

Dorsal Root Ganglion Neurons

The activity generated by cardiac sensory neurites associated with dorsal root ganglion afferent neurons differs in many respects from that generated by their nodose ganglion counterparts. First, in anesthetized animal models, during basal states dorsal root ganglion cardiac afferent neurons generate greater activity (~10 Hz) than do their nodose ganglion cardiac afferent neuronal (~0.1 Hz) counterparts. Second, whereas few nodose ganglion cardiac afferent neurons transduce mechanical stimuli, most (~95%) dorsal root ganglion cardiac afferent neurons are multimodal in nature (Table 3–1), transducing both mechanical and chemical stimuli.[47] As with nodose ganglion afferent neurons, sensory neurites associated with dorsal root ganglion afferent neurons are located primarily in the dorsal aspect of the atria and the outflow tracts of either ventricle. The sensory fields associated with a few of these afferent neurons are located in separate loci on a ventricle or even on an atrium and a ventricle.[34,47] When exposed to chemical stimuli, they can generate activity in excess of 100 Hz. Thus, the maximum activity generated by dorsal root ganglion cardiac afferent neurons can be an order magnitude greater than that achieved by their nodose ganglion counterparts during ischemic states.

Perhaps that is why symptoms arising from the ischemic myocardium are associated primarily with dorsal root rather than nodose ganglion afferent neurons (see Chapter 10).

Mechanical stimuli
The high-fidelity (fast-responding) mechanotransducing neurites associated with most dorsal root ganglion cardiac afferent neurons are uniquely orientated, in a functional sense, with respect to local atrial or ventricular muscle fascicles.[34,47,61] Such sensory transduction displays limited memory, generating phasic rather than tonic activity in response to local muscle fascicle deformation (Table 3–1). As shown in Figure 3–2, the activity generated by some fast-responding dorsal root afferent neurons delineates a range of regional ventricular pressure generation by producing either increasing or decreasing exponentials of activity or information in a quadratic fashion in response to similar alterations in regional ventricular pressure.[47] These data indicate that information provided by this relatively limited population of cardiac afferent neurons permits maximal resolution of the entire pressure range developed within a ventricle to spinal cord neurons. As increasing receptor field strain elicited during

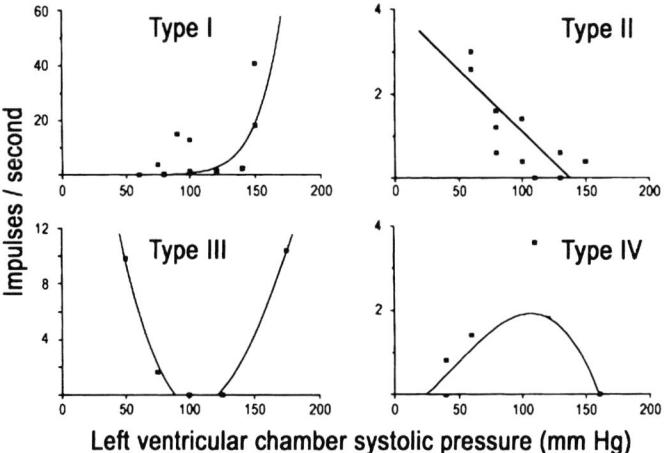

FIGURE 3–2 Activity generated by four different types of left ventricular mechanosensory neurites associated with dorsal root ganglion afferent neurons (c-class) as related to left ventricular chamber systolic pressure. Type 1: activity increases as chamber systolic pressure increases. Type II: activity decreases as chamber systolic pressure increases. Type III: activity is greatest when chamber pressure is lower and higher, being minimum when pressure is in the physiological range. Type IV: activity is maximal at normal systolic pressure, becoming reduced as chamber systolic pressure decreases or increases.

ventricular premature contractions can become the optimum stimulus for dorsal root ganglion afferent neuronal activation,[31] the relative magnitude of the inputs from mechanical versus chemical stimuli determines which modality exerts the greatest influence on the information they transduce to spinal cord neurons at any given time.[34,47]

Chemical stimuli
With respect to alterations in the chemical milieu of the heart, most dorsal root ganglion cardiac afferent neurons transduce multiple chemicals.[47] The total power content in the spectral domain of their activity depends on the relative content of each modality they are capable of transducing (Fig. 3–3). For instance, spectral analysis of the activity patterns generated by individual canine dorsal root ganglion cardiac afferent neurons indicates that they transduce purinergic agents in varied domains of their power spectra (adenosine peaks generated from 0.2 to 40 Hz; ATP from 0.2 to 5 Hz).[11] Substance P has also been shown to activate ventricular sensory neurites in the 0.2 to 18 Hz ranges of their activity spectra. Thus, transient regional myocardial ischemia may result in these afferent neurons generating activity in multiple (i.e., 0.4 to 30 Hz) components of their power spectra. Not all of these afferent neurons respond with the same activity spectral peaks to myocardial ischemia. Further investigations will be required to reveal the activity profiles that different cardiac afferent neurons generate in response to a cardiac event being transduced.

Despite limited knowledge concerning transduction properties, these preliminary data indicate that individual cardiac afferent neurons transduce selective chemical signals in specific activity domains so that multiple chemicals can be transduced simultaneously to spinal cord neurons by individual cardiac afferent neurons. Presumably, second-order neurons in the spinal cord are able to resolve such varied information content. Chemically induced afferent neuronal responses take time to develop and to resolve once the chemical stimulus has been removed; this may account for the fact that gradually evolving and long-lasting symptoms can occur in humans after relatively brief periods of compromised coronary arterial blood supply (Chapter 10).

Intrathoracic Extracardiac Afferent Neurons

The sensory neurites associated with somata in intrathoracic extracardiac ganglia[44] are concentrated in the atria and cranial aspects of either ventricle.[6,7] On the basis of physiological evidence, varied populations of cardiac afferent neurons in stellate, middle cervical, and mediastinal ganglia transduce local mechanical events.[6,7,12,16] The information they transduce

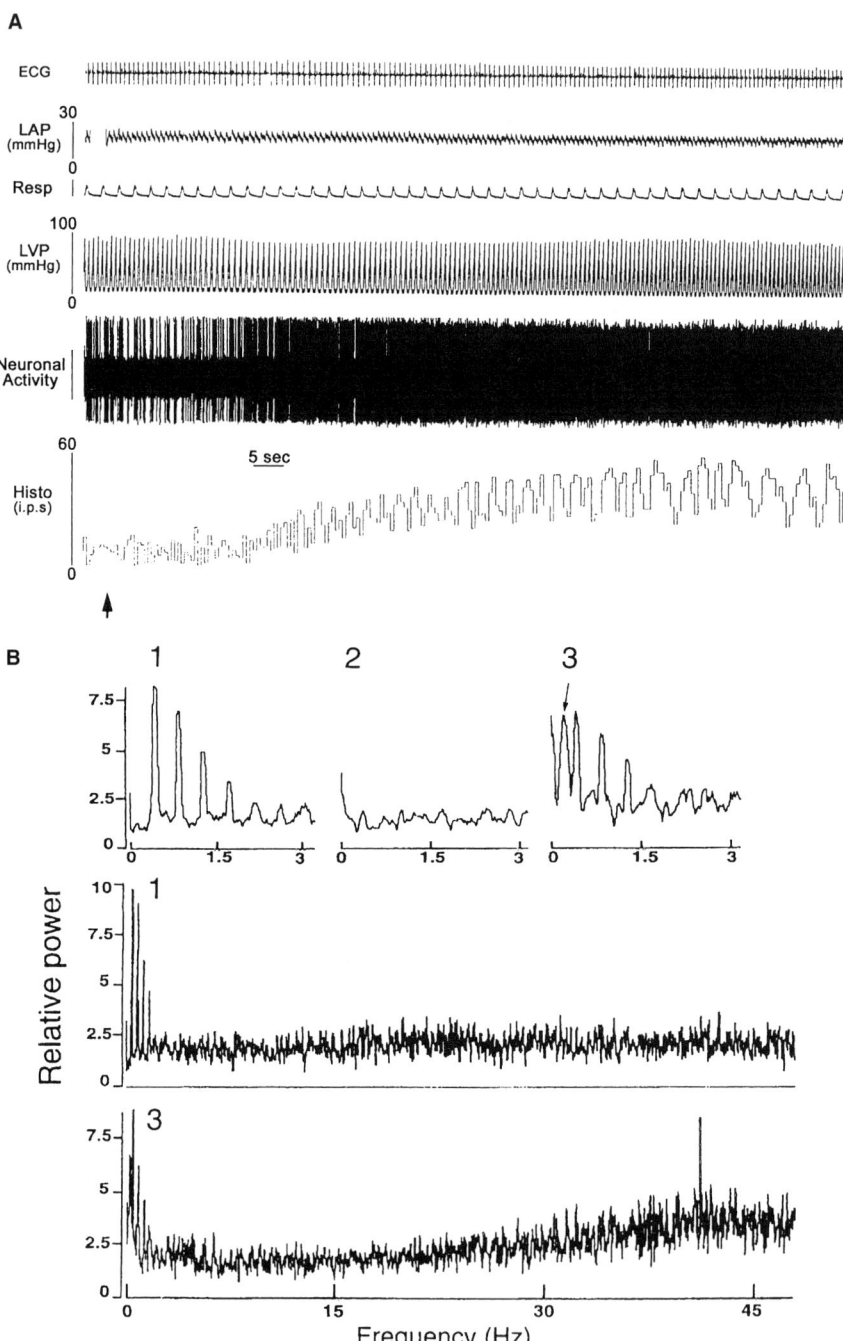

is relatively noise-free in physiological states, being primarily related to sensory field deformation.[3,5] That phase-related activity is generated by such atrial mechanosensory neurons in the presence of atrial fibrillation (Fig. 3–4) may reflect their capacity to transduce rhythmic sensory field deformation within restricted atrial regions even though the whole atrium generates uncoordinated contractile behavior. Accurate transduction of regional deformation is also displayed by ventricular endocardial mechanosensory neurites associated with intrathoracic afferent neurons (Fig. 3–5). The activity patterns generated by this population of cardiac afferent neurons can be best described as a linear function reflective of regional muscle fascicle deformation (Fig. 3–6). Thus the intrathoracic neuronal hierarchy transduces very precise information concerning the mechanical status of selected cardiac regions throughout each cardiac cycle.[3]

Another population of intrathoracic extracardiac neurons receives inputs solely from aortic mechanosensory afferent neurons.[5] The sensory neurites of these afferent neurons are concentrated in a contiguous band along the inner curvature of the aorta (Fig. 3–1). Aortic mechanosensory neurites associated with individual afferent neurons transduce regional wall deformation (as represented by aortic diameter) in an exponential manner (Fig. 3–7B–D). Their transduction capabilities reflect aortic wall deformation with such precision that when the action potentials generated by multiple aortic mechanosensory afferent axons are recorded simultaneously at slow heart rates, they generate four bursts of activity during each cardiac cycle that are synchronous with the four aortic pressure waves occurring in such a state (Fig. 3–7A). During normal pressure states, their grouped activity is maximal during peak (systolic) aortic pressure,

◂─────────────

FIGURE 3–3 Activity generated by a dorsal root ganglion afferent neuron associated with a c-class axon arising from multimodal sensory neurites in the right ventricular conus epicardium. **A.** The activity generated by this afferent neuron increased when its sensory neurites were exposed to adenosine (10 μM; applied topically at arrow below), displaying concomitant respiratory-related activity at that time (c.f., bottom line: histogram of neuronal activity with respiratory phase related behavior). **B.** During control states, this afferent neuron generated multiple, low-frequency components in the power spectrum of its activity (B1); that behavior disappeared when respiration ceased (B2). During topical application of adenosine, novel activity was generated at low- (0.03 Hz; B3 above) and high- (38 Hz; B3 below) frequency spectral peaks. These data demonstrate the capacity of individual cardiac afferent neurons to simultaneously transduce multiple sensory stimuli in differing spectral frequency domains. ECG, lead II of the electrocardiogram; LAP, left atrial pressure; Resp, enodtracheal pressure; LVP, left ventricular chamber pressure; neuronal activity, activity generated by identified unit; Histo, activity histogram.

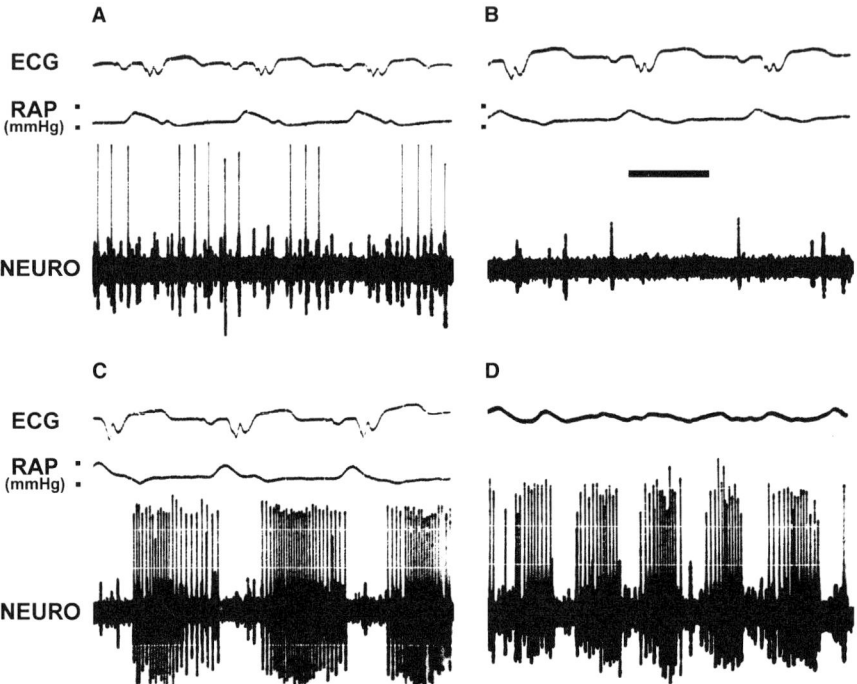

FIGURE 3–4 Activity generated by right atrial mechanosensory neurites associated with an afferent axon (Aδ-class afferent axon) in a dog's mediastinal (recurrent cardiac) nerve. **A.** In control states, three to four action potentials were generated during diastole in each atrial pressure cycle. **B.** When the pericardium was opened, right atrial systolic pressure (RAP) fell minimally such that this unit no longer generated activity. **C.** Right atrial systolic pressure increased following isoproterenol administration, as did the number of action potentials per atrial cycle. **D.** Following cardiac fibrillation (note disorganized ECG), rhythmic activity continued to be generated, presumably because of local rhythmic contractile behavior of its sensory field. RAP, right atrial chamber pressure; dots beside right atrial pressure traces in A–C, 10 mmHg; Neuro, neurograms of afferent axonal activity. Horizontal bar in B = 200 ms. (same timescale for each panel).

during the subsequent aortic dicrotic pressure notch, and during the two smaller reflectance-induced diastolic pressure waves.[55]

The precision of this mechanosensory transduction becomes further evident during pulsus alternans. In this state, aortic mechanosensory neurites are activated only during those cardiac cycles in which blood is expelled from the left ventricle into the aorta to distend that vessel.[6] In contrast, ventricular mechanosensory neurons are activated during each cardiac cycle during pulsus alternans, a responsive reflective of local ventricular deformation. Presumably, this is why intrathoracic local circuit neurons receiv-

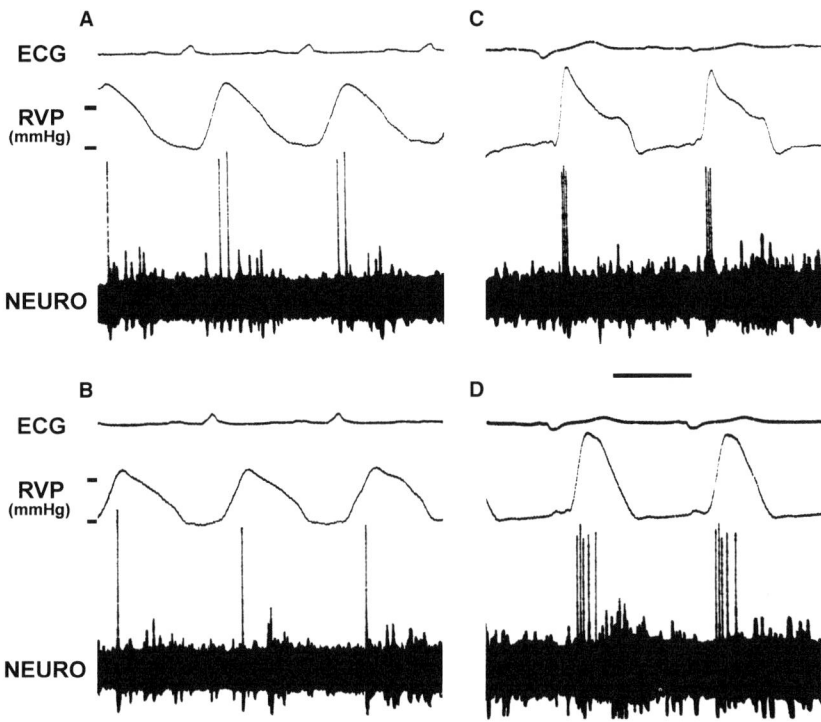

FIGURE 3–5 Activity generated by a c-class axon in a canine mediastinal (right cranial vagal) nerve that was associated with sensory neurites in the endocardium of the right ventricular conus. **A.** During control states, two action potentials were generated during isovolumetric contraction. **B.** Opening the pericardium slightly reduced right ventricular systolic pressure (15–12 mmHg) so that only one action potential was generated per cardiac cycle. **C.** Soon after administering isoproterenol (1 μg/kg i.v.), right ventricular systolic pressure increased to 32 mmHg; three action potentials were generated during each isovolumetric contraction as the configuration of systolic events changed. **D.** Later on, five action potentials were generated during isovolumetric contraction. Vertical bars beside right ventricular pressure (RVP) traces = 20 mmHg; Neuro, neurograms of afferent axonal activity; horizontal bar between C & D = 500 ms. (same timescale for each panel).

ing aortic mechanosensory inputs become active only during those cardiac cycles that produce flow out of the ventricle during pulses alternans (every second beat), whereas those transducing ventricular mechanical events generate action potential during each cardiac cycle in such a state.[6,7] In other words, different populations of intrathoracic local circuit neurons can transduce cardiovascular mechanical status differentially.[12]

Many cardiac sensory neurites associated with intrathoracic, extracardiac afferent neurons also transduce chemicals such as adenosine, pep-

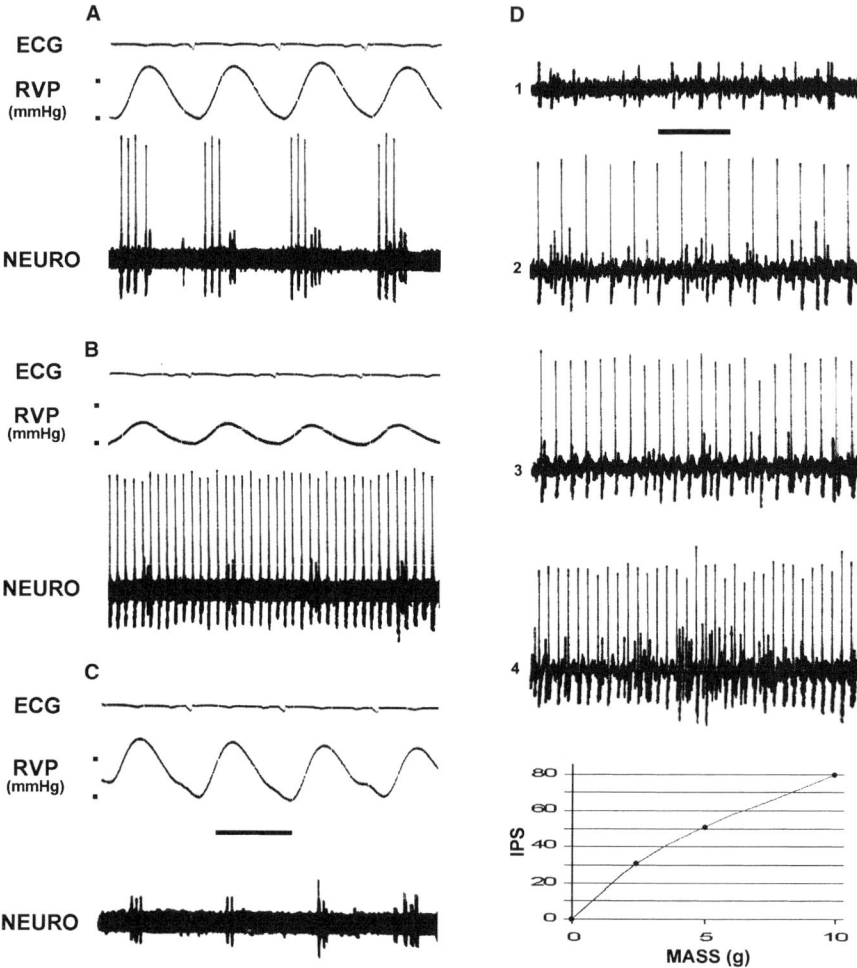

FIGURE 3–6 Activity generated by a c-class axon associated with sensory neurites in the right ventricular papillary muscle in a canine right recurrent cardiac nerve. **A.** In control states, three to four action potentials were generated during isovolumetric contraction. **B.** Occluding the superior vena cava reduced right ventricular systolic pressure (28–10 mm Hg) such that activity became continuous. **C.** Partially occluding the pulmonary artery increased right ventricular systolic pressure to 30 mmHg, eliminating activity. **D.** When the heart was fibrillated and emptied of blood, increasing mass was applied to the cordae tendinea of the right ventricular papillary muscle; activity increased (IPS = impulses per second) in a linear fashion as mass increased from 0 grams (D1) to 2.5 (D2), 5 (D3), and 10 (D4) grams (plotted lower right). Dots beside right ventricular pressure (RVP) traces in A–C = 0 and 20 mmHg; horizontal bars in C and D = 200 ms; Neuro, neurograms of afferent axonal activity.

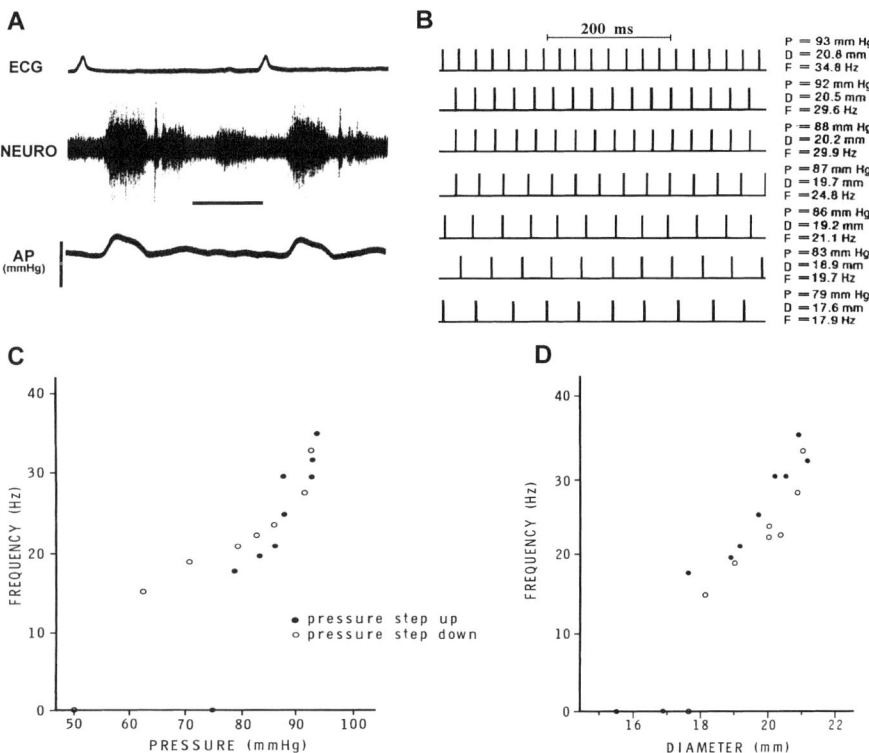

FIGURE 3–7 **A.** Action potentials recorded from multiple afferent axons (Aδ-class) in a canine dorsal cardiopulmonary nerve associated with aortic arch mechanosensory neurites displayed four waves of activity per cardiac cycle. Group activity recorded in situ was maximal during peak systolic aortic pressure (AP), just after the dicrotic notch and during the two subsequent smaller reflected pressure waves (vertical calibration bar beside aortic pressure, AP = 0–100 mmHg; horizontal time bar = 500 ms). Neuro, neurogram of afferent axonal activity. **B.** The activity generated by one afferent axon associated with aortic mechanosensory neurites in situ recorded after the heart was fibrillated and the aorta distended with blood to different pressure levels. Activity is plotted as frequency versus either aortic pressure **(C)** or diameter **(D)**. The frequency of axonal activity (F) increased or decreased logarithmically as aortic pressure (P) and, consequently, diameter (D) increased or decreased, respectively. The frequency of activity was relatively similar at a given aortic diameter, regardless of whether aortic pressure increased (pressure step up) or decreased (pressure step down) incrementally.

tides, and purinergic agents.[13,52] A small population of intrathoracic extracardiac afferent neurons is associated with sensory neurites in the interventricular septum and aortic root that only transduce chemical stimuli (Fig. 3–1). During physiological states these chemosensory neurons generate relatively constant activity that of necessity does not reflect re-

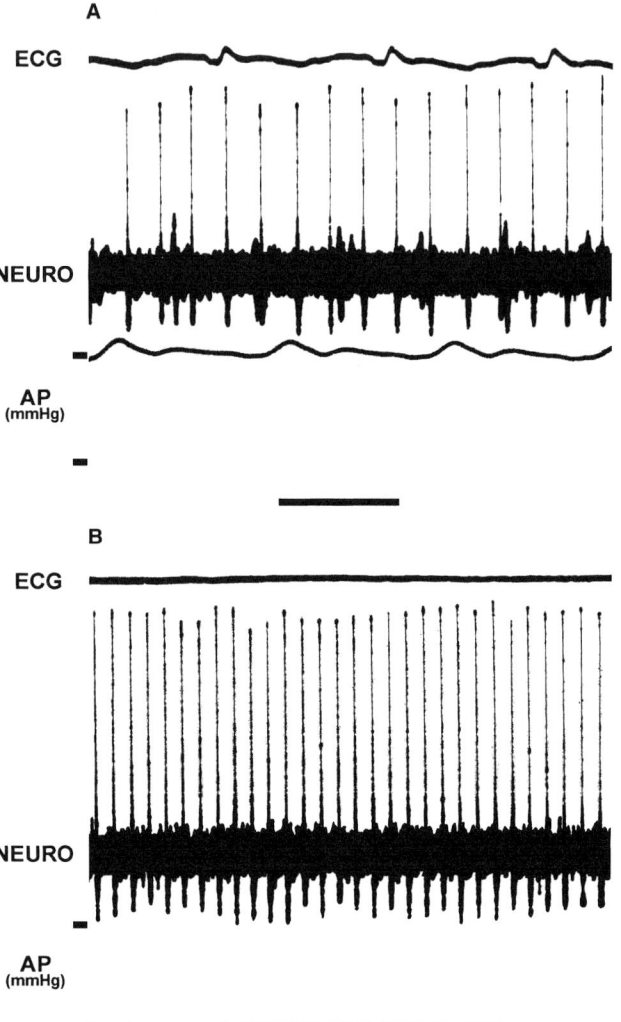

FIGURE 3–8 Activity generated by chemosensory neurites in the cranial interventricular septum associated with an afferent axon (Aδ-class) in a canine ventral medial cardiopulmonary nerve. **A.** During control states, action potentials were generated with relatively consistent interspike intervals (35 ips). **B.** Once the heart was fibrillated, activity increased to 70 ips. This axon did not respond to local tissue distortion. The upper trace in each panel represents a lead II of the ECG and the lowest trace aortic pressure (AP; short horizontal calibration bars = 0 and 100 mmHg). Neuro, neurograms of afferent axonal activity; Long horizontal calibration bar between A and B = 500 ms.

gional mechanics.[3,5] Their activity increases when the milieu surrounding their associated sensory neurites becomes hypoxic (Fig. 3–8).

Intrinsic Cardiac Afferent Neurons

Despite the fact that unipolar neurons have been identified within mammalian intrinsic cardiac ganglia for some time,[66] only recently has their transduction capabilities begun to be studied.[2,74] In accordance with anatomic evidence, it has been estimated that about 10% of the somata within the mammalian intrinsic cardiac nervous system are sensory in nature.[29,44,66,85] Sensory neurites associated with these neurons are located in atrial and ventricular tissues.[13,14,37] Most are multimodal in nature, transducing ion channel–modifying agents and chemicals such as α- and β-adrenoceptor agonists, peptides (i.e., bradykinin and substance P), purinergic agents (adenosine and ATP), and nitric oxide donors.[74] A relatively small population of intrinsic cardiac afferent neurons solely transduces regional cardiac mechanical deformation; these produce high-frequency, phasic activity reflective of local muscle fascicle deformation,[2] displaying a capacity to respond rapidly to local deformation during each cardiac cycle.

THE CARDIOVASCULAR AFFERENT NEURONAL HIERARCHY

Data presented in this chapter indicate that the heart and major intrathoracic vessels are richly innervated by afferent neurons located at each "level" of the cardiac neuroaxis.[13–16,23,29,47,75,76,82] These neurons are ultimately responsible for the genesis of multiple reflexes that regulate cardiac efferent postganglionic neuronal function.[4,9,17,58] The shortest latencies of the cardiovascular vagovagal reflexes that involve medullary neurons are in the 100 ms range. The shortest latencies of cardiocardiac reflexes involving spinal cord neurons are in the 200–500 ms range; the shortest latencies displayed by intrathoracic cardiocardiac feedback loops are in the 40 ms range.[4] In other words, the distance between target organ sensory neurites and their associated somata predicates to a large extent the latency of second-order neuronal activation involved in such cardiovascular–cardiac reflexes (Table 3–1). Data derived from the canine model suggest that many intrathoracic afferent neurons generate phasic (fast-responding) reflexes, indicative of the mechanical milieu of the heart. Needs change tonic (slow-responding) transduction of the cardiovascular chemical milieu determines to a great extent the information content transferred to cardiac myocytes via longer-latency reflexes involving centrally located neurons.

Fast-responding Afferent Neurons

We postulate that short-latency (30–80 ms) intrathoracic reflexes are required to modulate cardiac efferent neuronal outflows to the sinoatrial node on a beat-to-beat basis, as well as to coordinate regional contractile behavior within and among chambers.[62] Short-latency reflexes necessitate the processing of sensory-specific, high-fidelity information generated by fast-responding mechanosensory afferent neurons. Such information is needed to influence cardiac efferent neurons selectively throughout each cardiac cycle. The general characteristics of the fast-responding sensory neurons that influence rapidly responding autonomic efferent postganglionic neurons are summarized in Table 3–2.

Fast-responding afferent neurons are associated with mechanosensory neurites orientated relatively parallel to local muscle fascicles.[3,27,54,59] Their sensory fields are associated primarily in the sinoatrial nodal region, the dorsal atria, the endocardium of the ventricular outflow tracts (Fig. 3–5), or the papillary muscles of either ventricle (Fig. 3–6). The activity pattern of each is unique, reflective of their local sensory field deformation.[5] The most obvious example of such unique behavior is represented by mechanosensory neurites located in the main papillary muscle of the right ventricle, ones that are associated with C-fiber afferent axons;[3] they transduce local deformation in a relatively linear fashion (Fig. 3–6D). This papillary muscle stretches as intracavity pressure increases when the outflow tract of that chamber becomes partially obstructed. The activity generated by this population of mechanosensory afferent neurons decreases as right ventricular chamber systolic pressure increases, because length changes that this papillary muscle normally undergoes become reduced with the greater load. When right ventricular systolic pressure falls in response to partially obstructing flow into that chamber, the activity that these afferent neurons generate increases, since papillary muscle contraction can more easily overcome the lesser tension exerted on its chordae, thereby generating greater length change.[5] These data indicate that the transduction of local muscle fascicle deformation by endocardial mechanosensory neurons does not necessarily reflect chamber pressure development, but rather depends on the local deformation that their sensory neurites undergo. Afferent neurons associated with mechanosensory neurites in ventricular endocardial outflow tracts transduce local deformation in an exponential fashion, thus their activity reflects chamber pressure development (Fig. 3–5), as chamber pressure development reflects development of wall tension. Taken together, these data emphasize not only the degree of precision with which ventricular mechanosensory afferent neurons can transduce regional deformation to second-order neurons but also the fact that their behavior reflects local sensory neurite deformation rather than chamber pressure development.[3,4,47]

Many fast-responding intrathoracic cardiac afferent neurons retain their function after their chronic decentralization, whether they are located in intrinsic cardiac[2] or intrathoracic extracardiac[8] ganglia. Furthermore, chronically decentralized intrathoracic cardiac mechanosensory neurons can influence intrathoracic local circuit neurons for up to 2 seconds after their inputs terminate.[8] Short-term memory function displayed by intrathoracic local circuit neurons depends on the transduction of the cardiac milieu to affect cardiac efferent neurons not only during that cardiac cycle but also for the next several cardiac cycles. Because intrathoracic reflexes can exert considerable influence over regional cardiac dynamics,[9] the fidelity of such information transduction can affect both the temporal and spatial coordination of cardiac efferent postganglionic neurons regulating peristaltic contractile waves that normally progress from the inflow to the outflow tracts of either ventricle.[18,62]

Aortic mechanosensory neurites associated with afferent neurons in intrathoracic extracardiac ganglia generate activity in an exponential manner reflective of regional aortic pressure change (Fig. 3–7C). This population transduces aortic wall deformation with sufficient precision that their grouped activity reflects not only aortic wall deformation (Fig. 3–7D) but also the pulse wave that courses along the aorta wall. The latter presumably occurs because aortic mechanosensory neurites are arranged anatomically as a continuous, longitudinal band along the inner arch of the aorta, the only location where an uninterrupted sensory array can exist (Fig. 3–1). This anatomical arrangement permits populations of sensory neurites to transduce aortic wall deformation as related to local intravascular pressure, as well as pulse waves that travel along the thoracic aorta wall. The fidelity of such transduction ensures rapid, sequential information fed with precision to adjacent intrathoracic local circuit neurons[6,7] to exert short-latency control over intrathoracic cardiac sympathetic efferent postganglionic neurons.[4]

Slow-responding Afferent Neurons

As sensory neurites associated with most cardiac afferent neurons are multimodal in nature, much of the activity that they generate reflects the relatively slowly varying local chemical signals. Their "noisy" activity patterns limit the dynamic resolution of their information content, transducing longer-term alterations in their milieu. Since the somata of many slow-responding cardiac afferent neurons are distant from the target organ (Table 3–2), they cannot, by nature of their anatomy, transduce alterations in the cardiac milieu rapidly to second-order neurons. Thus the activity patterns they generate are primarily reflective of longer-duration events.

These afferent neurons function as leaky integrators, exhibiting memory capabilities that reflect past as well as current events.[51] Chemosensory afferent neurons feed information to intrathoracic extracardiac local circuit neurons and central interneurons that in turn modulate cardiac sympathetic efferent neurons over relatively long time scales. It is therefore hypothesized that one of the primary functions of these slow-responding sensory neurons is to supply inputs to longer-latency cardiac–cardiac control loops. Slow-responding, cardiac chemosensory afferent neurons generate complex activity patterns that can reflect the mechanical state of their interstitial milieu when mechanical alterations are of a significant enough magnitude to impinge on their sensory neurite transduction. Thus their underlying tonic activity, indicative of the interstitial chemical environment, can become phasic with respect to the cardiac cycle when inputs from an enhanced mechanical milieu reach sufficient levels.[34,47]

Sensory neurites associated with most ventricular afferent neurons transduces multiple chemicals, that can initiate cardio-cardiac reflexes. For instance, nitric oxide affects cardiac sensory neurite signaling. This may be one mechanism whereby nitrate therapy affects the neurocardiological status of patients with heart failure. That catecholamines released from sympathetic efferent postganglionic nerve terminals influence the transduction capabilities of adjacent cardiac sensory neurites suggests yet another feedback mechanism within the cardiac nervous system, one that may act to amplify local sympathetic efferent neuronal efficacy.[75]

After these chemosensory neurites are exposed to a chemical, the activity that many generate may not return to previous levels; frequently, it remains in an enhanced or depressed state reflective of events in the immediate past.[75] Such thresholded adaptation represents yet another characteristic of chemically transducing cardiac afferent neurons, one that should be considered when assessing neurocardiological responses to alterations in the chemical milieu of the heart. In sum, these different populations of cardiac afferent neurons generate short-term (heart rate variability) and relatively long-term (cardiac output variability) cardiac feedback control loops according to their transduction capabilities and functional anatomy.

CARDIOVASCULAR SENSORY TRANSDUCTION AND CARDIAC CONTROL

Cardiac sensory neurites transduce local mechanical deformation as well as alterations in their local chemical milieu in the neonatal period.[28] The varied mechanosensory and chemosensory information that cardiac sensory neurons provide to intrathoracic local circuit neurons and central interneurons may indeed form the basis for the ontogeny of the cardiac efferent nervous system (Chapter 8).

As described above, each of the differing populations of sensory neurons involved in cardiac regulation display unique transduction characteristics suited to the cardiocardiac reflexes that they subserve (Table 3–2). Extrathoracic reflex inputs to the heart are also dependent upon carotid artery mechanosensory inputs.[12] Medullary inputs arising from fast-responding afferent neurons, in particular those associated with mechanosensory neurites on major cervical and intrathoracic arteries, activate parasympathetic efferent preganglionic neurons with relatively short-duration latencies (about 100 ms duration). They also initiate spinal cord sympathetic efferent neuronal reflexes, some of which have latencies of activation longer than 250 ms.[4] Slow-responding, chemosensory cardiac afferent neurons appear to be primarily involved in longer-latency cardiovascular–cardiac reflexes. Thus, centrally mediated cardiocardiac reflexes display varied latencies of activation that reflect on the population of second-order central neurons they involve.[4] Some of these reflexes sustained relatively long-duration reflex activation of cardiac efferent neurons.[17] Chemosensory transduction sufficient to activate dorsal root ganglion cardiac afferent neurons to levels around 100 Hz apparently recruits previously inactive components within the cardiac neuronal hierarchy, perhaps accounting for cardiac sensory information affecting the sensorium (Chapter 7). In sum, central and intrathoracic cardiovascular–cardiac reflexes display a range of responses reflective of their afferent inputs and the neuronal networks they involve that together coordinate parasympathetic[53] and sympathetic[62] efferent postganglionic neuronal outputs to the heart.

We propose a broad grouping of cardiac sensory transduction into two functional categories (fast and slow responding) to depict spatially derived cardiac sensory transduction that initiates varied cardiovascular–cardiac reflexes as time-dependent signals (Table 3–2). As mentioned above, the relative distance between sensory neurites and their somata apparently represents an important determinant of this categorization. The somata of many cardiac afferent neurons located on or adjacent to the target organ display a capacity for high-frequency (phasic) transduction, thereby supplying information rapidly to target organ efferent neurons. In this manner, high-fidelity information content can exert rapid control over cardiac efferent neurons coordinating regional contractile patterns. Cardiac afferent neuronal somata located relatively distant from their sensory neurites (nodose and dorsal root ganglia) take longer to influence cardiac efferent neurons via interconnecting central interneurons.[4] Most of these cardiac afferent neurons display slow-responding sensory transduction,[51] as that is what is required for longer-latency feedback control. It should be noted that many of the latter can generate high-frequency, phasic activity (Fig. 3–3) when exposed to sufficient mechanical deformation such that mechanosensory information reaches a level that can be transduced simultaneous with chemosensory information.[34]

Tonic cardiovascular control also depends on the constant monitoring of arterial pressure via selective populations of neurons associated with mechanosensory neurites in the adventitia of major vessels. In addition to the aortic mechanosensory afferent neurons depicted above, the sensory neurites of other afferent neurons are concentrated in the adventitia of the bifurcation of the common carotid arteries (carotid sinus baroreceptors). One type of carotid artery baroreceptor is associated with rapidly conducting myelinated axons (2.5–60 m/second); these respond to local stretch secondary to distention of the arterial wall during each cardiac cycle. During normal arterial pressures, these A-type baroreceptors generate short bursts of activity during each pressure pulse (Chapter 6). Usually their discharge patterns are quite regular with respect to arterial dynamics because their activity encodes mean arterial pressure as well as the rate of rise and amplitude of the arterial pressure pulse. Most C-type carotid artery baroreceptors, by contrast, become active at higher pressures than the A-type baroreceptors, their discharge pattern usually being sparse and irregular. Thus, most C-type carotid artery baroreceptors are not activated at normal arterial pressures.[1] The relationship between the degree of their sensory neurite stretch and the frequency of discharge they produce defines overall carotid artery baroreceptor sensitivity. This is not a fixed relationship, but can be modified acutely or chronically in the presence of sustained arterial pressure changes (see Chapter 6).

Mathematical Model of Varied Cardiac Afferent Neuronal Transduction

This chapter has woven physiology and control theory together to highlight the main features of cardiovascular sensory determinants (see Table 3–2). The function of the entire cardiac neuronal hierarchy can be resolved into two basic issues: *(1)* the neuronal cell types (and their different functional capabilities) that make up the components of each level of this hierarchy; and *(2)* the type and time scale of information transduction as represented by distances and numbers of synapses involved. The emphasis will shift in this section to how the division of cardiac sensory neurons into two broad categories relates to understanding neural control of cardiac output, since that is the ultimate purpose of the cardiac neuronal hierarchy. The cardiac nervous system is mainly responsible for two things: *(1)* the efficient (coordinate) expelling of blood from the heart over short timescales (control exerted during each cardiac cycle and for a few subsequent beats) and *(2)* deterministic regulation of variations in cardiac output over timescales of minutes to hours that keep the individual alive and functioning adequately to meet daily demands. The efficient pumping of blood during each cardiac cycle requires precise coordination of regional cardiac dynamics. Precise control is essentially reflex based and, as such, requires little memory. We propose that the control of cardiac output over longer timescales, for instance during flight or fight, is much more complex, being dependent upon memory.

Cardiovascular sensory neurites are the primary source of information for this neuronal hierarchy, as they sense the ongoing status of the cardiac and vascular milieu. Each neuron in the relatively limited populations of cardiac afferent neurons depicted above receives inputs from multiple sensory neurites within specific sensory field(s) (Fig. 3–1). Together, sensory neurites perform the fundamental job of transducing a continuously varying local mechanical and/or chemical milieu directly or indirectly to cardiac efferent neurons. It is clear that cardiac neuronal feedback requires an understanding of not only sensory neurite function but also the anatomy of the arrays of sensory neurites associated with individual cardiac afferent neurons. Although we currently know little about either, it does appear that the transduction capabilities of cardiac sensory neurites fall roughly into two broad categories: fast- and slow-responding ones that generate phasic or tonic activity patterns, respectively (Table 3–2). This categorization leads directly to one principal on which the functional organization of the cardiac neuronal hierarchy depends: the physical distance between the somata of cardiac afferent neurons and their sensory neurites is important with respect to the type of information transduced throughout the cardiac neuroaxis.

As depicted above, the somata of cardiac afferent neurons located on or near the heart are primarily involved in control loops that have short latencies of activation (i.e., 40 ms). In that scenario, mechanosensitive cardiac afferent neurons can interact directly with cardiac efferent neurons with minimal intervening "computation" taking place. Their sensory neurites register information via *working memory* to directly influence their somata and, consequently, cardiac motor neurons. The sensory neurons involved display a clear relationship between the activity they generate and cardiac variables such as heart rate and regional strain along the major vector of their local muscle fascicles (Figs. 3–4 to 3–6). These fast-responding afferent neurons encode short time scale information required for fast reflex coordination of regional cardiac behavior and involve *short-term memory* for control of regional cardiac function.[4] These short-latency control loops ensure that phase shifts initiated by random, local-length variations that influence sensory neurites transducing the mechanical milieu do not factor into the control of intra- and interbeat regulation.

We further hypothesize that fast-responding sensory neurites provide input to short-latency reflexes that act to coordinate regional contractile function to maintain a balance between cardiac electrical and mechanical events (Table 3–2). Mechanosensory neurites located in atrial or ventricular endocardial tissues transduce regional deformation with surprising fidelity (Figs. 3–4 to 3–6). Since their sensory fields occupy limited cardiac regions, the activity that they generate can accurately reflect the varied dynamics of differing ventricular regions.[3,5] These data indicate that intrathoracic afferent neurons associated with fast-responding atrial or ventricular mechanosensory neurites transduce with fidelity the varied forces generated within different cardiac regions to influence selective populations of intrathoracic efferent neurons innervating specific cardiac regions.

Slow-responding cardiac afferent neurons, by contrast, generate noisy activity that bears little observable relationship to regional cardiac mechanics.[5,15] Slow-responding cardiac afferent neurons are by nature incapable of providing control during the timescales required for rapid coordination of regional contractile function. Rather, they are suited to control cardiac output over timescales of minutes to hours involving *longer-term memory*.[17] These, along with afferent neurons with sensory neurites in extracardiac tissues, feed information to higher computational centers. Neurons in the higher computational centers in turn regulate central neuronal outputs that influence local computation within the *little brain* on the heart.[10] We propose that these afferent neurons serve a major role in long-term regulation of cardiac output. These issues raise two fundamental questions: *(1)* What do slow-responding sensory neurites transduce? *(2)* Why are inputs from higher computational centers typically rerouted through the intrinsic cardiac nervous system? The answer to both of these questions hinges on understanding the role of noise in thresholded biological systems.

Before proceeding further, we must distinguish the main source of noise affecting slow-responding cardiac sensory neurites. It has been postulated that noise influences the initiation of action potentials by sensory neurites through fluctuations in local ionic current, even though such noise operates at frequencies high enough (very short timescales of variation) to exert no discernible influence.[75] Sensory neurites associated with individual cardiac afferent somata are randomized temporally with respect to their varying lengths and spatially with respect to their locations within the myocardium. Thus, the sensory neurites associated with individual cardiac afferent neuronal somata reduce a time-varying local chemical signal to a single, fluctuating activity pattern carried by an individual axon. The spatiotemporal transduction characteristics displayed by the various sensory neurites associated with each chemosensory neuron produces a relatively slow time-dependent signal derived primarily from alterations in their chemical milieu with, in many instances, superimposed fast fluctuations arising from their mechanical milieu.[51] The simplest mathematical construct for the production of such a noisy signal is by the superposition of many clean sinusoids with differing amplitudes but randomized phases among their varied sensory neurites. Each sinusoid models a clean sensory neurite signal, while random phase shifts are due to the random spatiotemporal source of inputs to each afferent neuron.

As to the first question, of determining the noisy inputs that some cardiac sensory neurites are transducing, we must first consider that control based on such inputs operates over the timescale of seconds to minutes. Therefore, such a signal can be modeled as the sum of a slow control signal that varies over a timescale of many seconds as well as a fast portion that operates over a timescale of seconds.[51] In this model, the noisy input signals that arise from an array of cardiac sensory neurites associated with individual afferent neurons are reduced to a slowly varying, aperiodic signal generated by an axon with superimposed noisy variations that depend on the relatively slowly varying local chemical milieu. Fast variations in the activity that they generate arise from rapidly occurring alterations in the local mechanical milieu. From a modeling perspective, noisy variations serve to amplify slowly varying signals that sum to evoke action potentials that would not have been generated in the absence of noisy variations. A corollary of this is the fact that slowly varying suprathreshold inputs to cardiac sensory neurites by themselves would rapidly adapt out. With the addition of noisy, low-amplitude signals, spatially localized adaptations are minimized and thus signal strength from slow-responding afferent neurons can be maintained. The generation of signals by cardiac chemosensory afferent neurons is fundamental to the long-term regulation of cardiac output.

From a practical perspective, this means that the cardiac neuronal hierarchy is dependent to a considerable extent on slowly varying input signals derived from very low concentrations of multiple, local chemicals liberated in the myocardial interstitium.[75] Furthermore, the transduction of cardiovascular sensory information initiating such reflexes can remodel (resetting of sensory input function) during the evolution of pathological states (see Cardiac Sensory Transduction in Diseased States, below). The basis of any noise amplification relates to the fact that cardiac afferent neurons are thresholded so that they only generate action potentials when chemical stimuli reach a stimulus threshold. It is intuitively obvious that slowly varying subthreshold signals, i.e., those too low to evoke a response in the absence of noise, evoke a response if noisy variations become superimposed on them. It is also evident that the timescale of these variations is important. If they operate over too short a timescale, they become "averaged out" to exert no effect, while variations with too long a timescale are interpreted as part of the control (background) information. Specifically, when cardiac afferent neurons are modeled using the FitzHugh-Nagumo canonical equations it is found that they respond primarily to noisy variations in their chemical milieu occurring over the recovery variable timescale.[51]

One conclusion derived from the FitzHugh-Nagumo model is that a fixed amount of input in the presence of relatively small noisy inputs is responsible for the average activity generated by individual cardiac afferent neurons.[51] For example, if the time between action potentials generated by cardiac sensory neurites is much longer than the recovery timescale following their activation, then, on average, a small fraction of the input is responsible for their activity. Hence, little or no direct correlation can be expected between the firing rate of cardiac chemosensory afferent neurons and signals arising from the normal myocardial milieu, even in the presence of adequate control. A result of this observation is that control based on subthreshold noisy signals does not rely on the precise timing of any action potential. With respect to this population of afferent neurons, it is only the average firing rate within a specific timescale that is required for the transduction of information to second-order neurons. In light of this discussion, it is understandable that one answer to the question posed at the beginning of this section is that noisy input signals to slow-responding sensory neurons are transduced as slowly varying subthreshold signals.

Reflex regulation of cardiac function is the result of the interplay between peripheral and central feedback control loops. In basal conditions, slow-responding cardiac afferent neurons provide information to peripheral and central neurons in the hierarchy to principally exert long-term control of cardiac output. Mechanosensory inputs provide dynamic information to peripheral neuronal elements within this hierarchy (intrinsic cardiac and extracardiac intrathoracic ganglia) to coordinate regional contractile function and heart rate. During stress, transduction by fast- and slow-responding cardiac afferent neurons becomes altered such that, if of sufficient magnitude, additional elements of the neural hierarchy for cardiac control become activated. If the change in their milieu is sufficient (e.g., during myocardial ischemia), the subsequent enhancement of sensory information may reach higher centers to affect conscious perception (e.g., etiology of angina of cardiac origin) and thereby evoke additional effects on cardiac control via suprabulbar neurons (e.g., those in the limbic system, hypothalamus, etc.; see Chapter 7). The input signals responsible for these effects are likely provided by multimodal, slow-responding cardiac afferent neurons.

The second question is, why are the inputs to intrathoracic cardiac efferent neurons from higher computational centers that receive tonic information from cardiovascular sensory neurons typically rerouted through local circuit neurons on the heart? In the simplest model, the *little brain* on the heart consists of redundantly connected populations of excitatory and inhibitory neurons.[10] Such neural networks, as modeled by the Wilson and Cowan equations, can generate a variety of behaviors.[52] Experimental evidence indicates that they may interact in a hysteretic fashion. A key feature of a hysteretic population of neurons is its ability to display memory.[8] Hysteretic systems display almost constant activity relating to inputs from excitatory and inhibitory neurons, referred to as hysteretic "states." The most important feature of these states is that they are stable over a wide input range. Thus, any shift to a new state reflective of altered sensory inputs only occurs when these inputs exceed or go below critical values. This feature provides two functions: memory and an excellent noise filter. Memory is achieved since inputs are heeded only when they exceed limits (low or high level limits) of critical values; thus inputs long past can influence the present. Noise filtering by local circuit neurons is achieved via the same smoothing action imposed by the critical value limits on the primary sensory inputs. This "state filter" may be required since the responses of cardiac efferent neurons to noisy sensory inputs would otherwise be simply too erratic for the desired precise control of regional cardiac function.

The intervention of the little brain on the heart ensures that signals arising from noisy afferent neuronal inputs, as well as those from higher computational centers, are filtered appropriately so that not too much credence is given to the immediate past. Thus, cardiac afferent information is processed in the context of the past sensory events by means of memory. The damping influence imposed by the local circuit neurons results in a directionally appropriate and coordinated control of neural effector outputs to the different regions of the heart. Our answer to the second question posed above is then, local computation at the level of the heart ensures that noisy signals returning to the heart are relatively consistent and proportional. This is desirable for the proper control of cardiac efferent neurons, while maintaining memory of the past (i.e., long-term memory) for control stability.

So far our discussion has focused on memory and noise reduction for the precise control of cardiac efferent neurons receiving multiple cardiovascular sensory inputs. Next we should consider how noisy sensory inputs to populations of local circuit neurons are useful for cardiac control. A hysteretic system is thresholded and, as such, when it goes to a new state it stays there until the inputs exceed a threshold.[52] Dropping back to the old state occurs only when its inputs are reduced to a level much below that which previously caused a shift to the new state. For slowly responding cardiac afferent neurons, the ongoing activity they display relates to the level of input they receive, but this changes over time. For instance, many cardiac chemical transducing afferent neurons that display relatively low levels of spontaneous activity in an anesthetized preparation respond to a chemical stimulus with activity enhancement. Cardiac afferent neurons displaying relatively high levels of spontaneous activity, by contrast, may respond to the same chemical with reduced activity.[75] These varied sensory responses, impinging as they do on local circuit neurons, contribute in large part to the long-term memory that these neural networks display. Thus, the activity generated by the chemosensory neurites associated with individual cardiac afferent neurons following exposure to a chemical frequently returns to a different state than the one that existed before exposure to that chemical.[75] This characteristic, which may be equated with relatively long-term memory, implies that cardiac chemosensory transduction is constantly in flux, reflective of events in the present as well as in the recent past.

Intrathoracic local circuit neurons receive convergent inputs from not only cardiovascular afferent neurons but also neurons in higher centers of the neural hierarchy as well as in other intrathoracic ganglia. As such, they constitute the primary processing component of the peripheral neuronal hierarchy. For these neurons, there are no so-called critical levels within which such state shifts occur. Rather, a full range of inputs is available for control. Furthermore, the noise level need not be tuned but simply set to a value that is high enough to evoke a response but not so high that aimless cycling occurs between states.[52] Noisy, superimposed variations allow very minor input alterations to be used for control.[51] However, there is a twofold price to pay for such reliance. It is possible to cycle aimlessly between states. For example, a dangerous state occurs in the presence of excessive memory, as modeled by the Wilson and Cowan equations. During high sensory inputs and high noise levels, it is easier to enter an excited state than to leave it. Such excessive memory is pathological, since its forcing of cardiac efferent neurons would be difficult to halt. When any component of this complex neuronal hierarchy receives excessive sensory inputs the consequences may be devastating with respect to increasing activation of populations of intrinsic cardiac neurons, thereby leading to cardiac mechanical (Chapter 4) or electrical (Chapter 11) dysfunction. Therefore, the evolution (and treatment) of cardiac pathology must be considered in terms of not only myocyte function but also how this neuronal hierarchy adapts or maladapts to altered cardiac status.

Cardiac Sensory Transduction in Diseased States

Myocardial Ischemia

The mechanical and chemical milieu of the heart becomes modified in the presence of a compromised coronary arterial blood supply. Many of the cardiac afferent neurons located throughout the cardiac neuronal hierarchy transduce ischemia-induced alterations in regional cardiac mechanics[34] and/or the local chemical milieu.[24,65] Although the mechanism underlying the genesis of symptoms and cardiovascular reflexes that are initiated during myocardial ischemia await full delineation, considerable progress has been made in identifying afferent neuronal sensory transduction in this state.[33,73]

With respect to the transduction of myocardial ischemia, about 80% of dorsal root ganglion cardiac afferent neurons do so,[47] while fewer of their nodose ganglion counterparts do.[15] In some instances, the activity generated by cardiac afferent neurons that influence central neurons becomes enhanced in the ischemic state just before the onset of ventricular fibrillation (Fig. 3–9). These data indicate that cardiac afferent neurons are capable of transducing subtle changes in the ischemic myocardial milieu before gross alterations in cardiac function become manifest. Many of the afferent neurons in intrathoracic extracardiac and intrinsic cardiac ganglia transduce the ischemic myocardium.[12] Thus, afferent neuronal inputs to second-order neurons in various regions of the entire cardiac neuroaxis may increase in the ischemic state. The subsequent resultant excessive activation of cardiac adrenergic efferent neurons may be involved in the genesis of ventricular tachydysrhythmias (Chapter 11) or even fibrillation.[10,49] These data are in accord with the finding that remodeling of the cardiac

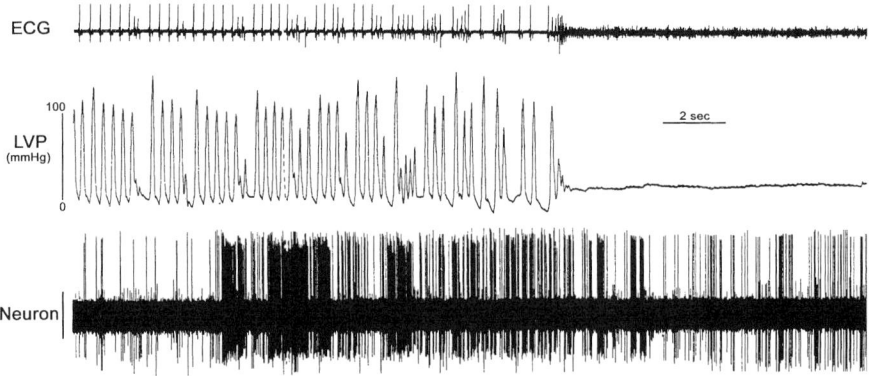

FIGURE 3–9 Activity generated by a few right nodose ganglion afferent neurons associated with chemosensory neurites in the ventral left ventricular epicardium during and after coronary artery occlusion. Their activity (as indicated by the multiple action potential heights) was enhanced by the occlusion, increasing even more during reperfusion that began 10 seconds before the start of this continuous record. Their activity increased even more a few seconds before the spontaneous occurrence of ventricular fibrillation. The traces represent an ECG, left ventricular chamber pressure (LVP), and afferent neuronal activity (neuron).

neuronal hierarchy secondary to cardiac surgical interventions may be involved in the genesis of postoperative cardiac electrical instability.[32]

When the blood flow in a coronary artery that perfuses an intrinsic cardiac ganglionated plexus becomes compromised, the function of its neurons is affected.[46] Over time, local ischemia may even induce pathological changes within the intrinsic cardiac nervous system.[43] Also, the activity generated by some intrinsic cardiac neurons is modified when distant ventricular tissues undergo ischemic changes, reflecting alterations in their sensory inputs from the ischemic territory.[12] Thus cardiovascular reflexes and symptoms attending myocardial ischemia involve a number of neuronal factors, including the status of the blood supply to the somata of intrinsic cardiac neurons compared to that of regional sensory neurites.

Transient coronary artery occlusion enhances the local release of chemicals such as adenosine,[35,67] bradykinin,[39] and substance P[36] from ischemic myocardium. Although not all authors are in agreement,[60] it now appears evident that adenosine-sensitive dorsal root[48] and nodose[76] ganglion cardiac afferent neurons transduce myocardial ischemia. Adenosine is known to play a key role in the genesis of symptoms attending myocardial ischemia (see Chapter 10); peptides such as substance P apparently play modulator roles in these events.[38] This concept is supported by the fact that local application of an adenosine receptor blocking agent to ventricular sensory neurites obtunds their capacity to transduce local ischemia.[76] Their capacity to transduce local ischemia to central neurons is apparently dependent to a large extent on the capacity of their sensory neurite adenosine A_1 and A_2 receptors[48,76] to affect their second messenger systems.[68]

Two of the major sequellae of ventricular ischemia are cardiac arrhythmias and cardiac failure. Early on in heart failure the capacity of cardiac sensory neurites to transduce their local milieu remains, even though overall cardiac control becomes obtunded.[87] As heart failure progresses, concomitant depression of ventricular mechanical function will induce a reduction in mechanosensory information transduced to second-order neurons. Severe cardiac failure will also be attended by alterations in the chemical milieu, thereby enhancing cardiac chemotransduction to second-order neurons. These complex changes in cardiac sensory transduction will presumably induce remodeling of the entire cardiac neuronal hierarchy, a subject that awaits full delineation.

Cardiac Arrhythmias

Excessive inputs to the cardiac neuronal hierarchy arising from cardiac chemotransduction can destabilize the hierarchy's capacity to modulate regional cardiac function, perhaps leading to excessive activation of its sympathetic efferent neurons to induced cardiac dysrhythmias (Chapter 11). One consequence of regional ventricular ischemia is the genesis of cardiac arrhythmias. It has been known for some time that the activity generated by cardiac mechanosensory neurites becomes altered in the presence of atrial or ventricular arrhythmias.[34,56,61,79] The activity generated by atrial mechanosensory neurons increases when there is atrial arrhythmias or fibrillation. When atrial fibrillation occurs, some atrial mechanosensory afferent neurons generate cyclic activity reflective of localized rhythmic mechanical events of their sensory milieu (Fig. 3–4D). Although the activity generated by most ventricular wall mechanosensory neurites increases in the presence of ventricular ectopic beats[34] when ventricular fibrillation occurs the activity that they generate decreases (Fig. 3–6D). Thus, most ventricular mechanosensory neurites generate reduced activity with ventricular fibrillation while most atrial neurites generate more activity in the presence of atrial fibrillation.[11] Alterations in cardiac sensory transduction that occur with altered cardiac electrical events should be placed in the context of the smoothing function that second-order neurons normally exert in such a state to minimize any deleterious affects that the resultant excessive activation or autonomic efferent neurons might induce.

Perspectives

Information fed forward by fast responding cardiac afferent neurons reflective of the local mechanical milieu of the heart influence cardiac efferent neurons directly throughout each cardiac cycle to exert rapid control over heart rate and regional contractility. In this scenario, fast-responding cardiac sensor neurons initiate fast-responding (short-loop) reflexes that coordinate regional cardiac contractile patterns. The slower-responding chemosensory cardiac afferent neurons apparently act to stabilize cardiac efferent neuronal function over longer timescales, "smoothing out" the influence exerted by their varied inputs via intermediary neurons (local circuit ones in the periphery and interneurons in the central nervous system). We hypothesize that inputs from slow-responding cardiac afferent neurons are coordinated within various components of the cardiac neuronal hierarchy with fast-responding ones that generate the short-latency intrathoracic reflexes to control heart rate and regional contractility on a beat-to-beat basis. Our understanding of the complex neuronal hierarchy that encodes sensory information reflective of the cardiac milieu needs full clarification before novel therapeutic strategies can be devised to target the varied components of the cardiac neuronal hierarchy during the evolution of cardiovascular disease.

ACKNOWLEDGMENTS

Much of the work presented in this chapter was performed with the assistance of Richard Livingston. The Medical Research Council of Canada, the Nova Scotia Heart and Stroke Foundation, the Canadian National Sciences and Research Council, and the National Institutes of Health (USA) provided financial support for this work.

REFERENCES

1. Andresen MC and Kunze DL. Nucleus tractus solitarius: gateway to neural circulatory control. *Annu Rev Physiol* 56:93–116, 1994.
2. Ardell JL, Butler CK, Smith FM, Hopkins DA, and Armour JA. Activity of in vivo atrial and ventricular neurons in chronically decentralized canine hearts. *Am J Physiol* 260 (*Heart Circ Physiol* 29):H713–H721, 1991.
3. Armour JA. Physiological behavior of thoracic cardiovascular receptors. *Am J Physiol* 225:177–185, 1973.
4. Armour JA. Instant-to-instant reflex cardiac regulation. *Cardiology* 61:309–328, 1976.
5. Armour JA. Thoracic and cardiovascular afferent nerves. In: Randall WC, ed. *Neural Regulation of the Heart*. New York: Oxford University Press, 1977, pp 13–42.
6. Armour JA. Activity of in situ middle cervical ganglion neurons in dogs using extracellular recording techniques. *Can J Physiol Pharmacol* 63:704–716, 1985.

7. Armour JA. Activity of in situ stellate ganglion neurons of dogs recorded extracellularly. *Can J Physiol Pharmacol* 64:101–111, 1986.
8. Armour JA. Neuronal activity recorded extracellularly in chronically decentralized in situ canine middle cervical ganglia. *Can J Physiol Pharmacol* 64:1038–1046, 1986.
9. Armour JA. Cardiac effects of electrically induced intrathoracic autonomic reflexes. *Can J Physiol Pharmacol* 66:714–720, 1988.
10. Armour JA. Anatomy and function of the intrathoracic neurons regulating the mammalian heart. In: Zucker IH and Gilmore JP, eds. *Reflex Control of the Circulation.* Boca Raton, FL: CRC Press, 1991, pp 1–37.
11. Armour JA. The role of peripheral autonomic neurons with P_1- and P_2-purinoreceptors in cardiac regulation. In: Burnstock G, Dobson JG, Liang BT, and Linden J, eds. *Cardiovascular Biology of Purines*, Norwell, MASS: Kluwer Academic Press, MA, 1998, pp 326–341.
12. Armour JA, Collier K, Kimber G, and Ardell JL. Differential selectivity of cardiac neurons in separate intrathoracic ganglia. *Am J Physiol* 274:R939–R949, 1998.
13. Armour JA and Hopkins DA. Activity of in situ canine left atrial neurons. *Am J Physiol* 259:H1207–H1215, 1990.
14. Armour JA and Hopkins DA. Activity of in vivo canine ventricular neurons. *Am J Physiol* 258:H320–H336, 1990.
15. Armour JA, Huang MH, Pelleg A, and Sylvén C. Responsiveness of in situ canine nodose ganglion cardiac afferent neurons to epicardial mechanoreceptor and/or chemoreceptor stimuli. *Cardiovasc Res* 28:1218–1225, 1994.
16. Armour JA and Janes RD. Neuronal activity recorded extracellularly from in situ mediastinal ganglia. *Can J Physiol Pharmacol* 66:119–127, 1988.
17. Armour JA and Pace JB. Cardiovascular effects of thoracic afferent nerve stimulation in conscious dogs. *Can J Physiol Pharmacol* 60:1193–1199, 1982.
18. Armour JA, Pace JB, and Randall WC. Interrelationship of architecture and function of the right ventricle. *Am J Physiol* 218:174–179, 1970.
19. Arndt JO, Brambling P, Hindorf K, and Röhnelt R. The afferent discharge pattern of atrial mechano-receptors of the cat during sinusoidal stretch of atrial strip in situ. *J Physiol* 240:33–52, 1974.
20. Baker DG, Coleridge HM, and Coleridge JCG. Vagal afferent C fibers from the ventricle. In: *Cardiac Receptors.* Hainsworth R, Kidd C, and Linden RJ, eds. London: Cambridge University Press, 1979, pp 117–137.
21. Baker D, Coleridge HM, Coleridge JCG, and Nerdum T. Search for cardiac nociceptor: stimulation by bradykinin of sympathetic afferent nerve endings in the heart of cat. *J Physiol* 306:519–536, 1980.
22. Blomquist TM, Priola DV, and Romero AM. Source of intrinsic innervation of canine ventricles: a functional study. *Am J Physiol* 252:H638–H644, 1987.
23. Bosnjak Z and Kampine JP. Cardiac sympathetic afferent cell bodies are located in the peripheral nervous system of the cat. *Circ Res* 64:554–562, 1989.
24. Brown AM. Excitation of afferent cardiac sympathetic nerve fibers during myocardial ischemia. *J Physiol* 190:35–53, 1967.
25. Butler CK, Smith FM, Cardinal R, Murphy DA, Hopkins DA, and Armour JA. Cardiac responses to electrical stimulation of discrete loci in canine atrial or ventricular ganglionated plexi. *Am J Physiol* 259:H1365–H1373, 1990.
26. Castillo-Melendez M, Krstew E, Lawrence AJ, and Jarrott B. Presynaptic

adenosine A2a receptors on soma and central terminals of rat vagal afferent neurons. *Brain Res* 652:137–144, 1994.
27. Chapman KM and Pankhurst JH. Strain sensitivity and directionality in cat atrial mechanosensitive nerve endings in vitro. *J Physiol* 259:405–426, 1976.
28. Chen RP-C, Thompson GW, and Armour JA. Transduction capabilities of neonatal ventricular afferent neurons in situ. *Auton Neurosci:* 87:1–8, 2001.
29. Cheng Z, Powley TL, Schwaber JS, and Doyle FJ. Vagal afferent innervation of the atria of the rat heart reconstructed with confocal microscopy. *J Comp Neurol* 381:1–17, 1997.
30. Coleridge HM, Coleridge JCG, and Kidd C. Cardiac receptors in the dog, with particular reference to two types of afferent endings in the ventricular wall. *J Physiol* 174:323–339, 1964.
31. Coleridge JCG, Hemmingway A, Holmes RL, and Linden RJ. Location of atrial receptors in the dog: a physiological and histological study. *J Physiol* 136:174–197, 1957.
32. Davis Z, Jacobs HK, Bonilla J, Anderson RR, Thomas C, and Forst W. Retaining the aortic fat pad during cardiac surgery decreases postoperative atrial fibrillation. *Heart Surg Forum* 3:108–112, 2000.
33. Foreman RD. Mechanisms of cardiac pain. *Annu Rev Physiol* 61:143–167, 1999.
34. Foreman RD, Blair RW, Holmes HR, and Armour JA. Correlation of activity generated by sympathetic afferent ventricular mechanosensory neurites with sensory field deformation in the normal and ischemic myocardium. *Am J Physiol* 276:R976–R989, 1999.
35. Fox AC, Reed GE, Meilman H, and Silk BB. Release of nucleosides from canine and human hearts as an index of prior ischemia. *Am J Cardiol* 43:52–59, 1979.
36. Franco-Cereceda A. Calcitonin gene-related peptide and tachykinins in relation to local sensory control of cardiac contractility and coronary vascular tone. *Acta Physiol Scand* 569(Suppl):2–63, 1988.
37. Gagliardi M, Randall WC, Beiger D, Wurster RD, Hopkins DA, and Armour JA. Activity of in vivo canine cardiac plexus neurons. *Am J Physiol* 255:H789–H800, 1988.
38. Gaspardone A, Crea F, Tomai F, Lamele M, Crossman DC, Pappagallo M, Versaci F, Chiariello L, and Gioffre PA. Substance P potentiates the algogenic affects of intraarterial infusion of adenosine. *J Am Coll Cardiol* 24:477–482, 1994.
39. Hashimoto K, Hirose M, Furukawa S, Hayakawa H, and Kimura E. Changes in hemodynamics and bradykinin concentration in coronary sinus blood in experimental coronary artery occlusion. *Jpn Heart J* 18:679–689, 1977.
40. Hillarp N-A. Peripheral autonomic mechanisms. In: Field J, ed. *Handbook of Physiology, Section I: Neurophysiology.* Washington, DC: American Physiological Society, 1960, pp 979–1006.
41. Hopkins DA and Armour JA. Ganglionic distribution of afferent neurons innervating the canine heart and physiologically identified cardiopulmonary nerves. *J Auton Nerv Syst* 26:213–222, 1989.
42. Hopkins DA, Gootman PM, Gootman N, and Armour JA. Anatomy of medullary and peripheral autonomic neurons innervating the neonatal porcine heart. *J Auton Nerv Syst* 64:74–84, 1997.
43. Hopkins DA, MacDonald SE, Murphy DA, and Armour JA. Pathology of intrinsic cardiac neurons associated with ischemic human hearts. *Anat Rec* 259: 424–436, 2000.

44. Horackova M and Armour JA. Role of peripheral autonomic neurons in maintaining adequate cardiac function. *Cardiovasc Res* 30:326–335, 1995.
45. Huang H-S, Pan H-L, Stahl GL, and Longhorst JC. Ischemia- and reperfusion-sensitive cardiac sympathetic afferents: influence of H_2O_2 and hydroxyl radicals. *Am J Physiol* 269:H888–H901, 1995.
46. Huang MH, Ardell JL, Hanna B, Wolf S, and Armour JA. Effects of transient coronary artery occlusion on canine intrinsic cardiac neuronal activity. *Integr Physiol Behav Sci* 28:5–21, 1993.
47. Huang MH, Negoescu RM, Horackova M, Wolf S, and Armour JA. Polysensory response characteristics of dorsal root ganglion neurones that may serve sensory functions during myocardial ischemia. *Cardiovasc Res* 32:503–515, 1996.
48. Huang MH, Sylvén C, Horackova M, and Armour JA. Ventricular sensory neurons in canine dorsal root ganglia: effects of adenosine and substance P. *Am J Physiol* 269:R318–R324, 1995.
49. Huang MH, Wolf SG, and Armour JA. Ventricular arrhythmias induced by chemically modified intrinsic cardiac neurons. *Cardiovasc Res* 28:636–642, 1994.
50. Katz DM and Karten HJ. Substance P in the vagal sensory ganglia. Localization in cell bodies and pericellular arborizations. *J Comp Neurol* 193:549–564, 1980.
51. Kember GC, Fenton GA, Armour JA, and Kalyaniwalla N. A competition model for aperiodic stochastic resonance in a Fitz-Hugh Nagumo model of cardiac sensory neurons. *Phys Rev E* 63:1–6, 2001.
52. Kember GC, Fenton GA, Collier K, and Armour JA. Stochastic resonance in a hysteretic population of cardiac neurons. *Phys Rev E* 61:1816–1824, 2000.
53. Levy MN and Warner MR. Parasympathetic effects on cardiac function. In: Armour JA and Ardell JL, eds. *Neurocardiology*. New York: Oxford University Press, 1994, pp 53–76.
54. Linden RJ and Kappagoda CT. *Atrial Receptors*. Cambridge, UK: Cambridge University Press, 1982.
55. MacDonald DA. *Blood Flow in Arteries*. London: Arnold, 1960.
56. Malliani A. Cardiovascular sympathetic afferent fibers. *Rev Physiol Biochem Pharmacol* 94:11–74, 1982.
57. Middlekauff HR, Rivkees SA, Raybould HE, Bitticaca B, Goldhaber JI, and Weiss JN. Localization and functional effects of adenosine A_1 receptors on cardiac vagal afferents in adult rats. *Am J Physiol* 274:H441–H447, 1998.
58. Minsi AJ and Thames MD. Reflexes from ventricular receptors with vagal afferents. In: Zucker IH and Gilmore JP, eds. *Reflex Control of the Circulation*. Boca Raton, FL: CRC Press, 1991, pp 359–406.
59. Paintal AS. A study of right and left atrial receptors. *J Physiol* 120:596–610, 1953.
60. Pan H-L and Longhurst JC. Lack of a role of adenosine in activation of ischemically sensitive cardiac sympathetic afferents. *Am J Physiol* 269:H106–H113, 1995.
61. Peters SR, Kostreva DR, Armour JA, Zuperku EJ, Igler FO, Coon RL, and Kampine JP. Cardiac, aortic, pericardial and pulmonary vascular receptors in the dog. *Cardiology* 65:85–100, 1980.
62. Randall WC, Armour JA, Geis WP, and Lippincott DP. Regional cardiac distribution of sympathetic nerves. *Fed Proc* 31:1199–1208, 1972.

63. Randall WC, Wurster RD, Randall DC, and Xi-Moy SX. From cardioaccelerator and inhibitory nerves to a heart brain: an evolution of concepts. In: Shepherd JT, Vatner SF, eds. *Nervous Control of the Heart*. Amsterdam: Harwood Academic Publishers, 1996, pp 173–200.
64. Ranson SW. Afferent paths for visceral reflexes. *Physiol Rev* 1:477–522, 1921.
65. Recordati G, Schwartz PJ, Pagani M, Malliani A, and Brown AM. Activation of cardiac vagal receptors during myocardial ischemia. *Experientia* 27:1423–1424, 1971.
66. Robb JS. *Comparative Basic Cardiology*. New York: Grune & Stratton, 1965.
67. Rubio R, Berne RM, and Katori M. Release of adenosine in reactive hyperemia of the dog heart. *Am J Physiol* 216:56–62, 1969.
68. Selbie LA and Hill SJ. G-protein-coupled-receptor cross-talk: the fine tuning of multiple receptor-signaling pathways. *Trends Pharmacol Sci* 19:87–93, 1998.
69. Schultz HD and Ustinova EE. Blockade of capsaicin receptors abolishes free radical–induced activation of cardiac afferents in rats. *Cardiovasc Res* 38:348–355, 1998.
70. Schultz HD, Wang W, Ustinova EE, and Zucker IH. Enhanced responsiveness of cardiac vagal chemosensitive endings to bradykinin in heart failure. *Am J Physiol* 273:R637–R645, 1997.
71. Sleight P and Widdicombe JG. Action potentials in fibres from receptors in the epicardium and myocardium of the dog's left ventricle. *J Physiol* (Lond) 181:235–258, 1965.
72. Sun S-Y, Wang W, and Schultz HD. Activation of cardiac afferents by arachidonic acid: relative contributions of metabolic pathways. *Am J Physiol (Heart and Circ Physiol)* 281:H93–H104, 2001.
73. Sylvén C. Angina pectoris. Clinical characteristics, neurophysiological and molecular mechanisms. *Pain* 36:145–167, 1989.
74. Thompson GW, Collier K, Ardell JL, Kimber G, and Armour JA. Functional interdependence of neurons in a single canine intrinsic cardiac ganglionated plexus. *J Physiol* 528:561–571, 2000.
75. Thompson GW, Horackova M, and Armour JA. Chemotransduction properties of nodose ganglion cardiac afferent neurons in guinea-pigs. *Am J Physiol* 279:R433–R439, 2000.
76. Thompson GW, Horackova M, and Armour JA. Role of P_1 purinergic receptors in myocardial ischemia sensory transduction. *Cardiovasc Res* 53:888–901, 2002.
77. Thorén P. Activation of left ventricular receptors with nonmedullated vagal afferent fibers during occlusion of a coronary artery of a cat. *Am J Cardiol* 37:1046–1051, 1976.
78. Thorén P. Characteristics of left ventricular receptors with nonmedullated vagal afferents in cats. *Circ Res* 40:415–421, 1977.
79. Thorén P. Role of cardiac vagal c-fibers in cardiovascular control. *Rev Physiol Biochem Pharmacol* 86:1–94, 1979.
80. Ustinova EE and Schultz HD. Activation of cardiac vagal afferents by oxygen-derived free radicals in rats. *Circ Res* 74:895–903, 1994.
81. Ustinova EE and Schultz HD. Activation of cardiac vagal afferents by ischemia and reperfusion: prostaglandins versus oxygen-derived free radicals. *Circ Res* 74:904–911, 1994.
82. Vance WH and Bowker RC. Spinal origins of cardiac afferents from the region of the left anterior descending artery. *Brain Res* 258:96–100, 1983.

83. Weinreich D, Koschorke GM, Undem BJ, and Taylor GE. Prevention of the excitatory actions of bradykinin by inhibition of PGI_2 formation in nodose neurones of the guinea-pig. *J Physiol* 483:735–746, 1995.
84. White JC. Cardiac pain: anatomic pathways and physiologic mechanisms. *Circulation* 16:644–655, 1954.
85. Yuan B-X, Ardell JL, Hopkins DA, and Armour JA. Gross and microscopic anatomy of canine intrinsic cardiac neurons. *Anat Rec* 239:75–87, 1994.
86. Yuan B-X, Hopkins DA, Ardell JL, and Armour JA. Differential cardiac responses induced by nicotinic sensitive canine intrinsic atrial and ventricular neurons. *Cardiovasc Res* 27:760–769, 1993.
87. Zucker IH. Baro and cardiac reflex abnormalities in chronic heart failure. In: *Reflex Control of the Circulation*. Zucker IH and Gilmore JP, eds. Boca Raton, FL: CRC Press, 1991, pp 849–873.
88. Zweier JL, Flaherty JT, and Weisfeld ML. Direct measurement of free radical generation following reperfusion of ischemic myocardium. *Proc Natl Acad Sci USA* 84:1404–1407, 1987.

4

Intrathoracic Neuronal Regulation of Cardiac Function

JEFFREY L. ARDELL

Regional control of cardiac function depends on the coordination of activity generated by neurons within intrathoracic autonomic ganglia and the central nervous system. The hierarchy of nested feedback loops there provides precise beat-to-beat control of regional cardiac function. Contrary to classical teaching, work from our laboratory and a number of others using electrophysiological and neuropharmacological techniques applied from the level of whole organ to that of neurons recorded in vitro, indicates that intrathoracic autonomic ganglia act as more than simple relay stations for autonomic efferent neuronal control of the heart.[4] Within the hierarchy of intrathoracic ganglia and nerve interconnections, complex processing of information depends on the spatial and temporal summation of varied sensory inputs (Chapter 3) and on inputs from central neurons (Chapters 5–7).[15] Neurons within intrathoracic autonomic ganglia are likewise modulated by circulating hormones, chief among them being circulating epinephrine and angiotensin II (Chapters 2 and 12).[74]

The progressive development of heart disease is associated with adaptation of these neurohumoral control mechanisms. This adaptation or remodeling likely involves various components of the cardiac neuroaxis (afferent, local circuit–processing, and efferent neurons), hormones, receptors, and signal transduction pathways within neural and myocyte end effectors. We hypothesize that differences exist in autonomic control of the heart before any overt signs of cardiovascular disease occur and that such differences critically influence the onset of cardiac disease and subsequent events. We further hypothesize that differential remodeling of the cardiac neuronal hierarchy (central and peripheral) for reflex control of the heart occurs during the evolution of heart disease. Understanding the neuronal reorganization and remodeling that occur within the peripheral autonomic nervous system and the interactions that occur between this neural remodeling and the remodeling of the myocardium will lead to novel approaches to the development of therapy directed at treating heart disease.

ANATOMICAL ORGANIZATION OF THE INTRATHORACIC NERVOUS SYSTEM

With respect to neural control of the heart, the intrathoracic ganglia and their interconnections form the final common pathway for autonomic modulation of cardiac function. Although recent studies have identified some of the anatomical and functional characteristics of intrathoracic autonomic neurons,[15,26,29,160] we are just beginning to understand how interactions among the network of neurons within the thorax act to regulate regional cardiac function. Data summarized here indicate that intrathoracic autonomic ganglia contain a heterogeneous population of cell types that include afferent, efferent, and local circuit neurons. Yet, as a group, the intrathoracic reflexes mediated within the peripheral autonomic nervous system function in a coordinated fashion, with central neurons located in the spinal cord (Chapter 5), brain stem (Chapter 6), and supraspinal (Chapter 7) regions to regulate cardiac output on a beat-to-beat basis. Relevant aspects of this peripheral nervous system are discussed below.

Afferent Neurons

Cardiac afferent neurons

Cardiovascular afferent neurons provide the autonomic nervous system with information about blood pressure, blood volume, and blood gases as well as the mechanical and chemical milieu of the heart (Chapter 3). With respect to sensory inputs from cardiopulmonary regions, the nodose and dorsal root ganglia are classically recognized as providing sensory inputs to brain stem and spinal cord neurons, respectively.[71] Recent data have indicated that intrathoracic extracardiac (i.e., stellate and middle cervical ganglia) and intrinsic cardiac ganglia also contain afferent neurons whose sensory neurites lie variously within the heart, lungs, and great thoracic vessels.[5,9,12,37,48] Additional sensory inputs for the control of cardiac autonomic efferent neurons arise from baroreceptors and chemoreceptors located along the aortic arch, carotid arteries, and carotid bodies,[41,46,72,162] as well as from other afferent neural elements within the central nervous system (CNS), especially the hypothalamus.[110] General characteristics of cardiac sensory neural transduction will be discussed first. Then each major group of cardiac afferent neurons will be considered in turn.

Overview of cardiac sensory neuronal transduction. It has been known for some time that cardiac sensory neurites (nerve endings) are associated with somata located in ganglia relatively distant from the heart—in nodose and dorsal root ganglia.[96,148,155] Recently, it has become evident that cardiac sensory neurites are also associated with somata located in intrathoracic ganglia, including those on the heart.[5] The relative distance between these sensory neurites and their associated somata represents a major determinant of their function (see Chapter 3). The somata of many cardiac afferent neurons located near or on the target display high-frequency (phasic) activity that directly affects target organ efferent neurons. The optimum stimulus for these afferents is primarily mechanical. In this manner, high-fidelity information content can exert rapid control over efferent neurons adjacent to or on the heart that modulate regional cardiac function. In contrast, it is hypothesized that cardiac afferent neuronal somata located relatively distant from their sensory neurites (i.e., in nodose or dorsal root ganglia) are involved in longer-latency influences on second-order neurons in the cardiac neuroaxis.[8] Slow-responding cardiac afferent neurons generally transduce alterations primarily in the local chemical milieu and thus by nature are generally not responsive to regional alterations that occur on a short timescale. These relatively distant cardiac afferent neurons are involved in relatively long-latency cardio-cardiac reflexes. Their activity reflects an integration of past stimuli (memory) with the current sensory milieu.[87] As discussed in detail in Chapter 3, these afferents can be functionally classified as fast responding and slow responding. That two broad categories of cardiac afferent neurons exist suggests unique transduction capabilities; cardiac information provided to second-order cardiac neuroaxis neurons depends not only on the location of their sensory neurites but also on the location of their somata.

Nodose ganglia afferent neurons. Some nodose ganglion somata receive afferent inputs from sensory neurites located in atrial and ventricular tissues. These sensory neurites preferentially sense chemical stimuli, with a few responding to mechanical stimuli or both modalities.[23,145,147] The response characteristics to induced stimuli are likewise divergent with mechanical stimuli exerting short-lived effects, while the augmentation in activity elicited by chemical stimuli far outlast the stimulus applied.[23,146] While inputs from these receptors contribute to overall cardiovascular regulation, they are not normally perceived.[60]

Dorsal root ganglia afferent neurons. The cell bodies of dorsal root ganglia afferent neurons that receive inputs from cardiac sensory neurites are located in C6–T6 dorsal root ganglia.[71] The sensory neurites of most of these afferent neurons transduce chemical and mechanical stimuli.[77] The inputs from this subpopulation of cardiac afferent neurons subserve normal cardiovascular regulation as well as nociception when excessively activated.[60,141]

Intrathoracic afferent neurons. Functional and anatomical data indicate that intrathoracic autonomic ganglia contain afferent soma.[26,48,160] The sensory neurites associated with these afferent neurons are variously located in atrial, ventricular, major vascular, and pulmonary tissues. Most are responsive to mechanical and chemical stimuli.[20] These afferent neurons continue to influence intrathoracic efferent postganglionic outflows to the heart even after long-term decentralization of intrathoracic ganglia.[5,9,12] It has been proposed that such intrathoracic afferent neurons provide inputs to the intrathoracic short-loop feedback control circuits that involve intrinsic cardiac and intrathoracic extracardiac neurons.[4,15,20] These intrathoracic neural circuits, acting in concert with CNS-mediated reflexes, dynamically control regional cardiac function throughout each cardiac cycle.

Aortic and carotid artery baroreflexes. Stretch receptors, sensitive to changes in vessel size, are located on thoracic and cervical arteries and are concentrated on the aortic arch and the carotid sinus. They provide inputs to neurons within the medulla and spinal cord proportional to systemic arterial blood pressure.[41,46,162] Inputs from these sensory neurites course centrally in the IXth and Xth cranial nerves to synapse with neurons located in the nucleus of the medullary solitary tract.[72] Via multisynaptic connections, they modulate the activity of cardiac parasympathetic efferent preganglionic neurons located primarily in the nucleus ambiguus.[72] They also influence sympathetic efferent neuronal outflow to the heart via brain stem projections to the intermediolateral (IML) region of the spinal cord.[59] Involvement of the baroreflex represents a negative feedback system that modulates cardiac function and peripheral vascular tone in response to everyday stressors (see Chapter 6).[125]

Efferent Neurons

Sympathetic efferent neurons
The somata of sympathetic preganglionic efferent preganglionic neurons which regulate the heart are located within the IML cell column of the spinal cord, projecting axons via the rami T1–T5 to synapse with sympa-

thetic postganglionic neurons contained within various intrathoracic extracardiac and intrinsic cardiac ganglia.[13] Activation of these sympathetic efferent projections augments heart rate, changes patterns and speed of impulse conduction through the heart, and increases contractile force in atrial and ventricular tissues.[7,120,122] Classically, the somata of sympathetic efferent postganglionic neurons that innervate the heart have been thought to be restricted to the stellate ganglia.[88] However, most cardiac sympathetic efferent postganglionic somata are located in thoracic middle cervical, mediastinal, and intrinsic cardiac ganglia.[13,15,21,22,63] A subpopulation of intrinsic cardiac neurons express the catecholaminergic phenotype; these neurons thus contain the necessary enzymes to convert L-Dopa to dopamine and norepinephrine.[31] The intrinsic cardiac nervous system also contains a separate population of small intensely fluorescent (SIF) cells that display tyrosine hydrolyase immunoreactivity.[106,107] Some of these cells project to adjacent principal intrinsic cardiac neurons.[136] Thus, there are sympathetic efferent postganglionic somata that project axons to various cardiac effector tissues localized in intrathoracic extracardiac and intrinsic cardiac ganglia.

Parasympathetic efferent neurons
The somata of cardiac parasympathetic efferent preganglionic neurons within the brain stem are located primarily within the nucleus ambiguous, with lesser numbers being located in the dorsal motor nucleus and regions in between.[72,102,117] Axons from these preganglionic soma project via the Xth cranial nerve to synapse with parasympathetic efferent postganglionic neurons located within various intrinsic cardiac ganglia.[34,35] Activation of parasympathetic efferent neurons depresses heart rate, slows the speed of impulse conduction through the heart, induces major suppression of atrial muscle contractile force, and evokes moderate negative inotropic effects on ventricular contractile force.[3,93,121]

Local Circuit Neurons

A subpopulation of neurons contained within extracardiac and intrinsic cardiac intrathoracic autonomic ganglia function to interconnect neurons within individual ganglia and between neurons in separate intrathoracic ganglia; these are called *local circuit neurons*.[3,13,15] Preliminary data indicate that these neurons are involved in processing of cardiovascular afferent information to coordinate sympathetic and parasympathetic efferent outflows to cardiac effector sites.[20] Interactions within this neuron population form the substrate for generation of the basal activity of cardiac neurons within peripheral autonomic ganglia, especially when intrathoracic ganglia are disconnected from the influence of central neurons.[5]

Neurohumoral Interactions Contributing to Cardiac Control

Figure 4–1 summarizes our current working hypothesis for neurohumoral interactions involved in control of cardiac function. Recent data indicate that a hierarchy of peripheral autonomic neurons function interdependently via nested feedback loops to regulate cardiac function on a beat-to-beat basis. This figure summarizes our emerging concept of neural control of the heart as mediated by intrathoracic extracardiac and intracardiac neurons that are continuously influenced by descending projections from

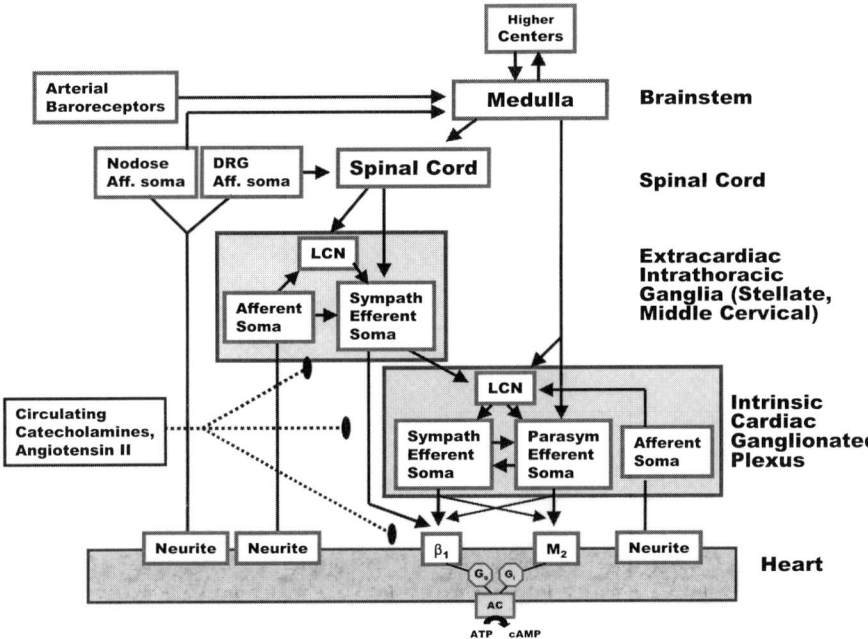

FIGURE 4–1 Schematic of proposed neural interactions occurring within the intrathoracic autonomic ganglia and between these peripheral networks and the central nervous system (CNS). Within the intrinsic cardiac ganglia are included sympathetic (Sympath) and parasympathetic (Parasym) efferent neurons, local circuit neurons (LCN), and afferent neurons. Contained within the extracardiac intrathoracic ganglia are sympathetic efferent neurons, local circuit neurons, and afferent (Aff.) neurons. These intrinsic cardiac and extracardiac networks form separate and distinct nested feedback loops that act in concert with CNS feedback loops involving the spinal cord and medulla to regulate cardiac function on a beat-to-beat basis. These nerve networks are also influenced by circulating humoral factors including catecholamines and angiotensin II. AC, adenylate cyclase; β_1, β_1-adrenergic receptor; DRG, dorsal root ganglia; G_i, inhibitory guanine nucleotide binding protein; G_s, stimulatory guanine nucleotide binding protein; M_2, muscarinic receptor. (Adapted from Armour et al.[20])

higher centers in the spinal cord, brain stem, and suprabulbar regions. Each successive synaptic relay point within this autonomic outflow, from the brain stem to the heart, is in turn influenced by afferent feedback from cardiac, intrathoracic vascular, and pulmonary sensory neurites. Accumulating evidence suggests that there may be at least four functionally distinct neuronal types within the intrinsic cardiac nerve plexus; parasympathetic postganglionic efferent neurons,[1,36,58,62] local circuit neurons,[21,22,63,157] adrenergic postganglionic efferent neurons,[27,104–106,159] and afferent neurons.[5,21,22,63] Local circuit and cardiac afferent neurons also lie within intrathoracic extracardiac ganglia, along with sympathetic postganglionic efferent neurons.[15,19] With respect to intrathoracic autonomic ganglia, cholinergic and adrenergic efferent neurons in these ganglia represent the output elements that project axons to cardiac electrical and mechanical tissues. Local circuit neurons interconnect adjacent neurons within one ganglion or link neurons in separate clusters of intrathoracic ganglia.[14,157] These interneurons are presumably involved in coordination of neuronal activity within these peripheral autonomic ganglia, likely providing the underling inputs necessary for the maintenance of basal autonomic neuronal discharge. Intrathoracic afferent neurons provide mechanosensitive and chemosensitive inputs from cardiopulmonary regions directly to intrinsic cardiac and extracardiac neurons, forming the basis of the intrathoracic neural feedback system.[5,76] Superimposed on activities generated by neurons in peripheral autonomic ganglia are efferent inputs from preganglionic neurons in the brain stem and spinal cord that together exert tonic influences on regional cardiac tone.[6,7,72] The CNS preganglionic inputs are in turn influenced by inputs from higher centers in the CNS[110] and by afferent feedback from peripheral cardiopulmonary afferent neurons.[10–12]

INTERACTIONS AMONG PERIPHERAL AUTONOMIC NEURONS

Cardiac performance is continuously modulated by both sympathetic and parasympathetic efferent neuronal inputs. The change induced in any regional cardiac function ultimately depends on the intrinsic characteristics of the cardiac end-effector being innervated, the level of central efferent neuronal inputs to intrathoracic neurons, and the interactions that occur between peripheral autonomic neurons and cardiac myocytes.

Interactions at the Organ Level

Sympathetic and parasympathetic efferent postganglionic nerve endings lie in close proximity to each other in the heart.[26,105,106,113,160] Interactions among sympathetic and parasympathetic efferent projections involve pre- and postjunctional mechanisms at these end-effectors. Postjunctional interactions involve modulation of adenylate cyclase via G protein–coupled receptor systems.[39,40,85,92] Myocardial β-adrenergic receptors are coupled to and stimulate adenylate cyclase via stimulatory guanine nucleotide binding protein (G_s).[40] Cardiomyocyte M_2 muscarinic receptors are coupled to and inhibit adenylate cyclase via inhibitory guanine nucleotide binding protein (G_i).[40] The interactions between these two receptor-coupled systems at the adenylate cyclase level ultimately determine the rate of formation of the second messenger cAMP.[39,40,85,92] The interactions that occur at the cardiac end-effectors also involve modulation of neurotransmitter release from prejunctional synaptic terminals. Neuronal release of the principal mediators norepinephrine and acetylcholine, along with the co-release of various neuropeptides (e.g., neuropeptide Y and vasoactive intestinal peptide), act on specific receptors associated with sympathetic or parasympathetic efferent axon terminals.[32,93,123,128] These mechanisms act to modulate subsequent neurotransmitter release.

Interactions within the Intrinsic Cardiac Nervous System

Recent studies indicate that peripheral sites separate from the end-effectors contribute to autonomic interactions for the control of cardiac function. Stimulation of parasympathetic and/or sympathetic efferent projections to the heart activates subpopulations of intrinsic cardiac neurons.[21,22,63] With respect to control of chronotropic function, disruption of the right atrial ganglionated plexus (RAGP) eliminates direct vagal projections to the sinoatrial node;[103] yet sympathetic efferent neuronal control of chronotropic function and the vagal inhibition of the sinus tachycardia induced by sympathetic efferent neurons are maintained (see Fig. 4–2).[103] We have proposed that such residual interactions depend on neural interactions occurring within various components of the intrinsic cardiac nervous system.[103,118] Whether such intraganglionic interactions play correspondingly important roles in modulation of dromotropic and inotropic function has yet to be determined.

Interneuronal interactions within the intrinsic cardiac nervous system depend in large part on common shared afferent inputs as well as interconnections mediated via local circuit neurons. To evaluate these interactions, we recorded activity from separate populations of neurons in the ventral RAGP.[143] This ganglionated plexus is primarily but not exclusively associated with control of the sinoatrial (SA) node.[6] In basal states, the coherence of activity generated by the two populations of RAGP neu-

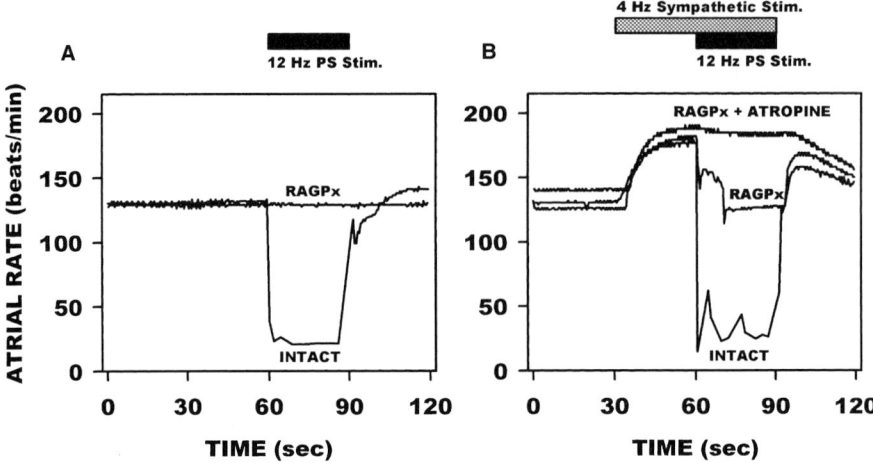

FIGURE 4–2 Atrial rate response to parasympathetic (**A**), sympathetic, (**B**), and concurrent sympathetic–parasympathetic stimulation (**B**) before (intact) and after surgical ablation of the ventral right atrial ganglionated plexus (RAGPx). Solid bars indicate duration of 12 Hz parasympathetic (PS) stimulation (stim.); crosshatched bar represents duration of 4 Hz stimulation of both stellate ganglia (sympathetic stim.). Note that after RAGPx ablation, vagal stimulation no longer slows atrial rate (A), but the tachycardia to sympathetic stimulation remains (B). When parasympathetic stimulation is superimposed on a background of sympathetic-induced tachycardia, the atrial rate rapidly returns to baseline. This residual sympathetic–parasympathetic interaction was eliminated by the muscarinic antagonist atropine (RAGPx + atropine). (Adapted from McGuirt et al.[103])

rons fluctuated with a periodicity of 30–50 seconds, with an average peak coherence of 0.88 ± 0.03.[143] Coherence was increased in conjunction with the enhanced neuronal activity evoked during exposure of their ventricular sensory inputs to mechanical and chemical stimuli (see Fig. 4–3).[143] Although we have yet to determine the role that common shared afferent inputs and local circuit neuronal interconnections play in coordinating activity between atrial and ventricular intrinsic cardiac ganglia, data indicate that coupled behavior can be displayed by different populations of target organ neurons.

Interactions within the Intrathoracic Nervous System

Coordination of autonomic outflows from intrathoracic neurons to cardiomyocytes depends in part on sharing of inputs from higher centers along with interactions among and between various peripheral ganglia. The interactions within and between intrathoracic ganglia involve local

Neuronal Regulation of Cardiac Function

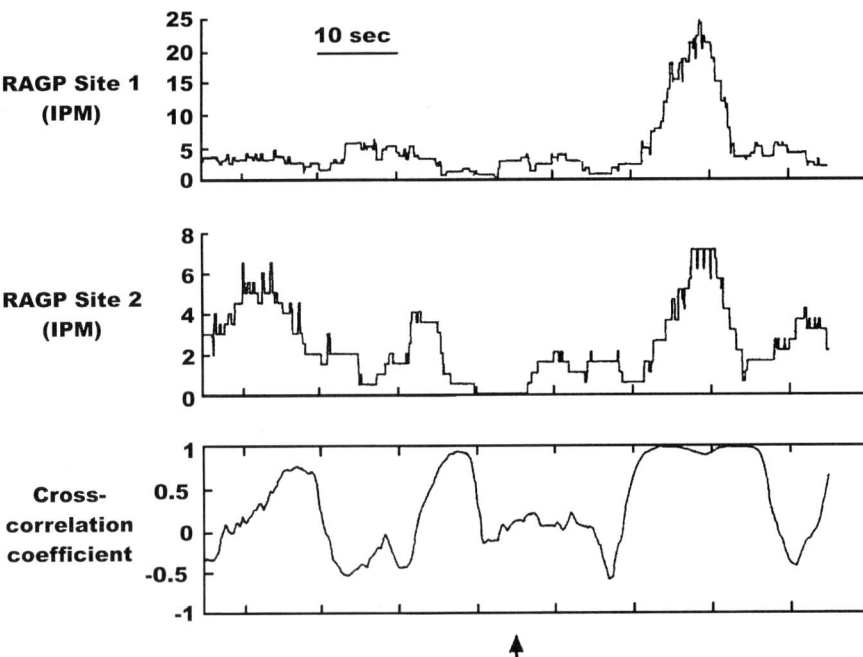

FIGURE 4-3 Activity generated by two different populations of intrinsic cardiac neurons (ICN) contained within the right atrial ganglionated plexus (RAGP). Arrow indicates application of veratridine to the epicardium of the left ventricle. At baseline, note the cycling of activity with a periodicity of 20 seconds. In the unstressed condition, this bursting is usually associated with increased coordination of activity between the two populations of neurons (see bottom trace). When an afferent stress is imposed to the ICN, as with application of epicardial veratridine, activity increased in both sites and the coherence of activity generated by these two populations of neurons approached unity. IPM, impulses per minute. (Adapted from Thompson et al.[143])

circuit neurons. As illustrated in Figure 4-4, disconnecting the intrathoracic nervous system from the CNS (decentralization) modifies but does eliminate afferent-mediated intrathoracic reflex modulation of autonomic ganglia function.[20] Activities generated by neurons in intrinsic cardiac ganglia demonstrate no consistent short-term relationship to neurons in extracardiac ganglia.[20] Yet the sharing of cardiopulmonary afferent information acting through both intrathoracic and brain stem–spinal cord feedback loops permits an overall coordination of effector control.[20] Together, these nested feedback control systems allow for a redundancy in neural control of the heart while at the same time maintaining the flexibility to differentially modulate regional cardiac function.[3]

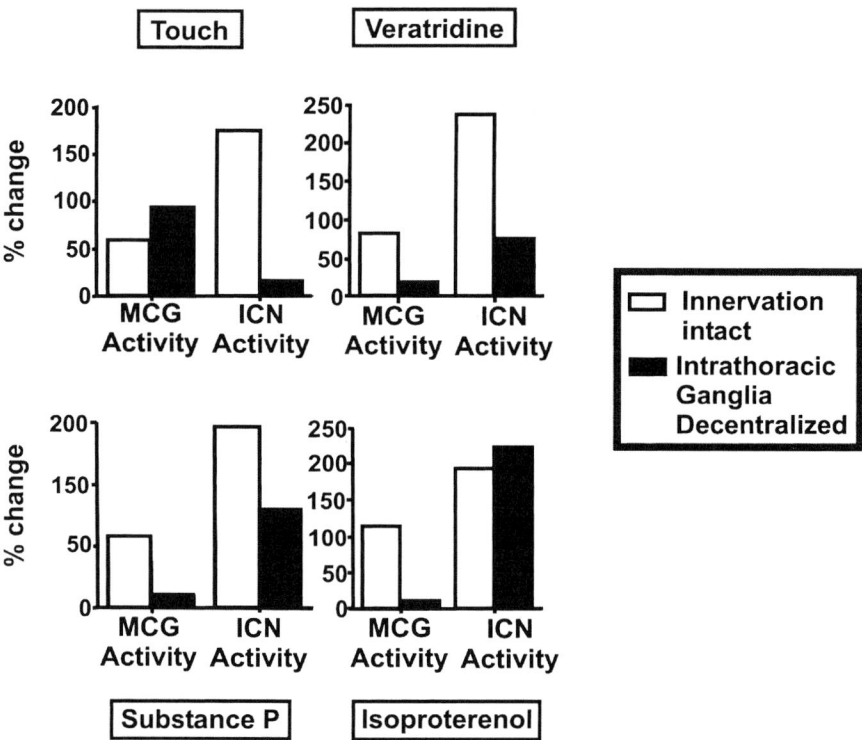

FIGURE 4–4 Effects of activating left ventricular (LV) sensory neurites on intrathoracic intrinsic cardiac (ICN) and extracardiac (MCG, middle cervical ganglia) neural activity before (open bars) and after (filled bars) decentralizing the intrathoracic nervous system from the central nervous system. Neural activity is presented as percent change from baseline. With innervation intact, activation of LV epicardial sensory neurites with mechanical stimuli (touch), chemical stimuli (veratridine and substance P), or intravenous isoproterenol evoked reflex-mediated increases in neuronal activities in both intrinsic cardiac and extracardiac ganglia. Decentralization of the intrathoracic nervous system from the central nervous system modified but did not eliminate reflex responses to subsequent cardiac afferent stimulations. These residual responses reflect the continued functioning of the nested intrathoracic feedback loops depicted in Figure 4–1. (Adapted from Armour et al.[20])

NEUROHUMORAL INTERACTIONS IN CONTROL OF CARDIAC FUNCTION

Angiotensin II–Sympathetic Efferent Neuronal Interactions

Angiotensin II (ANG II) exerts a major influence on cardiac control via its direct effects on the sympathetic nervous system. Cardiac ANG II production is up-regulated in congestive heart failure, with associated increases in neural release of catecholamines into the cardiac interstitium (Chapter 12). An intrinsic ANG I–converting enzyme-dependent angiotensin system exists in cardiac sympathetic ganglia, which can be activated by increased preganglionic stimulation.[89] Exogenous administration of ANG II to discrete populations of intrathoracic (extracardiac and intrinsic cardiac) sympathetic neurons leads to an increased release of norepinephrine (NE) and epinephrine (EPI) into the cardiac interstitial fluid space (ISF).[56] The level of NE liberated into the ISF during exogenous ANG II administration is equivalent to ISF NE content achieved during high-level electrical stimulation of the stellate ganglia (see Fig. 4–5). However, stellate ganglion stimulation causes significant NE spillover into coronary sinus blood; ANG II does not. Despite the fact that left ventricular myocardial EPI content is approximately 40-fold lower than that of NE (6 ± 1 vs. 237 ± 33 ng/g), equivalent levels of EPI and NE are released into the ventricular ISF upon activation of cardiac adrenergic efferent neurons either by electrical stimulation or locally administering ANG II.[56] Yet in neither case did significant amounts of EPI spill over into the coronary sinus blood.[56] These results suggest that catecholamine release and up-

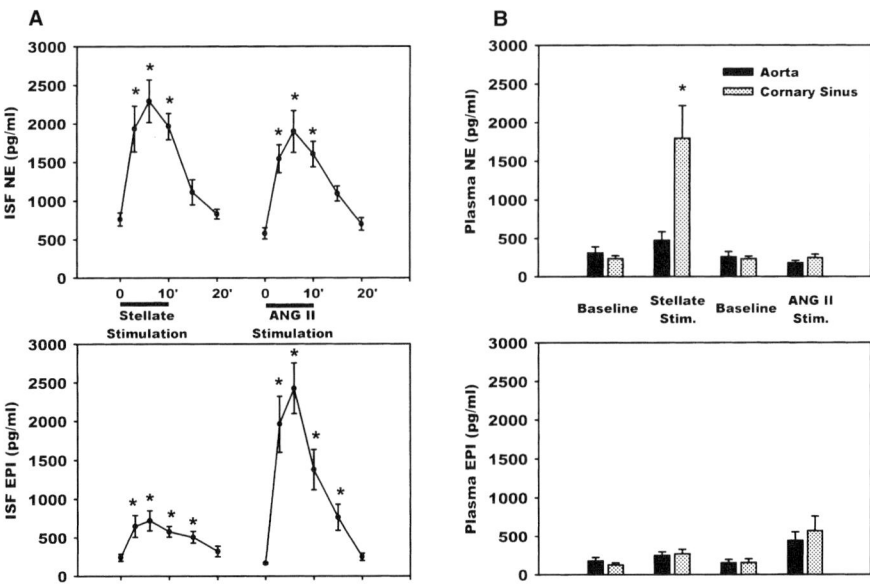

FIGURE 4–5 Cardiac interstitial fluid (ISF) (**A**), and aorta and coronary sinus norepinephrine (NE) and epinephrine (EPI) levels (**B**) in response to 10 minutes of stellate stimulation (4 Hz) and 10 minutes of angiotensin II (ANG II) infusion (100 μM, 1 ml/min) into the blood supply for the right atrial ganglionated plexus (RAGP). The ISF fluids were sampled using the microdialysis technique. *$P < 0.05$ vs. baseline values.

take mechanisms within the myocardium can be differentially affected, depending on how the sympathetic efferent nervous system is modified. They also demonstrate that measurement of circulating catecholamines provides an inadequate index of cardiac catecholamine release. Furthermore, ANG II can act at multiple levels within the neurohumoral hierarchy to modulate cardiac adrenergic efferent neuronal outflow.

Epinephrine Influences Sympathetic Efferent Neuronal Function

Ventricular EPI derives mainly from the uptake of circulating EPI by cardiac adrenergic efferent neurons, the principal source for circulating EPI being the adrenal medulla.[33,115] Epinephrine is stored in synaptic vesicles of nerves; it is co-released with NE during activation of sympathetic efferent nerve terminals.[33,95,128,130] Epinephrine released in this manner into the ISF can directly activate cardiac myocyte β_1-adrenergic receptors, thereby augmenting cardiac chronotropism and inotropism. Neurally released EPI can likewise activate adrenergic receptors on intrinsic cardiac adrenergic efferent neurons to modulate their release of NE into the interstitium.[16] In dogs with intact cardiac innervation, chronic adrenalectomy exerts no effect on ventricular NE content or the transcardiac NE gradient in the basal state; ventricular and plasma EPI content, however, falls below detectable levels in such a state.[115] Moreover, in adrenalectomized dogs, heart rate and blood pressure responses to electrical stimulation of a stellate ganglion become blunted.[115] Exogenous infusion of EPI increases myocardial EPI content significantly,[57,114,115] while enhancing NE release.[38] These partly restore heart rate and blood pressure responses elicited by stellate ganglion stimulation in dogs subjected to prior adrenalectomy.[115] The effect of short-term EPI administration on enhancing sympathetic efferent neuronal control of the heart has been ascribed to the fact that the EPI released from synaptic vesicles act on pre-synaptic β_2-adrenoreceptors to initiate a positive feedback mechanism that enhances local release of NE from cardiac sympathetic efferent postganglionic nerves.[38,115]

INTRATHORACIC NEURONS AND THE ROLE OF CHOLINERGIC AND NONCHOLINERGIC RECEPTORS IN CARDIAC CONTROL

Electrophysiology of Intrathoracic Neurons

Cardiac neurons generate spontaneous activity in situ, frequently exhibiting activity that is temporally related to cardiac or respiratory dynamics.[21,22,63] Of the neurons that display cardiac-related activity, many are affected by mechano- or chemosensory inputs from the heart.[22,63] Trains of electrical stimuli delivered to axons in the T1–T5 ventral roots activate a substantial population of stellate and middle cervical neurons.[10,11] These data indicate a convergence of preganglionic inputs onto the extracardiac postganglionic soma. In contrast, trains of electrical stimuli delivered to the vagosympathetic trunks or stellate ganglia activate a much smaller population of intrinsic cardiac neurons,[21,22,63] indicating that summation of inputs is required to modify the activity generated by neurons on the heart. Intrinsic cardiac neurons normally generate low-level activity consistent with a nerve network that functions as a "low pass filter," thereby minimizing the potential for imbalances within autonomic efferent neuronal inputs to the heart, a process which by itself could be arrhythmogenic.[81] Disruption of descending projections into intrathoracic autonomic ganglia elicits changes in neuronal membrane properties and synaptic efficacy (Fig. 4–6).[109,138,139] The net result of this neural remodeling is that the residual neural control of cardiac function becomes even more dependent on peripheral reflex control.

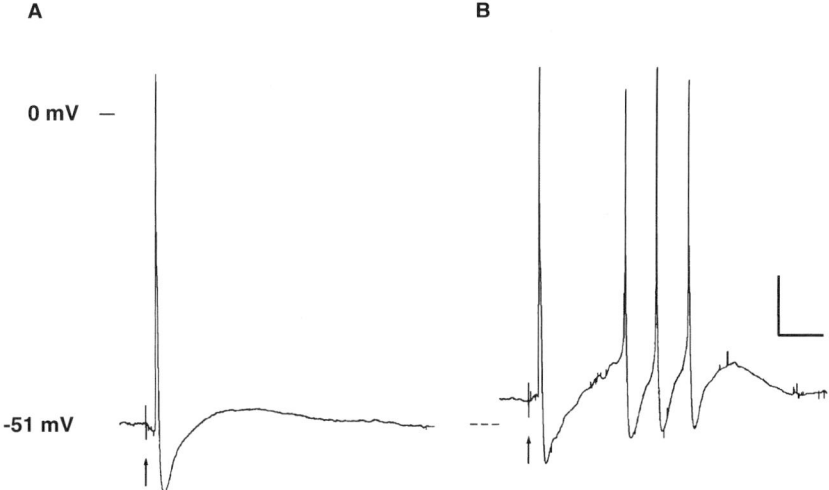

FIGURE 4–6 Effects of muscarine on orthodromic activation of a decentralized intrinsic cardiac neuron. An interganglionic nerve connected to the ganglion under study was stimulated with single pulse (at arrows; stimulus parameters set to produce supra-threshold postsynaptic response: 0.5 ms pulse duration, 3.2 mA; artifact truncated for clarity). **A.** Each stimulus applied to the nerve evoked one action potential (AP) prior to application of muscarine. **B.** Similar stimuli applied to the same nerve 30 seconds after local application of muscarine (100 μM; 50 ms) evoked multiple APs. Vertical bar represents 10 mV; horizontal bar represents 50 ms. (Adapted from Smith et al.[138])

Cholinergic Mechanisms

Synaptic transmission in autonomic ganglia principally involves the release of acetylcholine. Nicotinic and muscarinic cholinergic receptors have been associated with intrathoracic autonomic neurons.[2,65,79,137,158] Blockade of nicotinic receptors attenuates but does not eliminate activity generated by the intrinsic cardiac neurons.[21,22,63] Muscarinic blockade attenuates excitatory and inhibitory synaptic function within intrinsic cardiac ganglia as well.[158] These data indicate that acetylcholine exerts both mediator and modulator effects at synapses within intrathoracic autonomic ganglia.

Noncholinergic Mechanisms

Blockade of nicotinic and muscarinic cholinergic receptors attenuates but does not eliminate the activity generated by neurons within the intrathoracic autonomic ganglia.[5,14] This indicates that non-nicotinic putative neurotransmitters act as mediators for synaptic transmission within the intrathoracic neuronal system. Anatomical and physiological studies have identified multiple putative neurotransmitters associated with mammalian intrinsic cardiac neurons, including purinergic agents,[50,80] catecholamines,[31,84] angiotensin II,[74] calcitonin gene–related peptide,[69,94,153,154] neuropeptide Y,[51,64,140,153] substance P,[30,70,149] neurokinins,[69,144] endothelin,[18] and vasoactive intestinal peptide.[52,66,140,152–154] Direct application of various neurotransmitters adjacent to neurons in intrathoracic cardiac ganglia modifies the activities they generate, often resulting in concomitant changes in cardiac pacemaker and/or contractile behavior.[27,78–80] Various neurotransmitters may also function as neuromodulators. For example, substance P modulates the efficacy of intrinsic cardiac neurons to cholinergic activation[161] (Fig. 4–7). The precise role of these noncholinergic neurotransmitters in control of normal and diseased hearts remains largely unknown.

THE ROLE OF HOMOGENETITY OF NERVE FUNCTION IN CARDIAC CONTROL

Intrathoracic autonomic ganglia are capable of complex signal processing involving afferent, local circuit, as well as parasympathetic and sympathetic efferent neurons. While the physiological properties of extracardiac autonomic ganglia tend to amplify CNS and afferent feedback inputs, those of the intrinsic cardiac nervous system act to limit cardiac excitability. As such, the final common pathway of cardiac control—the intrinsic cardiac nervous system—may normally function as a low pass

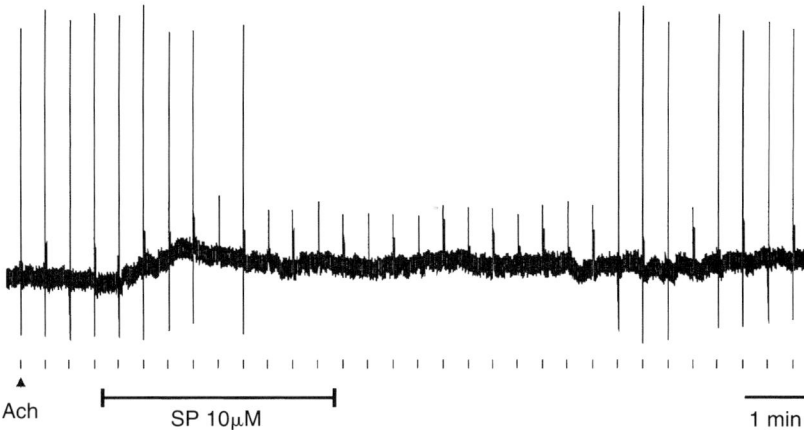

FIGURE 4–7 Inhibition of acetylcholine (ACh)-evoked responses by substance P (SP). Top trace shows intracellular recording from an intracardiac neuron and bottom marks indicate times when 28 ms puffs of ACh (10 mM) were given by local pressure injection. Local application of ACh-evoked action potentials. These ACh evoked potentials were blocked during bath application of 10 μM substance P (see horizontal bar). (Adapted from Zhang et al.[161])

filter to minimize transient neuronal imbalances arising from separate sympathetic and parasympathetic efferent neuronal inputs to the heart. Local afferent feedback mechanisms also exist within the intrathoracic ganglia that mediate local cardiocardiac reflexes at sites separate from the CNS. These intrathoracic reflexes allow for rapid changes in efferent outflow to the heart and help to maintain the homogeneity in controlling regional cardiac function. The synaptic events underlying such intraganglionic interactions apparently involve multiple neurotransmitters that interact with various neuronal receptors to exert rapid-acting neuronal membrane conductance changes and/or longer-term modulation of synapses within the intrathoracic cardiac nervous system. How the interplay among the various intrathoracic, spinal cord, and brain stem neurons ultimately affects regional cardiac function remains unknown. An equally important question concerns how these interactions are modified in specific cardiac disease states. Multiple lines of evidence indicate that if this neural hierarchy is disrupted, cardiac control is compromised, sometimes with lethal consequences.

Functional Interdependence for Control of Chronotropic and Inotropic Function

Cardiac vagal efferent neurons exert parallel and finely balanced control of cardiac chronotropic and dromotropic function. This coordination results in part via the bilateral convergence of descending parasympathetic efferent neuronal projections onto discrete aggregates of intrinsic cardiac neurons, with a potential contribution mediated via local circuit neuronal interconnects between intrinsic cardiac ganglia.[103,118,143] For chronotropic control, intrinsic cardiac neurons contained within the ventral right atrial[6] and posterior atrial[118] ganglionated plexuses predominate. Control of atrioventricular (AV) conduction is localized primarily in the inferior vena cava–inferior atrium ganglionated plexus.[6] In response to autonomic activation, induced electrically[103,112] or reflexive,[111] 1:1 AV conduction is maintained via the neural hierarchy and especially by its peripheral interactions. If specific end-effectors are compromised (e.g., sinus node disease)[97] or neuronal elements within the peripheral neural hierarchy become disrupted (e.g., ablation of one or more intrinsic cardiac ganglia),[112,118,119] control of cardiac electrical activity becomes unbalanced. This imbalance can have important implications in the genesis of cardiac arrhythmias. For example, the concurrent neural inputs to the SA and AV nodes limit AV conduction, so a premature atrial beat that is more than 10% greater than the existing heart rate is blocked.[101] If the inferior vena cava–inferior atrial ganglionated plexus is ablated, 1:1 AV conduction is maintained over a wide range of heart rates (Fig. 4–8)[112] and the protective effects of AV block are substantially attenuated. Conversely, in the context of sinus node disease, while chronotropic responses can be attenuated, vagal control of AV conduction can be hyperresponsive, thereby resulting in periodic AV block and an inappropriately low ventricular beating rate.[97]

Intrathoracic Nervous System and Cardiac Dysrhythmias

The neuronal heterogeneity depicted above can contribute to arrhythmia formation, even in the context of a normal myocardial electrical substrate. Neurons in the central and intrathoracic nervous systems have been implicated in the genesis of cardiac arrhythmias (see Chapters 7 and 11). Some studies have indicated that left-sided peripheral autonomic neurons show an increased propensity to elicit dysrhythmias when stimulated discretely.[132] As a matter of fact, neurons located on either side of the thorax do so (Chapter 11). In response to discrete electrical or chemical stimuli, the potential for arrhythmia formation increases when such stress in placed within more peripheral aspects of the cardiac neuronal hierarchy (Fig. 4–9)—e.g., chemical stimulation of a given intrinsic cardiac ganglionated plexus is more likely to induce abnormal atrial and/or ventricular rates than analogous stimuli of stellate or middle cervical ganglia.[42,74,81] These results likely reflect the filtering ability of the intrinsic cardiac nervous system to blunt erratic inputs arising from extracardiac neuronal sources. When the most peripheral elements of the hierarchy are

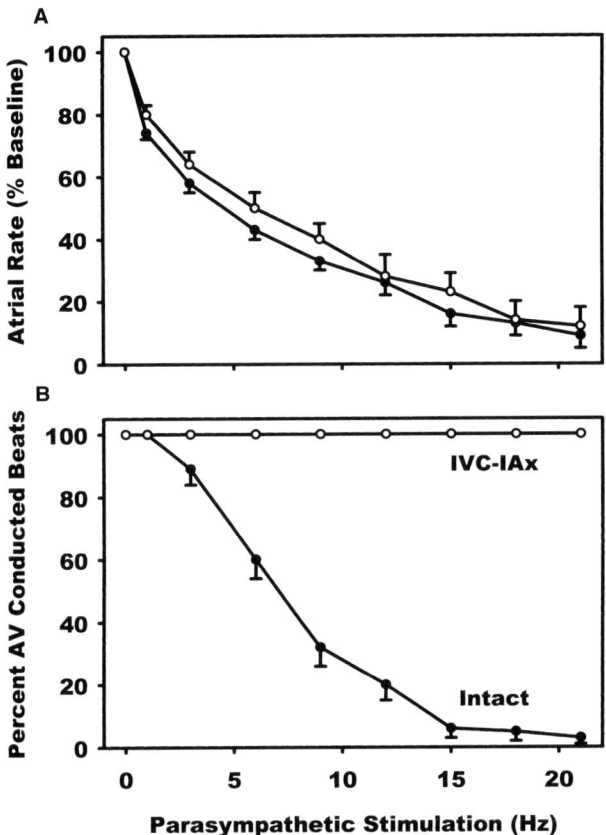

FIGURE 4–8 Chronotropic (**A**) and dromotropic response (**B**) to vagal stimulation prior to (open circles) and following (closed circles) surgical ablation of the inferior vena cava–inferior atrial ganglionated plexus (IVC-IAx). (Adapted from O'Toole et al.[112])

heterogeneously activated, there are minimal downstream mechanisms at the end-effectors to counteract autonomic imbalance. The potential for neuronal heterogeneity to contribute to arrhythmia formation is exacerbated when expressed against an underlying cardiac disease state.

NEURAL REMODELING IN HEART DISEASE

Myocardial Ischemia/Infarction

Myocardial ischemia and infarction can induce substantial changes in the intrathoracic neuronal networks and their reflex control of regional cardiac function.[19] Chen and co-workers[44,45,47] have recently proposed a hy-

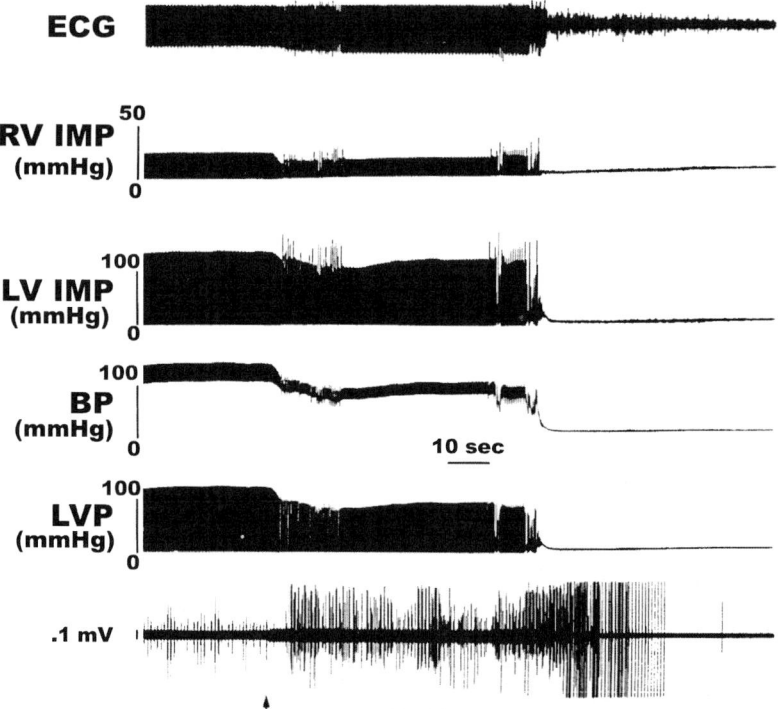

FIGURE 4–9 Administration of an H_1-histamine receptor antagonist (arrow) into the blood supply for the right atrial ganglionated plexus elicited changes in cardiac electrical and mechanical function and neural activity within the intrinsic cardiac nervous system (bottom trace). Induced arrhythmias degenerated into ventricular fibrillation, again in conjunction with the activation of a subpopulation of intrinsic cardiac neurons. ECG, electrocardiogram; RV IMP, right ventricular intramyocardial pressure; LV IMP, left ventricular intramyocardial pressure; BP, blood pressure; LVP, left ventricular pressure. (Adapted from Armour.[17])

pothesis of sudden cardiac death: Myocardial ischemia results in nerve injury, followed by sympathetic nerve sprouting and regional myocardial hyperinnervation. The coupling between augmented sympathetic nerve sprouting with electrically remodeled myocardium results in ventricular tachycardia or fibrillation as well as sudden cardiac death.[47] The results of these studies and others have indicated that the evolution of cardiac pathologies may be associated with a heterogeneous distribution of efferent projections to cardiac end-effectors.[91] Myocardial ischemia can also alter the neurochemical profile of these projections, for instance, modifying the expression of vasoactive intestinal polypeptide and calcitonin gene–related peptide by sympathetic efferent neurons.[124] Finally, the evolution of cardiac pathology can be associated with disruptions of the intrinsic cardiac nervous system[19,73] and its ability to process afferent information. Such changes could compromise the ability of the intrathoracic neuronal networks to maintain homeogeneity for reflex control of regional cardiac function. Neuronal remodeling, when coupled with the ischemic-induced heterogeneous electrical remodeling of cardiac myocytes,[75,116,156] creates a synergistic substrate for arrhythmia formation and sudden cardiac death.

Neurons in intrathoracic ganglia, including those on the heart, receive constant inputs from spinal cord neurons to modulate their behavior.[11,22,63] They also receive inputs from cardiac sensory neurites on an ongoing basis (Chapter 3). That is why the activity generated by most intrinsic cardiac neurons increases markedly in the presence of increased sensory inputs arising from the ischemic myocardium.[20] Excessive activation of limited populations of intrinsic cardiac neurons can induce cardiac dysrhythmias that lead to ventricular fibrillation.[81] Thus, therapies that act to stabilize heterogeneous-evoked activities within these cardiac reflex control circuits have obvious clinical importance.

Alterations in heart rate secondary to ventricular ischemia may be due in part to altered neural control of cardiac pacemaker cells. Myocardial ischemia can be attended by not only by tachycardia but also bradycardia. Activation of a sufficient population of nodose ganglion afferent neurons by exposing their sensory neurites to purinergic agents can result in the induction of bradycardia via medullary reflexes.[86] Bradycardia can also be induced when purinergic agents[80] activate sufficient populations of intrinsic cardiac neurons projecting axons to medullary neurons. In contrast, activation of cardiac sensory neurites associated with dorsal root ganglion neurons with adenosine can result in the reflex excitation of sympathetic efferent neurons that innervate the heart.[15] The details of the various reflex responses induced when specific populations of cardiac afferent neurons in nodose as opposed to dorsal root or intrathoracic ganglia are modified by local ischemia remain to be fully elucidated. Moreover, the way in which chronic ischemia remodels these peripheral and central mediated reflexes remains to be determined.

In the context of integrated physiology and pathophysiology, all things are not created equal. The different cardiac reflexes so mediated may have a profound impact on the progression of heart disease. For example, in a canine model with chronic ventral wall infarction and submaximal exercise accompanied by transient but complete circumflex coronary artery occlusion at the end of exercise, approximately 40% of animals developed ventricular fibrillation (VF).[131] Compared to the other 60% of animals, these VF "susceptible" animals exhibited depressed baroreflex sensitivity,[150] low variability in basal heart rate as determined by power spectral analysis[83] even before the myocardial infarction, and tachycardia during the transient coronary occlusion.[133] These results indicate that differences exist in autonomic control of the heart before any overt cardiovascular disease becomes evident. Such differences critically influence the outcome at the time of ischemic heart disease onset.

Congestive Heart Failure

Increases in the activities of both the renin–angiotensin and sympathetic nervous systems are pathognomonic of congestive heart failure. The increases in cardiac rate and contractility as well as total peripheral resistance that occur are initially compensatory in nature, increasing blood pressure and venous return (see Chapter 12). However, long-term activation of the renin–angiotensin and sympathetic nervous systems has adverse consequences that ultimately exacerbate the deleterious effects of

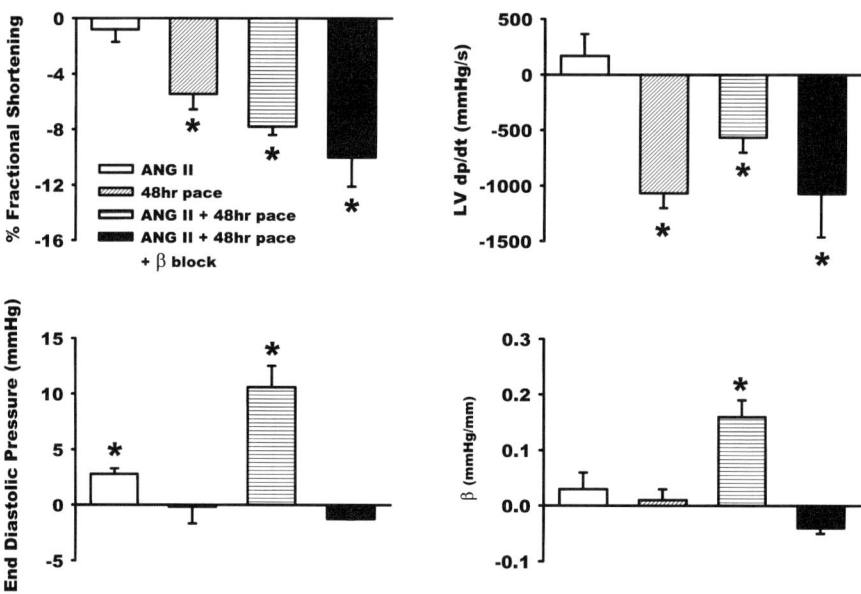

FIGURE 4–10 Change in systolic and diastolic function in response to 7-day treatment with angiotensin II (ANG II), 48 hours of tachycardia pacing (pace), ANG II treatment with the tachycardia pacing during the final 48 hours, and ANG II + tachycardia pacing with concurrent β-adrenergic receptor blockade. Note the synergism between pacing and ANG II to induce cardiac diastolic dysfunction, an effect that is blocked by β-adrenergic blockade. Myocardial damage with fibroblast/neutrophil infiltration from ANG II + 48 hour pace was also inhibited by β blockade. B (right panel), chamber stiffness. *$P < 0.05$ vs. baseline. (Adapted from Senzacki et al.[135])

heart failure. Angiotensin II can modulate cardiac interstitial fluid levels of norepinephrine and epinephrine, independent of its direct cardiomyocyte or systemic vascular effects.[56] Over time, this can result in a positive feedback cycle that can have deleterious effects on cardiac structure and function.[142] Senzaki et al.[134] showed that angiotensin II, when infused for 4 days followed by 48 hours of pacing (during continued angiotensin II infusion), markedly enhances LV dysfunction (Fig. 4–10). This effect can be prevented by pretreatment with a high dose of a selective β_1-receptor blocker.[135] Henegar et al.[68] showed that cardiac damage associated with increased angiotensin II could be minimized by β_1-adrenergic blockade or sympathectomy. These data suggest that the deleterious effects of exogenously administered angiotensin II are mediated by enhanced norepinephrine release secondary to activation of AT_1 receptors on cardiac adrenergic neurons. To understand the synergism between angiotensin II and the sympathetic nervous systems, future studies must focus on both the vascular and cardiac interstitial components of angiotensin II–generating mechanisms, their role in modulating catecholamine release, and the consequent postsynaptic interactions. For the development of future therapies, the progression of cardiac disease must be viewed in the context of myocyte remodeling (electrical and mechanical), matrix remodeling, and neurohumoral remodeling.

INTERACTIONS BETWEEN CENTRAL NERVOUS SYSTEM AND INTRATHORACIC NEURONAL NETWORKS: IMPLICATIONS FOR TREATMENT OF CARDIAC DISEASE

Myocardial ischemia reflects an imbalance in the supply/demand balance within the heart, with the resultant activation of cardiac afferent neurons and, consequently, the perception of symptoms such as angina pectoris (Chapter 10). In addition to such nociceptive responses, activated cardiac afferent neurons can elicit autonomic and somatic reflexes.[19,60] Pharmacological, surgical, and angioplasty therapies are commonly used to improve symptoms and cardiac function in patients with angina pectoris. While these treatments are usually successful, some patients still suffer from cardiac pain following these procedures.[98,129] Recently, epidural stimulation of the spinal cord (spinal cord stimulation [SCS]) has been suggested as an alternative to bypass surgery in high-risk patients.[100] With SCS, high-frequency, low-intensity electrical stimuli are delivered to the dorsal aspect of the T1–T2 segments of the thoracic spinal cord. This therapy decreases the frequency and intensity of anginal episodes.[53,67,127] Spinal cord stimulation reduces the magnitude and duration of ST segment alteration during exercise stress in patients with cardiac disease,[126] improves myocardial lactate metabolism,[99] and increases workload tolerance.[126] The mechanisms whereby this mode of therapy produces such beneficial effects are poorly understood.

Since intrathoracic neurons have been found to play important modulatory roles in cardiac regulation, we have begun to study SCS and its effects on the activity generated by intrinsic cardiac neurons.[61] Transient ventricular ischemia activates populations of neurons in intrathoracic ganglia, including those on the heart (Fig. 4–11).[19,76] Excessive focal activation of intrathoracic neural circuits can induce cardiac dysrhythmias, even in normally perfused hearts.[81] Spinal cord stimulation results in an immediate suppression in intrinsic cardiac neuronal activity. Suppressor effects are imposed on the intrinsic cardiac nervous system, regardless of whether SCS is applied immediately before, during, or after coronary artery occlusion (Fig. 4–11).[61] Furthermore, such suppression of intrinsic cardiac neuronal activity persists after cessation of the SCS.[25] That transection of the ansae subclavia eliminated these effects suggests that they primarily involve the sympathetic nervous system.[61]

The synaptic mechanisms and specific pathways mediating these re-

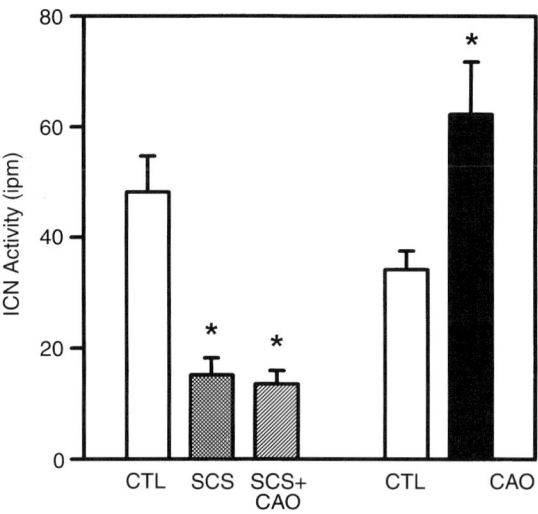

FIGURE 4–11 Change in intrinsic cardiac neuronal (ICN) activity induced by transient occlusion of the left anterior descending artery (CAO) and/or spinal cord stimulation (SCS) at 90% motor threshold. Note the augmentation in activity within the intrinsic cardiac neurons produced by CAO is attenuated by electrical stimulation of the dorsal aspects of the T1–T3 segments of the spinal cord. CTL, baseline control (Adapted from Foreman et al.[61])

sponses have yet to be determined. They likely involve both sympathetic afferent and efferent neurons. Spinal cord stimulation may activate sensory afferent fibers antidromically so that endorphins[54] or neuropeptides such as calcitonin gene–related peptide or substance P[24,27,49,69] are released locally in the intrinsic cardiac ganglia and myocardium. Opiates and neuropeptides can influence intrinsic cardiac neurons (see above). Spinal cord stimulation may also suppress intrinsic cardiac adrenergic efferent neurons as well as local circuit neurons as the result of altered sympathetic efferent preganglionic neuronal inputs. Activation of sympathetic efferent preganglionic axons can suppress many intrathoracic reflexes involved in cardiac regulation.[3,15] Thus these neurosuppressor effects may be due in part to activation of inhibitory synapses within intrathoracic ganglia.[43,108] Recent clinical experience with SCS highlights the dynamic interactions that can occur between central and intrathoracic neurons, demonstrating the potential for effective clinical treatment of cardiac pathology via modulation of the intrathoracic nervous system.

PERSPECTUS

Control of regional cardiac electrical and mechanical function depends on varied inputs arising from neurons in intrathoracic autonomic ganglia, the spinal cord, and brain stem, as well as the effects of circulating neurohumoral agents. Neural control of the heart relies on the coordination of the activities generated by the varied populations of neurons within intrathoracic autonomic ganglia and the CNS.[4] The hierarchy of nested feedback loops there provides precise beat-to-beat control over regional cardiac function. Within the hierarchy of intrathoracic ganglia (Fig. 4–1), complex processing takes place that involves the summation of preganglionic inputs from central neurons with those derived from cardiopulmonary sensory inputs.[13]

Excessive activation of the intrathoracic cardiac efferent nervous system, as occurs for example during myocardial ischemia, can provoke cardiac arrhythmias. These maladaptations likely involve changes within the cardiac nervous system in addition to alterations in cardiomyocyte function.[28,91] Differential adaptations of cardiomyocyte ion channels (e.g., I_K and I_{Ca}) and intercellular connections during the progression of heart disease have been termed electrical remodeling.[75,116,156] Recent data indicate that neurohumoral control mechanisms likewise reorganize during progression into certain cardiac diseases[142] and are referred to as *neurohumoral remodeling*.[47,91]

Changes in autonomic outflow accompany and influence the progression of cardiac disease. Sympathetic efferent neuronal activation contributes to sudden cardiac death in patients with ischemic and non-ischemic heart disease.[44,45,47] The Autonomic Tone and Reflexes After Myocardial Infarction (ATRAMI) study demonstrated that baroreflex sensitivity and heart rate variability predict risk for cardiovascular mortality and myocardial infarction.[90] Electrical stimulation of vagal efferent neurons suppresses the tendency toward ventricular fibrillation formation in dogs with depressed vagal reflex activity, as measured by baroreflex sensitivity.[151] Yet pharmacological agents that increase vagal efferent neuronal tone, such as a low-dose scopolamine, do not confer similar degrees of cardioprotection.[82] The mechanism(s) whereby activation of sympathetic efferent neurons and/or withdrawal of parasympathetic efferent neuronal tone increase the risk for sudden death are not clear. However, postinfarction heterogeneous remodeling of the cardiac neuronal hierarchy, including extracardiac sympathetic and intrinsic cardiac efferent neural elements, likely contributes to the resultant cardiac electrical instability.

After decades of progress, improvement in the management of cardiac arrhythmias appears to have leveled off. The problem of sudden cardiac death occurring as the result of an initial arrhythmic event has not been adequately addressed (except perhaps through palliative strategies which include public access defibrillators). This state of affairs is due in part to the fact that key pieces of information regarding cardiac arrhythmia formation are still missing, such as the ability to identify an apparently normal individual at risk before such an event occurs. While changes in myocardial electrical events have been well characterized in the diseased heart, information about the complex neuronal organization regulating cardiac rhythm remains limited. Comprehensive knowledge of the complex processing that occurs within the intrathoracic nervous system, as well as between peripheral and central cardiovascular neurons, should provide a basis for understanding the role that the cardiac nervous system plays in regulating the electrical behavior of not only the normal heart but also the diseased heart. A thorough understanding of this complex cardiac neuronal hierarchy should lay the foundation for novel therapeutic approaches to the effective treatment of cardiac arrhythmias, sudden cardiac death, and syncope of cardiac origin by targeting discrete populations of neurons that regulate regional cardiac behavior.

REFERENCES

1. Allen TGJ and Burnstock G. Intracellular studies of the electrophysiological properties of cultured intracardiac neurons of the guinea-pig. *J Physiol* 388: 349–366, 1987.

2. Allen TGJ and Burnstock G. M1 and M2 muscarinic receptors mediate excitation and inhibition of guinea-pig intracardiac neurons in culture. *J Physiol* 422:463–480, 1990.
3. Ardell JL. Structure and function of mammalian intrinsic cardiac neurons. In: Armour JA and Ardell JL, eds. *Neurocardiology*. New York: Oxford University Press, 1994, pp 95–114.
4. Ardell JL. Neurohumoral control of cardiac function. In: Sperelakis N, Kurachi Y, Terzic A and Cohen MV, eds. *Heart Physiology and Pathophysiology*. San Diego: Academic Press, 2001, pp 45–59.
5. Ardell JL, Butler CK, Smith FM, Hopkins DA, and Armour JA. Activity of in vivo atrial and ventricular neurons in chronic decentralized canine hearts. *Am J Physiol* 260:H713–H721, 1991.
6. Ardell JL and Randall WC. Selective vagal innervation of sinoatrial and atrioventricular nodes in canine heart. *Am J Physiol* 251:H764–H773, 1986.
7. Ardell JL, Randall WC, Cannon WJ, Schmacht DC, and Tasdemiroglu E. Differential sympathetic regulation of automatic, conductile and contractile tissue in dog heart. *Am J Physiol* 255:H1050–H1059, 1988.
8. Armour JA. Physiological behavior of thoracic cardiovascular receptors. *Am J Physiol* 225:177–185, 1973.
9. Armour JA. Synaptic transmission in chronically decentralized middle cervical and stellate ganglia of the dog. *Can J Physiol Pharmacol* 61:1149–1155, 1983.
10. Armour JA. Activity of in situ middle cervical ganglion neurons in dogs, using extracellular recording techniques. *Can J Physiol Pharmacol* 63:704–716, 1985.
11. Armour JA. Activity of in situ stellate ganglion neurons of dogs recorded extracellularly. *Can J Physiol Pharmacol* 64:101–111, 1986.
12. Armour JA. Neuronal activity recorded extracellularly in chronic decentralized in situ canine middle cervical ganglia. *Can J Physiol Pharmacol* 64:1038–1046, 1986.
13. Armour JA. Anatomy and function of the intrathoracic neurons regulating the mammalian heart. In: Zucker IH and Gilmore JP, eds. *Reflex Control of the Circulation*. Boca Raton, FL: CRC Press, 1991, pp 1–37.
14. Armour JA. Intrinsic cardiac neurons. *J Neuronal Cardiov Electrophysiol* 2:331–341, 1991.
15. Armour JA. Peripheral autonomic neuronal interactions in cardiac regulation. In: Armour JA and Ardell JL, eds. *Neurocardiology*. New York: Oxford University Press, 1994, pp 219–244.
16. Armour JA. Intrinsic cardiac neurons involved in cardiac regulation possess α_1, α_2, β_1 and β_2 adrenoreceptors. *Can J Physiol Pharmacol* 13:277–284, 1997.
17. Armour JA. Histamine-sensitive intrinsic cardiac and intrathoracic extracardiac neurons influence cardiodynamics. *Am J Physiol* 270:R906–R913, 1996.
18. Armour JA. Comparative effects of endothelin and neurotensin on intrinsic cardiac neurons in situ. *Peptides* 17:1047–1052, 1996.
19. Armour JA. Myocardial ischemia and the cardiac nervous system. *Cardiovasc Res* 41:41–54, 1999.
20. Armour JA, Collier K, Kember G, and Ardell JL. Differential selectivity of cardiac neurons in separate intrathoracic autonomic ganglia. *Am J Physiol* 274:R939–R949, 1998.

21. Armour JA and Hopkins DA. Activity of canine in situ left atrial ganglion neurons. *Am J Physiol* 259:H1207–H1215, 1990.
22. Armour JA and Hopkins DA. Activity of in vivo ventricular neurons. *Am J Physiol* 258:H326–H336, 1990.
23. Armour JA, Huang MH, Pelleg A, and Sylven C. Responsiveness of in situ canine nodose ganglion afferent neurons to epicardial mechanical or chemical stimuli. *Cardiovasc Res* 28:1218–1225, 1994.
24. Armour JA, Huang MH, and Smith FM. Peptidergic modulation of in situ canine intrinsic cardiac neurons. *Peptides* 14:191–202, 1993.
25. Armour JA, Linderoth B, Arora RC, DeJongste MJL, Ardell JL, Kingma JG, Hill M, and Foreman RD. Long-term modulation of the intrinsic cardiac nervous system by spinal cord neurons in normal and ischemic hearts. *Auton Neurosci* 95:71–79, 2002.
26. Armour JA, Murphy DA, Yuan BX, MacDonald S, and Hopkins DA. Gross and microscopic anatomy of the human intrinsic cardiac nervous system. *Anat Rec* 247:289–298, 1997.
27. Armour JA, Yuan BX, and Butler CK. Cardiac responses elicited by peptide administration to canine intrinsic cardiac neurons. *Peptides* 11:753–761, 1990.
28. Arora RC, Ardell JL, and Armour JA. Cardiac denervation and cardiac function. *Curr Interv Cardiol Rep* 2:188–195, 2000.
29. Arora RC, Waldmann M, Hopkins DA, and Armour JA. Porcine intrinsic cardiac ganglia. *Anat Rec* 271A:249–258, 2003.
30. Baluk P and Gabella G. Some intrinsic neurons of the guinea-pig heart contain substance P. *Neurosci Lett* 104:269–273, 1989.
31. Baluk P and Gabella G. Some parasympathetic neurons in the guinea-pig heart express aspects of the catecholaminergic phenotype in vivo. *Cell Tissue Res* 261:275–285, 1990.
32. Bartfai T, Iverfeldt K, Fisone G, and Serfozo P. Regulation of the release of coexisting neurotransmitters. *Annu Rev Pharmacol Toxicol* 28:285–310, 1988.
33. Berecek KH and Brody MJ. Evidence for a neurotransmitter role for epinephrine derived from the adrenal medulla. *Am J Physiol* 242:H593–H601, 1982.
34. Blinder KJ, Gatti PJ, Johnson TA, Lauenstein JM, Coleman WP, Gray AL, and Massari VJ. Ultrastructural circuitry of cardiorespiratory reflexes: there is a monsynaptic path between the nucleus of the solitary tract and vagal preganglionic motoneurons controlling atrioventricular conduction in the cat. *Brain Res* 785:143–157, 1998.
35. Blinder KJ, Johnson TA, and Massari VJ. Negative inotropic vagal preganglionic neurons in the nucleus ambiguus of the cat: neuroanatomical comparison with negative chronotropic neurons utilizing dual retrograde tracers. *Brain Res* 804:325–330, 1998.
36. Bluemel KM, Wurster RD, Randall WC, Duff MJ, and O'Toole MF. Parasympathetic postganglionic pathways to the sinoatrial node. *Am J Physiol* 259:H1504–H1510, 1990.
37. Bosnjak ZJ and Kampine JP. Cardiac sympathetic afferent cell bodies are located in the peripheral nervous system of the cat. *Circ Res* 64:554–562, 1989.
38. Boudreau G, Péronnet F, de Champlain J, and Nadeau R. Presynaptic effects of epinephrine on norepinephrine release from cardiac sympathetic nerves in dogs. *Am J Physiol* 265:H205–H211, 1993.

39. Brodde O-E. Beta-adrenoceptors in cardiac disease. *Pharmacol Ther* 60:405–430, 1993.
40. Brodde O-E and Zerkowski H-R. Neural control of cardiac myocyte function. In: Armour JA and Ardell JL, eds. *Neurocardiology*. New York: Oxford University Press, 1994, pp 193–218.
41. Brown AM. Cardiac reflexes. In: Berne RM, Sperelakis N, and Geiger SR, eds. *Handbook of Physiology, The Cardiovascular System, Section 2, Vol.1, The Heart*. Bethesda, MD: American Physiological Society (Williams and Wilkins), 1979, pp 677–689.
42. Butler CK, Smith FM, Nicholson J, and Armour JA. Cardiac effects induced by chemically activated neruons in canine intrathoracic ganglia. *Am J Physiol* 259:H1108–H1117, 1990.
43. Butler CK, Watson-Wright WM, Wilkinson M, Johnston DE, and Armour JA. Cardiac effects produced by long-term stimulation of thoracic autonomic ganglia or nerves: implications for interneuronal interactions within the thoracic autonomic nervous system. *Can J Physiol Pharmacol* 66:175–184, 1988.
44. Cao J-M, Chen LS, KenKnight BH, Ohara T, Lee M-H, Tsai J, Lai WW, Karagueuzian HS, Wolf PL, Fishbein MC, and Chen P-S. Nerve sprouting and sudden cardiac death. *Circ Res* 86:816–821, 2000.
45. Cao J-M, Fishbein MC, Han JB, Lai WW, Lai AC, Wu T-J, Czer L, Wolf PL, Denton TA, Shintaku P, Chen P-S, and Chen LS. Relationship between regional hyperinnervation and ventricular arrhythmia. *Circulation* 101:1960–1969, 2000.
46. Chapleau MW, Cunningham JT, Sullivan MJ, Wachtel RE, and Abboud FM. Structural versus functional modulation of the arterial baroreflex. *Hypertension* 26:341–347, 1995.
47. Chen P-S, Chen LS, Cao JM, Sharifi B, Karagueuzian HS, and Fishbein MC. Sympathetic nerve sprouting, electrical remodeling and the mechanisms of sudden cardiac death. *Cardiovasc Res* 50:409–416, 2001.
48. Cheng Z, Powley TL, Schwaber JS, and Doyle FJ. Vagal afferent innervation of the atria of the rat heart reconstructed with confocal microscopy. *J Comp Neurol* 381:1–17, 1997.
49. Croom JE, Foreman RD, Chandler MJ, and Barron KW. Cutaneous vasodilation during dorsal column stimulation is mediated by dorsal roots and CGRP. *Am J Physiol* 272:H950–H957, 1997.
50. Crowe R and Burnstock G. Fluorescent histochemical localization of quinacrine-positive neurons in the guinea-pig and rabbit atrium. *Cardiovasc Res* 16:384–390, 1982.
51. Dalsgaard CJ, Franco-Cereceda A, Saria A, Lundberg JM, Theodorsson-Norheim E, and Hökfelt T. Distribution and origin of substance P- and neuropeptide Y-immunoreactive nerves in the guinea-pig heart. *Cell Tissue Res* 243:477–485, 1986.
52. Della NG, Papka RE, Furness JB, and Costa M. Vasoactive intestinal peptide-like immunoreactivity in nerves associated with the cardiovascular system of guinea-pigs. *Neuroscience* 9:605–619, 1983.
53. Eliasson T, Augustinsson LE, and Mannheimer C. Spinal cord stimulation in severe angina pectoris: presentation of current studies, indications and clinical experience. *Pain* 65:169–179, 1996.

54. Eliasson T, Mannheimer C, Waagstein F, Andersson B, Bergh CH, Augustinsson LE, Hedner T, and Larson G. Myocardial turnover of endogenous opoids and CGRP in the human heart and the effects of spinal cord stimulation on pacing-induced angina pectoris. *Cardiology* 89:170–177, 1998.
55. Ellison JP and Hibbs RG. An ultrastructural study of mammalian cardiac ganglia. *J Mol Cell Cardiol* 8:89–101, 1976.
56. Farrell DM, Wei CC, Tallaj J, Ardell JL, Armour JA, Hageman GR, Bradley WE, and Dell'Italia LJ. Angiotensin II modulates catecholamine release into interstitial fluid of canine ventricle in vivo. *Am J Physiol (Heart Circ Physiol)* 281:H813–H822, 2001.
57. Fedida D. Modulation of cardiac contractility by α_1 adrenoceptors. *Cardiovasc Res* 27:1735–1742, 1993.
58. Fee JD, Randall WC, Wurster RD, and Ardell JL. Selective ganglionic blockade of vagal inputs to sinoatrial and/or atrioventricular regions. *J Pharmacol Exp Ther* 242:1006–1012, 1987.
59. Foreman RD. Spinal cord neuronal regulation of the cardiovascular system. In: Armour JA and Ardell JL, eds. *Neurocardiology*. New York: Oxford University Press, 1994, pp 245–276.
60. Foreman RD. Mechanisms of cardiac pain. *Annu Rev Physiol* 61:143–167, 1999.
61. Foreman RD, Linderoth B, Ardell JL, Barron KW, Chandler MJ, Hull SS, Ter-Horst GJ, DeJongste MJL, and Armour JA. Modulation of intrinsic cardiac neurons by spinal cord stimulation: implications for therapeutic use in angina pectoris. *Cardiovasc Res* 47:367–375, 2000.
62. Furukawa Y, Wallick DW, Carlson MD, and Martin PJ. Cardiac electrical responses to vagal stimulation of fibers to discrete cardiac regions. *Am J Physiol* 258:H1112–H1118, 1990.
63. Gagliardi M, Randall WC, Bieger D, Wurster RD, Hopkins DA, and Armour JA. Activity of in vivo canine cardiac plexus neurons. *Am J Physiol* 255:H789–H800, 1988.
64. Gu J, Polak JM, Allen JM, Huang WM, Sheppard MN, Tatemoto K, and Bloom SR. High concentrations of a novel peptide, neuropeptide Y, in the innervation of mouse and rat heart. *J Histochem Cytochem* 32:467–472, 1984.
65. Hancock JC, Hoover DB, and Hougland MW. Distribution of muscarinic receptors and acetylcholinesterase in the rat heart. *J Auton Nerv Syst* 19:59–66, 1987.
66. Hassall CJS and Burnstock G. Intrinsic neurons and associated cells of the guinea-pig heart in culture. *Brain Res* 364:102–113, 1986.
67. Hautvast RW, DeJongste MJL, Staal MJ, Van Gilst VH, and Lie KI. Spinal cord stimulation in chronic intractable angina pectoris: a randomized, controlled efficacy study. *Am Heart J* 136:114–120, 1998.
68. Henegar JR, Brower GL, Kabour A, and Janicki JS. Catecholamine response to chronic ANG II infusion and its role in myocyte and coronary vascular damage. *Am J Physiol* 269:H1564–H1569, 1995.
69. Hoover DB, Chang Y, Hancock JC, and Zhang L. Actions of tachykinins within the heart and their relevance to cardiovascular disease. *Jpn J Pharmacol* 84:367–373, 2000.
70. Hoover DB and Hancock JC. Distribution of substance P binding sites in guinea-pig heart and pharmacological effects of substance P. *J Auton Nerv Syst* 23:189–197, 1988.

71. Hopkins DA and Armour JA. Ganglionic distribution of afferent neurons innervating the canine heart and cardiopulmonary nerves. *J Auton Nerv Syst* 26:213–222, 1989.
72. Hopkins DA and Ellenberger HH. Cardiorespiratory neurons in the medulla oblongata: input and output relationships. In: Armour JA and Ardell JL, eds. *Neurocardiology*. New York: Oxford University Press, 1994, pp 277–308.
73. Hopkins DA, MacDonald S, Murphy DA, and Armour JA. Pathology of intrinsic cardiac neurons from ischemic human hearts. *Anat Rec* 259:424–436, 2000.
74. Horackova M and Armour JA. ANG II modifies cardiomyocyte function via extracardiac and intracardiac neurons: in situ and in vitro studies. *Am J Physiol* 272:R766–R775, 1997.
75. Huang B, El-Sherif T, Gidh-Jain M, Qin D, and El-Sherif N. Alterations of sodium channel kinetics and gene expression in the postinfarction remodeled myocardium. *J Cardiovasc Electrophysiol* 12:226–238, 2001.
76. Huang MH, Ardell JL, Hanna BD, Wolf SG, and Armour JA. Effects of transient coronary artery occlusion on canine intrinsic cardiac neuronal activity. *Integr Physiol Behav Sci* 28:5–21, 1993.
77. Huang MH, Horackova M, Negoescu RM, Wolf SG, and Armour JA. Polysensory response characteristics of dorsal root ganglion neurons that may serve sensory functions during myocardial ischemia. *Cardiovasc Res* 32:503–515, 1996.
78. Huang MH, Smith FM, and Armour JA. Amino acids modify activity of canine intrinsic cardiac neurons involved in cardiac regulation. *Am J Physiol* 264:H1275–H1282, 1993.
79. Huang MH, Smith FM, and Armour JA. Modulation of in situ canine intrinsic cardiac neuronal activity by nicotinic, muscarinic and β-adrenergic agonists. *Am J Physiol* 265:R659–R669, 1993.
80. Huang MH, Sylven C, Pelleg A, Smith FM, and Armour JA. Modulation of in situ canine intrinsic cardiac neuronal activity by local applied adenosine, ATP or analogues. *Am J Physiol* 265:R914–R922, 1993.
81. Huang MH, Wolf SG, and Armour JA. Ventricular arrhythmias induced by chemically modified intrinsic cardiac neurones. *Cardiovasc Res* 28:636–642, 1994.
82. Hull SS, Vanoli E, Adamson PB, De Ferrari GM, Foreman RD, and Schwartz PJ. Do increases in markers of vagal activity imply protection from sudden cardiac death? The case of scopolamine. *Circulation* 91:2516–2519, 1995.
83. Hull SS, Vanoli E, Adamson PB, Verrier RL, Foreman RD, and Schwartz PJ. Exercise training confers anticipatory protection from sudden death during acute myocardial ischemia. *Circulation* 89:548–552, 1994.
84. Jacobowitz D. Histochemical studies of the relationship of chromaffin cells and adrenergic nerves fibers to the cardiac ganglia of several species. *J Pharmacol Exp Ther* 158:227–240, 1967.
85. Jakobs KH, Minuth M, Bauer S, Grandt R, Greiner C, and Zubin P. Dual regulation of adenylate cyclase. A signal transduction mechanism of membrane receptors. *Basic Res Cardiol* 81:1–9, 1986.
86. Katchanov G, Xu J, Clay A, and Pelleg A. Electrophysiological–anatomic correlates of ATP-triggered vagal reflex in the dog. IV. Role of LV vagal afferents. *Am J Physiol (Heart Circ Physiol)* 272:H1898–H1903, 1997.

87. Kember G, Fenton GA, Armour JA, and Kalyaniwalla N. Competition model for aperiodic stochastic resonance in a FitzHugh-Nagumo model of cardiac sensory neurons. *Phys Rev E Stat Nonlin Soft Phys* 63:1–6, 2001.
88. Kuntz A. *The Autonomic Nervous System*. Philadelphia: Lea and Febiger, 1934.
89. Kushiku K, Yamada H, Shibata K, Tokunaga R, Katsuragi T, and Furukawa T. Upregulation of immunoreactive angiotensin II release and angiotensinogen mRNA expression by high-frequency preganglionic stimulation at the canine cardiac sympathetic ganglia. *Circ Res* 88:110–116, 2001.
90. La Rovere MT, Bigger JT, Marcus FI, Mortara A, and Schwartz PJ. Baroreflex sensitivity and heart-rate variability in prediction of total cardiac mortality after myocardial infarction. ATRAMI (Autonomic Tone and Reflexes After Myocardial Infarction). *Lancet* 351:478–484, 1998.
91. Lathrop DA and Spooner PM. On the neural connection. *J Cardiovasc Electrophysiol* 12:841–844, 2001.
92. Levitzki A. Regulation of adenylate cyclase by hormones and G-proteins. *FEBS Lett* 211:113–118, 1987.
93. Levy MN and Warner MR. Parasympathetic effects on cardiac function. In: Armour JA and Ardell JL, eds. *Neurocardiology*. Oxford University Press, 1994, pp 53–76.
94. Lundberg JM, Franco-Cereceda A, Hua X, Hokfelt T, and Fisher JA. Coexistence of substance P and calcitonin gene-related peptide-like immunoreactivities in sensory nerves in relation to cardiovascular and bronchoconstrictor effects of capsaicin. *Eur J Pharmacol* 108:315–319, 1985.
95. Majewski M, Rand MJ, and Tung LH. Activation of prejunctional β-adrenoceptors in rat atria by adrenaline applied exogenously or released as a cotransmitter. *Br J Pharmacol* 73:669–679, 1981.
96. Malliani A. Cardiovascular sympathetic afferent fibers. *Rev Physiol Biochem Pharmacol* 94:11–74, 1982.
97. Mangrum JM and DiMarco JP. The evaluation and management of bradycardia. *N Engl J Med* 342:703–709, 2000.
98. Mannheimer C, Camici P, Chester MR, Collins A, DeJongste MJL, Eliasson T, Follath F, Hellemans I, Herlitz J, Lüscher T, Pasic M, and Thelle D. The problem of chronic refractory angina. Report from the ESC joint study group on the treatment of refractory angina. *Eur Heart J* 23:355–370, 2002.
99. Mannheimer C, Eliasson T, Andersson B, Bergh CH, Augustinsson LE, Emanuelsson H, and Waagstein F. Effects of spinal cord stimulation in angina pectoris induced by pacing and possible mechanisms of action. *BMJ* 307:477–480, 1993.
100. Mannheimer C, Eliasson T, Augustinsson LE, Blomstrand C, Emanuelsson H, Larsson S, Norrsell H, and Hjalmarsson A. Electrical stimulation versus coronary bypass surgery in severe angina pectoris. The ESBY study. *Circulation* 97:1157–1163, 1998.
101. Martin P. Paradoxical dynamic interaction of heart period and vagal activity on atrioventricular conduction in the dog. *Circ Res* 40:81–89, 1977.
102. Massari VJ, Johnson TA, and Gatti PJ. Cardiotopic organization of the nucleus ambiguus? An anatomical and physiological analysis of neurons regulating atrioventicular conduction. *Brain Res* 679:227–240, 1995.
103. McGuirt AS, Schmacht DC, and Ardell JL. Autonomic interactions for control of atrial rate are maintained after SA nodal parasympathectomy. *Am J Physiol* 272:H2525–H2533, 1997.

104. Moravec M, Courtalon A, and Moravec J. Intrinsic neurosecretory neurons of the rat heart atrioventricular junction: possibility of local neuromuscular feed back loops. *J Mol Cell Cardiol* 18:357–367, 1986.
105. Moravec M and Moravec J. Intrinsic innervation of the atrioventricular junction of the rat heart. *Am J Anat* 171:307–319, 1984.
106. Moravec M and Moravec J. Adrenergic neurons and short proprioceptive feedback loops involved in the integration of cardiac function in the rat. *Cell Tissue Res* 258:381–385, 1989.
107. Moravec M, Moravec J, and Forsgren S. Catecholaminergic and peptidergic nerve components of intramural ganglia in the rat heart. *Cell Tissue Res* 262:315–327, 1990.
108. Murphy DA, O'Blenes S, Nassar BA, and Armour JA. Effects of acutely raising intracranial pressure on cardiac sympathetic efferent neuron function. *Cardiovasc Res* 30:716–724, 1995.
109. Murphy DA, Thompson GW, Ardell JL, McCraty R, Stevenson R, Sangalang VE, Cardinal R, Wilkinson M, Craig S, Smith FM, Kingma JG, and Armour JA. The heart reinnervates after transplant. *Ann Thorac Surg* 69:1769–1781, 2000.
110. Oppenheimer SM and Hopkins DA. Suprabulbar neuronal regulation of the heart. In: Armour JA and Ardell JL, eds. *Neurocardiology*. New York: Oxford University Press, 1994, pp 309–342.
111. O'Toole MF, Wurster RD, Phillips JG, and Randall WC. Parallel baroreceptor control of sinoatrial rate and atrioventricular conduction. *Am J Physiol (Heart Circ Physiol)* 246:H149–H153, 1984.
112. O'Toole MF, Ardell JL, and Randall WC. Functional interdependence of discrete vagal projections to the SA and AV nodes. *Am J Physiol* 251:H398–H404, 1986.
113. Pauza DH, Skripka V, Pauziene N, and Stropus R. Anatomical study of the neural ganglionated plexus in the canine right atrium: Implications for selective denervation and electrophysiology in the sinoatrial node in dog. *Anat Rec* 255:271–294, 1999.
114. Péronnet F, Boudreau G, de Champlain J, and Nadeau RA. Effect of increases in myocardial epinephrine content on epinephrine release from the dog heart. *Can J Physiol Pharmacol* 71:884–888, 1993.
115. Péronnet F, Boudreau G, de Champlain J, and Nadeau RA. Effect of changes in myocardial epinephrine stores on plasma norepinephrine gradient across the dog heart. *Am J Physiol* 266:H2404–H2409, 1994.
116. Pinto JM and Boyden PA. Electrical remodeling in ischemia and infarction. *Cardiovasc Res* 42:284–297, 1999.
117. Plecha DM, Randall WC, Geis GS, and Wurster RD. Localization of vagal preganglionic somata controlling sinoatrial and atrioventricular nodes. *Am J Physiol* 255:R703–R708, 1988.
118. Randall DC, Brown DR, Li SG, Olmstead ME, Kilgore JM, Sprinkle AG, Randall WC, and Ardell JL. Ablation of posterior atrial ganglionated plexus potentiates sympathetic tachycardia to behavioral stress. *Am J Physiol* 275:R779–R787, 1998.
119. Randall DC, Randall WC, Brown DR, Yingling JD, and Raisch RM. Heart rate control of awake dog after selective SA-nodal parasympathectomy. *Am J Physiol* 262:H1128–H1135, 1992.
120. Randall WC. Efferent sympathetic innervation of the heart. In: Armour JA

and Ardell JL, eds. *Neurocardiology*. New York: Oxford University Press, 1994, pp 77–94.
121. Randall WC and Ardell JL. Nervous control of the heart: anatomy and pathophysiology. In: Zipes DP and Jalife J, eds. *Cardiac Electrophysiology: From Cell to Bedside*. Philadelphia: W.B. Saunders, 1990, pp 291–299.
122. Randall WC, Armour JA, Geis GS, and Lippincott DB. Regional cardiac distribution of sympathetic nerves. *Fed Proc* 31:1199–1208, 1972.
123. Rigel DF. Effects of neuropeptides on heart rate in dogs: comparison of VIP, PHI, NPY, CGRP, and NT. *Am J Physiol* 255:H311–H317, 1988.
124. Roudenok V, Gutjar L, Antipova V, and Rogov Y. Expression of vasoactive intestinal polypeptide and calcitonin gene-related peptide in human stellate ganglia after acute myocardial infarction. *Ann Anat* 183:341–344, 2001.
125. Rowell RB. *Human Cardiovascular Control*. New York: Oxford University Press, 1993.
126. Sanderson JE, Brooksby P, Waterhouse D, Palmer RB, and Neubauer K. Epidural spinal electrical stimulation for severe angina: a study of its effects on symptoms, exercise tolerance and degree of ischemia. *Eur Heart J* 13:628–633, 1992.
127. Sanderson JE, Ibrahim B, Waterhouse D, and Palmer RB. Spinal cord stimulation for intractable angina: long-term clinical outcome and safety. *Eur Heart J* 15:810–814, 1994.
128. Schmidt HH, Schurr C, Hedler L, and Majewski M. Local modulation of noradrenaline release in vivo: presynaptic β_2-adrenoceptors and endogenous adrenaline. *J Cardiovasc Pharmacol* 6:641–649, 1984.
129. Schoebel FC, Frazier OH, Jessurun GAJ, DeJongste MJL, Kadipasaoglu KA, Jax TW, Heintzen MP, Cooley DA, Strauer BE, and Leschke M. Refractory angina pectoris in end-stage coronary artery disease: evolving therapeutic concepts. *Am Heart J* 134:587–602, 1997.
130. Schwartz DD and Eikenburg DC. Cardiovascular responsiveness to sympathetic activation after chronic epinephrine administration. *J Pharmacol Exp Ther* 238:148–154, 1986.
131. Schwartz PJ, Billman GE, and Stone HL. Autonomic mechanisms in ventricular fibrillation induced by myocardial ischemia during exercise in dogs with a healed myocardial infarction: an experimental preparation for sudden cardiac death. *Circulation* 69:790–800, 1984.
132. Schwartz PJ, La Rovere MT, and Vanoli E. Autonomic nervous system and sudden cardiac death. Experimental basis and clinical observations for post-myocardial infarction risk stratification. *Circulation* 85:I77–I91, 1992.
133. Schwartz PJ, Vanoli E, Stramba-Badiale M, De Ferrari GM, Billman GE, and Foreman RD. Autonomic mechanisms and sudden death. New insights from analysis of baroreflexes in conscious dogs with and without myocardial infarction. *Circulation* 78:969–979, 1988.
134. Senzaki H, Gluzband YA, Pak PH, Crow MT, Janicki JS, and Kass DA. Synergistic exacerbation of diastolic stiffness from short-term tachycardia-induced cardiodepression and angiotensin II. *Circ Res* 82:503–512, 1998.
135. Senzaki H, Paolocci N, Gluzband YA, Lindsey ML, Janicki JS, Crow MT, and Kass DA. β-blockade prevents sustained metalloproteinase activation and diastolic stiffening induced by angiotensin II combined with evolving cardiac dysfunction. *Circ Res* 86:807–815, 2000.

136. Shvalev VN and Sosunov AA. A light and electron microscopic study of cardiac ganglia in mammals. *Z Mikrosk Anat Forsch* 99:676–694, 1985.
137. Smith FM, Hopkins DA, and Armour JA. Electrophysiological properties of in vitro intrinsic cardiac neurons in the pig (*Sus scrofa*). *Brain Res Bull* 28: 715–725, 1992.
138. Smith FM, McGuirt AS, Hoover DB, Armour JA, and Ardell JL. Chronic decentralization of the heart differentially remodels canine intrinsic cardiac neuron muscarinic receptors. *Am J Physiol (Heart Circ Physiol)* 281:H1919–H1930, 2001.
139. Smith FM, McGuirt AS, Leger J, Armour JA, and Ardell JL. Effects of chronic cardiac decentralization on functional properites of canine intracardiac neurons in vitro. *Am J Physiol (Regul Integr Comp Physiol)* 281:R1474–R1482, 2001.
140. Sternini C and Brecha N. Distribution and colocalization of neuropeptide Y- and tyrosine hydroxylase-like immunoreactivity in the guinea-pig heart. *Cell Tissue Res* 241:93–102, 1985.
141. Sylven C. Angina pectoris. Clinical characteristics, neurophysiological and molecular mechanisms. *Pain* 36:145–167, 1989.
142. Tallaj J, Wei CC, Hankes GH, Holland M, Rynders P, Dillon AR, Ardell JL, Armour JA, Lucchesi PA, and Dell'Italia LJ. β_1-adrenergic receptor blockade attenuates angiotensin II-mediated catecholamine release into the cardiac interstitium in mitral regurgitation. *Circulation* 108:225–230, 2003.
143. Thompson GW, Collier K, Ardell JL, Kember G, and Armour JA. Functional interdependence of neurons in a single canine intrinsic cardiac ganglionated plexus. *J Physiol* 528:561–571, 2000.
144. Thompson GW, Hoover DB, Ardell JL, and Armour JA. Canine intrinsic cardiac neurons involved in cardiac regulation possess NK1, NK2 and NK3 receptors. *Am J Physiol* 275:R1683–R1689, 1998.
145. Thompson GW, Horackova M, and Armour JA. Chemotransduction properties of nodose ganglion cardiac afferent neurons in guinea-pigs. *Am J Physiol (Regul Integr Comp Physiol)* 279:R433–R439, 2000.
146. Thompson GW, Horackova M, and Armour JA. Role of P_1 purinergic receptors in myocardial ischemia sensory transduction. *Cardiovasc Res* 53:888–901, 2002.
147. Thoren P. Characteristics of left ventricular receptors with nonmedullated vagal afferents in cats. *Circ Res* 40:415–421, 1977.
148. Thoren P. Role of cardiac vagal c-fibers in cardiovascular control. *Rev Physiol Biochem Pharmacol* 86:1–94, 1979.
149. Urban L and Papka RE. Origin of small primary afferent substance P–immunoreactive nerve fibers in the guinea-pig heart. *J Auton Nerv Syst* 12: 321–331, 1985.
150. Vanoli E and Adamson PB. Baroreflex sensitivity: methods, mechanisms and prognostic value. *PACE* 17:434–445, 1994.
151. Vanoli E, DeFerrari GM, Stramba-Badiale M, Hull SS, Foreman RD, and Schwartz PJ. Vagal stimulation and prevention of sudden death in conscious dogs with a healed myocardial infarction. *Circ Res* 68:1471–1481, 1991.
152. Weihe E, Reinecke M, and Forssmann WG. Distribution of vasoactive intestinal polypeptide–like immunoreactivity in the mammalian heart: Interrelation with neurotensin- and substance P–like immunoreactive nerves. *Cell Tissue Res* 236:527–540, 1984.

153. Wharton J and Gulbenkian S. Peptides in the mammalian cardiovascular system. *Experientia* 43:821–832, 1987.
154. Wharton J, Polak JM, Gordon L, Banner NR, Springall DR, Rose M, Khagani A, Wallwork J, and Yacoub MH. Immunohistochemical demonstration of human cardiac innervation before and after transplantation. *Circ Res* 66:900–912, 1990.
155. White JC. Cardiac pain: anatomical pathways and physiologic mechanisms. *Circulation* 16:644–655, 1954.
156. Wijffels M, Kirchhof C, Dorland R, Power J, and Allessie MA. Electrical remodeling due to atrial fibrillation in chronically instrumented conscious goats. Roles of neurohumoral changes, ischemia, atrial stretch and high rate of electrical activation. *Circulation* 96:3710–3720, 1997.
157. Xi X, Randall WC, and Wurster RD. Morphology of intracellularly labeled canine intracardiac ganglion cells. *J Comp Neurol* 314:396–402, 1991.
158. Xi-Moy SX, Randall WC, and Wurster RD. Nicotinic and muscarinic synaptic transmission in canine intracardiac ganglion cells innervating the sinoatrial node. *J Auton Nerv Syst* 42:201–214, 1993.
159. Yuan BX, Ardell JL, Hopkins DA, and Armour JA. Differential cardiac responses induced by nicotine sensitive canine atrial and ventricular neurons. *Cardiovasc Res* 27:760–769, 1993.
160. Yuan BX, Ardell JL, Hopkins DA, Losier AM, and Armour JA. Gross and microscopic anatomy of the canine intrinsic cardiac nervous system. *Anat Rec* 239:75–87, 1994.
161. Zhang L, Tompkins JD, Hancock JC, and Hoover DB. Substance P modulates nicotinic responses of intracardiac neurons to acetylcholine in the guinea pig. *Am J Physiol (Regul Integr Comp Physiol)* 281:R1792–R1800, 2001.
162. Zucker IH, Wang W, Brandle M, and Schultz HD. Baroreflex and cardiac reflex control of the circulation in pacing-induced heart failure. In: Spinale FG, ed. *Pathophysiology of Tachycardia-Induced Heart Failure*. Armonk, NY: Futura Publishing Company, 1996, pp. 193–226.

5
Integrative Control of Cardiac Function by Cervical and Thoracic Spinal Neurons

ROBERT D. FOREMAN, MIKE J.L. DEJONGSTE,
AND BENGT LINDEROTH

Angina pectoris is regarded as a warning signal for jeopardized cardiac tissue and elicits a very strong emotional component. This type of pain, in general, is a treatable symptom, however, in some patients angina becomes refractory to conventional therapies. For these patients, chest pain associated with angina does not serve as a useful warning signal. Furthermore, these patients need to adapt their lifestyle accordingly and are often forced to severely restrict their physical activity. The exact mechanisms and neural network behind the manifestation of angina pectoris are obscure.

This chapter will begin with a brief summary of the modern concepts of the neural mechanisms behind angina pectoris. Our main aim, however, is to discuss the integrative action of high cervical and thoracic cardiovascular regulatory systems in normal and in ischemically compromised hearts. Chemical activation of neurons in the upper cervical segments of the spinal cord reduces activity of spinal neurons in T1–T5 segments in animals and electric activation of the dorsal spinal cord reduces the number of episodes of angina pectoris in humans. Furthermore, vagal afferent stimulation activates neurons of the upper cervical segments and suppresses the activity of upper thoracic spinal neurons. This intriguing upper cervical region is positioned between the supraspinal nuclei and the thoracic spinal circuitry (Fig. 5–1). As a consequence, neurons in the C1–C2 segments could serve as a filter, an integrator, or as a relay for afferent information since they also receive inputs from vagal afferents from the heart. We will also discuss interdependent interactions

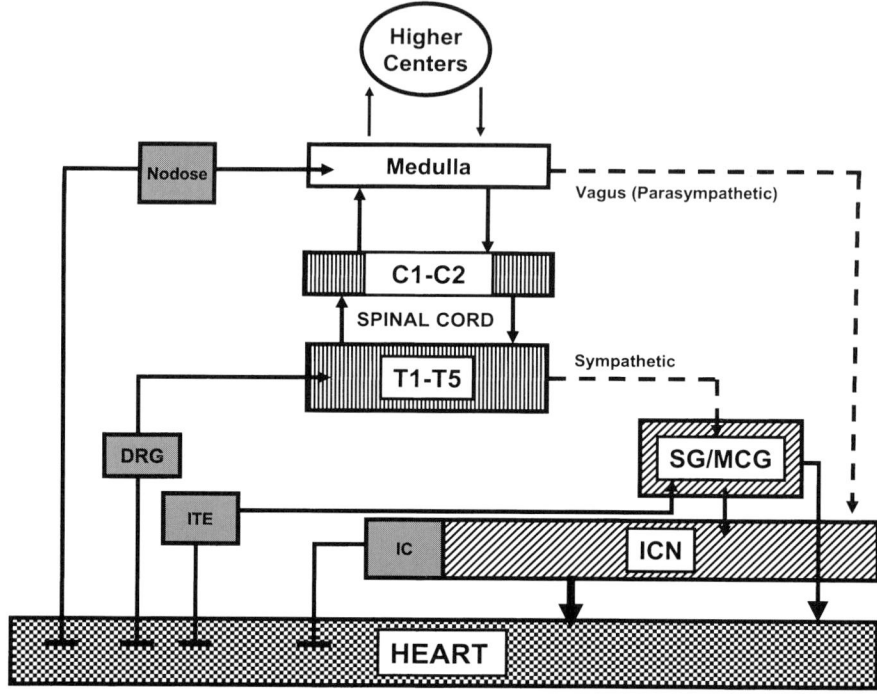

FIGURE 5–1 Schematic diagram outlining the major elements of the neuronal hierarchy that controls the heart. This figure summarizes the emerging concept of interdependent interactions occurring between the central nervous system and periphery for such cardiac control. The black arrows depict interactions between the different levels within the neural hierarchy. The dashed lines represent vagal (parasympathetic) efferent (medulla) and sympathetic efferent (T1–T5 spinal cord) inputs to the intrathoracic ganglia and to the heart. The gray lines, stippled boxes, and arrows illustrate afferent feedbacks derived from cardiac sensory neurites. For spinal control mechanisms, both cervical (C1–C2) and thoracic (T1–T5) neurons are involved. The peripheral aspects of the cardiac neuronal hierarchy are represented by the intrinsic cardiac nervous system (ICN) and extracardiac ganglia (SG/MCG). The solid arrows between the ganglia and the heart illustrate the direct and successive synaptic relays within this autonomic neuronal hierarchy to the heart. Note that ICN and SG/MCG contain afferent and efferent neurons, as well as local circuit neurons. The hierarchy of peripheral autonomic nested feedback loops functions in an interdependent manner to regulate regional cardiac function on a beat-to-beat basis. DRG, dorsal root ganglia; IC, intrinisic cardiac afferents; ITE, intrathoracic extracardiac afferents; SG, stellase ganglia; MCG, middle cervical ganglia.

between the spinal cord and intrathoracic nervous system both in the framework of overall integrated cardiac control and as an example of therapy specifically targeted at parts of the cardiac nervous system in heart disease.

ANGINA PECTORIS AND MYOCARDIAL ISCHEMIA

In stressed normal hearts, lactate and other metabolic substances are usually produced at increasing rates before oxygen supply and demand become metabolically imbalanced. The cardiorespiratory threshold that ultimately limits the exercise is determined by the onset of unpleasant sensations such as fatigue, shortness of breath, muscle tension, and weakness induced by these metabolically active substances.[66]

In contrast, patients with advanced coronary artery disease during exercise often experience a crushing, constrictive, suffocating discomfort usually in the upper substernal area, sometimes radiating to adjacent areas (predominantly left side) such as arms, neck, throat, and the lower jaw before they feel fatigue or shortness of breath. This momentary "pain" was first recognized as a clinical identity by Heberden, who defined the "agchonè" (the Greek root means "a rope to hang") on the chest ("pectoris"), as "a strangling sensation with a feeling of anxiety."[58] Only a century ago was angina pectoris linked to myocardial ischemia.[67] Given a normal arterial oxygen content within a wide arterial pressure range, the oxygen supply to the myocardium can be augmented six to eightfold through an autoregulatory response to meet the increased demand.[93] However, patients with a critical atherosclerotic stenosis (i.e., >75% narrowing) in one or more coronary arteries are not able to sufficiently adapt the oxygen supply to meet the increased metabolic demand of cardiomyocytes during exercise. The subsequent myocardial ischemia produces a metabolic imbalance between glucose oxidation and glycolysis and is responsible for alteration in excitation–contraction coupling with evolving (regional) contraction failure. In the ischemic heart, both in stable circumstances and predominantly during physical exercise, the "anginal warning signal" is transmitted to the central nervous system through afferent neural pathways[118] by local induction of the release of a variety of compounds such as potassium, lactate, adenosine, bradykinin, and prostaglandins,[105,127] which are able to sensitize and excite high-threshold nerve endings in the myocardium.[87] The provoked visceral nociception is characterized by its vaguely located "emotionally charged" distribution and by the influence of emotions on the experience of the anginal pain. In this respect, it is worth noting that mental stress appears to produce myocardial ischemic alterations similar to those from physical exercise.[37]

Finally, the released metabolic compounds also affect the responsiveness of motor neuron commands. The reactivity of motor neurons, depending on impulses relayed by the spinothalamic tract to medullary neurons of the cardiorespiratory centers, is influenced by central (i.e., reflexes in the spinal cord) and peripheral factors (e.g., receptors in the muscles).[12] The reduced responsiveness during exercise in cardiovascularly compromised patients is associated with activation of the sympathetic nervous system, resulting in a paradoxical reaction to limited exercise with increased heart rate and ventilation frequency.[49]

The Clinical Problem: Refractory Angina Pectoris

Typically, chronic stable angina can be treated with revascularization procedures such as percutaneous transluminal angioplasty or coronary artery bypass surgery and/or with medications such as angiotensin-converting enzyme (ACE) inhibitors, β blockers, and calcium channel blockers. However, a significant number of patients have chronic refractory angina pectoris—i.e., they do not get sufficient pain relief or restoration of function even from available surgical and optimal medical treatment.[39,63] On the basis of conservative criteria, it has been estimated that approximately 100,000 patients per year in the North America and an equal number in Europe are diagnosed as suffering from this chronic condition.[102] To standardize adjunct treatments and therapeutically assess these patients, an algorithm has been developed by the European Society of Cardiology Joint Study Group. This group, Kim et al.,[68] Mannheimer et al.,[89] and Mulcahy et al.[103] concluded that at present electrical neuromodulation may be one of the best available adjunct therapies for refractory angina.

Electrical Heart Neuromodulation: Transcutaneous Electrical Nerve Stimulation and Spinal Cord Stimulation

Electrical neuromodulation of the heart encompasses both the delivery of high-frequency, low-amplitude pulses to the chest wall via electrodes glued to the skin (transcutaneous electrical nerve stimulation [TENS]) and to the dorsal column surface of the spinal cord via an epidurally placed cathode lead that is advanced up to the T1–T2 segments (spinal cord stimulation [SCS]; Fig. 5–2). Both therapies have proven to be strikingly effective with more than 80% of patients experiencing pain relief.[44] A very important point is that patients who receive SCS therapy still experience the pain when severe ischemia occurs at a high work load and experience the warning of an impending myocardial infarction even when the stimulator is active.[4,57,65,104,120] Thus, the "angina" warning system is still intact, even though the angina threshold is raised.[57] This therapy, as judged by many researchers and clinicians is safe, minimally invasive, reversible,

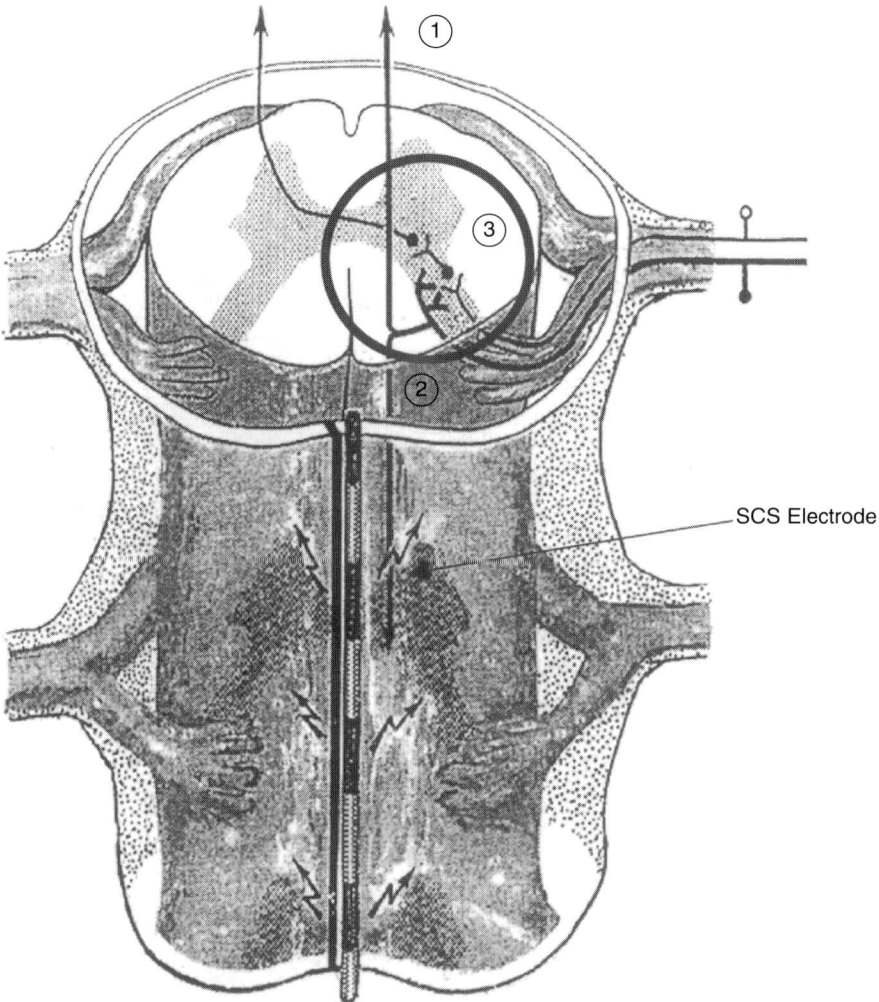

FIGURE 5–2 The Gate Control concept for suppression of pain with spinal cord stimulation (SCS). The mulipolar electrode, applied to the dorsal epidural surface, activates transmission of orthodromic (1) and antidromic (2) impulses in fibers of the dorsal columns. The orthodromic activity elicits paraesthesias in patients. Antidromic impulses are carried via dorsal column fiber collaterals to the dorsal horn below the cathode(s) where they excite neurons of the outer laminae. The activity in these neurons most likely invokes the "gate mechanism" (encircled; 3) that produces inhibitions of impulses in the small-diameter fiber systems the subserve nociception. (Redrawn after Linderoth and Meyerson.[80])

and cost-effective.[4,45,65,97,120] The present state of knowledge about physiological mechanisms involved in the beneficial effects of SCS as well as its utilization as a tool to study the neural control of the heart will be further discussed later in this chapter.

Processing of Cardiac Nociceptive Stimuli

Episodes of myocardial ischemia activate cardiac afferent neurons whose fibers course in both sympathetic[16,17] and vagus nerves (see Chapter 3).[131] Angina pectoris that often occurs during ischemic episodes is attributed to activation of sympathetic afferent fibers that enter the T1–T6 spinal cord segments.[71,140] Stimulation of these afferent fibers in acute animal experiments excites spinal neurons that are found primarily in the dorsal horns of the upper thoracic segments.

Responses of T1–T4 Spinal Neurons

Current knowledge about spinal processing of cardiac sensory information is based largely on recordings of extracellular potentials from individual neurons. An important component is how the central nervous system processes cardiac afferent activity being transmitted via the sympathetic and vagal afferent fibers. This section highlights the contributions of information transmitted in the sympathetic afferent fibers to thoracic spinal neurons, while a subsequent section will address the sympathetic and vagal inputs to the cervical as well as thoracic segments (Fig. 5–3).

The classical concept of acute cardiac nociception is based on a serial neuronal system that transmits information from cardiac afferents to spinal neurons. The transfer of information is mediated by classical neurotransmitters, such as excitatory amino acids, that induce membrane potential changes within a time span of milliseconds to seconds. Thus, nociceptive stimulation of cardiac afferents evokes discharge rates of spinal neurons that increase as long as the nociceptors are stimulated.[11,145] It is generally assumed that impulses of spinal neurons responding to cardiac stimuli constitute a simple renewal process with a very high number of degree of freedom.[126] In Foreman's[47] electrophysiological studies designed to study cardiac nociception, nociceptive responses of spinal neurons were determined on the basis of mean discharge rates of single neurons. In support of this classical concept, it was shown that discharge rates are often correlated in a generally linear manner to the intensity of noxious stimulation, and antinociception is consequently defined as a reduction in discharge rates of nociceptive neurons.[145]

Integrative Control of Cardiac Function 159

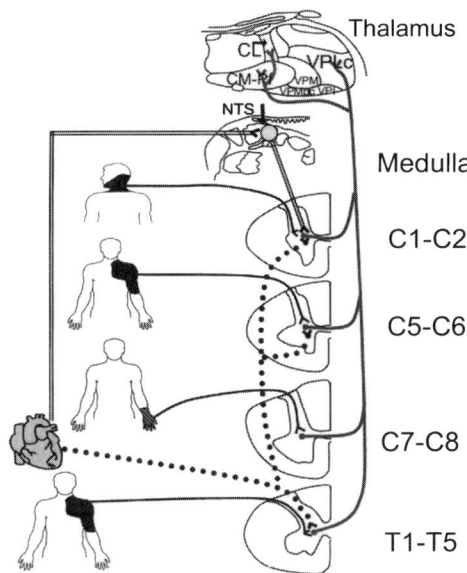

FIGURE 5-3 Schematic diagram outlining the neural organization to explain referred pain associated with angina pectoris. The spinothalamic tract (STT) cells in the cervical (C) and thoracic (T) areas are represented as a solid grey line connecting the segments of the thalamus. The STT ends in the lateral (VPLc) and medial (CM-Pf) nuclei of the thalamus. Solid black lines from figurines represent somatic afferent nerves. The dashed lines are cardiac afferent fibers that enter the T1–T5 spinal segments and the ascending pathway that bypasses C7–C8 segments and enters upper cervical segments. The long open lines are the vagal afferent fibers that synapse in the nucleus tractus solitarius (NTS) of the medulla, and the fibers sending information from the NTS to the C1–C2 STT cells. The black areas on the figurines represent primarily muscle input from the chest and upper arm and neck and jaw. The stippled area is the cutaneous input from the hand and distal arm. CL, nucleus, centralis lateralis; CM-Pf, centrum medianum parafascicular nucleus; VPI, ventral posteroinferior nucleus; VPLc, ventral posterolateral nucleus, caudal part; VPM, ventral posteromedial nucleus; VPMpc, ventral posteromedial nucleus, parvocellular part. (Redrawn from Foreman.[47])

Sympathetic afferents from the heart convey noxious[9,16,83,133,134] and mechanical,[21,88] presumably innocuous, information via the dorsal roots primarily to the upper thoracic segments.[61,71,107] Both centrally projecting as well as non-projecting upper thoracic neurons respond to noxious stimuli applied to the heart.[2,3,13,14,59,111,139] These same neurons receive nociceptive somatic inputs from the upper chest and triceps region of the forelimb.[2,3,13,14,59,111] It has also been shown that parasternal and forelimb dermal neurostimulation, conveying impulses via somatic afferents to the upper spinal cord, induces neuronal activity in the spinothalamic tract (STT).[40] This convergence of visceral and somatic input onto a common pool of STT cells provides a mechanism to explain pain referral to somatic structures in angina pectoris.[47] A typical example of an upper thoracic cell responding to somatic and noxious chemical stimulation of the heart is shown in Fig. 5–4. The marked increase in spontaneous activity and in the chemically evoked responses after rostral C1 spinal transection demonstrated that this cell was tonically inhibited by pathways descending from the upper cervical and supraspinal regions. The presence of tonic modulation supports the idea that there is a hierarchy of control or modulation from the upper cervical spinal cord. Intrapericardial injections of algogenic chemicals generally increased the activity of T3–T4 spinal neurons, but the activity decreased in a few cells.[111] Mechanical stimulation of the somatic fields on the chest and forelimbs activated afferent fibers that converged onto T3–T4 spinal neurons.

Stimulation of the heart with algogenic chemicals provides a simple but efficient method for activating cardiac afferent neurons. Coronary artery occlusion in rats (Fig. 5–5) also serves as a stimulus to activate spinal neurons or spinal reflexes and elicits responses in T3 spinal neurons. It remains to be elucidated whether the results of coronary artery experiments are comparable to the results of the experiments using algogenic chemical stimulation of cardiac afferent afferent neurons.

In addition to electrophysiological studies, c-*fos* studies have been performed to identify cells in the upper thoracic spinal cord that respond to noxious cardiac stimulation.[40] The early gene c-*fos* serves as a marker of

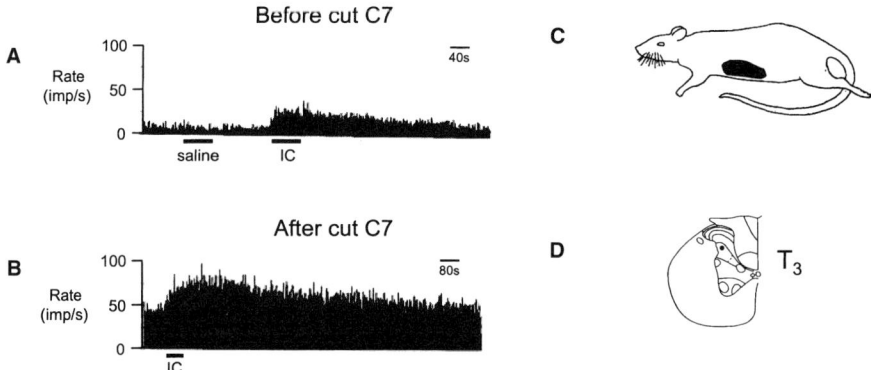

FIGURE 5–4 Responses of a T3 spinal neuron to visceral and somatic stimulation. **A,B.** Responses of the cell to saline (**A**) and to intrapericardial injections of algogenic chemicals (IC) before (**A**) and after (**B**) spinal cord transaction at the C7 segment. imp/s, impulses per second. **C.** Location of the somatic receptive field is represented by the black ellipse on the rat figurine. **D.** A cross section of the spinal cord with the black dot marking the location of the recording site for this cell. (Redrawn from Qin et al.[111])

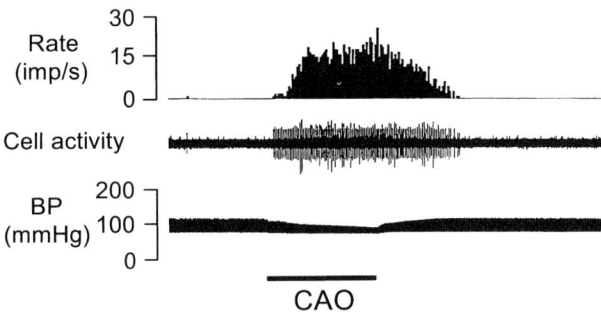

FIGURE 5–5 Response of a T3 deeper spinal neuron to occlusion of the left coronary artery (CAO). The top trace is the rate of cell discharges in impulses per second (imp/s). The second trace shows the raw record of the individual extracellular action potentials (cell activity). The third trace is blood pressure (BP) in mmHg. The horizontal bar represents the period for CAO. The occlusion was maintained for 1 minute.

neuronal activity to study the mediation of either cardiac noxious stimuli, dermal neurostimulation, or both. It should be noted that c-*fos* is not a marker of pain itself, but may reflect cell activity and cannot distinguish whether the activity produces inhibitory or excitatory effects. Finally, c-*fos* also gives an impression about the populations of cells that may be responding, which may be more difficult to determine when a single cell at a time is studied.

An intriguing finding was the expression of c-*fos* at the upper thoracic spinal level after nociceptive stimulation of the heart. Pericardial capsaicin injection, as a cardiac noxious stimulus, also induced c-*fos* expression in lamina III and IV of the dorsal horns at these levels.[1a] These laminae, plus the deeper laminae V and VII, are the locations of the cells of origin of the STT. The laboratory of Foreman[47] has shown in anaesthetised primates that the firing of STT cells after various stimuli increased after intracardiac infusion of bradykinin. Since cells were found with c-*fos* expression, it may be that capsaicin is able to activate cardiac receptors in the same way as bradykinin does. Furthermore, Bolser et al.[15] demonstrated that cardiac nervous stimulation with either bradykinin or capsaicin injections into the pericardium activated spinoreticular neurons. However, capsaicin stimulation excited and inhibited the activity of equal numbers of cells that did not project supraspinally, whereas bradykinin predominately excited spinal neurons. Thus, the fewer cells observed in the spinal cord of capsaicin-activated c-*fos* studies compared to the bradykinin-induced activity might be due to activation of different populations of cells with these two chemicals. In addition, the use of anaesthetised and vagotomised animals might also be contributing factors to the differences.

Responses of C1–C2 Neurons

Commonly, pain resulting from ischemic heart disease is referred to the chest, left arm, and sometimes the right arm.[119] Less frequently, pain is referred to the neck and jaw regions. Surgical sympathectomies in humans commonly abolish or relieve angina pectoris;[82,140,141] however, sympathectomy occasionally unmasked pain referred to the neck and jaw or revealed stress-induced pain in these regions. The more rostral location of this pain led investigators to suggest that vagal afferent fibers may be involved in the transmission of nociceptive information from the thoracic region and also from other regions. A proposal was made that nociceptive vagal information might converge onto STT cells of the upper cervical segments receiving somatic information from the neck and jaw region. Results of a study in primates showed that stimulation of cardiac receptors with algogenic chemicals injected into the pericardial sac predominately increased activity of the C1–C2 STT neurons (Fig. 5–3).[26] Nerve ablation experiments demonstrate that interruption of ipsilateral vagal fibers significantly reduces the mean increase in activity of 80% of the C1–C2 STT cells in response to intrapericardiac algogenic chemicals. These results support the idea that cardiac vagal afferents transmit most of the nociceptive information to C1–C2 STT neurons. In addition, noxious somatic input most commonly from the neck, jaw, ear, and upper arm regions converges onto these STT cells.[24,26] Thus, these results are consistent with the suggestion that activation of cardiac vagal fibers might lead to production of referred pain sensation, particularly in neck and jaw regions. These results also indicate that nociceptive information from the heart could modulate the activity of upper cervical segments.

UPPER CERVICAL MODULATION OF THORACIC SPINAL CORD ACTIVITY

Within the hierarchy for cardiac control, we suggest that neurons of the upper cervical segments modulate information processing in the spinal neurons of the upper thoracic segments. This suggestion is based on results of both human and animal studies. In human studies, SCS of the upper cervical segments relieves pain in patients with angina pectoris.[53] Preliminary experimental studies in our laboratory have shown that SCS applied to the upper cervical segments of the spinal cord in rats suppressed the activity of spinal neurons in the T3–T4 segments (Fig. 5–6). Further evidence for upper cervical modulation of the thoracic spinal cord comes from a preliminary study indicating that chemical stimulation of

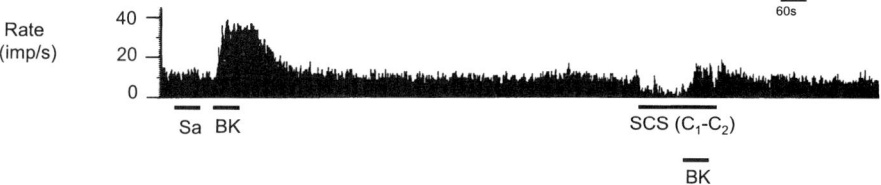

FIGURE 5–6 Effects of upper cervical (C1–C2) spinal cord stimulation (SCS) on responses of a T3 cell to intrapericardial injections of bradykinin (BK). Saline (Sa) was used as a control. The first BK injection is the SCS control. Electrical stimulation (250 µA, 250 µs, and 50 Hz) of the ipsilateral C1–C2 dorsal columns applied prior to the second intrapericardial injection of BK markedly reduced the evoked responses. Horizontal lines are the period of the stimulus.

cells in the C1–C2 segments also reduced upper thoracic spinal neuronal activity. These preliminary results are reinforced by an earlier study demonstrating that chemical stimulation of C1–C2 cells suppresses activity of lumbosacral spinal neurons even after the spinal cord was transected at the spinomedullary junction.[109]

C1 Modulation of Upper Thoracic Cell Activity

We originally assumed that supraspinal pathways were necessary for descending inhibitory effects of visceral afferents on sensory neurons. However, based on the evidence from a previous study,[109] it was hypothesized that cell bodies located in the gray matter of C1–C2 spinal segments can modulate nociceptive cardiac-evoked activity of spinal neurons in the upper thoracic spinal cord (Fig. 5–7). To address this hypothesis, effects of glutamate activation of cell bodies in the upper cervical spinal cord on the activity of cells in the T3–T4 spinal cord evoked by injections of bradykinin (BK) into the pericardial sac were examined. Glutamate has been used to activate cell bodies in the cervical spinal cord in previous studies.[109,121,123] Glutamate (1 M) was absorbed onto filter paper pledgets (2 × 2 mm), which were placed on the dorsal surface of the C1–C2 segments. Saline control pledgets were applied at the same sites before and after glutamate. Saline elicited no responses. In pilot experiments, evoked activity was recorded from a T3 cell to glutamate before (Fig. 5–8) and after rostral C1 transections. These transections were made to demonstrate that supraspinal pathways were not necessary to elicit the effects from C1 cell activation. The preliminary results showed that chemical stimulation of C1 cell bodies with glutamate suppressed the evoked responses of T3 cells to algogenic chemical stimulation of cardiac afferent fibers (Fig. 5–8). After accounting for the reduction in the spontaneous activity after glutamate application, the

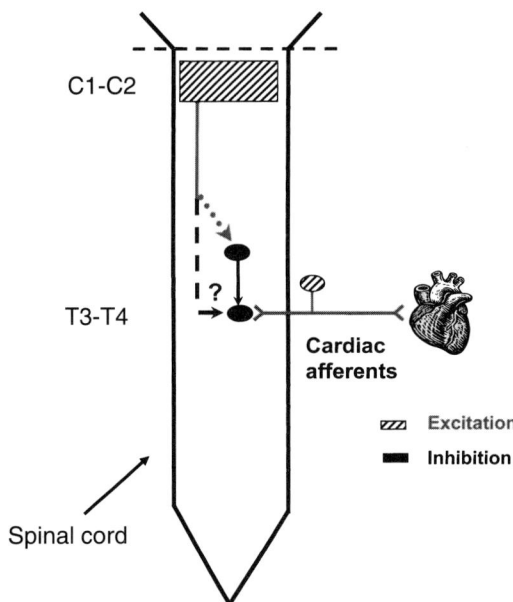

FIGURE 5–7 Schematic diagram of the possible pathway for upper cervical modulation of the activity of thoracic spinal neurons. The cross-hatched box represents the propriospinal neurons projecting to the thoracic segments. The activity of T3–T4 spinal neurons evoked by activation of cardiac afferents is modulated by propriospinal neurons, represented by the lines between the cervical and thoracic segments. It is hypothesized that either these projections directly inhibit the T3–T4 spinal neurons or such inhibition is mediated via an intervening inhibitory interneuron.

evoked response was much smaller than the control response. Supraspinal pathways were not required because the effects remained after rostral C1 spinal transaction. These preliminary results suggest that cells in the upper cervical segments may serve as an important relay in the hierarchy of cardiac control that modulates the activity of cells in thoracic segments.

C1–C3 Descending Propriospinal Neurons

Since activation of cardiopulmonary afferent and vagal afferent fibers excite C1–C3 neurons and suppress activity of thoracic spinothalamic tract cells and spinal neurons, propriospinal neurons should be available to transmit the information from the cervical to the thoracic spinal cord. To identify the propriospinal neurons, extracellular activity of C1–C3 neurons was antidromically activated by stimulating their axons most commonly in the ipsilateral ventrolateral quadrant of the thoracic spinal cord (Fig. 5–9).[25,144] Stimulation of the cardiopulmonary afferent fibers and vagal afferent fibers above but not below the heart increased the activity of the propriospinal neurons. This study demonstrates an electrophysiological basis for the transmission of information from the cervical to thoracic spinal cord as has been observed clinically.[53]

Some anatomical studies have been performed to identify projections and locations of C1–C3 descending propriospinal neurons. In monkeys,

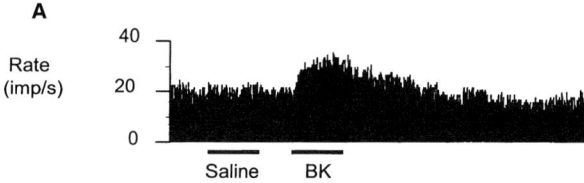

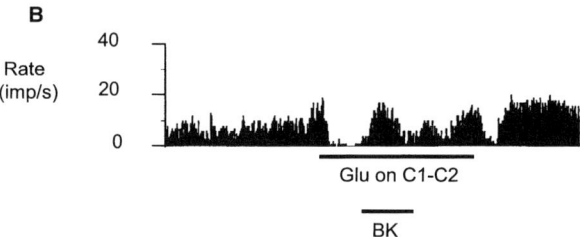

FIGURE 5–8 Responses of T3 cell to application of glutamate on the dorsal surface of the C1–C2 segments. **A.** Responses were evoked by intrapericardial injections of bradykinin (BK). Saline was used as the control. **B.** Pledgets of glutamate placed on the C1–C2 dorsal spinal cord decreased the discharge rate of the cell for the 3-minute period during which it was applied. Background activity recovered after glutamate was removed. imp/s, impulses per second.

horseradish peroxidase (HRP) injected in thoracic spinal cord labeled C1–C2 cells in the lateral cervical nucleus, the central gray region, lamina I, and lateral regions of laminae V–VIII.[20] In rats, fluorogold or HRP injected in lumbosacral segments labeled C1–C2 cells primarily in laminae V and X, the lateral cervical nucleus, and the ventral horn.[100] Similar distributions of C1–C3 neurons were found in cats after HRP injections in upper lumbar segments.[94,143] Recording sites marked by lesions in our electrophysiological study described above were located in laminae that were labeled in various anatomical studies; however, lesions also were found in lamina IV.

VAGAL MODULATION AND THE SPINAL HIERARCHY

An interesting finding is the differential processing of cardiac vagal afferent information in the cervical and thoracic spinal cord. We have shown in previous studies that electrical and chemical stimulation of vagal afferent fibers primarily excites neurons of the C1 and C2 segments (cf Fig.

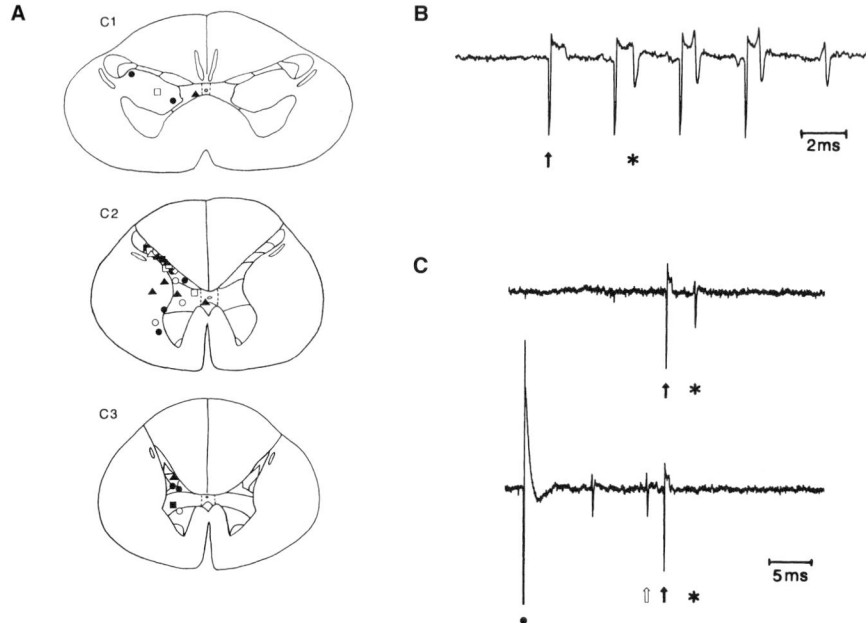

FIGURE 5–9 Locations of recording sites and identification of descending propriospinal neurons. **A.** The various symbols represent the lesion sites of C1–C3 descending propriospinal neurons that were located histologically ($n = 30$). Spinal cord drawings are based on Apkarian and Hodge.[4a] **B.** An example of antidromic activation of a left C1 neuron from an electrode in left ventrolateral quadrant of the T4 segment. Antidromic impulses followed a high-frequency train stimulus (333 Hz). Arrow, first of four stimulus artifacts; *, first of four antidromic impulses. **C.** *Top:* Stimulus artifact (black arrow) followed by antidromic impulse. *Bottom:* Antidromic impulse was blocked (*) when it collided with an orthodromic impulse produced by electrically stimulating the stellate ganglion. Open arrow, orthodromic impulse; ●, stimulus artifact from cardiopulmonary sympathetic afferent stimulation stimulation. (Redrawn from Chandler et al.[25])

5–3).[26,110] It should be pointed out that these cervical cells also receive input that is carried to the thoracic spinal cord via the sympathetic afferents. However, vagal information elicits larger (evoked) responses. In contrast to excitation of upper cervical spinal neurons, vagal input from the cardiopulmonary region generally reduces neuronal activity in sensory cells of rats, cats, and monkeys in segments below C3 (Fig. 5–10);[1,23,60,115,130] vagal facilitation of responses to noxious inputs is reported only at low-stimulus intensities.[115,117] Antinociceptive effects of vagal stimulation were also found in the tail-flick response in rats,[112–114] and vagotomy attenuates opioid-mediated and stress-induced analgesia.[85,86] Thus the mechanisms are complex.

Vagal Modulation of T3–T4 Neurons via C1–C2 Segments

Electrical stimulation of the vagal afferent neurons, in general, suppresses the activity of the upper thoracic spinal neurons (Fig. 5–10). We also have shown that electrical and chemical stimulation of vagal afferent neurons excites upper cervical spinal neurons. Previous studies have demonstrated the importance of the vagus for the balance that is necessary for cardiac regulation following a myocardial infarction.[29,38,46,70,72,73,124,125] However, it has not yet been elucidated whether elimination of the vagus and chemical disruption of upper cervical cell activity will affect the

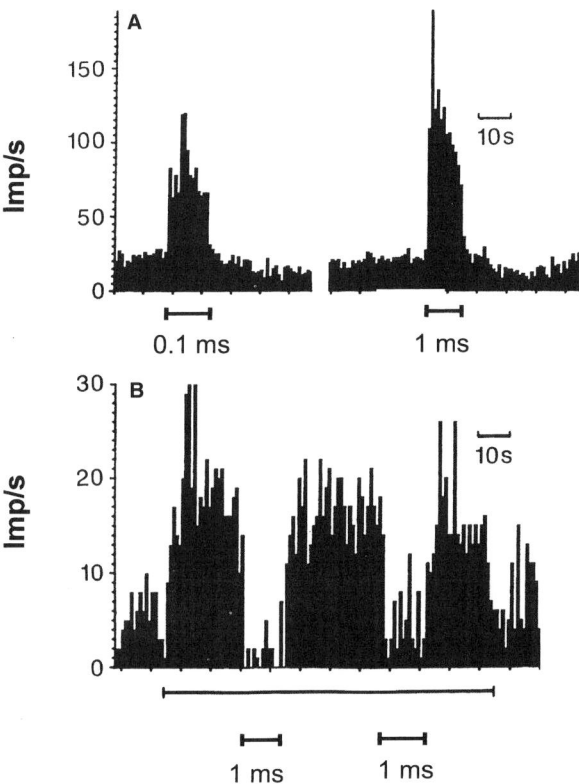

FIGURE 5–10 Effects of vagal afferent stimulation on the activity of a spinothalamic tract cell in the C1–C2 segments (**A**) and a spinothalamic tract cell in the C4 segment (**B**) in the same experiment. The thoracic vagus above the heart was stimulated electrically (30 V, 0.1 ms or 1 ms, and 10 Hz). The impulses of the spinothalamic tract cells were led through a ratemeter to produce the discharge patterns in impulses/second (Imp/s). The short horizontal bars represent the duration of vagal stimulation and the values below them represent the duration of each stimulus pulse. The long horizontal bar in B represents stimulation of the somatic receptive field by brushing the hair to increase the background activity.

coherence and correlation of activity (or independence) of different populations of neurons within and between segments of the spinal cord.

We propose that at least part of the vagal inhibitory effects of the upper thoracic neurons might depend on the C1–C2 relay. Our preliminary results support this possibility. We have demonstrated that disruption of C1–C2 neurons with the excitotoxin ibotenic acid eliminated the suppressor effects of vagal stimulation on thoracic spinal neurons. Vagal suppression of evoked activity of thoracic spinal neurons resulting from intrapericardial injections of algogenic chemicals was also attenuated or eliminated after ibotenic acid administration on the cord. We propose that the inhibitory effects of vagal modulation on the neuronal networks of the thoracic spinal cord depend in part on activation of relays in the upper cervical spinal cord.

The Role of Vagal Activation Reconsidered

Propriospinal neurons in the upper cervical segments are excited by vagal stimulation.[24,25,144] These results demonstrate that direct descending pathways from supraspinal nuclei to the thoracic, as well as lumbosacral, segments are not required to produce the suppressive effects of vagal stimulation. In fact, it is possible that vagal stimulation evokes activity in the subcoeruleus/parabrachial (SC/PB) pathway, which then excites the propriospinal neurons of the upper cervical segments.[116] In addition to the SC/PB pathway, a portion of vagal afferent information might be transmitted directly to C1–C2 segments[95] or be relayed via axons that project directly from the NTS to the upper cervical segments.[101] One important notion from this discussion is that neurons of the upper cervical segments can modulate the activity of thoracic cells receiving cardiac afferent input especially from vagal afferent stimulation.

So what is the role of the vagal afferent fibers in producing the inhibitory effects on sensory processing and sympathetic efferent activity? Contrary to the idea that activation of vagal afferent fibers may induce visceral pain, except in the neck and jaw regions, vagal afferent neurons may serve as an important rapid-signaling pathway for communicating the immunological changes from the periphery to the areas in the brain that respond to infection and inflammation.[28,43,51,52,84] In turn, mediators of inflammation then induce the production of vasoactive neurohumoral compounds.[42] Acute inflammatory reactions in animal models are induced by injecting the endotoxin lipopolysaccharide (LPS) intraperitoneally or intravenously.[36,132] The inflammatory reaction systemically causes the release of interleukin (IL)-1, IL-6, IL-1β, and tumor necrosis factor-α (TNF-α), which is a potent mediator of the systemic responses. The release of these inflammatory cytokines triggers several systemic responses that include altered pain sensitivity and metabolism, hyperthermia, and increased release of adrenocorticotropin (ACTH), glucocorticoids, and liver acute-phase proteins.[10,129,138] An important point is that at least some of the systemic responses to inflammation depend on the integrity of the vagal afferent pathway. The evidence shows that some of the inflammatory cytokines resulting from LPS injections systemically activate the vagal afferents.[18,43,51] Furthermore, vagal afferent neuron stimulation is required to induce the increased expression of mRNA and protein levels of IL-1β in the hypothalamus and activate the hypothalamus–pituitary–adrenal axis.[54,55,62]

In addition, the activation of this vagal pathway to supraspinal structures, such as the hypothalamus and the amygdala, stimulates descending antinociceptive pathways that may provide projections of a visceral organ against local inflammatory reactions resulting from intraperitoneal LPS administration.[28] It is thus possible that vagal activation resulting from the release of cytokines might inhibit the activity of spinothalamic tract cells and spinal neurons in the thoracic segments as well as in the lumbosacral segments. To support this idea, preliminary studies have shown that after LPS administration into the intrapericardial space, evoked thoracic cell activity to intrapericardial injections of bradykinin is gradually reduced over a 4-hour period. However, the suppressed evoked responses are reversed after bilateral cervical vagotomy. Thus, the vagal afferent neuron pathway to supraspinal structures could be important for eliciting the activation of immune responses resulting from systemic infections and inflammation and might not be the pathway that contributes to the perception of angina pectoris.

SPINAL CORD STIMULATION AND THE NEURAL HIERARCHY OF CARDIAC CONTROL

On the basis of the Gate-Control Model provided by Melzack and Wall,[96] electrical stimulation of the spinal cord (SCS) has been applied to relieve a variety of chronic pain conditions.[75,99,106] Conceivably, since the electrodes are applied onto the surface of the dorsal dura mater overlying the spinal cord (see Fig. 5–2), the dorsal columns are certainly activated, as indicated by the evoked paresthesiae experienced by the patient (thus the early label DCS). There are also many observations of autonomic effects of SCS: increased peripheral microcirculation, increased skin temperature, and depression of autonomic reflexes.[77,80] After three decades of clinical use, the common experience is that neuropathic pain of peripheral origin remains the typical indication for treatment with SCS.[98,99] Pain conditions of a predominantly nociceptive origin and "mixed pain syndromes" seemed to respond much less. However, since the late 1970s, SCS has also been found effective for pain in tissue ischemia;[99] this was first discovered in patients with occlusive arterial disease in their legs.[30] The stimulation-induced effects of this type of pain, however, seem to be related to a direct effect on the ischemic state, with a secondary and slower relief of the ischemic pain.[77]

Spinal Cord Stimulation in Cardiac Pain

Since the mid-1980s, cardiac pain has been successfully treated both with TENS[90] and subsequently by SCS with electrode positioning at a high thoracic (T1–T2) level.[39,63] Spinal cord stimulation was initially met with skepticism, especially by cardiologists, who questioned if a technique eliminating the angina signaling severe coronary ischemia[4,65,91] could be a therapy to recommend. After several studies demonstrating that SCS cannot eliminate signs of critical cardiac ischemia, does not increase the number of arrhythmic episodes,[41,44] does not impair left ventricular function, and produces fewer side effects than many pharmaceutical regimens,[44] this therapy has been adopted in several cardiology centers, specifically with the advent of newer adjunct treatments like laser and gene therapy.[68,89] In Europe, SCS has been used in angina therapy for more than a decade. At present approximately 3000 cases have been implanted for this indication worldwide. It is estimated that since 2002, approximately 400 or more new implants are performed annually in Europe alone.

Clinical Outcome

Paradoxically enough, SCS for treatment of angina pectoris has proved to be much more effective and dependable than in neuropathic pain conditions. The success rate for relieving angina pectoris is often in the range of 80% or greater after several years of follow-up.[39,44,63] In fact, a randomized, prospective study of 104 patients with a high surgical risk showed that SCS is equally effective as bypass surgery in eliminating angina at half-year follow-up but that the thoracic surgery carried significantly more instances of morbidity and even mortality.[92] Besides the reduction in angina pectoris, clinical studies have shown that myocardial ischemia is reduced following SCS.[39,91]

Technique

The procedure for SCS to alleviate angina pectoris involves the insertion, under local anesthesia, of a multipolar lead through a Tuohy needle puncturing the epidural space at approximately the T5–T6 level.*[99] The lead is then advanced rostrally up to the T1–T2 segments and placed midline or just to the left of midline (depending on the distribution of the patient's angina). The SCS is turned on (typical stimulation parameters: 50–100 Hz; 0.2–0.4 ms; and intensity to produce comfortable parethesias) and tests are run to confirm that paresthesias evoked by activation of the stimulator is sensed in the somatic regions where the patients usually experience the angina pectoris. A pulse-generator is then implanted subcutaneously and connected to the electrode system (Fig. 5–11). The patients manage stimulation themselves using a simple remote control.

A typical therapeutic patient regimen would be low-amplitude stimulation three times a day for 1 hour in addition to strong stimulation (3–4 minutes) during an angina attack.[39] The protocols vary considerably among different centers and some centers recommend at least 6–8 hours of stimulation time per day.

An important finding for mechanisms discussed in this chapter is that human studies have shown SCS of the C1–C2 spinal segments to relieve pain symptoms as well as T1–T2 SCS in patients with chronic refractory angina pectoris.[53] The challenge now is to determine the underlying mechanisms that produce the anginal pain relief experienced with SCS applied to these different regions and to relate this to present knowledge of the spinal control hierarchy.

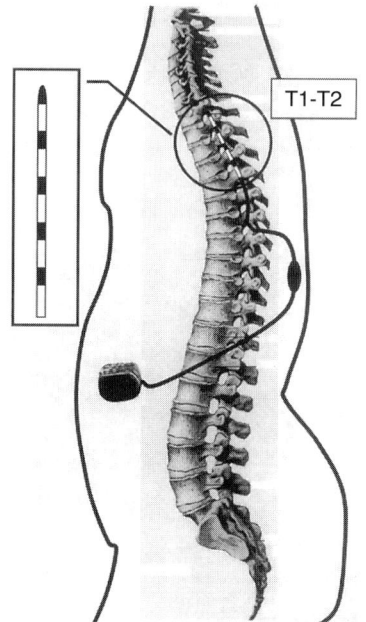

FIGURE 5–11 Spinal cord stimulation system implanted for therapy of refractory angina pectoris. Active poles of the electrode were positioned at the T1–T2 level after puncture of the epidural space at about T6. Subcutaneous extension wires connect the electrode to the pulse generator implanted on the anterior abdominal wall.

Previous Conceptions of Physiological Mechanisms

According to the Gate Theory of Melzack and Wall,[96] all types of nociceptive transmission in the spinal dorsal horn are equally inhibited by the simultaneous activation of large myelinated fibers (e.g., in the dorsal columns, which antidromically would "close the gate"). This proved not to be the case, since acute nociception was not blocked (e.g., a patient would still feel a pinch applied to a leg, but experience relief of a neuropathic pain component).[77] Attenuation of nociceptive pain conditions with SCS seems to rest on fundamentally different physiological mechanisms from those needed to eliminate neurogenic pain.[77,80]

Suppression of Central Sensitization

In neuropathic pain, both peripheral and central neuronal sensitization contributes to the translation to chronicity of the condition.[33,77,98] In conditions with long-lasting neuropathic symptoms following peripheral nerve injury in experimental animals, hypersensitization of central neurons (i.e., wide dynamic range (WDR) cells in the dorsal horns) has been observed.[142] Such conditions also increased release of excitatory transmitters and glutamate in the dorsal horn of rats.[34,35,81] Spinal cord stimulation–induced release of GABA has been shown in the dorsal horn and an inhibitory effect on release of excitatory amino acids seems to be relayed via activation of the $GABA_B$ receptors.[35] Most likely it is this sequence of events that is mirrored in the inhibition by SCS of hyperactive dorsal horn WDR neurons in neuropathic rats.[142] Many other inhibitory circuits in the spinal cord are probably simultaneously activated, which explains why similarly identical clinical cases may respond differently. Few of these systems have as yet been explored.[35,77,79] However, in ischemic pain states there are many indicators of the activation of mechanisms different from those probably involved in neuropathic pain.[7,8,80]

Spinal Cord Stimulation Mechanisms in Ischemia

Experimental studies have confirmed the notion of sympathetic inhibition as one factor behind increased peripheral perfusion. They have also indicated that SCS acts predominantly on sympathetic efferent neurons innervating the peripheral vasculature that transmits via ganglionic nicotinic receptors and acts mainly on α_1-adrenoreceptors at the neuroeffector junction.[76–79] The hypothesis of a possible antidromic component in the effect was first substantiated for near–motor threshold stimulation amplitudes in the studies by Croom et al.[31,32] and was later confirmed for lower SCS amplitudes by Tanaka et al.[128] The current concept holds that at least two complementary mechanisms exist, with the relative participation of the two mechanisms being dependent on the activity level of the sympathetic system.

For more complex vascular beds (e.g., the cardiac circulation), two main hypotheses have been presented: *(1)* SCS alters coronary blood flow by redistribution from a well-perfused ischemic area, and *(2)* SCS decreases cardiac oxidative metabolism (i.e., ischemia is resolved without a demonstrable flow increase).[77] It is still debatable whether total coronary blood flow increases following SCS. In this respect, only Chauhan et al.[27] observed an increase in total coronary blood flow during 5 minutes of TENS. As indicated by positron emission tomography (PET) studies, however, an increase in total coronary blood flow is not required for redistribution of coronary blood flow, and the stimulation-induced flow changes are better described as a "homogenization" of the cardiac circulation.[56] An experimental study on healthy canines with acute ischemia during SCS therapy failed to confirm the clinical findings using PET.[69] There are several studies, however, both clinical and experimental, which demonstrate that the myocardial ischemia in apparently normal and failing hearts may be counteracted by SCS.[39] Since we presently lack firm indicators of a general flow increase or redistribution to ischemic areas, a protective effect by SCS on the cardiomyocytes (e.g., a decrease in oxygen-dependant metabolism) constitutes a strong alternative. There are indications that SCS may induce protective effects in tissues totally deprived of their oxygen supply by shutting off circulation[50] and that this effect may depend on actions of substances such as calcitonin gene–related peptide (CGRP).[50] In addition, the induction of heat shock proteins (HSP) by SCS has been suggested as a protective mechanism.[40]

Recent studies with microdialysis of ischemic and nonischemic coronary tissue during ischemia and SCS have demonstrated a release in the interstitial fluid of the catecholamines, norepinephrine, and epinephrine without affecting left ventricular function (Ardell JL et al., unpublished results). Since Vegh and Parratt[136] showed that both the infusion and local release of endogenous norepinephrine in the canine heart can reduce arrhythmias in the face of ischemic challenge, it is possible that similar mechanisms might also be functioning when SCS is applied during myocardial ischemia. The resultant effects may be related to presynaptic inhibition of local norepinephrine release or mechanisms that invoke preconditioning effects.[137] In pharmacologically induced preconditioning, adenosine and opioids influence the G protein–coupled receptors, which in turn up-regulate protein kinase C; this is thought to phosphorylate the ATP-sensitive K channel, a key player in preconditioning.[136] Since adenosine has strong vasodilatory effects and is involved in pain transmission, this substance may couple the involved neural and cardiac interactions via inhibition of norepinephrine.[19,108] Moreover, dipyridamole, an adenosine reuptake inhibitor, has been found to blunt the effect of SCS.[56] Finally, the intake of caffeine, an adenosine-receptor antagonist, has been observed to impair the effects of neuromodulation.[122] Thus, several observations indicate that SCS, without evoking ischemia, could activate a preconditioning-like mechanism protecting the heart from the consequences of severe myocardial ischemia.

Exploring the Neurocardiac Hierarchy with Spinal Cord Stimulation

Recent experimental observations have indicated a hierarchy of control mechanisms that permits central spinal processing of afferent and efferent autonomic inputs to influence intrinsic cardiac as well as intrathoracic, extracardiac neuronal integration and local neural coordination without necessarily involving the higher brain centers (see Fig. 5–1).[74] We have proposed that under normal, physiological conditions, stimuli applied to the heart do not elicit marked changes in cardiac efferent neuronal activity because central neurons can suppress excessive cardiac sensory information processing. Experimental evidence shows that the central nervous system maintains a tonic inhibitory influence over intrathoracic cardiopulmonary–cardiac reflexes.[5] On the basis of this evidence, it seems probable that disease processes could upset the balance between the central and peripheral neuronal processing of cardiac sensory information.

Recent studies further support the hypothesis that in the hierarchy of cardiac control, activation of spinal neuronal circuits can modulate the intrathoracic cardiac nervous system. Recent canine studies have shown that electrical activation of the dorsal columns at the T1–T2 segments significantly reduces activity generated by the intrinsic cardiac neurons in their basal conditions, as well as when activated in the presence of regional ventricular ischemia.[48] In this study, the dorsal spinal cord at the T1–T2 was stimulated with "clinical parameters" and at an intensity of 90% of motor threshold.[48] Using these parameters, SCS effectively reduced intrinsic cardiac neuronal activity by approximately 77%, whether it was applied before, during, or following the onset of a 2-minute coronary artery occlusion (see Chapter 4, Fig. 4–1). Transection of the subclavian ansae eliminated the suppressor effects of SCS on intrinsic cardiac neural activity, indicating that the responses were due primarily to the influence of spinal cord neurons acting via the sympathetic nervous system. In a follow-up study, SCS for 17 minutes in the face of left anterior coronary ar-

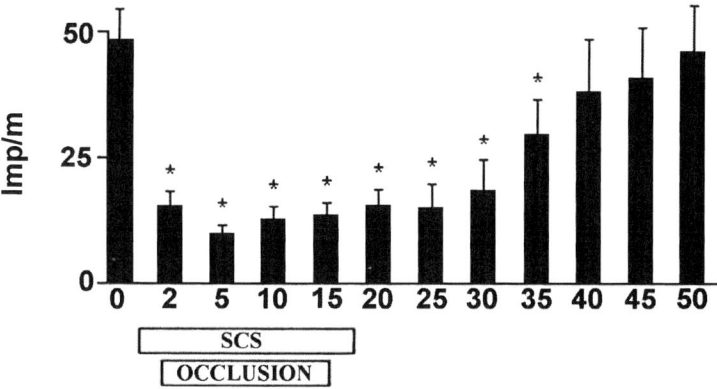

FIGURE 5–12 Histogram showing neuronal activity averaged before, during, and after coronary artery occlusion occurring in the presence of spinal cord stimulation (SCS). SCS (T1–T3) was applied for 17 minutes and the coronary artery occlusion was sustained for 15 minutes. Neuronal activity was significantly suppressed *($P < 0.05$) during SCS and the firing frequency was reduced for up to 45 minutes after termination of SCS. (Redrawn from Armour et al.[6])

tery occlusion for 15 minutes suppressed intrinsic cardiac neuronal activity (-76%) throughout the stimulation period, and suppression could persist for at least 45 minutes after SCS was terminated (Fig. 5–12).[6] This observation, supported by clinical studies, indicates that a cardioprotective benefit may persist even after SCS therapy is discontinued.[64]

Furthermore, it has also been demonstrated that SCS not only modulates the intrinsic cardiac nervous system but it also modifies the cardiac nociceptive activity of spinothalamic tract neurons within the T3–T4 segments (Fig. 5–13).[22] However, in contrast to the long-lasting effects of SCS on the activity of the intrinsic cardiac neurons, the evoked activity of spinothalamic tract cell neurons was suppressed only during SCS.

In summary, SCS may depend on the hierarchical control of the spinal cord to influence the function of the final common neuronal pathway of the heart, the intrinsic cardiac nervous system, in the presence of ischemic challenge. These observations suggest that SCS could limit myocardial ischemia by modifying local regulation of the heart and inhibit local circuits that could otherwise induce arrhythmias leading to more generalized ischemic threats. In either case, effects of SCS on the activity of the intrinsic cardiac nervous system support the important concept of a regulatory hierarchy for cardiac function. We believe that the activity elicited at each level in the hierarchy, from the brain stem to the spinal cord, and further

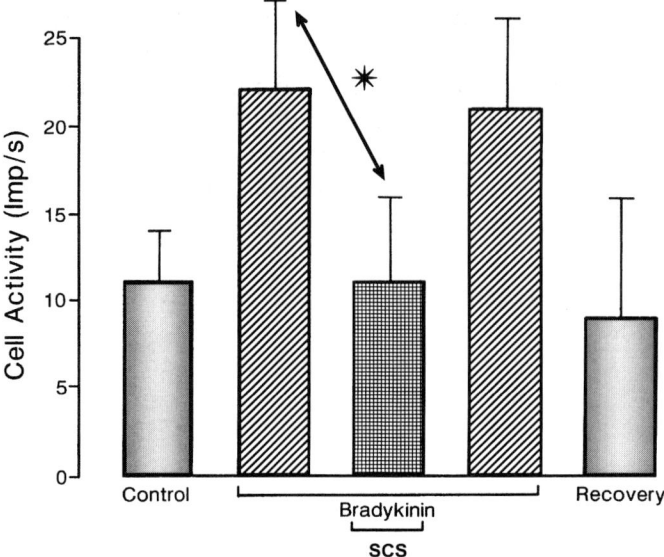

FIGURE 5–13 Summary of responses of T3 spinothalamic tract cells to intrapericardial injections of bradykinin (BK) during spinal cord stimulation (SCS). Electrical stimulation (250 µA, 250 µs, and 50 Hz) of the ipsilateral C1–C2 dorsal columns applied during intrapericardial injections of BK markedly reduced the evoked responses. Arrow represents the significant difference between BK responses before and during SCS application *($P < 0.05$). Horizontal lines are the periods of the stimulus. (Redrawn from Chandler et al.[22]).

to the intrathoracic neurons, is eventually transmitted to the intrinsic cardiac nervous system (see Fig. 5–1 and Chapter 4, Fig. 4–1). Very little information has been published to address underlying mechanisms that could explain how the central and cardiac nervous systems interact to maintain adequate efferent neuronal input to the heart. Disease processes could change the balance between the central and peripheral neurons involved in such regulation. A disturbance in the fine balance within the whole cardiac neuroaxis might result in dramatic changes in cardiac efferent neuronal outflow. As a result, these disturbances could lead to the development of dysrhythmias that might progress to ventricular fibrillation.

CONCLUSIONS

We have presented experimental evidence of a hierarchy in the upper spinal cord, encompassing levels C1–C2 and T1–T4, for the control of cardiac function. Vagal afferents might have a pivotal function in this control system. Electric activation of either the C1–C2 or upper thoracic spinal levels, or stimulation of the vagal nerves, may modulate nociceptive afferent neurons from the heart. Furthermore, and maybe even more interesting, spinal stimulation can control the intrinsic cardiac neurons in both normal conditions and states of acute ischemia. In this way, SCS could serve as a cardioprotective adjunct to pharmacotherapy, reducing the probability that local coronary ischemia, via intrinsic activation, will lead to generalized and potentially life-threatening dysrhythmias. There are also recent studies indicating that SCS could induce protective changes at both cellular and subcellular levels to reduce cell death in the face of critical and persistent cardiac ischemia. Further exploration of the hierarchical organization of spinal control of cardiac function seems important to develop new, effective, and tolerable therapies for patients with ischemically compromised hearts who do not benefit from the standard revascularization procedures aided by optimal pharmacotherapy.

REFERENCES

1a. Albutaihi IA, Hautvast RW, DeTongote MT, Ter Horst GJ, Staal MJ: Cardiac nocoception in rats: neuronal pathways and the influence of dermal neurostimulation on conveyance to the central nervous system. *J Molec Neurosci* 20:43–52, 2003.
1. Ammons WS, Blair RW, and Foreman RD. Vagal afferent inhibition of spinothalamic cell responses to sympathetic afferents and bradykinin in the monkey. *Circ Res* 53:603–612, 1983.
2. Ammons WS, Girardot MN, and Foreman RD. Effects of intracardiac bradykinin on T2–T5 medial spinothalamic cells. *Am J Physiol* 249:R147–R152, 1985.
3. Ammons WS, Girardot MN, and Foreman RD. T2–T5 spinothalamic neurons projecting to medial thalamus with viscerosomatic input. *J Neurophysiol* 54:73–89, 1985.
4. Anderson C, Hole P, and Oxhoj H. Does pain relief with spinal cord stimulation for angina conceal myocardial infarction? *Br Heart J* 71:419–421, 1994.
4a. Apkarian AV and Hodge CJ. Primate spinothalamic pathways: I. A quantitative study of the cells of origin of the spinothalamic pathway. *J Comp Neurol* 288:447–473, 1989.
5. Armour JA. Synaptic transmission in the chronically decentralized middle cervical and stellate ganglia of the dog. *Can J Physiol Pharmacol* 61:1149–1155, 1983.
6. Armour JA, Linderoth B, Arora RC, DeJongste MJ, Ardell JL, Kingma JG Jr, Hill M, and Foreman RD. Long-term modulation of the intrinsic cardiac nervous system by spinal cord neurons in normal and ischemic hearts. *Auton Neurosci* 95:71–79, 2002.
7. Augustinsson LE, Linderoth B, Eliasson T, and Mannheimer C. Spinal cord stimulation in peripheral vascular disease and angina pectoris. In: Gilden-

berg PH and Tasker R, eds. *Textbook of Stereotactic and Functional Neurosurgery*. New York: McGraw-Hill, 1997, pp. 1973–1978.

8. Augustinsson LE, Linderoth B, and Mannheimer C. Spinal cord stimulation in different ischemic conditions. In: Illis LS, ed. *Spinal Cord Dysfunction III: Functional Stimulation*. New York: Oxford University Press, 1992, pp. 270–293.
9. Baker DG, Coleridge HM, Coleridge JC, and Nerdrum T. Search for a cardiac nociceptor: stimulation by bradykinin of sympathetic afferent nerve endings in the heart of the cat. *J Physiol* 306:519–536, 1980.
10. Baumann H and Gauldie J. The acute phase response. *Immunol Today* 15:74–80, 1994.
11. Besson JM and Chaouch A. Peripheral and spinal mechanisms of nociception. *Physiol Rev* 67:67–186, 1987.
12. Bigland-Ritchie B, Jones DA, and Woods JA. Excitation frequency and muscle fatigue: electrical responses during human voluntary and stimulated contractions. *Exp Neurol* 64:414–427, 1979.
13. Blair RW, Weber RN, and Foreman RD. Characteristics of primate spinothalamic tract neurons receiving viscerosomatic convergent inputs in T3–T5 segments. *J Neurophysiol* 46:797–811, 1981.
14. Blair RW, Weber RN, and Foreman RD. Responses of thoracic spinothalamic neurons to intracardiac injection of bradykinin in the monkey. *Circ Res* 51:83–94, 1982.
15. Bolser DC, Chandler MJ, Garrison DW, and Foreman RD. Effects of intracardiac bradykinin and capsaicin on spinal and spinoreticular neurons. *Am J Physiol* 257:H1543–H1550, 1989.
16. Brown AM. Excitation of afferent cardiac sympathetic nerve fibres during myocardial ischaemia. *J Physiol* 190:35–53, 1967.
17. Brown AM and Malliani A. Spinal sympathetic reflexes initiated by coronary receptors. *J Physiol* 212:685–705, 1971.
18. Bucinskaite V, Kurosawa M, Miyasaka K, Funakoshi A, and Lundeberg T. Interleukin-1beta sensitizes the response of the gastric vagal afferent to cholecystokinin in rat. *Neurosci Lett* 229:33–36, 1997.
19. Burgdorf C, Richardt D, Kurz T, Seyfarth M, Jain D, Katus HA, and Richardt G. Adenosine inhibits norepinephrine release in the postischemic rat heart: the mechanism of neuronal stunning. *Cardiovasc Res* 49:713–720, 2001.
20. Burton H and Lowey AD. Descending projections from the marginal cell layer and other regions of the monkey spinal cord. *Brain Res* 116:485–491, 1976.
21. Casati R, Lombardi F, and Malliani A. Afferent sympathetic unmyelinated fibres with left ventricular endings in cats. *J Physiol* 44:81–87, 1979.
22. Chandler MJ, Brennan TJ, Garrison DW, Kim KS, Schwartz PJ, and Foreman RD. A mechanism of cardiac pain suppression by spinal cord stimulation: implications for patients with angina pectoris. *Eur Heart J* 14:96–105, 1993.
23. Chandler MJ, Hobbs SF, Bolser DC, and Foreman RD. Effects of vagal afferent stimulation on cervical spinothalamic tract neurons in monkeys. *Pain* 44:81–87, 1991.
24. Chandler MJ, Zhang J, and Foreman RD. Vagal, sympathetic and somatic sensory inputs to upper cervical (C1–C3) spinothalamic tract neurons in monkeys. *J Neurophysiol* 76:2555–2567, 1996.
25. Chandler MJ, Zhang J, Qin C, and Foreman RD. Spinal inhibitory effects of cardiopulmonary afferent inputs in monkeys: neuronal processing in high cervical segments. *J Neurophysiol* 87:1290–1302, 2002.

26. Chandler MJ, Zhang J, Qin C, Yuan Y, and Foreman RD. Intrapericardiac injections of algogenic chemicals excite primate C1–C2 spinothalamic tract neurons. *Am J Physiol (Regul Integr Comp Physiol)* 279:R560–R568, 2000.
27. Chauhan A, Mullins PA, Thuraisingham SI, Taylor G, Petch MC, and Schofeld PM. Effect of transcutaneous electrical nerve stimulation on coronary blood flow. *Circulation* 89:694–702, 1994.
28. Coelho AM, Fioramonti J, and Bueno L. Systemic lipopolysaccharide influences rectal sensitivity in rats: role of mast cells, cytokines, and vagus nerve. *Am J Physiol (Gastrointest Liver Physiol)* 279:G781–G790, 2000.
29. Cole CR, Blackstone EH, Pashkow FJ, Snader CE, and Lauer MS. Heart-rate recovery immediately after exercise as a predictor of mortality. *N Engl J Med* 341:1351–1357, 1999.
30. Cook AW, Oygar A, Baggenstos P, Pacheco S, and Kleriga E. Vascular disease of extremities. Electric stimulation of spinal cord and posterior roots. *NY State J Med* 76:366–368, 1976.
31. Croom JE, Foreman RD, Chandler MJ, and Barron KW. Cutaneous vasodilation during dorsal column stimulation is mediated by dorsal roots and CGRP. *Am J Physiol* 272:H950–H957, 1997.
32. Croom JE, Foreman RD, Chandler MJ, and Barron KW. Reevaluation of the role of the sympathetic nervous system in cutaneous vasodilation during dorsal spinal cord stimulation: are multiple mechanisms active? *Neuromodulation* 1:91–101, 1998.
33. Cui JG. *Spinal Cord Stimulation in Neuropathy. Experimental Studies of Biochemistry and Behavior*. Stockholm, Sweden: Karolinska Institutet, 1999.
34. Cui JG, Linderoth B, and Meyerson BA. Effects of spinal cord stimulation on touch-evoked allodynia involve GABAergic mechanisms. An Experimental study in the mononeuropathic rat. *Pain* 66:287–295, 1996.
35. Cui JG, O'Connor WT, Ungerstedt U, Meyerson BA, and Linderoth B. Spinal cord stimulation attenuates augmented dorsal horn release of excitatory amino acids in mononeuropathy via a GABAergic mechanism. *Pain* 73:87–95, 1997.
36. Dantzer R. How do cytokines say hellow to the brain? Neural versus humoral mediation. *Eur Cytokine Netw* 5:271–273, 1994.
37. Deanfield JE, Shea M, Kensett M, Horlock P, Wilson RA, de Landsheer XM, and Selwyn AP. Silent myocardial ischemia due to mental stress. *Lancet* 2(8410):1001–1005, 1984.
38. De Ferrari GM, Mantica M, Vanoli E, Hull SS, and Schwartz PJ. Scopolamine increases vagal tone and vagal reflexes in patients after myocardial infarction. *J Am Coll Cardiol* 22:1327–1334, 1993.
39. DeJongste MJ. Spinal cord stimulation for ischemic heart disease. *Neurol Res* 22:293–298, 2000.
40. DeJongste MJ, Hautvast RW, Ruiters MH, and Ter Horst GJ. Spinal cord stimulation and the induction of c-fos and heat shock protein in the central nervous system of rats. *Neuromodulation* 2:27–32, 1998.
41. DeJongste MJ, Nagelkerke D, Hooyschuur CM, Journee HL, Meyler PW, Staal MJ, de Jonge P, and Lie KI. Stimulation characteristics, complications, and efficacy of spinal cord stimulation systems in patients with refractory angina: a prospective feasibility study. *Pacing Clin Electrophysiol* 17:1751–1760, 1994.

42. DeJongste MJ and Ter Horst GJ. Mediators of Inflammation in patients with coronary artery disease. In: Ter Horst GJ, ed. *The Nervous System and the Heart*. Totowa, NJ: Humana Press, 1999, pp 467–490.
43. Ek M, Kurosawa M, Lundeberg T, and Ericsson A. Activation of vagal afferents after intravenous injection of interleukin-1beta: role of endogenous prostaglandins. *J Neurosci* 18:9471–9479, 1998.
44. Eliasson T, Augustinsson LE, and Mannheimer C. Spinal cord stimulation in severe angina pectoris: presentation of current studies, indications and clinical experience. *Pain* 65:169–179, 1996.
45. Eliasson T, Jern S, Augustinsson LE, and Mannheimer C. Safety aspects of spinal cord stimulation in severe angina pectoris. *Coron Artery Dis* 5:845–850, 1994.
46. Ferrell TG, Odemuyiwa O, Bashir Y, Cripps TR, Malik M, Wad DE, and Camm AJ. Prognostic value of baroreflex sensitivity testing after acute myocardial infarction. *Br Heart J* 67:129–137, 1992.
47. Foreman RD. Mechanisms of cardiac pain. *Annu Rev Physiol* 61:143–167, 1999.
48. Foreman RD, Linderoth B, Ardell JL, Barron KW, Chandler MJ, Hull SS Jr, TerHorst GJ, DeJongste MJ, and Armour JA. Modulation of intrinsic cardiac neurons by spinal cord stimulation: implications for its therapeutic use in angina pectoris. *Cardiovasc Res* 47:367–375, 2000.
49. Gadevia SC, Kinlan KJ, and McKenzie DK. Respiratory sensations, cardiovascular control, kinaesthesia, and transcranial stimulations during paralysis in humans. *J Physiol* 470:85–107, 1993.
50. Gheradini G, Lundeberg T, Cui JG, Eriksson SV, Trubek S, and Linderoth B. Spinal cord stimulation improves survival in ischemic skin flaps: an experimental study of the possible mediation via the calcitonin gene-related peptide. *Plast Reconstruct Surg* 103:1221–1228, 1999.
51. Goehler LE, Gaykema RP, Hammack SE, Maier SF, and Watkins LR. Interleukin-1 induces c-fos immunoreactivity in primary afferent neurons of the vagus nerve. *Brain Res* 804:306–310, 1998.
52. Goehler LE, Gaykema RP, Nguyen KT, Lee JE, Tilders FJ, Maier SF, and Watkins LR. Interleukin-1beta in immune cells of the abdominal vagus nerve: a link between the immune and nervous systems? *J Neurophysiol* 19:2799–2806, 1999.
53. Gonzalez-Darder JM, Canela P, and Gonzalez-Martinez V. High cervical spinal cord stimulation for unstable angina pectoris. *Stereotact Funct Neurosurg* 56:20–27, 1991.
54. Hansen MK, Nguyen KT, Goehler LE, Gaykema RP, Fleshner M, Maier SF, and Watkins LR. Effects of vagotomy on lipopolysaccharide-induced brain interleukin-1beta protein in rats. *Auton Neurosci* 85:119–126, 2000.
55. Hansen MK, Taishi P, Chen Z, and Krueger JM. Vagotomy blocks the induction of interleukin-1beta (IL-1beta) mRNA in the brain of rats in response to systemic IL-1beta. *J Neurophysiol* 18:2247–2253, 1998.
56. Hautvast RW, Blanksma PK, DeJongste MJ, Pruim J, van der Wall EE, Vaalburg W, and Lie KI. Effect of spinal cord stimulation on myocardial blood flow assessed by positron emission tomography in patients with refractory angina pectoris. *Am J Cardiol* 77:462–467, 1996.
57. Hautvast RW, Ter Horst GJ, DeJong BM, DeJongste MJ, Blanksma PK, Paans

AM, and Korf J. Relative changes in regional cerebral blood flow during spinal cord stimulation in patients with refractory angina pectoris. *Eur J Neurosci* 9:1178–1183, 1997.
58. Heberden W. Some account of a disorder of the breast. *Med Trans Coll Physicians (Lond)* 2:59, 1772.
59. Hobbs SF, Chandler MJ, Bolser DC, and Foreman RD. Segmental organization of visceral and somatic input onto C3–T6 spinothalamic tract cells of the monkey. *J Neurophysiol* 68:1575–1588, 1992.
60. Hobbs SF, Oh UT, Chandler MJ, and Foreman RD. Cardiac and abdominal vagal afferent inhibitino of primate T9–S1 spinothalamic cells. *Am J Physiol* 257:R889–R895, 1989.
61. Hopkins DA and Armour JA. Ganglionic distribution of afferent neurons innervating the canine heart and cardiopulmonary nerves. *J Auton Nerv Syst* 26:213–222, 1989.
62. Hosoi T, Okuma Y, and Nomura Y. Electrical stimulation of afferent vagus nerve induces IL-1beta expression in the brain and activates HPA axis. *Am J Physiol (Regul Integr Comp Physiol)* 279:R141–R147, 2000.
63. Jessurun GA, DeJongste MJ, and Blanksma PK. Current views on neurostimulation in the treatment of cardiac ischemic syndromes. *Pain* 66:109–116, 1996.
64. Jessurun GA, DeJongste MJ, Hautvast RW, Tio RA, Brouwer J, van Lelieveld S, and Crijns HJ. Clinical follow-up after cessation of chronic electrical neuromodulation in patients with severe coronary artery disease: a prospective randomized controlled study on putative involvement of sympathetic activity. *Pacing Clin Electrophysiol* 22:1432–1439, 1999.
65. Jessurun GA, Ten Vaarwerk IA, DeJongste MJ, Tio RA, and Staal MJ. Seqeulae of spinal cord stimulation for refractory angina pectoris. Reliability and safety profile of long-term clinical application. *Coron Artery Dis* 8:33–38, 1997.
66. Jones NL and Killian KJ. Exercise limitation in health and disease (review). *N Engl J Med* 2000:633–641, 2002.
67. Keefer CS and Resnik WH. Angina pectoris; a syndrome caused by anoxemia of the myocardium. *Arch Intern Med* 41:769, 1928.
68. Kim MC, Kini A, and Sharma SK. Refractory angina pectoris: mechanism and therapeutic options. *J Am Coll Cardiol* 39:923–934, 2002.
69. Kingma JG Jr, Linderoth B, Ardell JL, Armour JA, DeJongste MJ, and Foreman RD. Neuromodulation therapy does not influence blood flow distribution or left-ventricular dynamics during acute myocardial ischemia. *Auton Neurosci* 91:47–54, 2001.
70. Kleiger RE, Miller JP, Bigger JT Jr, and Moss AJ. Decreased heart rate variability and its association with increased mortality after acute myocardial infarction. *Am J Cardiol* 59:256–262, 1987.
71. Kuo DC, Oravitz JJ, and DeGroat WC. Tracing of afferent and efferent pathways in the left inferior cardiac nerve of the cat using retrograde and transganglionic transport of horseradish peroxidase. *Brain Res* 321:111–118, 1984.
72. La Rovere MT, Pinna GD, Hohnloser SH, Marcus FI, Mortara A, Nohara R, Bigger JT, Jr, Camm AJ, and Schwartz PJ. Baroreflex sensitivity and heart rate variability in the identification of patients at risk for life-threatening arrhythmias: implications for clinical trials. *Circulation* 103:2072–2077, 2001.

73. La Rovere MT, Specchia T, Mortara A, and Schwartz PJ. Baroreflex sensitivity, clinical correlates, and cardiovascular mortality among patients with a first myocardial infarction. A prospective study. *Circulation* 78:816–824, 1988.
74. Lathrop DA and Spooner PM. On the neural connection. *J Cardiovasc Electrophysiol* 12:841–844, 2001.
75. Linderoth B. Spinal cord stimulation in ischemic pain. In: Horsch S and Claeys L, eds. *Spinal Cord Stimulation: An Innovative Method in the Treatment of PVD and Angina*. Darmstadt, Germany: Steinkopff Verlag, 1995, pp 19–35.
76. Linderoth B, Fedorcsak I, and Meyerson BA. Peripheral vasodilation after spinal cord stimulation: animal studies of putative effector mechanisms. *Neurosurgery* 28:187–195, 1991.
77. Linderoth B and Foreman RD. Physiology of spinal cord stimulation. Review and update. *Neuromodulation* 2;150–164, 1999.
78. Linderoth B, Gunasekera L, and Meyerson BA. Effects of sympathectomy on skin and muscle microcirculation during dorsal column stimulation: animal studies. *Neurosurgery* 29:874–879, 1991.
79. Linderoth B, Herregodts P, and Meyerson BA. Sympathetic mediation of peripheral vasodilation induced by spinal cord stimulation. Animal studies of the role of cholinergic and adrenergic receptor subtypes. *Neurosurgery* 35:711–719, 1994.
80. Linderoth B and Meyerson BA. Dorsal column stimulation: modulation of somatosensory and autonomic function. In: McMahon SB and Wall PD, eds. *The Neurobiology of Pain*. London: Academic Press, 1995, pp 263–277.
81. Linderoth B, Stiller C-O, Gunasekera L, O'Connor WT, Franck J, Gazelius B, and Brodin E. Release of neurotransmitters in the CNS by spinal cord stimulation. Survey of the present state of knowledge and recent experimental studies. *Stereotact Funct Neurosurg* 61:157–170, 1993.
82. Lindgren I and Olivecrona H. Surgical treatment of angina pectoris. *J Neurosurg* 4:19–39, 1947.
83. Lombardi F, Bella P, Della R, Casati R, and Malliani A. Effects of intracoronary administration of bradykinin on the impulse activity of afferent sympathetic unmyelinated fibers with left ventricular endings in the cat. *Circ Res* 48:69–75, 1981.
84. Maier SF, Goehler LE, Fleshner M, and Watkins LR. The role of vagus nerve in cytokine-to-brain communication. *Ann NY Acad Sci* 840:289–300, 1998.
85. Maixner W and Randich A. Role of the right vagal nerve trunk in antinociception. *Brain Res* 298:374–377, 1984.
86. Maixner W, Touw KB, Brody MJ, Gebhart GF, and Long JP. Factors influencing the altered pain perception in the spontaneously hypertensive rat. *Brain Res* 237:137–145, 1982.
87. Malliani A. The elusive link between transient myocardial ishemia and pain. *Circulation* 73:201–204, 1986.
88. Malliani A, Recordati G, and Schwartz PJ. Nervous activity of afferent cardiac sympathetic fibres with atrial and ventricular endings. *J Physiol* 229:457–469, 1973.
89. Mannheimer C, Camici PG, Chester M, Collins A, DeJongste MJ, Elisson T, Follath F, Hellemans I, Herlitz J, Luscher TF, Pasic M, and Thelle DS. The problem of chronic refractory angina. *Eur Heart J* 23:355–370, 2002.

90. Mannheimer C, Carlson CA, Emanuelsson H, Vedin A, Waagstein F, and Wilhelmson C. The effects of transcutaneous electrical nerve stimulation in patients with severe angina pectoris. *Circulation* 71:308–316, 1985.
91. Mannheimer C, Eliasson T, Andersson B, Bergin CH, Augustinsson LE, Emanuelsson H, and Waagstein F. Effects of spinal cord stimulation in angina pectoris induced by pacing and possible mechanisms of action. *BMJ* 21:307(6902):477–480, 1993.
92. Mannheimer C, Eliasson T, Augustinsson LE, Blomstrand C, Emanuelsson H, Larsson S, Norrsell H, and Hjalmarsson A. Electrical stimulation versus coronary artery bypass surgery in severe angina pectoris: the ESBY study. *Circulation* 97:1157–1163, 1998.
93. Maseri A. The coronary circulation. In: *Ischemic Heart Disease*. New York: Churchill Livingston, 1995, p. 71.
94. Matsushita M, Ikeda M, and Hosoya Y. The location of spinal neurons with long descending axons (long descending propriospinal tract neurons) in the cat: a study with the horseradish peroxidase technique. *J Comp Neurol* 184: 63–80, 1979.
95. McNeill DL, Chandler MJ, Fu QG, and Foreman RD. Projection of nodose ganglion cells to the upper cervical spinal cord in the rat. *Brain Res Bull* 27: 151–155, 1991.
96. Mezack R and Wall PD. Pain mechanisms: a new theory. *Science* 150:971–979, 1965.
97. Merry AF, Smith WM, Anderson DJ, Emmens DJ, and Choong CK. Cost-effectiveness of spinal cord stimulation in patients with intractable angina. *N Z Med J* 114:179–181, 2001.
98. Meyerson BA and Linderoth B. Mechanisms of spinal cord stimulation in neuropathic pain. Invited review. *Neurol Res* 22:285–292, 2000.
99. Meyerson BA and Linderoth B. Spinal cord stimulation. In: Loeser JD, ed. *Bonica's Management of Pain*. Philadelphia: Lippincott Williams & Wilkins, 2000, pp 1857–1876.
100. Miller KE, Douglas VD, Richards AB, Chandler MJ, and Foreman RD. Propriospinal neurons in the C1–C2 spinal segments project to the L5–S1 segments of the rat spinal cord. *Brain Res Bull* 47:43–47, 1998.
101. Mtui EP, Anwar M, Gomez R, Reis DJ, and Ruggiero DA. Projections from the nucleus tractus solitarii to the spinal cord. *J Comp Neurol* 337:231–252, 1993.
102. Mukherjee D, Bahtt D, and Roe MT. Direct myocardial revascularization and angiogenesis: how many patients might be eligible? *Am J Cardiol* 84:598–600, 1999.
103. Mulcahy D, Knight C, Stables R, and Fox K. Lasers, burns, cuts, tingles, and pumps: a consideration of alternative treatments for intractable angina. *Br Heart J* 71:406–408, 1994.
104. Murray S, Carson KG, Ewings PD, Collins PD, and James MA. Spinal cord stimulation significantly decreases the need for acute hospital admission for chest pain in patients with refractory angina pectoris. *Heart* 82:89–92, 1999.
105. Nerdrum T, Baker DG, Coleridge HM, and Coleridge JC. Interaction of bradykinin and prostaglandin E1 on cardiac pressor reflex and sympathetic afferents. *Am J Physiol* 250:R815–R822, 1986.

106. North RD and Linderoth B. Spinal cord stimulation for chronic pain. In: Schmidek HH, ed. *Schmedik and Sweet's Operative Neurosurgical Techniques.* Philadelphia: W.B. Saunders, 2000, pp 2407–2422.
107. Oldfield BJ and McLachlan EM. Localization of sensory neurons traversing the stellate ganglion of the cat. *J Comp Neurol* 182:915–922, 1978.
108. Pernow J. Adenosine as an important mediator of post-ischaemic neuronal stunning. *Cardiovasc Res* 49:693–694, 2001.
109. Qin C, Chandler MJ, Miller KE, and Foreman RD. Chemical activation of cervical cell bodies: effects on responses to colorectal distension in lumbosacral spinal cord of rats. *J Neurophysiol* 82:3423–3433, 1999.
110. Qin C, Chandler MJ, Miller KE, and Foreman RD. Responses and afferent pathways of superficial and deeper C(1)–C(2) spinal cells to intrapericardial algogenic chemicals in rats. *J Neurophysiol* 85:1522–1532, 2001.
111. Qin C, Chandler MJ, Miller KE, and Foreman RD. Chemical activation of cardiac receptors affects activity of superficial and deeper T3–T4 spinal neurons in rats. *Brain Res* 959:77–85, 2003.
112. Randich A and Aicher SA. Medullary substrates mediating antinociception produced by electrical stimulation of the vagus. *Brain Res* 445:68–76, 1988.
113. Randich A and Maixner W. Interactions between cardiovascular and pain regulatory systems. *Neurosci Biobehav Rev* 8:343–367, 1984.
114. Ren K, Randich A, and Gebhart GF. Vagal afferent modulation of a nociceptive reflex in rats: involvement of spinal opioid and monoamne receptors. *Brain Res* 446:285–294, 1988.
115. Ren K, Randich A, and Gebhart GF. Vagal afferent modulation of spinal nociceptive transmission in the rat. *J Neurophysiol* 62:401–415, 1989.
116. Ren K, Randich A, and Gebhart GF. Electrical stimulation of cervical vagal afferents. I. Central relays for modulation of spinal nociceptive transmission. *J Neurophysiol* 4:1098–1114, 1990.
117. Ren K, Randich A, and Gebhart GF. Effects of electrical stimulation of vagal afferents on spinothalamic tract cells in the rat. *Pain* 44:311–319, 1991.
118. Rosen SD, Paulesu E, Frith CD, Frackowiak RSJ, Davies GJD, Jones T, and Camici PG. Central nervous pathways mediating angina pectoris. *Lancet* 344:147–150. 1994.
119. Sampson JJ and Cheitlin MD. Pathophysiology and differential diagnosis of cardiac pain. *Prog Cardiovasc Dis* 13:507–531, 1971.
120. Sanderson JE, Ibrahim B, Waterhouse D, and Palmer RB. Spinal electrical stimulation for intractable angina—long-term clinical outcome and safety. *Eur Heart J* 15:810–814, 1994.
121. Sandkuhler J, Stelzer B, and Fu QG. Characteristics of propriospinal modulation of nociceptive lumbar spinal dorsal horn neuron in the cat. *Neuroscience* 54:957–967, 1993.
122. Sawynok J. Adenosine receptor activation and nociception. *Eur J Pharmacol* 347:1–11, 1998.
123. Schramm LP and Livingstone RH. Inhibition of renal nerve sympathetic ativity by spinal stimulation in rat. *Am J Physiol* 252:R514–R525, 1987.
124. Schwartz PJ, La Rovere MT, and Vanoli E. Autonomic nervous system and sudden cardiac death. Experimental basis and clinical observations for post-myocardial infarction risk stratification. *Circulation* 85:177–191, 1992.
125. Schwartz PJ, Vanoli E, Stramba-Badiale M, De Ferrari GM, Billman GE, and

Foreman RD. Autonomic mechanisms and sudden death. New insights from analysis of baroreceptor reflexes in conscious dogs with and without a myocardial infarction. *Circulation* 78:969–979, 1988.
126. Steedman WM and Zachary S. Characteristics of background and evoked discharges of multireceptive neurons in lumbar spinal cord of cat. *J Neurophysiol* 63:1–15, 1990.
127. Sylven C. Angina pectoris: clinical characteristics, neurophysiological and molecular mechanisms. *Pain* 36:145–167, 1989.
128. Tanaka S, Barron KW, Chandler MJ, Linderoth B, and Foreman RD. Low intensity spinal cord stimulation may induce cutaneous vasodilation via CGRP release. *Brain Res* 896:183–187, 2001.
129. Ter Horst GJ, Nagel JG, DeJongste MJ, and Werf van der YD. Selective blood–brain barrier dysfunction after intravenous injections of rTNFa in the rat. In: Teelken A and Korf J, eds. *Neurochemistry and Neuroimmunology of EAE: Implicatons for Therapy of MS*. New York: Plenum Press, 1997, 141–146.
130. Thies R and Foreman RD. Descending inhibition of spinal neurons in the cardiopulmonary region by electrical stimulation of vagal afferent nerves. *Brain Res* 207:178–183, 1981.
131. Thoren PN. Activation of left ventricular receptors with non-medulled vagal afferent fibers during occlusion of coronary artery in the cat. *Am J Cardiol* 37:1046–1051, 1976.
132. Tilders FJ, DeRijk RH, Van Dam AM, Vincent VA, Schotanus K, and Persoons JH. Activation of the hypothalamus-pituitary-adrenal axis by bacterial endotoxins: routes and intermediate signals. *Psychoneuroendocrinology* 19:209–232, 1994.
133. Uchida U and Murao S. Afferent sympathetic nerve fibers originating in left atrial wall. *Am J Physiol* 227:753–758, 1974.
134. Uchida Y and Murao S. Excitation of afferent cardiac sympathetic nerve fibers during coronary occlusion. *Am J Physiol* 226:1094–1099, 1974.
135. Vance WH and Bowker RC. Spinal origins of cardiac afferents from the region of the left anterior descending artery. *Brain Res* 258:96–100, 1983.
136. Vegh A and Parratt JR. Noradrenaline, infused locally, reduces arrhythmia severity during coronary artery occlusion in anaesthetised dogs. *Cardiovasc Res* 55:53–63, 2002.
137. Vegh A and Parratt JR. The role of mitochondrial K(ATP) channels in antiarrhythmic effects of ischaemic preconditioning in dogs. *Br J Pharmacol* 137:1107–1115, 2002.
138. Watkins LR and Maier SF. Beyond neurons: evidence that immune and glial cells contribute to pathological pain states. *Physiol Rev* 82:981–1011, 2002.
139. Weber RN, Blair RW, and Foreman RD. Effects of cardiac administration of bradykinin on thoracic spinal neurons in the cat. *Exp Neurol* 78:703–715, 1982.
140. White JC. Cardiac pain. Anatomic pathways and physiologic mechnisms. *Circulation* 16:644–655, 1957.
141. White JC and Bland EF. The surgical relief of severe angina pectoris. *Medicine (Baltimore)* 27:1–42, 1948.
142. Yakhnitsa V, Linderoth B, and Meyerson BA. Spinal cord stimulation attenuates dorsal horn neuronal hyperexcitability in rat model of mononeuropathy. *Pain* 79:223–233, 1999.

143. Yezierski RP, Culberson JL, and Brown PB. Cells of origin of propriospinal connections to cat lumbosacral gray as determined with horseradish peroxidase. *Exp Neurol* 69:493–512, 1980.
144. Zhang J, Chandler MJ, and Foreman RD. Cardiopulmonary sympathetic and vagal afferents excite C1–C2 propriospinal cells in rats. *Brain Res* 969:53–58, 2003.
145. Zimmerman M. Encoding in dorsal horn interneurons receiving noxious and non noxious afferents. *J Physiol (Paris)* 73:221–232, 1977.

6

Central Nervous System Regulation of the Heart

MICHAEL C. ANDRESEN, DIANA L. KUNZE,
AND DAVID MENDELOWITZ

The neural mechanisms that control cardiac function have attracted considerable research interest over the past century, starting with the discoveries of the first neurotransmitter by Otto Loewi[103] and the earliest electroneurograms recording the discharge of single baroreceptor afferent axons by Lord Adrian.[1] Despite this long and distinguished history, fundamental gaps in our understanding persist—gaps that, if filled, might hold valuable keys to the development of important new therapeutic approaches to cardiovascular diseases.

Cardiovascular reflexes involving the brain stem modulate heart rate in a powerful manner. In the resting state, these reflexes actively depress heart rate. Furthermore, arterial baroreceptor reflexes involving the medulla function on a beat-to-beat basis. The general reflex pathways from arterial baroreceptors back to the heart and their performance characteristics are well established.[135] Notwithstanding this overall basic understanding, we know few details of how neural mechanisms within the varied components combine to give rise to the reflex's overall functional performance. Recent prospective clinical studies of the incidence of cardiac sudden death after coronary artery stenosis identify baroreflex sensitivity as a robust indicator to stratify mortality risk among these patients.[94] Despite compelling information concerning the importance of the baroreflex in humans and animal models,[17,93,95,145] our understanding of the determinants of baroreflex sensitivity remains quite limited.

The consensus view of the core circuit involved in this medullary reflex is that a pathway beginning with sensory neurites (nerve endings) located in key cardiovascular locations includes afferent neuronal somata that project to brain stem neurons in the nucleus of the solitary tract (NTS). In the NTS, these afferent projections contact neurons that relay information to other brain stem and central neurons. Some of the outputs from the former converge on neurons in autonomic premotor nuclei. The goal of this chapter is to review the basic framework of brain stem autonomic neuronal regulation of cardiac function and then highlight studies of key cellular and molecular mechanisms contributing to baroreflex performance. Improved understanding of these brain stem mechanisms and their modulation will help to identify ways of exerting specific control over baroreflex sensitivity, thus forming the basis of novel therapeutic strategies to help reduce the risk of cardiac disease, including cardiac dysrhythmia formation and sudden cardiac death.

Clearly, much of the control of regional cardiodynamics is reflex in nature, although paracrine and endocrine regulation contribute to the long-term stability of the cardiovascular system. This chapter focuses on some of the basic tenets of these control mechanisms and will highlight new initiatives that promote our understanding of this field and, as such, can yield novel insights into cardiac control. Perhaps the most fundamental autonomic regulatory reflex is the baroreflex controlling heart rate (Fig. 6–1). Among major cardiovascular targets, the heart is unique in that it receives dual autonomic regulation supplied by sympathetic and parasympathetic efferent neurons. The general organization of the basic neural pathways of these autonomic divisions begins with initial steps that are generally similar for both sympathetic and parasympathetic efferent neuronal pathways. Sensory information derived from arterial baroreceptors enters the central nervous system (CNS) to modulate neurons in the NTS. Cranial afferent neurons with sensory neurites in other visceral organs also synapse in the NTS. These sensory inputs loosely sort into viscerotopic representations across this nucleus.[3,104,135,156] Beyond this afferent processing stage in the NTS, parasympathetic and sympathetic neuronal pathways diverge.

In operating as a classic negative feedback system, the baroreflex is initiated by a rise in arterial blood pressure that activates arterial baroreceptor sensory neurites associated with afferent neurons in the nodose ganglia that project to NTS neurons (Fig. 6–1). Neurons in the NTS in turn activate cardioinhibitory vagal preganglionic neurons located primarily in the nucleus ambiguus (NA) and sympathoinhibitory neurons located in the caudal ventrolateral medulla (CVLM). The premotor sympathoexcitatory neurons are distributed primarily within the rostral portions of the ventrolateral medulla (RVLM). Medullary cardiac parasympathetic efferent preganglionic neurons project directly to the parasympathetic efferent postganglionic neurons located throughout the atrial and ventricular ganglionated plexuses (Chapter 4). The RVLM sympathetic premotor neurons, by contrast, project to sympathetic preganglionic neurons in the

Central Nervous System Regulation of the Heart

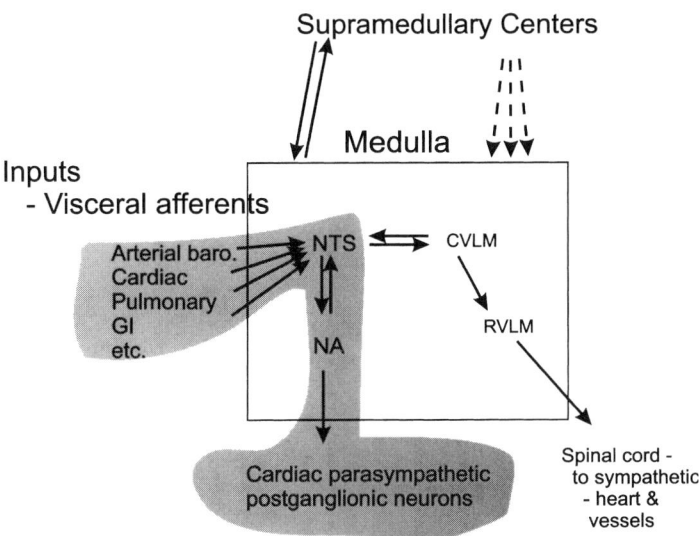

FIGURE 6–1 General schema of organization of baroreflex control of central autonomic outflow to the cardiovascular system. CVLM, caudal ventrolateral medulla; GI, gastrointestinal; NA, nucleus ambiguus; NTS, nucleus of the solitary tract; RVLM, rostral ventrolateral medulla.

intermediolateral cell column of the spinal cord, including those in the caudal cervical and cranial thoracic levels that project to the heart (Chapter 5). Thus, all of the required neural circuitry for cardiovascular baroreflexes is present in the medulla. That the gain or sensitivity of the heart rate baroreflex in resting, conscious animals is affected by midcollicular decerebration[18,140] indicates that supramedullary brain structures contribute important modulatory inputs to this reflex. Despite this finding, the core, competent baroreflex circuit appears to reside below the pons.[98,104]

The shortest anatomical pathway (thus likely involving the fewest number of synapses) and therefore the simplest one for this cardiac parasympathetic circuit involves at a minimum the following: *(1)* afferent neurons associated with cardiovascular mechanoreceptors, *(2)* second-order NTS neurons, *(3)* cardiac parasympathetic preganglionic motorneurons located primarily in the NA, and *(4)* parasympathetic postganglionic neurons intrinsic to the heart.[3,111] This minimal baroreflex pathway is subject to the influences of a wide variety of other neurons within the brain stem and elsewhere. This short reflex loop presumably is responsible for the initiation of fast-responding reflexes[91] that enable cardiac parasympathetic efferent postganglionic neurons to adjust cardiac performance within each cardiac cycle.[157]

This chapter reviews a series of recent experimental initiatives taken to understand the components of this the simplest of cardiovascular reflexes. It will focus on the first three main neurons in the four-neuron minimal loop of the cardiovascular baroreflex. Other chapters cover the transduction of cardiac sensory information (Chapter 3) and the function of the intrinsic cardiac nervous system positioned at the final interface of the cardiac myocytes that include cardiac parasympathetic postganglionic neurons (Chapter 4). This chapter focuses on the processes of translating and transforming arterial baroreceptor information into a CNS output to the peripheral cardiac nervous system.

Primary Afferent Neurons of the Baroreflex

Morphology and Discharge Patterns of Arterial Baroreceptors

Tonic cardiovascular regulation depends on the constant monitoring of arterial pressure, as well as cardiac rate and force. A primary responsibility for this function resides in the arterial baroreceptors. *Baroreceptors* comprise sensory nerve endings that lie in the adventitial layer of major arteries primarily at the bifurcation of the common carotid arteries, the arch of the thoracic aorta, or other major intrathoracic arteries (Chapter 3). The A-type baroreceptors have rapidly conducting myelinated fibers (2.5–60 m/second). These respond to local stretch secondary to distention of the arterial wall in each cardiac cycle, generating short bursts of impulses during the rising phase of the pressure pulse (Chapter 3). Thus, their impulses reflect mean arterial pressure as well as the frequency and amplitude of the pressure pulse.[9,12] Many of these arterial mechanosensory neurites have a branching morphology with lanceolate endings.[88] Other baroreceptors end in a "club-like structure." C-type arterial mechanoreceptors are associated with unmyelinated axons with conducting velocities <2.5 m/second. C-type sensory endings generally consist of small-diameter neurites that form nets within the adventitia. These C-type baroreceptors generally produce low-frequency activity that corresponds generally to mean arterial pressure. As such, C-type baroreceptors respond with less precision to the arterial pressure pulse than do mechanosensory neurites associated with A-type axons.[168,182] The threshold for C-type baroreceptor activation is, on average, higher than that of A-type arterial baroreceptor neurons, so that most C-type baroreceptors are not activated by normal arterial pressures. As discussed below, these two groups of baroreceptors appear to play different roles in cardiovascular reflex control.

Arterial Baroreceptor Transduction

The transduction of a mechanical stretch to an electrical signal by the sensory neuron is presumed to occur through stretch-activated, nonselective cation channels in their sensory terminals; such channel activity has not yet been directly measured. Although extensive morphological studies have been conducted at the electron microscopic level, we do not know precisely where the transduction process takes place in A- or C-type sensory endings.[88] Activation of the cation channels would be expected to produce depolarization that leads to the generation of an action potential, the number and frequency of which relate to the degree of stretch of sensory neurites associated with each mechanosensory neuron. This activity is then conducted via nodose and petrosal ganglia afferent neurons to NTS neurons, thereby providing information to other central neurons regarding ongoing arterial pressure and heart rate. The relationship between the amplitude of sensory terminal stretch and the frequency of discharge that they generate describes *baroreceptor sensitivity*. This is not a fixed relationship, but is plastic in that it can be modified over an appropriate range in the face of sustained blood pressure changes.[89,122] Under physiological conditions, this is important for the maintenance of rapid control over heart rate and blood pressure. There is also evidence that baroreceptor sensitivity changes occur during development, aging, or in the presence of pathological states.[4]

Ion Channels Underlying the Genesis of Baroreceptor Activity

At least 15 voltage-gated ion channels have been identified that underlie the electrical activity generated by mechanosensory sensory neurons (D.L. Kunze, unpublished data). The expression of specific channels differs between A-type and C-type afferent neurons with regard to the type and/or magnitude of their response characteristics. The most obvious difference is the presence of a tetrodotoxin (TTX)-resistant sodium current in the C-type neurons that tends to broaden their action potentials, presenting the possibility for a greater calcium influx during action potential generation; this may account for differences contributed by calcium-activated potassium currents in C-type as compared to A-type sensory neurons. The presence of TTX-resistant sodium currents in C-type baroreceptors offers one explanation for the relatively diverse discharge properties of these sensory neurons compared to the greater uniformity displayed among A-type baroreceptors.[102,144] The I_h current contributes to the resting potential of the cell and is much larger in A- than in C-type neurons.[40] The functional significance of this difference in I_h current is not clear. Furthermore, C-type afferent neurons have transient outward potassium currents that are not present in A-type afferent neurons. Recently, mathematical modeling has been used to link the properties of the various individual isolated ionic currents observed in a single cell type to the cellular discharge properties displayed by the mechanosensory neurites associated with A- and C-type neurons.[143] Major differences in encoding properties based on the relative expression of these ion channels closely parallels the known discharge characteristics of baroreceptor subtypes recorded in situ. Understanding the role of specific ion channels in coding their discharge properties becomes important in light of recent studies in the somatosensory system where it has been demonstrated that the expression of specific channels can be altered by axotomy, growth factors, increased activity, and exposure to inflammatory agents.[53,59,61,130,174] Such transduction processing by baroreceptors would lead to changes in their discharge properties and thus the information they transduce to neurons in the NTS.

What role do channels play in cardiovascular function in disease states? Mutated forms of several of the channels present in baroreceptors are responsible for cardiac and neural pathologies. Despite this, surprisingly little attention has been paid to the consequences of these mutations in cardiac neuronal control. One exception is a study of the cardiovascular consequences of removal of the calcium channel responsible for the "N"-type calcium current. Although these currents are expressed in many neurons, they are known to contribute the calcium that enters to mediate synaptic transmission between the baroreceptor afferent neuron and second-order neurons in the NTS.[114] Mice lacking the α_{1B} subunit display a selective deficit in N-type calcium channel activity, and these mice have elevated arterial pressure and heart rates, with reduced sensitivity to carotid artery occlusion.[79] Little is known about the precise mechanisms responsible for these reduced baroreflex sensitivity or whether baroreceptor afferents in these mice contribute to the cardiovascular changes.

Transmitters and Transmitter Receptors on Sensory Terminals

A- and C-type baroreceptor neurons are diverse with respect to their capacity to generate basic pressure-related discharge patterns. For instance, baroreceptor C fibers, but not most A-type fibers, express capsaicin-sensitive VR1 receptors involving nonselective cation channels.[14,25,44,54] The properties of this receptor/channel would be expected to confer both temperature and hydrogen ion sensitivity to C-type baroreceptor function. Some C-type fibers, but not A fibers, contain the neuropeptide substance P within their sensory neurites while another peptide, calcitonin gene-related peptide (CGRP), is present in subpopulations of C- and A-type axons associated with baroreceptor somata.[72] If analogies hold between the somatic and visceral sensory afferent nervous systems, these peptides are released from sensory terminals to directly or indirectly modify their discharge (Fig. 6–2).[16] Potential targets of peptides released locally from the somatic nervous system are endothelial cells of nearby blood vessels or mast cells. These "target cells" are then presumed to release substances such as ATP, histamine, and serotonin that feed back to modify the activity generated by these sensory neurites. Receptors for these substances have been documented on the soma of baroreceptor af-

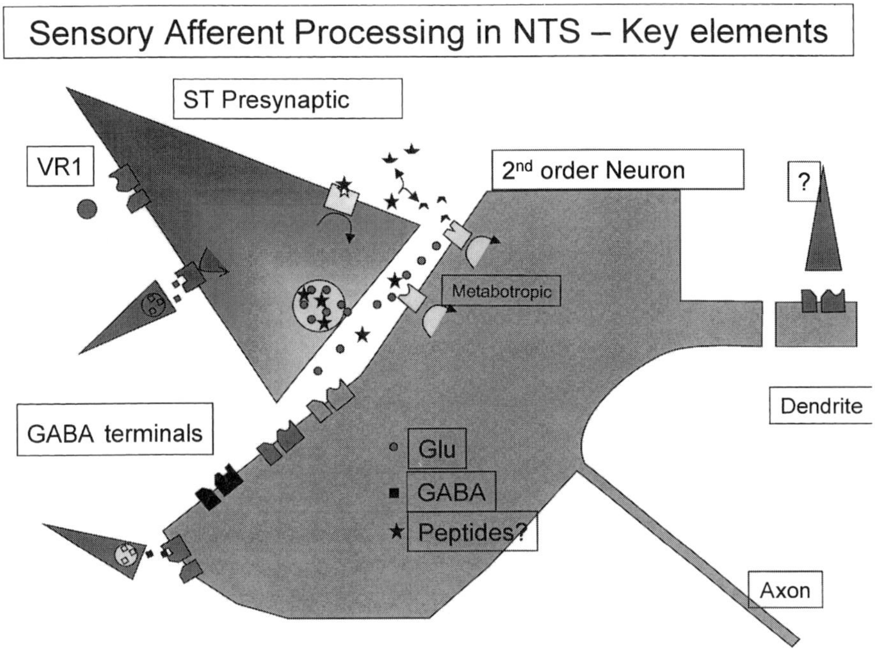

FIGURE 6–2 Schematic of the cellular basis of afferent baroreceptor processing. The triangle to the left represents the presynaptic terminal arising from the afferent neuron via the nodose ganglion and the solitary tract (ST). This presynaptic terminal contains a number of key elements that regulate the release of neurotransmitter(s) represented by a single large presynaptic vesicle that may contain more than one substance. The presynaptic terminals themselves have a variety of ion channels and receptors for different neurotransmitters. The second-order neurons have receptors for different neurotransmitters, including glutamate (Glu), GABA, and peptides. Together, the ion channels (agonist and voltage gated) and second-messenger systems (curved arrows) contribute to both pre- and postsynaptic processing that will determine the outflow of action potentials along the axon of the second-order nucleus of the solitary tract (NTS) neuron.

ferent neurons and thus are likely to be expressed on their sensory terminals. Electron microscopic studies of baroreceptor nerve terminals have shown that pericytes or Schwann cells ensheath much of the baroreceptor ending;[88] these are potential sites of interaction between the baroreceptor and other cells in its environment. One neurotransmitter that seems to modify both A- and C-type baroreceptors is norepinephrine. It has long been known that there are catecholamine receptors on baroreceptor sensory neurites and that many vascular regions containing baroreceptor are supplied with copious sympathetic efferent postganglionic neuronal innervation. These sympathetic endings may serve as a source of catecholamines that increase the threshold for baroreceptor discharge.[67,123,124,168] Another area of interest is the recent demonstration that inflammatory mediators released during immediate allergic reactions can produce profound effects on the excitability of visceral sensory neurites by unmasking their NK_2 receptor function.[180] Perhaps this is related to the fact that prostacyclin, acting at the baroreceptor terminals, modifies A-type baroreceptor discharge.[28] This also parallels findings in the somatosensory system.

The above discussion points out the many possibilities for modulation of baroreceptor discharge under a variety of physiological and pathological conditions. Many of the neurotransmitters and channels associated with their sensory neurites of baroreceptor neurons are also expressed within their medullary terminals, being prime targets for presynaptic modulation of transmitter release. Thus, many of the issues regarding the influences of ion channel integration on signal processing discussed above also apply to synaptic processing of baroreceptor inputs to NTS neurons. The interactions of these presynaptic inputs to postsynaptic neurons are the focus of the next section concerning the nature of information exchange between first-order sensory neurons and second-order NTS neurons along this baroreflex pathway.

NUCLEUS OF THE SOLITARY TRACT—SECOND-ORDER NEURONS IN THE BAROREFLEX

Key anatomical studies have shown that dorsal medial portions of the caudal NTS are the site of baroreceptor afferent neuronal contacts with CNS neurons.[30,34,113] The second-order neurons of the baroreceptor reflex lie generally within this medullary region and mark the first stage of these reflex pathways within the CNS. While the general location of these neurons has been known for some 20 years, the small size of these neurons and movement of the brain due to respiration and vascular pulses have made intracellular recordings limited in duration.[57,68,120] More recently, isolation of the medial NTS with portions of the solitary tract (ST) containing its afferent axonal inputs has allowed greater depth of study of the cellular mechanisms within the NTS.[7,13,15,22,26,66,118,132,150,184] Interesting distinctions are emerging among these cellular mechanisms, neurotransmitter receptors, and circuit organization of brain stem compared to cortical function.[3] The discussion below summarizes several recent issues that have emerged in this field to emphasize that knowledge of the mechanisms of cortical brain control may not always be readily relevant to brain stem physiology.

Afferent Neurotransmission in the Nucleus of the Solitary Tract

As in most parts of the CNS, glutamate is the major excitatory neurotransmitter in NTS (for a detailed review, see Andresen and Kunze[3]). Microinjection of glutamate or its receptor-specific analogs (e.g., NMDA, AMPA, and kainate) into the NTS evokes decreases in blood pressure and heart rate that mimic responses elicited by baroreceptor activation (e.g., aortic depressor nerve stimulation).[62,99,138,162] Conversely, injecting a broad-spectrum glutamate antagonist, such as kynurenate, into the NTS blocks these baroreflexes. While such findings are consistent with a major role of glutamate in the function of NTS neurons in cardiovascular regulation, direct evidence of the action and identification of specific neurons involved has yet to be elucidated.

With the difficulty of obtaining lengthy intracellular recordings in vivo, isolation of the medial NTS in horizontal slices along with their afferent axonal inputs in the ST has paved the way for studies of the cellular interactions occurring between first order afferent neurons and second-order neurons in the NTS.[118] Electrical stimuli delivered to the ST activate short-latency excitatory postsynaptic potentials in NTS neurons that rely on non-NMDA receptors to elicit them.[7] Since application of carbocyanine dyes to the aortic depressor nerve stains the central terminations of aortic mechanosensory neurons in the NTS, development of a thin horizontal slice of the NTS has led to voltage clamp studies directed at determining synaptic transmission arising from baroreceptor inputs to medial NTS neurons.[43] Neurons visualized through infrared illumination and differential interference contrast microscopy (IR-DIC) demonstrate fluorescent-labeled baroreceptor terminals on specific NTS neurons. Studies involving identified NTS neurons with sensory inputs from baroreceptor afferent neurons found that glutamate released from ST afferent axon terminals activates non-NMDA receptors on such neurons (Fig. 6–3).[43]

Patch voltage clamp recordings of medial NTS neurons demonstrate that the short-latency excitatory postsynaptic currents (EPSCs) induced

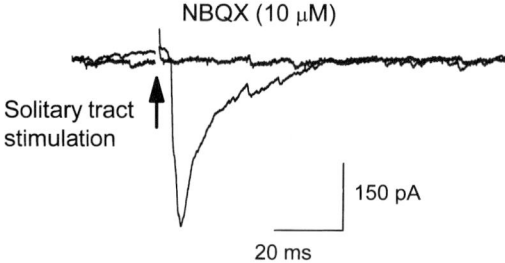

FIGURE 6–3 Glutamatergic transmission of solitary tract stimuli to medial NTS neuron. Patch recording of neuron voltage clamped to −70 mV. Single shocks (arrow) show excitatory postsynaptic current (EPSC) that is blocked in the presence of the non-NMDA receptor antagonist NBQX. This neuron displayed DiA-positive terminals on its soma that were characteristic of medial NTS neurons contacted by aortic baroreceptors.[43]

in this way vary little in latency from stimulus to stimulus (synaptic jitter; <150 μs calculated as the standard deviation of the latency). Thus glutamate appears to be the primary transmitter mediating aortic mechanosensory information at the level of the NTS. Interestingly, such synaptically released glutamate does not have access to NMDA receptors on most NTS second-order neurons.[43] The relative domination of the non-NMDA receptors and sparse representation of NMDA receptors associated with these second-order NTS neurons are quite different from the qualities associated with most CNS synapses. Recently, a small cohort of second-order NTS neurons has been identified that are preferentially contacted by capsaicin-resistant solitary tract afferents that give rise to EPSCs with a small-amplitude NMDA component.[83] As is to be expected from such synaptic characteristics, frequency-dependent depression is an important feature of these ST-NTS synapses and thus NTS afferent transmission for the most part lacks the cellular template responsible for long-term potentiation commonly associated with NMDA receptors.[119] Presumably, this is an important characteristic of their capacity to transfer information to other central neurons and it is intriguing that only select portions of these afferents activate NMDA receptors.

Gamma aminobutyric acid (GABA) is a major CNS inhibitory transmitter within the NTS.[170] $GABA_A$ receptors are generally located postsynaptically and coupled to chloride channels, while $GABA_B$ receptors are generally presynaptic in location. Both act to inhibit by inhibiting calcium channels and transmitter release and/or by activating potassium channels.[20,106,127,152,153] $GABA_A$ and $GABA_B$ binding is found in the NTS[170] and each affects blood pressure control.[46,185] GABA, when microinjected into the NTS, increases blood pressure primarily via $GABA_A$

receptors;[109] GABA$_A$ antagonists block these increases and enhance responses elicited by aortic depressor nerve (ADN) stimulation.[19,90]

Inhibitory transmission is commonly associated with second-order neurons in the medial NTS. Very effective short-loop, short-latency feedback inhibition within the medulla appears to be mediated by GABA acting on second-order neurons.[5,116] Interestingly, the basic coupling of pre- and postsynaptic GABA receptors to their effectors is fundamentally different in the brain stem and hippocampus.[164] In the hippocampus, pre- and postsynaptic GABA receptors are pharmacologically indistinguishable and coupled to a common population of ion channels. In the NTS, pre- and postsynaptic GABA receptors are coupled to different effectors.[21] Such local network connections are likely important in controlling information flow within the NTS. For instance, one important GABA pathway appears to be driven from aortic mechanosensory afferent neurons to second-order medial NTS neurons via two different synaptic mechanisms—an initial glutamatergic step followed by activation of the GABAergic neuron.[43] Such disynaptic pathways, in addition to being blocked by either non-NMDA glutamate antagonists or by GABA$_A$ antagonists, display the highly unreliable transmission of a multisynapse path.[43] The identification of these rapid feedback circuits in thin slices of NTS suggests that the key components of this potent inhibitory loop are highly localized and may arise from interneurons in close proximity to second-order neurons.

Despite the pre-eminence of glutamate as the primary neurotransmitter in the NTS, this region is rich in other neurotransmitters that affect second-order NTS neurons (for detailed references, see Andresen and Kunze[3] and Lawrence and Jarrott[96]). A fascinating new horizon of relatively unexplored mechanisms for NTS integration is indicated by the extensive anatomical presence of co- or accessory neurotransmitters within the NTS. Immunohistochemical studies indicate that NTS neurons are associated with a large number of potential neurotransmitters, including all major classes of biogenic amines and peptides.[170] The presence of many of these candidate transmitters is supported by microinjection studies indicating that placement of mimetic agonists in the NTS affects cardiovascular function. Many of these neurotransmitters, including neuropeptides, exert strong modulatory actions on target neurons, with effects extending beyond the time frame of fast neurotransmission induced by chemicals such as glutamate. Responses to application of chemicals such as ATP into the NTS[52,133,146–148] appear to follow the precedent of dorsal root ganglion afferent neurons and likely represent properties of nerve terminals arising from nodose ganglion neurons. Such modulators presumably alter ion channels and second-messenger enzymatic cascades within NTS neurons; few details on their functions are currently available. For the most part, these cotransmitters remain to be demonstrated at a cellular level and their affected neurons have yet to be identified. Accessory transmitters (cotransmitters) are particularly prominent in C-type neurons in the spinal cord.[97]

Of the dozens of neuropeptides identified to date, all are thought to use G protein–linked signal transduction pathways.[82] As such, peptidergic transmitters tend to have prolonged actions that primarily modulate sensitivity to other inputs rather than triggering excitation or inhibition of neuron discharge directly. G protein–linked receptors undergo endocytosis of the bound receptor complex. In the case of substance P, this endocytosis process can have a quite dramatic short-term impact on spinal neuronal morphology. Recent studies describe a massive but reversible restructuring of postsynaptic neurons in the dorsal horn within minutes of such stimulation.[107] The functional consequences of activating these neurons have not been studied. Clues suggest that peptides act in a way that is fundamentally different from amino acid neurotransmitters.[100] Despite intensive efforts, Iversen maintains that "there are few, if any, examples in which the physiological role of a particular peptide in an identified neural pathway can be described exactly."[82] Visceral sensory neurons are no exception to this view. Peptides and their receptors have been associated immunohistochemically with NTS neurons. They are known to influence NTS neuronal/reflex function and in many cases are released from sensory neuron sites.[170] Two key peptides associated with baroreflexes (neurons in the NTS and NA) are substance P and CGRP.[157]

Substance P has long been closely linked to afferent neurons via immunohistochemistry and its use-dependent release, as well as through depletion within areas of the NTS associated with the baroreflex.[65] Some substance P in the NTS originates from central efferent neuronal sources.[165] Substance P is localized to presynaptic sites on vagal efferent preganglionic neurons in the NA.[105] Experiments in the spinal cord point to an excess of substance P receptor sites, many of which are a considerable distance from transmitter release sites.[107] This and other evidence suggest that substance P has additional, spatially distant, extrasynaptic targets as well those juxtaposed to release sites. Depressor responses elicited by microinjections of substance P or the amino terminal fragment (sub-P1–7) into the NTS require an intact glutamatergic response;[69] such substance P microinjections enhance the baroreflex.[27,58] These data suggest that substance P acts in a modulatory way on the brain stem to facilitate the actions of the primary sensory transmitter, glutamate.[69]

Expression of these peptides in nodose ganglion afferent neurons is relatively unaffected by axotomy.[73] CGRP and substance P coexist in a large fraction of carotid sinus afferent neurons.[78] In the brain stem, A_2-

catecholamine neurons in the NTS receive many CGRP synaptic inputs.[63] Furthermore, the CGRP-induced presynaptic reductions in norepinephrine release from the medulla are compromised in the presence of hypertension.[169] The relation of these peptides to glutamate transmission in the NTS is unclear. Baroreflex studies suggest that CGRP acts centrally to facilitate autonomic cardiac reflexes.[129,154] In comparison, CGRP and substance P enhance the release of glutamate in spinal dorsal horn slices during dorsal root stimulation.[85]

The medullary brain slice approach has revealed new layers of the detailed functional organization of the NTS (Fig. 6–2). The ability to control the concentrations of various agents in tissue slices offers a greater specificity and higher resolution than is practical in intact preparations. In the NTS, short-latency excitatory postsynaptic potentials elicited by ST stimulation are blocked by non-NMDA antagonists, but are unaffected by NMDA receptor or channel antagonists.[7,8] Thus, baroreceptor as well as other fast sensory afferent synaptic transmission is mediated by glutamate acting at a non-NMDA receptor. Recent studies have identified a small component of the solitary tract afferent–activated EPSC that activates NMDA receptors on a subset of capsaicin-resistant second-order NTS neurons, and these are likely innervated selectively by A-type afferent axons.[83] NMDA responses are also apparent in other neurons within the NTS. Generally, only small NMDA currents (<15 pA) are evoked in most dissociated neurons from the medial NTS.[45,125] In the presence of non-NMDA antagonists, however, field stimulation of sites near the solitary tract elicits small, slow EPSPs in NTS neurons, a response that is enhanced by the omission of extracellular Mg^{2+} or blocked by the NMDA antagonist AP5.[23,29] Overall, these results are consistent with a relative predominance of NMDA receptors on interneurons within the NTS and their relative absence on cells receiving sensory inputs. This NTS organization may position the NMDA receptor at a point in the NTS circuitry to exert a particularly selective or powerful influence on selective pathways through NTS and on GABAergic inhibition. Importantly, through well-established mechanisms the NMDA receptor provides the potential for activity-dependent plasticity.

Nucleus Ambiguus—Cardiac Preganglionic Parasympathetic Neurons

Heart rate in healthy individuals is determined to a large extent by the tonic, reflex excitation of parasympathetic efferent neurons that innervate the heart. However, cardiac vagal efferent neuronal activity becomes diminished or even unresponsive in many disease states, including hypertension, heart failure, and sudden cardiac death.[95,137,171] A delay in the inhibitory actions of this autonomic motor system after exercise is a powerful predictor of overall mortality in such a state.[31] Restoration of normal cardiac vagal efferent neuronal activity suppresses ischemia and reperfusion-induced arrhythmias and decreases the risk of sudden death after myocardial infarction. These findings suggest that increasing cardiac vagal efferent neuronal activity may be an effective clinical target in treating some heart diseases.[48,95,137,171,179,181]

The reflex control of heart rate is dominated by the cardioinhibitory response elicited by parasympathetic efferent neurons. In conscious or anesthetized animals, there is a tonic level of parasympathetic efferent neuronal firing and relatively low sympathetic efferent neuronal activity at rest in humans,[134,161] dogs,[142] cats,[91] and rats.[32,160] During increases in arterial pressure, the initial reflex-induced slowing of the heart is caused primarily if not exclusively by increases in cardiac vagal nerve activity.[142,160,161] During decreases in arterial pressure, the baroreflex-induced tachycardia is caused mostly by decreases in parasympathetic neuronal activity in addition to increases in sympathetic efferent neuronal activity.[142,155,158] When both parasympathetic and sympathetic efferent neuronal activities are present, parasympathetic activity dominates in the control of heart rate. As a matter of fact, increases in parasympathetic efferent neuronal activity evoke a bradycardia that is more pronounced when there is a high level of sympathetic efferent neuronal firing.[101] When there is a moderate or high level of parasympathetic efferent neuronal tone, changes in sympathetic efferent neuronal firing elicit negligible changes in heart rate.[101]

There are a number of hypotheses concerning the mechanisms responsible for this interaction (Chapter 4). It has been proposed that the release of acetylcholine from parasympathetic efferent neurons might act presynaptically on sympathetic efferent nerve terminals to inhibit their release of norepinephrine.[137] Parasympathetic–sympathetic interactions might also be the result of postsynaptic competition between different guanine nucleotide-binding (G) proteins within the membranes of sinoatrial pacemaker cells that directly modulate calcium and potassium channels involved in cardiac pacemaker activity.[24,75,137]

It is widely accepted that parasympathetic efferent postganglionic neuronal activity originates primarily from their medullary inputs rather than from peripheral ganglia. Preganglionic cardiac vagal fibers are tonically active, with a firing pattern that is frequently pulse synchronous; it is most active during post-inspiration and reduced during inspiration.[64,91,105,155] Sectioning their preganglionic fibers, leaving only the postganglionic parasympathetic innervation intact, releases the heart from much of this tonic parasympathetic efferent neuronal inhibition.[74]

The origin within the central nervous system of the tonic cardiac vagal activity remains unknown. Presumably, some of it originates as a consequence of tonic inputs from cardiovascular sensory neurons. The intrinsic firing properties and voltage-gated currents in identified cardiac vagal neurons have been characterized in vitro.[81,110–112,117] These data demonstrate that, in the absence of synaptic activity, cardiac vagal neurons in the nucleus ambiguus (NA) are normally silent. Cardiac vagal neurons do not display pacemaker-like activity such as repetitive or phasic depolarizations or the genesis of spontaneous action potentials. However, only a small depolarizing current (100 pA) is needed to evoke repetitive firing in cardiac vagal efferent neurons; this activity occurs with little delay and minimal spike frequency adaptation during maintained depolarizing currents. The voltage-gated currents and firing characteristics of cardiac vagal efferent neurons enable them to follow fast synaptic drive closely, as well as to integrate long-lasting modulatory influences.

The absence of pacemaker activity in cardiac vagal neurons in vitro is consistent with results from in vivo studies. In the relatively few in vivo studies that have successfully identified and examined cardiac vagal neurons with extracellular electrodes, most of the neurons identified by antidromic stimulation did not generate spontaneous activity.[64,108,128] In the only in vivo study in which intracellular recordings were successful (and in only two neurons), cardiac vagal neurons were silent.[64] The lack of ongoing cardiac vagal activity in these anesthetized in vivo preparations is somewhat unexpected, since in conscious rats,[32,158,160] dogs,[142] cats,[91] or humans[134,161] there is a relatively high level of tonic cardiac vagal efferent neuronal activity. However, in the in vivo experiments, excitatory pathways to cardiac vagal neurons may have been inhibited because of the trauma of the acute open-chest surgery or the anesthesia that in general inhibits excitatory pathways.[175] The tonic ongoing parasympathetic activity present in unanesthetized animals is therefore likely initiated to a large extent by excitatory synaptic inputs that appear to be susceptible to trauma and/or anesthesia.

Three major synaptic inputs to cardiac vagal preganglionic neurons have been characterized recently. The neurotransmitters involved in these pathways are glutamate, GABA, and acetylcholine. The neural pathways, transmitters, and receptors that alter the activity of cardiac vagal efferent neurons are discussed below, along with the potential role of these inputs in mediating cardiovascular and cardiorespiratory homeostasis.

Glutamate

Stimulation of the NTS evokes a glutamatergic pathway that activates both NMDA and non-NMDA postsynaptic currents in cardiac vagal efferent neurons.[111,126] The NMDA antagonist AP5 blocks the long-lasting component and CNQX; a selective non-NMDA blocker abolishes the rapidly inactivating synaptic responses. Synaptic events can follow stimulation frequencies of 5–100 Hz, consistent with activation of a monosynaptic pathway. This monosynaptic projection from NTS to vagal cardiac efferent neurons in the NA most likely plays an essential role in cardiovascular reflex control. This pathway may constitute the essential link between increases in blood pressure and afferent baroreceptor neuronal activity, activation of neurons in the NTS, and the reflex compensatory decrease in heart rate initiated by increases in efferent cardioinhibitory vagal neuronal activity. This link from the NTS to cardiac vagal efferent neurons is the critical component in the baroreflex pathway, as discussed above.

GABA

Cardiac vagal efferent preganglionic neurons receive spontaneous GABAergic inhibitory postsynaptic currents (IPSCs) that can be blocked by the $GABA_A$ receptor antagonist bicuculline.[177] GABAergic synaptic currents in cardiac vagal preganglionic neurons can be consistently evoked upon stimulation of the NTS and these responses also can be blocked by bicuculline. It is possible that this inhibitory pathway from the NTS is involved in the patterning of cardiac vagal bursting activity that is pulse synchronous with the cardiac cycle. Opioids, which are known to excite efferent cardiac vagal neurons and evoke a bradycardia, act at least in part by disinhibition. μ-Opioid agonist and nociceptin inhibit the inhibitory GABAergic neurotransmission to efferent cardiac vagal neurons.[172,173]

It is also possible that GABAergic inputs to cardiac vagal efferent preganglionic neurons are involved in central cardiorespiratory interactions. There are two well-known physiological interactions between respiratory and cardiac vagal neurons. During each respiratory cycle, the heart beats more rapidly in inspiration and slows during post-inspiration. This is referred to as *respiratory sinus arrhythmia*, which benefits pulmonary gas exchange by improving ventilation-to-perfusion ratios within each respiratory cycle. It is present in healthy fetuses, newborns, and mature animals and humans[49,51,71,77,115,141,151] but becomes diminished in many disease states. In distressed fetuses and partially asphyxiated newborns, respiratory sinus arrhythmia is decreased; this is correlated (independent of heart or respiratory rate) with low Apgar scores and neonatal mortality.[39,115,141] It has been speculated that abnormality of cardiorespiratory control, such as a prolonged period of post-inspiration accompanied by a severe maintained decrease in heart rate, may be involved in sudden infant death syndrome (SIDS).[39,70,115,141,158] In infants that succumb to SIDS, a centrally mediated slowing of heart rate that precedes or accompanies apnea may be critically involved in its etiology.[115,141] Bradycardia is the most prevalent and predictive event in infants monitored for apparent life-threatening events.[33] As discussed below, both GABAergic and nicotinic receptors may be involved in generating cardiorespiratory interactions. Thus it is worth noting that the one of the most significant risk factors associated with SIDS is maternal cigarette smoking, as well as postnatal exposure to nicotine.[163]

While feedback from pulmonary stretch receptors and direct respiratory-related changes in venous return and cardiac stretch can evoke respiratory-related fluctuations in heart rate, the dominant source of respiratory sinus arrhythmia originates from the brain stem.[11] Respiratory sinus arrhythmia persists when the lungs are stationary (caused by muscle paralysis or constant flow ventilation). Furthermore, respiratory modulation of heart rate remains synchronized with brain stem respiratory rhythms even if artificial ventilation and chemoreceptor activation occur at different intervals.[36,50,77,151,158] In both animals and humans, respiratory sinus arrhythmia is mediated via cardiac vagal efferent neurons; respiratory sinus arrhythmia persists in experimental animals upon sectioning sympathetic pathways, as well as in quadriplegic patients with spinal cord injury inducing sympathetic efferent neuronal dysfunction.[36,50,77,80,151]

The respiratory system also influences heart rate by modulating the baroreceptor and chemoreceptor inputs to cardiac vagal efferent neurons. In both animals and humans, baroreceptor and chemoreceptor reflexes are inhibited during inspiration; they are facilitated during post-inspiration and expiration, as well as during a maintained phase of post-inspiration and apnea.[35,49,105,108] Respiratory modulation of both reflexes persists after pulmonary denervation and ventilatory paralysis. This finding suggests that this "gating" of the baroreceptor and chemoreceptor reflexes occurs within the brain stem.[36,139,158]

Cardiac vagal efferent neuronal activity (recorded from efferent axons in cardiac nerves) has pronounced respiratory modulation. Cardiac vagal efferent axons fire most rapidly in post-inspiration, often being silent during inspiration.[108,155] It appears likely that at least one source of these cardiorespiratory interactions involves an increase in GABAergic inputs to vagal efferent preganglionic neurons during inspiration.[64] Respiratory inputs do *not* seem to alter baroreceptor and chemoreceptor synapses at their first synapse in the NTS.[155,158] Rather, the few relevant data that do exist suggest that the cardiorespiratory interactions occur at the level of the NA.[64,155]

Acetylcholine

Acetylcholine is involved in mediating cardiorespiratory interactions and exciting cardiac vagal efferent neurons in the medulla via four mechanisms: *(1)* activating a direct ligand-gated postsynaptic nicotinic receptor, *(2)* enhancing postsynaptic non-NMDA currents, *(3)* presynaptically facilitating (via α_7 subunit–containing nicotinic receptors) excitatory glutamatergic transmission,[111,121,128,131,179] and *(4)* facilitating both inhibitory GABAergic and glycinergic activity to cardiac vagal efferent neurons.[178] Recent work has shown that the faclitation of glutamatergic neurotransmission by nicotinic cholinergic receptors is dependent on activation of pre- and postsynaptic P-type voltage-gated calcium channels.[179] The nicotinic facilitation of GABAergic and glycinergic neurotransmission to efferent cardiac vagal neurons is endogenously active and can be exaggerated by the acetylcholinesterase inhibitor neostigmine.[178]

One source of the cholinergic innervation of cardiac vagal efferent preganglionic neurons originates from inputs arising from superior laryngeal neurons. To test the hypothesis that superior laryngeal neurons synapse on cardiac vagal efferent neurons in the medulla, a novel Bartha strain of the pseudorabies rabies (PRV) that expresses green fluorescent protein (GFP) was used to visualize and thus record from neurons that synapse on and influence the vagal motor outflow to the heart. The Bartha strain of PRV, an attenuated swine α-herpes virus, can be used as a transsynaptic marker of neural circuits. Bartha PRV invades neuronal networks in the central nervous system through peripherally projecting axons, replicates in these parent neurons, and then travels retrogradely and transsynaptically to label second- and higher-order neurons in a time-dependent manner. To identify cardiac vagal efferent neurons and, in particular, neurons that synapse on them, a series of experiments was performed in which Bartha PRV-GFP was injected into the pericardial sac and tissues were collected for histochemical examination after different survival periods. After 2 days of survival, only cardiac vagal preganglionic neurons were labeled. The labeling pattern was identical to the population of such neurons labeled with conventional retrograde fluorescent tracers. To label superior laryngeal neurons, the fluorescent tracer DiI was applied to the superior laryngeal nerve 2 days prior to sacrifice. Superior laryngeal efferent neurons were identified anatomically in close proximity to cardiac vagal efferent preganglionic neurons that were labeled 2 days after injecting Bartha PRV-GFP into the pericardial sac; no superior laryngeal neurons contained the virus.

After establishing that Bartha PRV-GFP can be used to identify neurons in specific functional circuits for subsequent electrophysiological experiments, a second series of immunohistochemical experiments was performed in which animals were sacrificed 3 days after injecting the virus into the pericardial sac. DiI was applied to the superior laryngeal nerve of these animals 3 days prior to sacrifice. After 3 days, labeling was present in cardiac vagal efferent preganglionic neurons as well as in other neurons in the NA and additional brain stem regions that included the nearby periambigual area and the NTS. Within the NA, superior laryngeal motorneurons were colabeled with both DiI and PRV-GFP, demonstrating that they also innervate cardiac vagal efferent preganglionic neurons.

To recapitulate, cardiac vagal preganglionic neurons rely on synaptic neurotransmission to these neurons to control their firing. These neurons receive three major synaptic inputs—glutamatergic, GABAergic, and cholinergic. Stimulation of the NTS evokes a glutamatergic pathway that activates both NMDA and non-NMDA postsynaptic currents in these cardiac vagal neurons. Additionally, there is GABAergic innervation of cardiac vagal preganglionic neurons that can be activated by stimulating the NTS. Acetylcholine excites cardiac vagal preganglionic neurons via 3 mechanisms: *(1)* activating a direct ligand-gated postsynaptic nicotinic receptor, *(2)* enhancing postsynaptic non-NMDA currents, and *(3)* presynaptically facilitating (via α_7 subunit–containing nicotinic receptors) glutamate release. This enhancement by nicotinic cholinergic receptors is dependent on activation of presynaptic P-type voltage-gated calcium channels. Both the GABAergic and cholinergic inputs to these cardiac vagal preganglionic neurons are probably involved in cardiorespiratory interactions. The glutamatergic pathway from the NTS to cardiac vagal efferent postganglionic neurons is likely the essential link between increases in blood pressure and afferent baroreceptor neuronal activity, as the latter afferent neurons activate neurons in the NTS such that efferent cardioinhibitory vagal neurons become reflexly excited.

BASIS OF BAROREFLEX INTEGRATION—CLINICAL RELEVANCE OF SYSTEMS RESPONSES AND PLASTICITY

Baroreceptors and the Baroreflex

Considerable information is available about sensory transduction by arterial baroreceptors (for reviews see Andresen and Mendelowitz,[5] Andresen and Yang,[6] and Krauhs.[88]). The rat aortic depressor nerve is an ideal preparation for these studies as it contains afferent axons arising only from aortic baroreceptors. Aortic baroreceptors fall into the general functional classes outlined above for A- and C-type visceral sensory axons. There are relatively fewer studies of baroreceptors with C-type axons than those involving A-type axons.[166,167] Even though C-type baroreceptors are technically more difficult to record, they represent the overwhelming majority of baroreceptors.[2,45,56] A-type baroreceptors generate relatively high and regular discharge frequencies, whereas C-type baroreceptors generally display irregular and relatively low discharge activity rates. C-type aortic baroreceptors in rats have an average pressure threshold that is higher than that of A-type baroreceptors, although C-type thresholds overlap with the A-type range; roughly 25% of C-type baroreceptors are active at normal blood pressure.[168] C-type baroreceptors generate activity during each cardiac cycle in vivo that occurs either as a burst of action potentials synchronous with each pulse but at a lower frequency than those generated by A-type baroreceptors, or, more often, as only one or two action potentials loosely correlated to each pressure pulse.[183] These differences in transduction suggest that A- and C-type baroreceptors provide different information to medullary neurons. Despite the efforts of several research groups,[10,41,42,47,86,87,92,149,159] there is no consensus on which aspect of the discharge patterns is important for the baroreflex control.

A- versus C-type Baroreflex Responses

Studies have demonstrated differences in blood pressure and heart rate responses elicited following activation of A-type baroreceptors compared to that of C-type baroreceptors.[41,42] Graded, electrical stimuli recruit successively the A- and then the C-type axons in a nerve as the stimulus intensity increases. Using these methods, C-type baroreceptors appear to have proportionally greater reflex effects than the A-type ones.[54,55] At even low frequencies, C-type baroreceptor discharge has substantial reflex consequences (Fig. 6–4). Thus, cardiac baroreflex responses to aortic depressor nerve activation display an interesting interaction between A-type and C-type baroreceptor inputs during synchronous electrical activation. Currently virtually nothing is known about the mechanisms responsible for their functional differences.

Plasticity and Subtype Interactions: A- and C-type Sensory Synaptic Fields

Peripheral nerve damage induces specific changes in the organization of sensory neuronal inputs to the spinal cord.[37,38] Endings of deafferented neurons take on new receptive fields by expanding into adjacent regions that are innervated by intact afferent neurons. Central endings do not de-

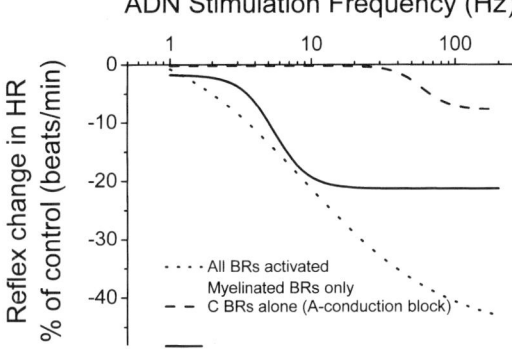

FIGURE 6-4 Aortic baroreflex response (BR) relations for heart rate (HR) for A- and C-type baroreceptor activation. Electrical activation of the aortic depressor nerve (ADN) at different frequencies yields characteristic response relations. If low intensities are used, only A-type axons are excited and only modest reflex responses are observed (dashed curve). High intensities activate all baroreceptor axons and produce much larger responses with a different frequency relation (dotted curve). If anodal current is used to block conduction of A-type axons, the resulting C-type relation suggests that C fibers produce substantial reflex bradycardia at modest and physiological frequencies of C-type baroreceptors (solid line). These curves are based largely on published studies in the rat.[55]

generate, but their peptide content may become depleted. Since TTX blockade of peripheral conduction fails to produce similar changes, nerve activity itself is unlikely to be responsible for such central neuronal reorganization.[176] Exposure of neonates to the vanilloid agonist capsaicin permanently destroys small sensory ganglion cells and within hours triggers massive degeneration of C-type axons and their central terminals; large A-type afferent neuronal somas are unaffected by this treatment.[60] Capsaicin depletes substance P and other C-type afferent markers to a degree comparable to axotomy, whereas A-input receptive fields expand greatly.[60] This central structural relationship has fostered the hypothesis that C-type sensory fibers influence central synaptic connectivity. Thus lesioning of C-fiber sensory neurons with capsaicin not only produces sensory deficits but changes the pattern of information processed via capsaicin-insensitive afferent neuronal pathways in addition to indirectly altering higher-order pathways (e.g., sympathetic efferent neurons).[60,76]

Recent experiments suggest that the postsynaptic representation of glutamate receptors on dorsal horn neurons may be different from sensory boutons, depending on whether boutons were associated with A- or C-type neurons.[136] The AMPA postsynaptic receptors at C-type synapses are more calcium permeable than those associated with A-type processes.

Such differentiation may also be present in the medulla and at the NTS. This idea is supported by the discovery of differential predominance of varieties of potassium channels on second-order NTS neurons innervated by capsaicin-resistant and -sensitive afferents.[14,44,83] This differentiation has a major impact on synaptic transmission, information transfer, and the plasticity displayed by these two afferent neuronal populations as well as by their pathway interactions very early within brain stem reflex pathways.

Parasympathetic Efferent Neuronal Control and the Origins of Tone

The arterial baroreflex is a powerful controller of heart rate via cardiac parasympathetic efferent neurons. Both A-type and C-type arterial baroreceptors are tonically active at resting blood pressures, generating activity primarily during each systole.[84] Recent findings suggest that the activity of the arterial baroreflex is a major determinant of the tonic activity generated by parasympathetic efferent neurons that target the heart. Because the baroreceptor loop is so activated during each cardiac cycle, parasympathetic efferent neuronal activity is sustained at a tonic level by this reflex drive during normal blood pressure states. Clearly, the multiple interneuronal interactions involved in this reflex loop, from the level of the baroreceptor afferent neurons to second- and higher-order neurons in the NTS that influence cardiac vagal efferent preganglionic neurons primarily in the NA, are responsible for the overall performance of this arterial baroreflex arc. Further advances in our understanding of these mechanisms may presage the development of novel therapeutic strategies to control cardiac performance during cardiovascular disease and thereby improve clinical outcomes.

REFERENCES

1. Adrian ED. The impulses produced by sensory nerve endings. Part I. *J Physiol (Lond)* 61:49–72, 1926.
2. Andresen MC, Krauhs JM, and Brown AM. Relationship of aortic wall baroreceptor properties during development in normotensive and spontaneously hypertensive rats. *Circ Res* 43:728–738, 1978.
3. Andresen MC and Kunze DL. Nucleus tractus solitarius: gateway to neural circulatory control. *Annu Rev Physiol* 56:93–116, 1994.
4. Andresen MC, Kuraoka S, and Brown AM. Baroreceptor function and changes in strain sensitivity in normotensive and spontaneously hypertensive rats. *Circ Res* 47:821–828, 1980.
5. Andresen MC and Mendelowitz D. Sensory afferent neurotransmission in

caudal nucleus tractus solitarius—common denominators. *Chem Senses* 21: 387–395, 1996.
6. Andresen MC and Yang M. Arterial baroreceptor resetting: contributions of chronic and acute processes. *Clin Exp Pharmacol Physiol* 15(Suppl):19–30, 1989.
7. Andresen MC and Yang M. Non-NMDA receptors mediate sensory afferent synaptic transmission in medial nucleus tractus solitarius. *Am J Physiol* 259:H1307–H1311, 1990.
8. Andresen MC and Yang M. Excitatory amino acid receptors and afferent synaptic transmission in the nucleus tractus solitarius. In: Barraco RA, ed. *Nucleus of the Solitary Tract.* Boca Raton, FL: CRC Press, 1994, pp 187–192.
9. Angell-James JE. The effects of altering mean pressure, pulse pressure and pulse frequency on the impulse activity in baroreceptor fibres from the aortic arch and right subclavian artery in the rabbit. *J Physiol (Lond)* 214:65–88, 1971.
10. Angell-James JE and Daly MdB. Comparison of the reflex vasomotor responses to separate and combined stimulation of the carotid sinus and aortic arch baroreceptors by pulsatile and non-pulsatile pressure in the dog. *J Physiol (Lond)* 209:257–293, 1970.
11. Anrep GV, Pascual W, and Rossler R. Respiratory variations of the heart rate: II. The central mechanisms of the respiratory arrhythmia and the interrelations between the central and reflex mechanisms. *Proc R Soc Lond* 119:218–231, 1935.
12. Arndt J, Dorrenhaus A, and Wiecken H. The aortic arch baroreceptor response to static and dynamic stretches in an isolated aorta-depressor nerve preparation of cats in vitro. *J Physiol (Lond)* 252:59–78, 1975.
13. Aylwin ML, Horowitz JM, and Bonham AC. Non-NMDA and NMDA receptors in the synaptic pathway between area postrema and nucleus tractus solitarius. *Am J Physiol* 44:H1236–H1246, 1998.
14. Bailey TW, Jin Y-H, Doyle MW, and Andresen MC. Vanilloid sensitive afferents activate neurons with prominent A-type potassium currents in nucleus tractus solitarius. *J Neurosci* 22:8230–8237, 2002.
15. Barnes KL, Knowles WD, and Ferrario CM. An in vitro slice preparation of the canine medulla for investigation of the neural actions of angiotensin. *Hypertension* 10:365, 1987.
16. Basbaum AI and Jessell TM. The perception of pain. In: Kandel ER, Schwartz JH, and Jessell TM, eds. *Principles of Neural Science.* New York: McGraw-Hill, 2000, pp 472–491.
17. Bigger JT, Jr., La Rovere MT, Steinman RC, Fleiss JL, Rottman JN, Rolnitzky LM, and Schwartz PJ. Comparison of baroreflex sensitivity and heart period variability after myocardial infarction. *J Am Coll Cardiol* 14:1511–1518, 1989.
18. Blake DW and Korner PI. Effects of ketamine and althesin anesthesia on baroreceptor—heart rate reflex and hemodynamics of intact and pontine rabbits. *J Auton Nerv Syst* 5:145–154, 1982.
19. Bousquet P, Feldman J, Bloch R, and Schwartz J. Evidence for a neuromodulatory role of GABA at the first synapse of the baroreceptor reflex pathway. Effects of GABA derivatives injected into the NTS. *Naunyn Schmiedebergs Arch Pharmacol* 319:168–171, 1982.
20. Bowery N. $GABA_B$ receptors and their significance in mammalian pharmacology. *Trends Pharmacol Sci* 10:401–407, 1989.

21. Brooks PA, Glaum SR, Miller RJ, and Spyer KM. The actions of baclofen on neurones and synaptic transmission in the nucleus tractus solitarii of the rat in vitro. *J Physiol (Lond)* 457:115–129, 1992.
22. Brooks PA and Spyer KM. Investigation of inositol hexakisphosphate actions in rat nucleus tractus solitarius in vitro. *Neurosci Lett* 105:120–124, 1989.
23. Brooks PA and Spyer KM. Evidence for NMDA receptor–mediated synaptic events in the rat nucleus tractus solitarii in vitro. *J Physiol (Lond)* 467:21P, 1993.
24. Brown AM. Regulation of heartbeat by G protein–coupled ion channels. *Am J Physiol* 259:H1621–H1628, 1990.
25. Caterina MJ and Julius D. The vanilloid receptor: a molecular gateway to the pain pathway. *Annu Rev Neurosci* 24:487–517, 2001.
26. Champagnat J, Siggins GR, Koda LY, and Denavit-Saubie M. Synaptic responses of neurons of the nucleus tractus solitarius in vitro. *Brain Res* 325: 49–56, 1985.
27. Chan JYH, Tsou M-Y, Len W-B, Lee T-Y, and Chan SHH. Participation of noradrenergic neurotransmission in the enhancement of baroreceptor reflex response by substance P at the nucleus tractus solitarii of the rat: a reverse microdialysis study. *J Neurochem* 64:2644–2652, 1995.
28. Chapleau MW, Li Z, Meyrelles SS, Ma X, and Abboud FM. Mechanisms determining sensitivity of baroreceptor afferents in health and disease. *Ann NY Acad Sci* 940:1–19, 2001.
29. Chen CY and Bonham AC. Non-NMDA and NMDA receptors transmit area postrema input to aortic baroreceptor neurons in NTS. *Am J Physiol* 275: H1695–H1706, 1998.
30. Ciriello J, Hochstenbach SL, and Roder S. Central projections of baroreceptor and chemoreceptor afferent fibers in the rat. In: Barraco RA, ed. *Nucleus of the Solitary Tract*. Boca Raton, FL: CRC Press, 1994, pp 35–50.
31. Cole CR, Blackstone EH, Pashkow FJ, Snader CE, and Lauer MS. Heart-rate recovery immediately after exercise as a predictor of mortality. *N Engl J Med* 341:1351–1357, 1999.
32. Coleman T. Arterial baroreflex control of heart rate in the conscious rat. *Am J Physiol* 238:H515–H520, 1980.
33. Cote A, Hum C, Brouillette RT, and Themens M. Frequency and timing of recurrent events in infants using home cardiorespiratory monitors. *J Pediatr* 132:783–789, 1998.
34. Czachurski J, Lackner K, Ockert D, and Seller H. Localization of neurones with baroreceptor input in the medial solitary nucleus by means of intracellular application of horseradish peroxidase in the cat. *Neurosci Lett* 28:133–137, 1982.
35. Davidson NS, Goldner S, and McCloskey DI. Respiratory modulation of barareceptor and chemoreceptor reflexes affecting heart rate and cardiac vagal efferent nerve activity. *J Physiol* 259:523–530, 1976.
36. De Burgh Daly M. Some reflex cardioinhibitory responses in the cat and their modulation by central inspiratory neuronal activity. *J Physiol* 439:559–577, 1991.
37. Devor M and Wall PD. Effect of peripheral nerve injury on receptive fields of cells in the cat spinal cord. *J Comp Neurol* 199:277–291, 1981.
38. Devor M and Wall PD. Plasticity in the spinal cord sensory map following peripheral nerve injury in rats. *J Neurosci* 1:679–684, 1981.

39. Divon MY, Winkler H, Yeh SY, Platt LD, Langer O, and Merkatz IR. Diminished respiratory sinus arrhythmia in asphyxiated term infants. *Am J Obstet Gynecol* 155:1263–1266, 1986.
40. Doan TN and Kunze DL. Contribution of the hyperpolarization–activated current to the resting membrane potential of rat nodose sensory neurons. *J Physiol* 514:125–138, 1999.
41. Douglas WW, Ritchie JM, and Schaumann W. Depressor reflexes from medullated and nonmedullated fibres in the rabbit's aortic nerve. *J Physiol (Lond)* 132:187–198, 1956.
42. Douglas WW and Schaumann W. A study of the depressor and pressor components of the cat's carotid sinus and aortic nerves using electrical stimuli of different intensities and frequencies. *J Physiol (Lond)* 132:173–186, 1956.
43. Doyle MW and Andresen MC. Reliability of monosynaptic transmission in brain stem neurons in vitro. *J Neurophysiol* 85:2213–2223, 2001.
44. Doyle MW, Bailey TW, Jin Y-H, and Andresen MC. Vanilloid receptors presynaptically modulate visceral afferent synaptic transmission in nucleus tractus solitarius. *J Neurosci* 22:8222–8229, 2002.
45. Drewe JA, Miles R, and Kunze DL. Excitatory amino acid receptors of guinea pig medial nucleus tractus solitarius neurons. *Am J Physiol* 259:H1389–H1395, 1990.
46. Durgam VR, Vitela M, and Mifflin SW. Enhanced gamma-aminobutyric acid-B receptor agonist responses and mRNA within the nucleus of the solitary tract in hypertension. *Hypertension* 33:530–536, 1999.
47. Ead HW, Green JN, and Neil E. A comparison of the effects of pulsatile and non-pulsatile blood flow through the carotid sinus on the reflexogenic activity of the sinus baroreceptors in the cat. *J Physiol (Lond)* 118:509–519, 1952.
48. Eckberg DL, Drabinsky M, and Braunwald E. Defective cardiac parasympathetic control in patients with heart disease. *N Engl J Med* 285:877–883, 1971.
49. Eckberg DL and Orshan CR. Respiratory and baroreceptor reflex interactions in man. *J Clin Invest* 59:780–785, 1977.
50. Elghozi JL, Girard A, and Laude D. Effects of drugs on the autonomic control of short-term heart rate variability. *Auton Neurosci* 90:116–121, 2001.
51. Elghozi JL, Laude D, and Girard A. Effects of respiration on blood pressure and heart rate variability in humans. *Clin Exp Pharmacol Physiol* 18:735–742, 1991.
52. Ergene E, Dunbar JC, O'Leary DS, and Barraco RA. Activation of P_2-purinoceptors in the nucleus tractus solitarius mediate depressor responses. *Neurosci Lett* 174:188–192, 1994.
53. Everill B and Kocsis JD. Reduction in potassium currents in identified cutaneous afferent dorsal root ganglion neurons after axotomy. *J Neurophysiol* 82:700–708, 1999.
54. Fan W and Andresen MC. Differential frequency–dependent reflex integration of myelinated and nonmyelinated rat aortic baroreceptors. *Am J Physiol* 275:H632–H640, 1998.
55. Fan W, Schild JH, and Andresen MC. Graded and dynamic reflex summation of myelinated and unmyelinated rat aortic baroreceptors. *Am J Physiol* 277:R748–R756, 1999.
56. Fazan VP, Salgado HC, and Barreira AA. A descriptive and quantitative light and electron microscopy study of the aortic depressor nerve in normotensive rats. *Hypertension* 30:693–698, 1997.

57. Felder RB and Mifflin SW. Modulation of carotid sinus afferent input to nucleus tractus solitarius by parabrachial nucleus stimulation. *Circ Res* 63:35–49, 1988.
58. Feldman PD. Neurokinin$_1$ receptor mediation of the vasodepressor effects of substance P in the nucleus of the tractus solitarius. *J Pharmacol Exp Ther* 273:617–623, 1995.
59. Fields RD. Effects of ion channel activity on development of dorsal root ganglion neurons. *J Neurobiol* 37:158–170, 1998.
60. Fitzgerald M. Capsaicin and sensory neurons—a review. *Pain* 15:109–130, 1983.
61. Fjell J, Cummins TR, Dib-Hajj SD, Fried K, Black JA, and Waxman SG. Differential role of GDNF and NGF in the maintenance of two TTX-resistant sodium channels in adult DRG neurons. *Brain Res Mol Brain Res* 67:267–282, 1999.
62. Florentino A, Varga K, and Kunos G. Mechanism of the cardiovascular effects of GABA$_B$ receptor activation in the nucleus tractus solitarii of the rat. *Brain Res* 535:264–270, 1990.
63. Fodor M, Gallatz K, and Palkovits M. Calcitonin gene-related peptide innervation of A2-catecholamine cells in the nucleus of the solitary tract of the rat. *Brain Res* 690:141–144, 1995.
64. Gilbey MP, Jordan D, Richter DW, and Spyer KM. Synaptic mechanisms involved in the inspiratory modulation of vagal cardio-inhibitory neurones in the cat. *J Physiol* 356:65–78, 1984.
65. Gillis RA, Helke CJ, Hamilton BL, Norman WP, and Jacobowitz DM. Evidence that substance P is a neurotransmitter of baro- and chemoreceptor afferents in nucleus tractus solitarius. *Brain Res* 181:476–481, 1980.
66. Glaum SR, Brooks PA, Spyer KM, and Miller RJ. 5-Hydroxytryptamine-3 receptors modulate synaptic activity in the rat nucleus tractus solitarius in vitro. *Brain Res* 589:62–68, 1992.
67. Goldman W and Saum WR. A direct excitatory action of catecholamines on rat aortic baroreceptors in vitro. *Circ Res* 55:18–30, 1984.
68. Granata AR and Kitai ST. Intracellular study of nucleus parabrachialis and nucleus tractus solitarii interconnections. *Brain Res* 492:281–292, 1989.
69. Hall ME, Greer RA, and Stewart JM. Effects of L-glutamate, substance P and substance P(1–7) on cardiovascular regulation in the nucleus tractus solitarius. *Regul Pept* 46:102–109, 1993.
70. Harper RM and Bandler R. Finding the failure mechanism in sudden infant death syndrome. *Nat Med* 4:157–158, 1998.
71. Hathorn MKS. Respiratory sinus arrhythmia in new-born infants. *J Physiol (Lond)* 385:1–12, 1987.
72. Helke CJ, O'Donohue TL, and Jacobowitz DM. Substance P as a baro- and chemoreceptor afferent neurotransmitter: immunocytochemical and neurochemical evidence in the rat. *Peptides* 1:1–9, 1980.
73. Helke CJ and Rabchevsky A. Axotomy alters putative neurotransmitters in visceral sensory neurons of the nodose and petrosal ganglia. *Brain Res* 551:44–51, 1991.
74. Heymans C and Neil E. *Reflexogenic Areas of the Cardiovascular System.* London: Churchill, 1958.
75. Hille B. *Ionic Channels of Excitable Membranes.* Sunderland, MA: Sinauer Associates, 1992.

76. Holzer P. Capsaicin: cellular targets, mechanisms of action, and selectivity for thin sensory neurons. *Pharmacol Rev* 43:143–201, 1991.
77. Hrushesky WJ. Quantitative respiratory sinus arrhythmia analysis. A simple noninvasive, reimbursable measure of cardiac wellness and dysfunction. *Ann N Y Acad Sci* 618:67–101, 1991.
78. Ichikawa H, Rabchevsky A, and Helke CJ. Presence and coexistence of putative neurotransmitters in carotid sinus baro- and chemoreceptor afferent neurons. *Brain Res* 611:67–74, 1993.
79. Ino M, Yoshinaga T, Wakamori M, Miyamoto N, Takahashi E, Sonoda J, Kagaya T, Oki T, Nagasu T, Nishizawa Y, Tanaka I, Imoto K, Aizawa S, Koch S, Schwartz A, Niidome T, Sawada K, and Mori Y. Functional disorders of the sympathetic nervous system in mice lacking the alpha 1B subunit (Cav 2.2) of N-type calcium channels. *Proc Natl Acad Sci U S A* 98:5323–5328, 2001.
80. Inoue K, Miyake S, Kumashiro M, Ogata H, and Yoshimura O. Power spectral analysis of heart rate variability in traumatic quadriplegic humans. *Am J Physiol* 258:H1722–H1726, 1990.
81. Irnaten M, Aicher SA, Wang J, Venkatesan P, Evans C, Baxi S, and Mendelowitz D. μ-Opioid receptors are located postsynaptically and endomorphin-1 inhibits voltage-gated calcium currents in premotor cardiac parasympathetic neurons in the rat nucleus ambiguus. *Neuroscience* 116:573–582, 2003.
82. Iversen LL. Neuropeptides: promise unfulfilled. *Trends Neurosci* 18:49–50, 1995.
83. Jin Y-H, Bailey TW, Doyle MW, Li BY, Chang KSK, Schild JH, Mendelowitz D, and Andresen MC. Ketamine differentially blocks sensory afferent synaptic transmission in medial nucleus tractus solitarius (mNTS). *Anesthesiology* 98:121–132, 2003.
84. Jones J and Thoren PN. Characteristics of aortic baroreceptors with nonmedullated afferents arising from the aortic arch of rabbits with chronic renovascular hypertension. *Acta Physiol Scand* 101:286–293, 1977.
85. Kangrga IM and Randic M. Tachykinins and calcitonin gene-related peptide enhance release of endogenous glutamate and aspartate from the rat spinal dorsal horn slice. *J Neurosci* 10:2026–2038, 1990.
86. Kendrick JE, Matson GL, Oberg B, and Wennergren G. The effect of stimulus pattern on the pressure response to electrical stimulation of the carotid sinus nerve of cats. *Proc Soc Exp Biol Med* 144:412–416, 1973.
87. Koizumi K and Sato A. Reflex activity of single sympathetic fibres to skeletal muscle produced by electrical stimulation of somatic and vago-depressor afferent nerves in the cat. *Pflugers Arch* 332:283–301, 1972.
88. Krauhs JM. Structure of rat aortic baroreceptors and their relationship to connective tissue. *J Neurocytol* 8:401–414, 1979.
89. Krieger EM, Salgado HC, and Michelini L. Resetting of the baroreceptors. In: Guyton AC and Hall JE, eds. *International Review of Physiology*. Baltimore: University Park Press, 1982, pp 119–147.
90. Kubo T and Kihara M. Evidence for gamma-aminobutyric acid receptor–mediated modulation of the aortic baroreceptor reflex in the nucleus tractus solitarii of the rat. *Neurosci Lett* 89:156–160, 1988.
91. Kunze DL. Reflex discharge patterns of cardiac vagal efferent fibres. *J Physiol (Lond)* 222:1–15, 1972.
92. Kunze DL. Regulation of activity of cardiac vagal motorneurons. *Fed Proc* 39:2513–2518, 1980.

93. La Rovere MT, Bigger JT, Jr., Marcus FI, Mortara A, Schwartz PJ, and ATRAMI Investigators. Baroreflex sensitivity and heart-rate variability in prediction of total cardiac mortality after myocardial infarction. *Lancet* 351:478–484, 1998.
94. La Rovere MT, Pinna GD, Hohnloser SH, Marcus FI, Mortara A, Norhara R, Bigger JT, Jr., Camm AJ, Schwartz PJ, and ATRAMI Investigators. Baroreflex sensitivity and heart rate variability in the identification of patients at risk for life-threatening arrhythmias: implications for clinical trials. *Circulation* 103:2072–2077, 2001.
95. La Rovere MT, Specchia G, Mortara A, and Schwartz PJ. Baroreflex sensitivity, clinical correlates, and cardiovascular mortality among patients with a first myocardial infarction. A prospective study. *Circulation* 78:816–824, 1988.
96. Lawrence AJ and Jarrott B. Neurochemical modulation of cardiovascular control in the nucleus tractus solitarius. *Prog Neurobiol* 48:21–53, 1996.
97. Lawson SN. Morphological and biochemical cell types of sensory neurons. In: Scott SA, ed. *Sensory Neurons: Diversity, Development, and Plasticity*. New York: Oxford University Press, 1992, pp 27–59.
98. Lee JS, Andresen MC, Morrow D, and Chang KSK. Isoflurane depresses baroreflex control of heart rate in decerebrate rats. *Anesthesiology* 96:1214–1222, 2002.
99. Leone C and Gordon FJ. Is L-glutamate a neurotransmitter of baroreceptor information in the nucleus of tractus solitarius? *J Pharmacol Exp Ther* 250:953–962, 1989.
100. Levine JD, Fields HL, and Basbaum AI. Peptides and the primary afferent nociceptor. *J Neurosci* 13:2273–2286, 1993.
101. Levy MN and Zieske H. Autonomic control of cardiac pacemaker activity and atrioventricular transmission. *J Appl Physiol* 27:465–470, 1969.
102. Li BY and Schild JH. Patch clamp electrophysiology in the nodose ganglia of the adult rat. *J Neurosci Methods* 115:157–167, 2002.
103. Loewi O. Über humorale Übertragbarkeit der Herznervenwirkung. *Pflugers Arch* 189:239–242, 1921.
104. Loewy AD. Central autonomic pathways. In: Loewy AD and Spyer KM, eds. *Central Regulation of Autonomic Functions*. New York: Oxford University Press, 1990, pp 88–103.
105. Loewy AD and Spyer KM. Vagal preganglionic neurons. In: Loewy AD and Spyer KM, eds. *Central Regulation of Autonomic Functions*. New York: Oxford University Press, 1990, pp 68–87.
106. MacDermott AB, Role LW, and Siegelbaum SA. Presynaptic ionotropic receptors and the control of transmitter release. *Annu Rev Neurosci* 22:443–485, 1999.
107. Mantyh PW, DeMaster E, Malhotra A, Ghilardi JR, Rogers SD, Mantyh CR, Liu H, Basbaum AI, Vigna SR, Maggio JE, and Simone DA. Receptor endocytosis and dendrite reshaping in spinal neurons after somatosensory stimulation. *Science* 268:1629–1632, 1995.
108. McAllen RM and Spyer KM. The baroreceptor input to cardiac vagal motoneurones. *J Physiol (Lond)* 282:365–374, 1978.
109. McWilliam PN and Shepheard SL. A GABA-mediated inhibition of neurones in the nucleus tractus solitarius of the cat that respond to electrical stimulation of the carotid sinus nerve. *Neurosci Lett* 94:321–326, 1988.

110. Mendelowitz D. Firing properties of identified parasympathetic cardiac neurons in nucleus ambiguus. *Am J Physiol* 271:H2609–H2614, 1996.
111. Mendelowitz D. Advances in parasympathetic control of heart rate and cardiac function. *News Physiol Sci* 14:155–161, 1999.
112. Mendelowitz D and Kunze DL. Identification and dissociation of cardiovascular neurons from the medulla for patch clamp analysis. *Neurosci Lett* 132:217–221, 1991.
113. Mendelowitz D, Yang M, Andresen MC, and Kunze DL. Localization and retention in vitro of fluorescently labeled aortic baroreceptor terminals on neurons from the nucleus tractus solitarius. *Brain Res* 581:339–343, 1992.
114. Mendelowitz D, Yang M, Reynolds PJ, and Andresen MC. Heterogeneous functional expression of calcium channels at sensory and synaptic regions in nodose neurons. *J Neurophysiol* 73:872–875, 1995.
115. Meny RG, Carroll JL, Carbone MT, and Kelly DH. Cardiorespiratory recordings from infants dying suddenly and unexpectedly at home. *Pediatrics* 93:44–49, 1994.
116. Mifflin SW and Felder RB. Synaptic mechanisms regulating cardiovascular afferent inputs to solitary tract nucleus. *Am J Physiol* 259:H653–H661, 1990.
117. Mihalevich M, Neff RA, and Mendelowitz D. Voltage-gated currents in identified parasympathetic cardiac neurons in the nucleus ambiguus. *Brain Res* 739:258–262, 1996.
118. Miles R. Frequency dependence of synaptic transmission in nucleus of the solitary tract in vitro. *J Neurophysiol* 55:1076–1090, 1986.
119. Milner B, Squire LR, and Kandel ER. Cognitive neuroscience and the study of memory. *Neuron* 20:445–468, 1998.
120. Miura M. Postsynaptic potentials recorded from nucleus of the solitary tract and its subjacent reticular formation elicited by stimulation of the carotid sinus nerve. *Brain Res* 100:437–440, 1975.
121. Morillo AM, Nunez-Abades PA, Gaytan SP, and Pasaro R. Brain stem projections by axonal collaterals to the rostral and caudal ventral respiratory group in the rat. *Brain Res Bull* 37:205–211, 1995.
122. Munch PA, Andresen MC, and Brown AM. Rapid resetting of aortic baroreceptors in vitro. *Am J Physiol* 244:H672–H680, 1983.
123. Munch PA and Brown AM. Sympathetic modulation of rabbit aortic baroreceptors in vitro. *Am J Physiol* 253:H1106–H1111, 1987.
124. Munch PA, Thoren PN, and Brown AM. Dual effects of norepinephrine and mechanisms of baroreceptor stimulation. *Circ Res* 61:409–419, 1987.
125. Nakagawa T, Shirasaki T, Tateishi N, Murase K, and Akaike N. Effects of antagonists on N-methyl-D-aspartate response in acutely isolated nucleus tractus solitarii neurons of the rat. *Neurosci Lett* 113:169–174, 1990.
126. Neff RA, Mihalevich M, and Mendelowitz D. Stimulation of NTS activates NMDA and non-NMDA receptors in rat cardiac vagal neurons in the nucleus ambiguus. *Brain Res* 792:277–282, 1998.
127. Nicoll RA, Malenka RC, and Kauer JA. Functional comparison of neurotransmitter receptor subtypes in mammalian central nervous system. *Physiol Rev* 70:513–551, 1990.
128. Nosaka S, Yamamoto T, and Yasunaga K. Localization of vagal cardioinhibitory preganglionic neurons with rat brain stem. *J Comp Neurol* 186:79–92, 1979.

129. Okamoto H, Hoka S, Kawasaki T, Sato M, and Yoshitake J. Effects of CGRP on baroreflex control of heart rate and renal sympathetic nerve activity in rabbits. *Am J Physiol* 263:R874–R879, 1992.
130. Okuse K, Chaplan SR, McMahon SB, Luo ZD, Calcutt NA, Scott BP, Akopian AN, and Wood JN. Regulation of expression of the sensory neuron–specific sodium channel SNS in inflammatory and neuropathic pain. *Mol Cell Neurosci* 10:196–207, 1997.
131. Pardini BJ, Lund DD, and Schmid PG. Organization of the sympathetic postganglionic innervation of the rat heart. *J Auton Nerv Syst* 28:193–202, 1989.
132. Paton JFR, Rogers WT, and Schwaber JS. Tonically rhythmic neurons within a cardiorespiratory region of the nucleus tractus solitarii of the rat. *J Neurophysiol* 66:824–838, 1991.
133. Phillis JW, Scislo TJ, and O'Leary DS. Purines and the nucleus tractus solitarius: Effects on cardiovascular and respiratory function. *Clin Exp Pharmacol Physiol* 24:738–742, 1997.
134. Pickering TG, Gribbin B, Petersen ES, Cunningham DJ, and Sleight P. Effects of autonomic blockade on the baroreflex in man at rest and during exercise. *Circ Res* 30:177–185, 1972.
135. Pilowsky PM and Goodchild AK. Baroreceptor reflex pathways and neurotransmitters: 10 years on. *J Hypertens* 20:1675–1688, 2002.
136. Popratiloff A, Weinberg RJ, and Rustioni A. AMPA receptor subunits underlying terminals of fine-caliber primary afferent fibers. *J Neurosci* 16:3363–3372, 1996.
137. Rardon DP and Bailey JC. Parasympathetic effects on electrophysiologic properties of cardiac ventricular tissue. *J Am Coll Cardiol* 2:1200–1209, 1983.
138. Reis DJ, Joh TH, Nathan MA, Renaud B, Snyder DW, and Talman WT. Nucleus tractus solitarii: catecholaminergic innervation in normal and abnormal control of arterial pressure. In: Meyer P and Schmitt H, ed. *Nervous System and Hypertension*. New York: John Wiley & Sons, 1979, pp 147–164.
139. Richter DW and Spyer KM. Cardiorespiratory control. In: Loewy AD and Spyer KM, eds. *Central Regulation of Autonomic Functions*. New York: Oxford University Press, 1990, pp 189–207.
140. Sapru HN, Gonzalez E, and Krieger AJ. Aortic nerve stimulation in the rat: cardiovascular and respiratory responses. *Brain Res Bull* 6:393–398, 1981.
141. Schechtman VL, Raetz SL, Harper RK, Garfinkel A, Wilson AJ, Southall DP, and Harper RM. Dynamic analysis of cardiac R-R intervals in normal infants and in infants who subsequently succumbed to the sudden infant death syndrome. *Pediatr Res* 31:606–612, 1992.
142. Scher A and Young A. Reflex control of heart rate in the unanesthetized dog. *Am J Physiol* 218:780–789, 1970.
143. Schild JH, Clark JW, Hay M, Mendelowitz D, Andresen MC, and Kunze DL. A- and C-type nodose sensory neurons: model interpretations of dynamic discharge characteristics. *J Neurophysiol* 71:2338–2358, 1994.
144. Schild JH and Kunze DL. Experimental and modeling study of Na^+ current heterogeneity in rat nodose neurons and its impact on neuronal discharge. *J Neurophysiol* 78:3198–3209, 1997.
145. Schwartz PJ, La Rovere MT, and Vanoli E. Autonomic nervous system and sudden death: experimental basis and clinical observations for post-myocardial infarction risk stratification. *Circulation* 85(Suppl I):77–91, 1992.

146. Scislo TJ, Augustyniak RA, Barraco RA, Woodbury DJ, and O'Leary DS. Activation of P_{2x}-purinoceptors in the nucleus tractus solitarius elicits differential inhibition of lumbar and renal sympathetic nerve activity. *J Auton Nerv Syst* 62:103–110, 1997.
147. Scislo TJ, Ergene E, and O'Leary DS. Impaired arterial baroreflex regulation of heart rate after blockade of P_2-purinoceptors in the nucleus tractus solitarius. *Brain Res Bull* 47:63–67, 1998.
148. Scislo TJ and O'Leary DS. Differential role of ionotropic glutamatergic mechanisms in responses to NTS P(2x) and A(2a) receptor stimulation. *Am J Physiol (Heart Circ Physiol)* 278:H2057–H2068, 2000.
149. Seagard JL, Hopp FA, Drummond HA, and Van Wynsberghe DM. Selective contribution of two types of carotid sinus baroreceptors to the control of blood pressure. *Circ Res* 72:1011–1022, 1993.
150. Shihara M, Hori N, Hirooka Y, Eshima K, Akaike N, and Takeshita A. Cholinergic systems in the nucleus of the solitary tract of rats. *Am J Physiol* 276:R1141–R1148, 1999.
151. Shykoff BE, Naqvi SS, Menon AS, and Slutsky AS. Respiratory sinus arrhythmia in dogs. Effects of phasic afferents and chemostimulation. *J Clin Invest* 87:1621–1627, 1991.
152. Sieghart W. Structure and pharmacology of gamma-aminobutyric acid$_A$ receptor subtypes. *Pharmacol Rev* 47:181–234, 1995.
153. Sigel E and Kannenberg K. GABA$_A$-receptor subtypes. *Trends Neurosci* 19:386, 1996.
154. Sirén A-L and Feuerstein G. Cardiovascular effects of rat calcitonin gene-related peptide in the conscious rat. *J Pharmacol Exp Ther* 247:69–78, 1988.
155. Spyer KM. Neural organisation and control of the baroreceptor reflex. *Rev Physiol Biochem Pharmacol* 88:24–124, 1981.
156. Spyer KM. The central nervous organization of reflex circulatory control. In: Loewy AD and Spyer KM, eds. *Central Regulation of Autonomic Functions*. New York: Oxford University Press, 1990, pp 168–188.
157. Spyer KM. Central nervous mechanisms contributing to cardiovascular control. *J Physiol (Lond)* 474:1–19, 1994.
158. Spyer KM and Gilbey MP. Cardiorespiratory interactions in heart-rate control. *Ann NY Acad Sci* 533:350–357, 1988.
159. Stegemann J and Tibes U. Sinusoidal stimulation of carotid sinus baroreceptors and peripheral blood pressure in dogs. *Ann NY Acad Sci* 156:787–795, 1967.
160. Stornetta RL, Guyenet PG, and McCarty RC. Autonomic nervous system control of heart rate during baroreceptor activation in conscious and anesthetized rats. *J Auton Nerv Syst* 20:121, 1987.
161. Sullebarger JT, Liang C-S, Woolf PD, Willick AE, and Richeson JF. Comparison of phenylephrine bolus and infusion methods in baroreflex measurements. *J Appl Physiol* 69:962–967, 1990.
162. Talman WT, Granata AR, and Reis DJ. Glutamatergic mechanisms in the nucleus tractus solitarius in blood pressure control. *Fed Proc* 43:39–44, 1984.
163. Taylor JA and Sanderson M. A reexamination of the risk factors for the sudden infant death syndrome. *J Pediatr* 126:887–891, 1995.
164. Thompson SM, Capogna M, and Scanziani M. Presynaptic inhibition in the hippocampus. *Trends Neurosci* 16:222–227, 1993.

165. Thor KB and Helke CJ. Serotonin and substance P–containing projections to the nucleus tractus solitarii of the rat. *J Comp Neurol* 265:275–293, 1987.
166. Thoren PN, Andresen MC, and Brown AM. Effects of changes in extracellular ionic concentrations on aortic baroreceptors with nonmyelinated afferent fibers. *Circ Res* 50:413–418, 1982.
167. Thoren PN, Andresen MC, and Brown AM. Resetting of aortic baroreceptors with non-myelinated afferent fibers in spontaneously hypertensive rats. *Acta Physiol Scand* 117:91–97, 1983.
168. Thoren PN, Saum WR, and Brown AM. Characteristics of rat aortic baroreceptors with nonmedullated afferent nerve fibers. *Circ Res* 40:231–237, 1977.
169. Tsuda K, Tsuda S, Goldstein M, and Masuyama Y. Effects of calcitonin gene-related peptide on [^{3}H]norepinephrine release in medulla oblongata of spontaneously hypertensive rats. *Eur J Pharmacol* 191:101–105, 1990.
170. Van Giersbergen PLM, Palkovits M, and De Jong W. Involvement of neurotransmitters in the nucleus tractus solitarii in cardiovascular regulation. *Physiol Rev* 72:789–824, 1992.
171. Vanoli E, De Ferrari GM, Stramba-Badiale M, Hull SS, Jr., Foreman RD, and Schwartz PJ. Vagal stimulation and prevention of sudden death in conscious dogs with a healed myocardial infarction. *Circ Res* 68:1471–1481, 1991.
172. Venkatesan P, Wang J, Evans C, Irnaten M, and Mendelowitz D. Endomorphin-2 inhibits GABAergic inputs to cardiac parasympathetic neurons in the nucleus ambiguus. *Neuroscience* 113:975, 2002.
173. Venkatesan P, Wang J, Evans C, Irnaten M, and Mendelowitz D. Nociceptin inhibits gamma-aminobutyric acidergic inputs to cardiac parasympathetic neurons in the nucleus ambiguus. *J Pharmacol Exp Ther* 300:78–82, 2002.
174. Voilley N, de Weille J, Mamet J, and Lazdunski M. Nonsteroid antiinflammatory drugs inhibit both the activity and the inflammation-induced expression of acid-sensing ion channels in nociceptors. *J Neurosci* 21:8026–8033, 2001.
175. Wakamori M, Ikemoto Y, and Akaike N. Effects of two volatile anesthetics and a volatile convulsant on the excitatory and inhibitory amino acid responses in dissociated CNS neurons of the rat. *J Neurophysiol* 66:2014–2021, 1991.
176. Wall PD, Mills R, Fitzgerald M, and Gibson SJ. Chronic blockade of sciatic nerve transmission by tetrodotoxin does not produce central changes in the dorsal of the spinal cord of the rat. *Neurosci Lett* 30:315–320, 1982.
177. Wang J, Irnaten M, and Mendelowitz D. Characteristics of spontaneous and evoked GABAergic synaptic currents in cardiac vagal neurons in rats. *Brain Res* 889:78–83, 2001.
178. Wang J, Wang X, Irnaten M, Venkatesan P, Evans C, Baxi S, and Mendelowitz D. Endogenous acetylcholine and nicotine activation enhances GABAergic and glycinergic inputs to cardiac vagal neurons. *J Neurophysiol* 89:2473–2478, 2003.
179. Waxman MB and Wald RW. Termination of ventricular tachycardia by an increase in cardiac vagal drive. *Circulation* 56:385–391, 1977.
180. Weinreich D, Moore KA, and Taylor GE. Allergic inflammation in isolated vagal sensory ganglia unmasks silent NK-2 tachykinin receptors. *J Neurosci* 17:7683–7693, 1997.
181. Whitescarver SA, Ott CE, and Kotchen TA. Parasympathetic impairment of baroreflex control of heart rate in Dahl S rats. *Am J Physiol* 259:R76–R83, 1990.

182. Yao T and Thoren PN. Adrenergic and pressure-induced modulation of carotid sinus baroreceptors in rabbits. *Acta Physiol Scand* 117:9–17, 1983.
183. Yao T and Thoren PN. Characteristics of brachiocephalic and carotid sinus baroreceptors with non-medullated afferents in rabbit. *Acta Physiol Scand* 117:1–8, 1983.
184. Yen JC, Chan JYH, and Chan SHH. Differential roles of NMDA and non-NMDA receptors in synaptic responses of neurons in nucleus tractus solitarii of the rat. *J Neurophysiol* 81:3034–3043, 1999.
185. Zhang J and Mifflin SW. Receptor subtype specific effects of GABA agonists on neurons receiving aortic depressor nerve inputs within the nucleus of the solitary tract. *J Auton Nerv Syst* 73:170–181, 1998.

7

Forebrain Control of Healthy and Diseased Hearts

DAVID F. CECHETTO

A number of parallels can be drawn between the anatomical and physiological characteristics of the visceral and somatic nervous systems. They both have ascending sensory pathways that terminate in either the marginal layers of the spinal cord[76] or the caudal medulla.[59] Their sensory information is relayed to the cortex, primarily via a crossed pathway from a lower brain stem site to the thalamus. Each has a topographically organized afferent pathway throughout the neuraxis such that much of this ascending sensory information has collateral pathways to other limbic or basal ganglia sites that participate in the integration of responses to peripheral stimuli. Furthermore, the descending pathways for visceral and somatic system control are similar in that there is a primary region in the frontal cortex of the brain with direct connections to the spinal cord, with multiple subcortical sites exerting very strong tonic control over the final common pathway. However, these two major brain systems diverge in one very important aspect. Perturbations in the autonomic control regions of the brain can, and often do, lead to death due to cardiac, gastric, vascular, or renal complications. Disruptions in specific regions of the somatic nervous system, by contrast, usually result in less life-threatening complications, such as paralysis.

Stroke has been shown to lead to death due to cardiac dysfunction as a result of lesions in critical components of the forebrain that control the autonomic nervous system. Emotional stress can have a major impact on cardiovascular function, an effect that must, by definition, originate in the forebrain. Recent investigations have elucidated the organization and function of the regions in the brain that are responsible for these effects. A clear understanding of the organization of the autonomic control system of the forebrain is critical for designing therapies for prevention of death due to autonomic failure. This chapter will first summarize the anatomy, physiology, and pharmacology of the higher brain centers involved in central autonomic control. Then the role of these centers in cardiovascular disease will be considered from the point of view of perturbations that are caused by conditions such as stroke and emotional stress.

ORGANIZATION OF THE FOREBRAIN IN CENTRAL AUTONOMIC CONTROL

In general, the organization of central autonomic control can be viewed as a series of reflex loops involving progressively higher centers in the brain. For example, the basic baroreceptor loop for reflex sympathetic efferent neuronal control involves inputs to the nucleus of the solitary tract,[66,113,114,115,171] with a subsequent relay of information to the ventral lateral medulla and possibly a secondary connection within the ventral lateral medulla, and finally a descending output to the sympathetic preganglionic neurons in the thoracic spinal cord (see Chapter 5). As will be seen from the following discussion, longer more complex loops exist in forebrain sites such as the hypothalamus,[64,169] amygdala,[82,86,228] even the cerebral cortex.[20,21,170,230,231] Thus, central autonomic neuronal control can, by and large, be viewed as a series of pathways bringing information to the forebrain sites where increasingly higher-level integration takes place. As a consequence, they influence relatively direct descending pathways to brain stem and spinal cord regions containing neurons that project to intrathoracic neurons control heart rate and contractility (Chapter 4).

Parabrachial Nucleus: Visceral Relay to the Forebrain

Visceral inputs, including those arising from cardiovascular, gastrointestinal, respiratory, and gustatory afferent neurons, have a primary termination in the nucleus of the solitary tract (Fig. 7–1). The nucleus of the solitary tract has extensive projections to the parabrachial nucleus of the pons. It has been shown that the parabrachial nucleus is primarily responsible for disseminating this information to multiple regions of the forebrain (Fig. 7–1).[44,45,158,183,205] Furthermore, the cardiovascular, gastrointestinal, respiratory, and the gustatory regions of the nucleus of the solitary tract[7,60,61,112–115,171] have a distinct pattern of termination in the pararachial nucleus.[101] The general visceral (including cardiovascular) afferent portion of the nucleus of the solitary tract projects to the external lateral, central, dorsal lateral, and the waist areas of the parabrachial nucleus. The rostral third of the nucleus of the solitary tract is the site of ter-

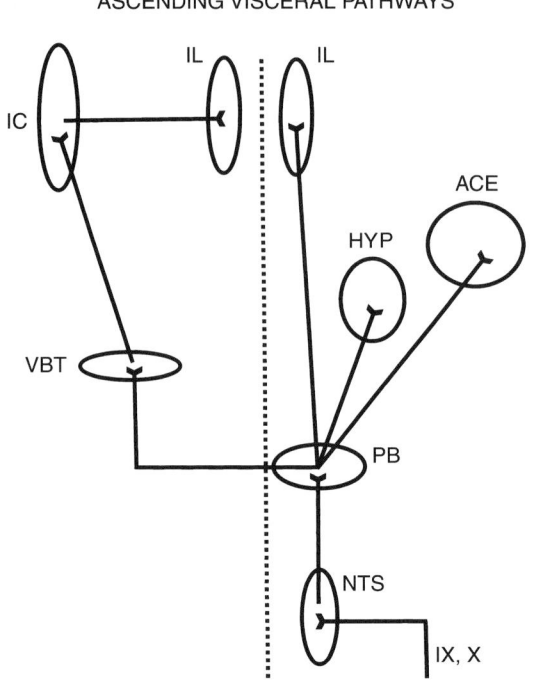

ASCENDING VISCERAL PATHWAYS

FIGURE 7–1 Pathways for visceral afferent information from the periphery ascending throughout the neuraxis. The dashed line indicates the midline of the central nervous system. ACE, central nucleus of the amygdala; HYP, hypothalamus; IC, insular cortex; IL, infralimbic cortex; IX, glossopharyngeal nerve; NTS, nucleus of the solitary tract; PB, parabrachial nucleus; VBT, ventral basal thalamus; X, vagus nerve.

mination of gustatory inputs.[95,96,225,243] Its neurons project primarily to the medial and ventral lateral subnuclei of the parabrachial nucleus.[101]

The parabrachial nucleus has topographically organized afferent and efferent connections to a number of forebrain sites, including the hypothalamus and amygdala.[80,149] The efferent projections from the parabrachial nucleus to the hypothalamus and amygdala would suggest that visceral information is relayed to these sites,[21,94] as has been confirmed by a number of electrophysiological investigations.[44,45,52,98] This has also been supported by the recent demonstration that electrical stimulation of the parabrachial nucleus elicits an ipsilateral increase in c-fos activity in areas of the hypothalamus and amygdala, including the paraventricular and supraoptic nuclei of the hypothalamus and the central nucleus of the amygdala.[134] An essential role for the parabrachial nucleus in relaying cardiovascular information to the amygdala has also been established.[44,45] As discussed below, the modality-specific transfer of visceral information to the cortex involves a relay in the ventral basal thalamus.[194]

The neurotransmitter mechanisms mediating the ascending visceral information through the parabrachial nucleus have also been elucidated. The relay of visceral information through the parabrachial nucleus is mediated by N-methyl-D-asparate (NMDA) receptors, while α_2 adrenergic and $GABA_A$ receptors contribute to the maintenance of tonic activity of neurons projecting to the ventral basal thalamus, the next step in the pathway to the visceral sensory cortex.[195] In addition, a number of peptides found in the parabrachial nucleus have been implicated in modulation of visceral information projecting to the forebrain. These peptides, including substance P, calcitonin gene–related peptide, somatostatin, neurotensin, and cholecystokinin, exert variable effects on the relay of visceral information such as inhibition or excitation of the signal or enhancing the signal to background firing ratio.[197] Finally, it has been shown that neuropeptides in the parabrachial nucleus interact with the primary neurotransmitters and their receptors to produce the modulatory effects.[196]

The parabrachial nucleus, in addition to relaying visceral information to the forebrain, also plays an integrative role in autonomic control. It projects signals to the sympathetic and parasympathetic efferent preganglionic neurons via direct connections to regions containing such neurons.[80,101,205] For example, stimulation of the lateral or medial parabrachial nucleus in the cat increases blood pressure, indicating its involvement in cardiovascular control.[53,54] Thus, the parabrachial nucleus serves as a higher-order reflex center for autonomic control of the cardiovascular system.

Thalamus: Cortical Relay Station

There was early evidence for general visceral inputs to the ventral basal thalamus.[1,2] Stimulation of the central end of the transected vagus results in short latency–evoked potentials in the ventral basal thalamus.[69] These potentials were recorded at a site corresponding to the medial part of the parvocellular ventral posterior thalamic nucleus. In addition, stimulation of the glossopharyngeal nerve results in evoked responses in the ventral basal thalamus.[26] Recording single neuronal activity delineated the organization of the visceral sensory modalities in the ventral basal thalamus. Gustatory-sensitive neurons are located in the most medial part of the ventral posterior thalamic nucleus.[1,20,50,85,135,160,162] Neurons responsive to general visceral activation, including baroreceptors, chemoreceptors, lung afferents, and gastric mechanoreceptors, are located immediately lateral to gustatory responsive ones.[43]

Retrograde tracing anatomical experiments have determined the organization of the parabrachial inputs to the ventral basal thalamus. Tracers injected into the medial portion of the paravocellular ventral posterior thalamic nucleus, the site of gustatory responsive neurons, resulted in retrograde labeling in many neurons in the contralateral external medial parabrachial subnucleus.[43] Injections more laterally in the parvocellular ventral posterior thalamic nucleus resulted in intense retrograde labeling of neurons in the contralateral external medial parabrachial subnucleus. These results were confirmed by anterograde tracer injections into the parabrachial nucleus.[43] The existence of a pathway mediating general visceral afferent vagal input from the left parabrachial nucleus and projecting to the right ventrobasal thalamus has recently been demonstrated physiologically.[194–196] Thus, there is a modality-organized input of vagal visceral information to the ventral basal thalamus that includes a midline crossing in the pathway from the parabrachial nucleus to the thalamus (Fig. 7–1). These visceral input regions of the thalamus project to visceroreceptive sites in the insular cortex,[17] as reviewed in detail in the following section.[6]

Some of the neurotransmitter mechanisms included in thalamic processing of visceral information have been delineated. The results of these experiments indicate that a non-NMDA excitatory amino acid receptor is necessary for the relay of visceral afferent information in the ventral basal thalamus, while muscarinic receptors may modulate visceral neuronal excitability in the parvocellular ventral posterior nucleus of the thalamus by an interaction between the inhibitory M_2 and excitatory M_3 or M_5 muscarinic receptor subtypes.[17] In addition to the vagal visceral input to the thalamus, there is also a sympathetic afferent input that appears to terminate in the thoracic region of the ventral posterior lateral nucleus.[2,145,173,219] This sympathetic afferent system arises from spinothalamic neurons receiving convergent visceral and somatic inputs.[9–13,22–25,76]

The paraventricular nucleus of the thalamus is the primary thalamic site of neurons that project efferent axons to the infralimbic region of the medial prefrontal cortex.[62,77,150] The infralimbic cortex, as discussed below, is the forebrain site considered to be the primary visceral motor cortex. Furthermore, the paraventricular nucleus of the thalamus has been demonstrated to be critical in relaying circadian information to the infralimbic cortex and other regions of the brain, since it also receives inputs from all major components of the circadian timing system, including the suprachiasmatic nucleus, the subparaventricular zone (the major terminal field of the suprachiasmatic nucleus), the intergeniculate leaflet, and the retina.[151,240,241] Thus, it has been suggested that the paraventricular nucleus of the thalamus functions as an output component to provide circadian timing information to regions of the brain, such as the infralimbic cortex, responsible for autonomic, hormonal, or behavioral control.[150,151]

Insular Cortex: Visceral Sensory Cortex

In 1869 Hughlings Jackson suggested that both voluntary and involuntary control was represented in the convolutions of the cerebrum.[102] The first demonstration of the likely location for this representation was provided in 1938, when it was shown that stimulation of the cervical vagus nerve in cats resulted in an increased cortical electrical activity in the orbitoinsular region.[16] This finding was confirmed in 1951 when it was demonstrated that stimulation of afferent axons in the vagus nerve elicits evoked potentials (8–10 ms delay) in the insular cortex.[69] Since these first two investigations indicating the possibility of autonomic inputs to the insular cortex, there have been a number of anatomical and electrophysiological studies demonstrating the organization of visceral inputs to this cortical region.[43] These studies have led to the concept that the insular cortex can be considered the visceral sensory cortex.

Previous studies have suggested the presence of a taste (special visceral) cortical area in the anterior insula in monkeys and humans (cf.[15,20,52]). Localization of a special visceral sensory, gustatory region in the cerebrum provides the most convincing evidence of visceral input to the insular cortex.[159,178,207,214,246] There are no data in the primate on the relationships of these cortical gustatory areas with areas activated by general visceral inputs. The extensive information obtained in the rat would suggest that there should be a representation of the thoracic and abdominal viscera in the insular cortex that is in close approximation to the gustatory representation.

Anatomical results in the rat have indicated the possibility that the insular cortex is organized in a viscerotopic manner.[202,210,211,217,235,237] Subsequent single-neuron recordings established that general visceral sensation is represented in the insular cortex[50,52] and that selective stimulation of visceral sensory modalities activates neurons in the insular cortex in a viscerotopic manner.[42,50,52] Neuronal recordings also demonstrated that gustatory inputs are located in a rostral dysgranular region of the insular cortex,[50,214,243] previously identified by other investigators.[128,163,245,248] General visceral inputs were primarily located more posteriorly and dorsally in the rat granular region of the insular cortex.[50] In the human, gustatory activation is located superior to general visceral inputs.[124]

The pathway for the flow of visceral afferent information to the insular cortex indicates that there are direct and indirect ipsilateral projections from the lateral parabrachial nucleus to the posterior granular and dysgranular insular cortex.[52,203,205] However, a substantial projection to the insular cortex from the contralateral parabrachial nucleus has also been shown.[50,149] The indirect parabrachial projections to the posterior (cardiovascular) rat insula synapse in the thalamus (the parvocellular ventral posterior thalamic nucleus described above) and are principally connected with the contralateral insula, although ipsilateral thalamoinsular projections have been noted, primarily from intralaminar thalamic nuclei.[50]

In summary, neurons in the cardiovascular region of the caudal medial nucleus of the solitary tract in the medulla project principally to the rostral lateral parabrachial nucleus.[101] There are bilateral (but principally ipsilateral) direct inputs from this parabrachial region to the posterior insula and bilateral (but principally contralateral) indirect inputs to the ventrobasal thalamus. From there, ipsilateral thalamoinsular afferent projections arise (Fig. 7–1).

In addition to receiving visceral afferent input, the insular cortex is also capable of generating substantial autonomic efferent responses via descending pathways[46] (Fig. 7–2). Ablation of the orbitoinsular region in cats results in the autonomic manifestations (piloerection, dilatation of the pupils, retraction of the nictitating membrane, panting, tachycardia) of rage,[39,122] suggesting that the insular cortex plays a role in the tonic regulation of autonomic (particularly sympathetic) efferent neuronal responses. Stimulation studies have supported this view. Electrical stimulation of the insular cortex in a variety of mammals elicits changes in blood pressure, heart rate, respiration, piloerection, pupillary dilatation, gastric motility, peristaltic activity, salivation, and adrenaline secre-

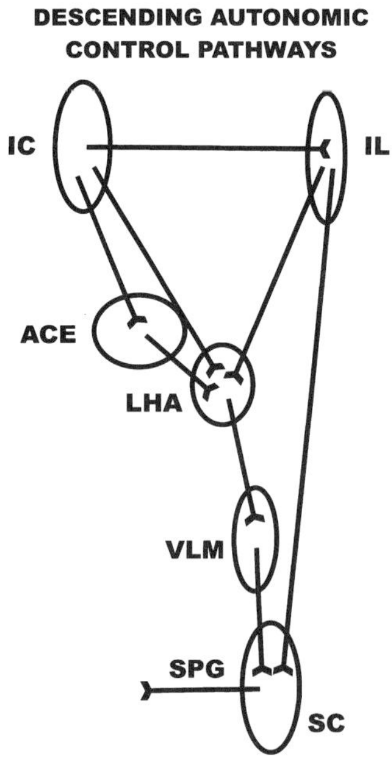

FIGURE 7–2 Pathways from the insular (IC) and infralimbic (IL) cortices for the control of sympathetic efferent neuronal activity. ACE, central nucleus of the amygdala; LHA, lateral hypothalamic area; SC, spinal cord; SPG, spinal preganglionic neuron; VLM, ventral lateral medulla.

tion.[47,68,93,103,110,174,176,189,235,237] These include increases or decreases in heart rate and arterial pressure when discrete sites of the insular cortex are stimulated.[48,165,249] Two distinct cardiovascular regions have been distinguished in the insular cortex of the rat. Increases in heart rate and arterial blood pressure are induced when the caudal posterior insular cortex is stimulated; bradycardia and depressor and bradycardia responses are obtained from the rostral posterior insular cortex.[165,249] The alterations in cardiovascular variables induced in this way can be relatively profound. In the anesthetized rat, it is possible to elicit severe arrhythmias resulting in complete cessation of heart activity in response to prolonged electrical microstimulation of the insular cortex.[170] Anatomical data also indicate that interrelationships between the insular cortex and the infralimbic cortex are important in the integrated response elicited from the forebrain (Fig. 7–3). The insular cortex provides very intense input to the infralimbic cortex.[62,249] These connections suggest that the insular cortex is a likely source of visceral sensory information to the infralimbic cortex. In fact, the infralimbic cortex may be an important site in the pathway by which the insular cortex can affect tonic regulation of the autonomic efferent nervous system.[52]

Infralimbic Cortex: Visceral Motor Cortex

A variety of autonomic responses can be elicited by stimulation of the medial prefrontal cortex (for review see Cechetto and Saper,[52]), including complete cessation of the heart function.[238] Although variable responses are obtained in different species and under different experimental conditions,[68,110,140,237] the main effects elicited from the infralimbic cortex are bradycardia accompanied by hypotension.[31–33,106] Sympathoexcitatory neurons in the ventrolateral medulla are inhibited by stimulation of the infralimbic cortex, suggesting that this area mediates infralimbic cortex cardiovascular responses.[230] Following infralimbic cortex lesions, baroreceptor gain is diminished.[231] Furthermore, inactivation of its neurons reverses renal hypertension.[218] Lesions of the infralimbic cortex interfere with the conditioned heart rate response[29,30,79] and significantly reduce sympathetic but not parasympathetic efferent neural tone regulating heart rate change evoked by a conditioned stimulus.[79]

The infralimbic cortex has extensive connections with both the limbic and autonomic nervous systems of the brain. These connections include inputs from the insular cortex, entorhinal cortices, hippocampus, amygdala, visceral relay nuclei of the thalamus, paraventricular nucleus of the thalamus, parabrachial nucleus, and the nucleus of the solitary tract.[62,80,186,202,205,217,228,229,249] The infralimbic cortex has descending projections to autonomic sites, including the insular cortex, central nucleus of the amygdala, ventral basal thalamus, anterior hypothalamus, lateral hypothalamic area, parabrachial nucleus, nucleus of the solitary tract and sympathetic preganglionic neurons in the interomedial lateral nucleus of the spinal cord.[105,155,185,220,222,249] A study of the infralimbic cortex by Takagishi and Chiba[220] supports the concept that the infralimbic cortex can be considered the "visceral motor cortex." Thus, infralimbic connectivity provides the anatomical substrate with physiological evidence for a critical role in autonomic control of cardiovascular function.

Amygdala: Cortical Collaborator in Autonomic Control

The amygdala plays an important role in the expression of emotional behavior,[111] integrating autonomic responses to emotional stimuli such as fear and anxiety.[48,67] In rabbits, lesions of the amygdala or injecting β-adrenergic antagonist or opiate agonists into the amygdala attenuate the bradycardia response induced by conditioned fear.[83,84,118] Furthermore, both the behavioral and autonomic concomitants of classical conditioning of fear to an acoustic stimulus sequentially involve the primary auditory sites in the brain stem, the auditory receptive region of the thalamus, and the amygdala.[82,108,136,138] In the rat and rabbit, lesions of the central nucleus of the amygdala abolish the behavioral and cardiovascular responses to auditory conditioned stimuli.[82,137] Lesions of the lateral hypothalamic area abolish only the cardiovascular but not the behavioral response to such stimuli.[137] This suggests an important interaction between neurons in the central nucleus of the amygdala and the lateral hypothalamic area in the elaboration of the cardiovascular response to conditioned stimuli.

Electrical stimulation of the amygdala increases heart rate and blood pressure in the awake rat, while it decreases these variables in anesthetized animals.[81,86] Similar changes in heart rate and arterial blood pressure have been demonstrated with microinjections of glutamate into the amygdala that activate cell bodies only and not fibers of passage.[107] This dependence on the state of consciousness of the animal was further indicated by the demonstration that the pressor response evoked by amygdalar stimulation becomes attenuated during sleep states.[78] In the monkey, amygdalar stimulation produces either tachycardia or bradycardia, depending on separate representations and projection pathways.[63] Ventricular fibrillation induced in stressed pigs by myocardial ischemia can be aborted by bilateral cooling of the central nucleus of the amygdala, but not by similar cooling of adjacent areas.[40]

The amygdala projects to autonomic neurons in the hypothalamus, parabrachial nucleus, nucleus of the solitary tract, and dorsal motor nucleus of the vagus, neurons involved in cardiovascular control.[65,104,148,149,177,201,203,206] Amygdalar outputs to the infralimbic and insular cortices are ipsilateral in nature, arising primarily from the basolateral nucleus.[8,62,130,131–133,177] The efferent outputs from the infralimbic and insular cortices terminate in the lateral basolateral and central nucleus of the amygdala.[105,185,190] Multiple baroceptor inputs to the central nucleus of the amygdala are present in the cat and likely in humans.[16,45] Thus, the amygdala is a critical site mediating emotional behavior effects on the cardiovascular system, with major inputs to and projections from the infralimbic and insular cortices (Fig. 7–3). The central nucleus of the amygdala also projects extensively to the medial dorsal nucleus of the thalamus,[130,181,191] which in turn projects back to the infralimbic and insular cortices.[131,182] Thus, there is a complete circuit from the insular and infralimbic cortices to the amygala, especially the basolateral nucleus, to the medial dorsal nucleus of the thalamus, and then back to the cortex (Fig. 7–3). It is likely that this circuit is responsible for the integration and even initiation of the autonomic responses associated with emotion and stress.

Lateral Hypothalamic Area: Mediator of Forebrain Autonomic Responses

The functional organization within the lateral hypothalamic area has been elucidated recently; pressor effects can be elicited mainly from the perifornical lateral hypothalamic area, whereas depressor effects are elicitable from the tuberal and posterior lateral hypothalamic area.[3,4] The latter two regions are directly connected with posterior insular and brain stem sites

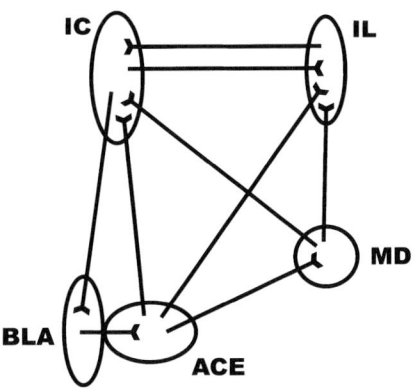

FIGURE 7–3 Pathways within the forebrain controlling the autonomic concomitants of stress and emotional behavior. ACE, central nucleus of the amygdala; BLA, basolateral nucleus of the amygdala; IC, insular cortex; IL, infralimbic cortex; MD, medial dorsal nucleus of the thalamus.

involved in cardiovascular function. The perifornical lateral hypothalamic area, by contrast, has little such direct connectivity.[3,4] All three areas, however, project directly to the intermediolateral cell column of the cervical and thoracic spinal cord from which cardiovascular sympathetic preganglionic neurons originate.[51]

Anatomical evidence clearly demonstrates specific projections from the cardiovascular response sites in the insular and infralimbic cortices to the lateral hypothalamus.[105,249] Synaptic blockade of the lateral hypothalamic area can completely abolish the sympathetic and cardiovascular effects of stimulation of the insular or infralimbic cortices.[37,47] The sympathetic and cardiovascular responses originating from the insular and infralimbic cortices are mediated by glutamate acting on NMDA receptors.[37,242] This suggests that the lateral hypothalamic area is an obligatory synapse for cardiovascular efferent neurons in the insular cortex (Fig. 7–2). Furthermore, neuropeptides such as dynorphin and neuropeptide Y modulate the cortical autonomic responses mediated by the lateral hypothalamic area.[169,242] When the GABA antagonist bicuculline is injected in the lateral hypothalamic area, heart rate and arterial blood pressure increase in cats[236] and rats[70,244] and the autonomic concomitants of the defense reaction are inhibited.[209] GABA mechanisms have also been shown to be involved in the autonomic responses originating from the insular and infralimbic cortices.[37,242]

The lateral hypothalamic area has descending projections to both the ventral lateral medulla and the interomedial lateral cell column of the spinal cord.[51] The autonomic response originating in the insular cortex and mediated by the lateral hypothalamic area have a functional synapse in the ventral lateral medulla, these synapses being mediated by glutamate acting on local α-amino-3-hydroxy-5-methylisoxazole-4-propionic acid (AMPA) or kainate receptors.[36]

Lateralization of Cardiovascular Function in the Forebrain

Stimulation and lesions studies in animals and humans have revealed some intriguing insights into the organization of the forebrain with respect to the lateralization of cardiovascular control. In humans, reversible anesthesia of the right hemisphere leads to a decrease in heart rate, whereas transient anesthesia of the left hemispshere has the opposite effect.[250] In stroke patients, changes in plasma catecholamines and circadian blood pressure correlated strongly with the percentage of insular infarction and the responses demonstrated a right hemispheric dominance for sympathetic efferent neuronal effects.[200] Stimulation of the right anterior insular cortex in humans elicits increases in heart rate and blood pressure, while left anterior insular stimulation decreases heart rate.[167] In the rat, lesions of the right posterior insular cortex lead to an increase in basal sympathetic tone and plasma catecholamines, while lesions of the left posterior insular cortex in the urethane anesthetized rat exert significantly less effect on sympathetic efferent neuronal tone and do not affect baseline arterial blood pressure.[90] In the rat, right hemispheric lesions result in an exaggerated cardiovascular response to environmental stress.[58] Thus, it appears that the right hemisphere, in particular the right insular cortex, exerts predominant effects on cardiovascular sympathetic efferent neuronal function, while the left hemisphere predominantly affects the parasympathetic efferent nervous system.

At first, it may seem a contradiction for both lesions and stimulation of the right hemisphere to elicit increases in sympathetic efferent neuronal tone and, consequently, arterial blood pressure. However, in an investigation using anesthetized Wistar rats, it was shown that injections of an excitatory amino acid agonist into the right insular cortex resulted in a significant increase in mean arterial pressure and sympathetic efferent nerve activity. In the conscious animal, when an excitatory amino acid agonist or a local anesthetic, lidocaine, was administered into the right insular cortex, significant increases in arterial blood pressure occurred.[34] These results, and those above, suggest that, in the conscious state, the right insular cortex exerts tonic inhibition over sympathetic efferent neuronal tone that can be abolished by lesions or inactivation, thereby leading to increases in sympathetic efferent neuronal tone. However, this proposed model indicates that the right insular cortex also has a pool of sympathoexcitatory neurons that are normally relatively quiescent; when activated, they unmask an additional increase in sympathetic efferent neuronal tone.[34]

Further lateralization is seen in forebrain cardiovascular control by an examination of the inputs to the insular cortex that affect cardiovascular reflex control. Clustering of baroreceptor-related cells within the right posterior insula have been shown in the rat.[251] In addition, right posterior insular lesions augment basal cardiovascular sympathetic efferent neuronal tone without affecting baroreceptor gain. Left posterior insular cortex lesions in the urethane-anesthetized rat significantly increased baroreceptor reflex gain without affecting baseline blood pressure.[252] Consistent with these findings, large left hemisphere lesions decreased baroreceptor sensitivity in the unanesthetized rat.[192,193]

Recent human functional magnetic resonance imaging (MRI) studies demonstrated a significant lateralization between the left and right insular cortex during baroreceptor activation.[124] One of the interesting aspects of this investigation was that the single left-handed subject studied had lateralization opposite to the right-handed individuals in the study; this finding suggests that handedness may be related to asymmetry in forebrain cardiovascular control sites. Recently, a prospective study of the North American Symptomatic Carotid Endarterectomy Trial revealed that handedness has a strong relationship with sudden cardiac death. In this study, the 5-year risk of death within 24 hours was 2.3% in left-handed or ambidextrous patients and 7.3% for right-handed patients (V. Hachinski).

Role of the Forebrain in Cardiovascular Disease

Behavioral and emotional factors play an important role in the pathogenesis of cardiovascular disease, including ventricular arrhythmia formation and sudden death.[72,234] In experimental animals, behavioral stress as well as cortical or diencephalic stimulation can result in a reduction of the ventricular fibrillation threshold.[109,233] Both the insular and infralimbic cortices exert relatively direct effects on subcortical autonomic control sites that modulate cardiac sympathetic–parasympathetic interactions that in turn can lead to life-threatening cardiac arrhythmias.[154] Stroke induced by middle cerebral artery occlusion in the cat and rat results in an increase in levels of arterial norepinephrine, sympathetic efferent nerve activity, myocytolysis, blood pressure and mortality.[35,38,49,91,213,234] Similar changes are observed in stroke patients.[153,161,166] In addition, cardiac arrhythmias have been implicated in sudden, unexpected epileptic death during seizures originating from limbic temporal lobe foci,[27,87,125,166] Thus, hemispheric stroke, epilepsy, and psychological stress can lead to cardiovascular dysfunction. Evidence indicates that forebrain sites, including the insular and infralimbic cortices and the amygdala, may be important for the onset of cardiovascular abnormalities associated with these conditions. These possibilities are reviewed below.

Cardiovascular Consequences of Stress

There is a considerable amount of clinical and experimental evidence implicating stress, anger, and anxiety in the occurrence of atherosclerosis, hypertension, myocardial ischemia and infarction, cardiac arrhythmia formation, and sudden cardiac death. This evidence clearly suggests that integration between the emotional and autonomic centers in the brain becomes involved. Coordination between the activities of neurons in autonomic control sites of the cerebral cortex and the limbic system is required for such a thesis.

Stress and cardiovascular changes in animals
References to the effects of stress on cardiovascular status can be found as far back as ancient times, in the work of the Arabian physician Avicenna, in which wolves were used to generate mental stress in lambs; in this situation of high stress, death would often occur (reviewed in Sudakov[216]). Since that time, numerous studies have demonstrated the relationship between acute mental stress and cardiovascular disturbances.[58,74,147,175] Grouping chickens with unfamiliar chickens induces coronary artery stenosis and increased incidence of myocardial infarction.[179,180] Mice reared in isolation and then placed in direct contact with other mice developed arteriosclerosis and hypertension.[100]

Much of the animal experimentation on the role of anger in cardiac susceptibility has been performed in the canine model. An anger-like state was shown to result in an augmentation of the beat-to beat fluctuations in the magnitude of the T wave of the ECG (T-wave alternans), an effect shown to be due to an increase in cardiac sympathetic efferent neuronal tone. Furthermore, induction of an anger-like state and coronary occlusion in the dog elicits an additive effect that results in increased T-wave alternans of the ECG.[156,157] Earlier investigations in the dog demonstrated a profound affect of either aversive stimuli or an anger-like state on the production of ventricular extra systoles and fibrillation.[141,232,234] These experimental results clearly indicate that in animal models of stress and anger, it is possible to substantially increase cardiac vulnerability, something that may be exaggerated by the presence of compromised coronary artery blood flow.

Similar results have been found in nonhuman primates.[97] Relocating monkeys within different colonies resulted in a greater incidence of atherosclerosis and myocardial infarction than that in the control animals in each colony.[116,117] Experimental evidence clearly demonstrates a link between mental stress and conditions such as hypertension, atherosclerosis, and myocardial infarction in animals, including nonhuman primates.

Stress and cardiovascular changes in humans, epidemiological studies
Reports exist of cardiovascular disturbances frequently following natural disasters, such as earthquakes and blizzards. The cause of such events is believed to be the sudden increase in stress elicited by such events.[88,129,139,226] Life stress due to events such as the death of a relative, war, or an accident is a contributing factor in the pathogenesis of cardiovascular disturbances.[73,146] In addition, several studies have reported episodes of anger or frustration in the period preceding myocardial infarction.[152,172,223]

Interviews of 1623 patients 4 days after the onset of cardiac symptoms determined that the risk of myocardial infarction was elevated during the first 2 hours after an outburst of anger.[147] In a prospective study, the risk of a fatal or nonfatal coronary event was 3.2 times higher among the men reporting the highest compared to the lowest level of anger on an anger content scale.[120] Similarly, the risk of fatal coronary heart disease or sudden cardiac death is elevated among patients with high levels of anxiety.[119,121] Thus, the relationship between stress and cardiovascular disturbances is well documented, although the nature of the response is not. Use of mental stress models in the laboratory more clearly identifies the cardiovascular responses to stressful situations.

Stress and cardiovascular reactivity in humans
Stress in the laboratory can be created through the use of tasks such as word–color interference (the Stroop test), mental arithmetic, or simulated public speaking. Using such techniques, researchers have shown significant increases in both blood pressure and heart rate in response to mental stress.[19,28,89,215,239] Some results demonstrate a link between type-A personality and clinical cardiovascular disturbances,[14,99,188] while other evidence indicates either a negative relationship between these factors[71,187] or no relationship at all.[41,208]

Steptoe and Ross[215] could not demonstrate a significant difference between cardiovascular reactivity responses of type-A and type-B subjects to three challenging tasks (mental arithmetic, word association, and digit-symbol substitution). Manuck and collaborators,[144] however, found significant differences in cardiovascular responses to the Stroop Word Color test in post–myocardial infarction patients. Furthermore, all cardiovascular reactors to the Stroop test suffered cardiovascular incidents (myocardial infarcts and/or stroke) in the 64 months following the test.[144] These results suggest that cardiovascular reactivity can be used as a predictor of future cardiovascular problems in the general population. In a recent investigation, cardiovascular reactivity assessed by measuring changes in the hemodynamics during a frustrating cognitive task, the Stroop Color Word test, demonstrated that a larger increase in systolic blood pressure is a significant predictor of atherosclerotic changes after controlling for age and initial plaque size.[18]

Cardiovascular consequences of stress
It is clear that the brain, in particular the forebrain, plays the primary role in mediating this effect of stress on the cardiovascular system.[49,141,164] Neuronal activity, associated with cardiovascular reactivity, could prove to be a useful predictor of future cardiovascular problems.

Autonomic control regions of the brain may respond differently in reactors and non-reactors, thus contributing to the different responses to mental stress. Manipulations of certain brain regions or autonomic nerves to the heart are sufficient to elicit fatal arrhythmias and other cardiovascular changes.[49,154,164,198,221,227] Cardiovascular complications have been observed in a variety of neurological conditions, including, stroke, head injury, brain tumor, epilepsy, and the Guillain-Barré syndrome.[27,49,125,154,164,221,227] In addition, neurogenic cardiovascular complications are seen under stressful conditions and in psychiatric diseases, and are believed to cause sudden, unexpected deaths.[154]

Several investigations have indicated that the insular cortex is a likely site mediating the cardiovascular consequences of stress. In the cat and rat, experimental lesions that include the insular cortex result in an increase in blood pressure, circulating norepinephrine levels, sympathetic efferent nerve activity, cardiac myocytolysis, and death, as is seen clinically.[35,38,91,213] As discussed above, the connections of the insular cortex with the adjacent somatosensory areas and limbic and cardiovascular control sites, such as those in the amygdala and hypothalamus, reflect the importance of the insular cortex in the integration of somatic and visceral functions in response to physical activities, behavioral changes, and different emotional states. Stimulation within the insular cortex produces changes in blood pressure and/or heart rate and even profound arrhythmias and death in asystole. Thus, various clinical studies have confirmed the importance of the insular cortex in mediating the cardiovascular alterations attending stroke.[126,199]

A number of lines of evidence have implicated the amygdala and its connectivity with the insular cortex in the cardiovascular consequences of stroke and stress.[6,56–58,249] Studies on fear and anxiety reactions demonstrate that the amygdala is central in integrating autonomic responses to emotional stimuli.[67,75,107,127,136–138] There are striking neurochemical changes in the amygdala following stroke associated with lesions of the insular cortex that mediate enhanced cardiovascular responses to stress.[5,56–58] Some insights into the relationship between the insular cortex and the amygdala in the generation of cardiovascular events in response to stress have been revealed using MRI studies in humans classified as reactors or non-reactors on the basis of their arterial blood pressure and heart rate response to a mentally stressful task, the Stroop test.[123] During such testing, non-reactors had a significant left-sided dominance in insular cortex activity that was not seen in the reactors, while reactors demonstrated significantly greater activation in the left amygdala. These results suggest that the loss of inhibition from the left insular cortex leads to an increased responsiveness of the left amygdala and the consequent exaggerated sympathetic efferent neuronal reactivity of reactors.[123]

Cardiovascular Consequences of Stroke

About 6% of patients die from sudden cardiac death following a stroke.[212] In addition, there are more arrhythmias and increased levels of cardiac enzymes and circulating catecholamine levels in stroke patients than in patients admitted with the initial diagnosis of stroke who turned out to have other pathological conditions.[153,161] The effect of stroke on the heart and the sometimes fatal complications attending this pathology remain relatively unknown and neglected. These complications are clinically important because they affect prognosis adversely.

Experimental studies
It has been shown that middle cerebral artery occlusion (MCAO) in animals results in an increase in blood pressure, circulating norepinephrine level, sympathetic efferent nerve activity, myocytolysis, and death if the insular cortex is included in the infarct.[38,49,91] An asymmetric effect can be shown, in that animals receiving an MCAO in the right hemisphere have greater increases in arterial pressure, sympathetic efferent nerve activity, QT intervals, and circulating norepinephrine levels than animals with left MCAO.[90] The aged brain is more vulnerable to ischemic insults and most strokes occur in older individuals.[142,184] In our stroke model, older animals had significantly increased mortality as well as elevated sympathetic efferent nerve activity, plasma norepinephrine concentration, and prolongation of the QT interval of the ECG prior to death.[92] Thus, it appears that there is impaired cardiovascular control in the elderly that may contribute to the higher mortality observed in elderly stroke patients.

Clinical studies
Clinical studies have confirmed the importance of the insular cortex in mediating the cardiovascular consequences of stroke.[126,199,200] Changes in circadian blood pressure, cardiac arrhythmias, and QTc interval prolongation correlate only with the extent of insular infarction, confirming our observations of right hemispheric dominance for sympathetic efferent neuronal responsiveness.[200] More recently, sympathetic- and parasympathetic-mediated heart rate variability was found to be reduced in stroke patients, particularly those suffering right MCA and insular cortical lesions. In a study of seven patients, two patients with left insular lesions and five patients with right insular lesions died suddenly. In contrast, there were no deaths among stroke patients who did not have insular cor-

tical involvement.[224] Clearly the insula, and particularly the right one, plays a crucial role in the mediation of the cardiac complications attending stroke.

PERSPECTIVES

Data presented in this chapter indicate that the insular and infralimbic cortices, as well as the amygdala, play major integrative roles in the control of the cardiovascular system. The interconnections among neurons in these sites and autonomic cardiovascular control neurons in the brain stem and spinal cord are relatively well established. Recently, very intriguing evidence has emerged regarding the relationship of the forebrain to the autonomic concomitants of emotional stress associated with cardiovascular dysfunction observed following stroke or stress. These studies leave a number of unanswered questions about the role of multiple neurotransmitters in the pathways involved, as well as the exact relationship of the pathways observed in animal models to those that may exist in humans. Although much remains to be done to fully elucidate forebrain control of the heart, findings accumulated to date point out the importance of central neurons not only in the maintainance of adequate cardiac function but also in the development of therapeutic strategies to manage many cardiac disease states.

REFERENCES

1. Ables MF and Benjamin RM. Thalamic relay nucleus for taste in albino rat. *J Neurophysiol* 23:376–382, 1960.
2. Aidar O, Geohagan WA, and Ungewitter LH. Splanchnic afferent pathways in the central nervous system. *J Neurophysiol* 15:131–138, 1952.
3. Allen GV and Cechetto DF. Functional and anatomical organization of cardiovascular pressor and depressor sites in the lateral hypothalamic area: I. Descending projections. *J Comp Neurol* 315:313–332, 1992.
4. Allen GV and Cechetto DF. Functional and anatomical organization of cardiovascular pressor and depressor sites in the lateral hypothalamic area. II. Ascending projections. *J Comp Neurol* 330:421–438, 1993.
5. Allen GV, Cheung RT, and Cechetto DF. Neurochemical changes following occlusion of the middle cerebral artery in rats. *Neuroscience* 68:1037–1050, 1995.
6. Allen GV, Saper CB, Hurley KM, and Cechetto DF. Organization of visceral and limbic connections in the insular cortex of the rat. *J Comp Neurol* 311:1–16, 1991.
7. Altschuler SM, Bao XM, Bieger D, Hopkins DA, and Miselis RR. Viscerotopic

representation of the upper alimentary tract in the rat: sensory ganglia and nuclei of the solitary and spinal trigeminal tracts. *J Comp Neurol* 283:248–268, 1989.
8. Amaral DG and Price JL. Amygdalo-cortical projections in the monkey (*Macaca fascicularis*). *J Comp Neurol* 230:465–496, 1984.
9. Ammons WS. Characteristics of spinoreticular and spinothalamic neurons with renal input. *J Neurophysiol* 58:480–495, 1987.
10. Ammons WS, Blair RW, and Foreman RD. Raphe magnus inhibition of primate T1–T4 spinothalamic cells with cardiopulmonary visceral input. *Pain* 20:247–260, 1984.
11. Ammons WS, Blair RW, and Foreman RD. Responses of primate T1–T5 spinothalamic neurons to gallbladder distension. *Am J Physiol* 247:R995–1002, 1984.
12. Ammons WS, Girardot MN, and Foreman RD. Effects of intracardiac bradykinin on T2–T5 medial spinothalamic cells. *Am J Physiol* 249:R147–R152, 1985.
13. Ammons WS, Girardot MN, and Foreman RD. T2–T5 spinothalamic neurons projecting to medial thalamus with viscerosomatic input. *J Neurophysiol* 54:73–89, 1985.
14. Anonymous. Ischemic heart disease and psychological patterns. Prevalence and incidence studies in Belgium and France. French-Belgian Collaborative Group. *Adv Cardiol* 29:25–31, 1982.
15. Augustine JR. The insular lobe in primates including humans. *Neurol Res* 7:2–10, 1985.
16. Bailey P and Bremer F. A sensory cortical representation of the vagus nerve with a note on the effects of the low blood pressure on the cortical electrogram. *J Neurophysiol* 1:405–412, 1938.
17. Barnabi F and Cechetto DF. Neurotransmitters in the thalamus relaying visceral input to the insular cortex in the rat. *Neurosci Abstr* 21:637–637, 2001.
18. Barnett PA, Spence JD, Manuck SB, and Jennings JR. Psychological stress and the progression of carotid artery disease. *J Hypertens* 15:49–55, 1997.
19. Becker LC, Pepine CJ, Bonsall R, Cohen JD, Goldberg AD, Coghlan C, Stone PH, Forman S, Knatterud G, Sheps DS, and Kaufmann PG. Left ventricular, peripheral vascular, and neurohumoral responses to mental stress in normal middle-aged men and women. Reference Group for the Psychophysiological Investigations of Myocardial Ischemia (PIMI) Study. *Circulation* 94:2768–2777, 1996.
20. Benjamin RM and Akert K. Cortical and thalamic areas involved in taste discrimination in the albino rat. *J Comp Neurol* 111:231–259, 1959.
21. Berkley KJ and Scofield SL. Relays from the spinal cord and solitary nucleus through the parabrachial nucleus to the forebrain in the cat. *Brain Res* 529:333–338, 1990.
22. Blair RW, Ammons WS, and Foreman RD. Responses of thoracic spinothalamic and spinoreticular cells to coronary artery occlusion. *J Neurophysiol* 51:636–648, 1984.
23. Blair RW, Weber RN, and Foreman RD. Characteristics of primate spinothalamic tract neurons receiving viscerosomatic convergent inputs in T3–T5 segments. *J Neurophysiol* 46:797–811, 1981.
24. Blair RW, Weber RN, and Foreman RD. Responses of thoracic spinothala-

mic neurons to intracardiac injection of bradykinin in the monkey. *Circ Res* 51:83–94, 1982.
25. Blair RW, Weber RN, and Foreman RD. Responses of thoracic spinoreticular and spinothalamic cells to intracardiac bradykinin. *Am J Physiol* 246:H500–H507, 1984.
26. Blomqvist AJ, Benjamin RM, and Emmers R. Thalamic localization of afferents from the tongue in squirrel monkey *Saimiri sciureus*. *J Comp Neurol* 118: 7788–7795, 1962.
27. Blumhardt LD, Smith PE, and Owen L. Electrocardiographic accompaniments of temporal lobe epileptic seizures. *Lancet* 1:1051–1056, 1986.
28. Boutcher SH and Nugent FW. Cardiac response of trained and untrained males to a repeated psychological stressor. *Behav Med* 19:21–27, 1993.
29. Buchanan SL and Powell DA. Cingulate cortex: its role in Pavlovian conditioning. *J Comp Physiol Psychol* 96:755–774, 1982.
30. Buchanan SL and Powell DA. Cingulate damage attenuates conditioned bradycardia. *Neurosci Lett* 29:261–268, 1982.
31. Buchanan SL, Powell DA, and Buggy J. 3H-2-deoxyglucose uptake after electrical stimulation of cardioactive sites in anterior medial cortex in rabbits. *Brain Res Bull* 13:371–382, 1984.
32. Buchanan SL, Valentine J, and Powell DA. Autonomic responses are elicited by electrical stimulation of the medial but not lateral frontal cortex in rabbits. *Behav Brain Res* 18:51–62, 1985.
33. Burns SM and Wyss JM. The involvement of the anterior cingulate cortex in blood pressure control. *Brain Res* 340:71–77, 1985.
34. Butcher KS and Cechetto DF. Autonomic responses of the insular cortex in hypertensive and normotensive rats. *Am J Physiol* 268:R214–R222, 1995.
35. Butcher KS and Cechetto DF. Insular lesion evokes autonomic effects of stroke in normotensive and hypertensive rats. *Stroke* 26:459–465, 1995.
36. Butcher KS and Cechetto DF. Neurotransmission in the medulla mediating insular cortical and lateral hypothalamic sympathetic responses. *Can J Physiol Pharmacol* 76:737–746, 1998.
37. Butcher KS and Cechetto DF. Receptors in lateral hypothalamic area involved in insular cortex sympathetic responses. *Am J Physiol* 275:H689–H696, 1998.
38. Butcher KS, Hachinski VC, Wilson JX, Guiraudon C, and Cechetto DF. Cardiac and sympathetic effects of middle cerebral artery occlusion in the spontaneously hypertensive rat. *Brain Res* 621:79–86, 1993.
39. Cannon WB and Britton SW. Studies on the conditions of activity in endocrine glands. XV. Pseudoaffective medulliadrenal secretion. *Am J Physiol* 72:283–294, 1925.
40. Carpeggiani C, Landisman C, Montaron MF, and Skinner JE. Cryoblockade in limbic brain (amygdala) prevents or delays ventricular fibrillation after coronary artery occlusion in psychologically stressed pigs. *Circ Res* 70:600–606, 1992.
41. Case RB, Heller SS, Case NB, and Moss AJ. Type A behavior and survival after acute myocardial infarction. *N Engl J Med* 312:737–741, 1985.
42. Cechetto DF. Central representation of visceral function. *Fed Proc* 46:17–23, 1987.
43. Cechetto, D. F. Supraspinal mechanisms of visceral representation. In: Gebhart GF, ed. *Visceral Pain* Seattle: IASP Press, 1995, pp 261–290.

44. Cechetto DF and Calaresu FR. Parabrachial units responding to stimulation of buffer nerves and forebrain in the cat. *Am J Physiol* 245:R811–R819, 1983.
45. Cechetto DF and Calaresu FR. Central pathways relaying cardiovascular afferent information to amygdala. *Am J Physiol* 248:R38–R45, 1985.
46. Cechetto DF and Chen SJ. Subcortical sites mediating sympathetic responses from insular cortex in rats. *Am J Physiol* 258:R245–R255, 1990.
47. Cechetto DF and Chen SJ. Hypothalamic and cortical sympathetic responses relay in the medulla of the rat. *Am J Physiol* 263:R544–R552, 1992.
48. Cechetto DF and Gelb AW. The amydala and cardiovascular control. *J Neurosurg Anasthesiol* 13:329–332, 2001.
49. Cechetto DF and Hachinski V. Cardiovascular consequence of experimental stroke. *Baillieres Clin Neurol* 6:297–308, 1997.
50. Cechetto DF and Saper CB. Evidence for a viscerotopic sensory representation in the cortex and thalamus in the rat. *J Comp Neurol* 262:27–45, 1987.
51. Cechetto DF and Saper CB. Neurochemical organization of the hypothalamic projections to the spinal cord in the rat. *J Comp Neurol* 272:579–604, 1988.
52. Cechetto DF and Saper CB. Role of the cerebral cortex in autonomic function. In: Loewy AD and Spyer KM, eds. *The Autonomic Nervous System: Central Regulation of Autonomic Function*. New York: Oxford University Press, 1990, pp 208–223.
53. Chamberlin NL and Saper CB. Topographic organization of cardiovascular responses to electrical and glutamate microstimulation of the parabrachial nucleus in the rat. *J Comp Neurol* 326:245–262, 1992.
54. Chamberlin NL and Saper CB. Topographic organization of respiratory responses to glutamate microstimulation of the parabrachial nucleus in the rat. *J Neurosci* 14:6500–6510, 1994.
55. Cheung RT and Cechetto DF. Neuropeptide changes following excitotoxic lesion of the insular cortex in rats. *J Comp Neurol* 362:535–550, 1995.
56. Cheung RT and Cechetto DF. Colchicine affects cortical and amygdalar neurochemical changes differentially after middle cerebral artery occlusion in rats. *J Comp Neurol* 387:27–41, 1997.
57. Cheung RT, Diab T, and Cechetto DF. Time-course of neuropeptide changes in peri-ischemic zone and amygdala following focal ischemia in rats. *J Comp Neurol* 360:101–120, 1995.
58. Cheung RT, Hachinski VC, and Cechetto DF. Cardiovascular response to stress after middle cerebral artery occlusion in rats. *Brain Res* 747:181–188, 1997.
59. Ciriello J and Calaresu FR. Projections from buffer nerves to the nucleus of the solitary tract: an anatomical and electrophysiological study in the cat. *J Auton Nerv Syst* 3:299–310, 1981.
60. Ciriello J, Hrycyshyn AW, and Calaresu FR. Horseradish peroxidase study of brain stem projections of carotid sinus and aortic depressor nerves in the cat. *J Auton Nerv Syst* 4:43–61, 1981.
61. Ciriello J, Hrycyshyn AW, and Calaresu FR. Glossopharyngeal and vagal afferent projections to the brain stem of the cat: a horseradish peroxidase study. *J Auton Nerv Syst* 4:63–79, 1981.
62. Conde F, Maire-Lepoivre E, Audinat E, and Crepel F. Afferent connections of the medial frontal cortex of the rat. II. Cortical and subcortical afferents. *J Comp Neurol* 352:567–593, 1995.

63. Cornish KG and Hall RE. Heart rate changes caused by chemical stimulation of amygdaloid body. *Physiol Behav* 22:947–954, 1979.
64. Dampney RA, Colman MJ, Fontes MA, Hirooka Y, Horiuchi J, Li YW, Polson JW, Potts PD, and Tagawa T. Central mechanisms underlying short- and long-term regulation of the cardiovascular system. *Clin Exp Pharmacol Physiol* 29:261–268, 2002.
65. Danielsen EH, Magnuson DJ, and Gray TS. The central amygdaloid nucleus innervation of the dorsal vagal complex in rat: a *Phaseolus vulgaris* leucoagglutinin lectin anterograde tracing study. *Brain Res Bull* 22:705–715, 1989.
66. Davies RO and Kalia M. Carotid sinus nerve projections to the brain stem in the cat. *Brain Res Bull* 6:531–541, 1981.
67. Davis M. The role of the amygdala in fear and anxiety. *Annu Rev Neurosci* 15:353–375, 1992.
68. Delgado JMR. Circulatory effects of cortical stimulation. *Physiol Rev* 4:146–171, 1960.
69. Dell P and Olson R. Projections thalamiques corticales et cerebelleuses des afferences viscerales vagales. *Comptes Rendus Soc Biol (Paris)* 145:1084–1088, 1951.
70. DiMicco JA and Abshire VM. Evidence for GABAergic inhibition of a hypothalamic sympathoexcitatory mechanism in anesthetized rats. *Brain Res* 402:1–10, 1987.
71. Dimsdale JE, Gilbert J, Hutter AM, Jr, Hackett TP, and Block PC. Predicting cardiac morbidity based on risk factors and coronary angiographic findings. *Am J Cardiol* 47:73–76, 1981.
72. Eliot RS and Buell JC. The role of the CNS in cardiovascular disorders. *Hosp Pract (Off Ed)* 18:189–189, 1983.
73. Engel GL. Sudden and rapid death during psychological stress. Folklore or folk wisdom? *Ann Intern Med* 74:771–782, 1971.
74. Folkow B, Hallback M, and Weiss L. Cardiovascular responses to acute mental "stress" in spontaneously hypertensive rats. *Clin Sci Mol Med Suppl* 45(Suppl 1):131s–133s, 1973.
75. Folkow B, Hallback-Nordlander M, Martner J, and Nordborg C. Influence of amygdala lesions on cardiovascular responses to alerting stimuli, on behaviour and on blood pressure development in spontaneously hypertensive rats. *Acta Physiol Scand* 116:133–139, 1982.
76. Foreman RD, Blair RW, and Weber RN. Viscerosomatic convergence onto T2–T4 spinoreticular, spinoreticular-spinothalamic, and spinothalamic tract neurons in the cat. *Exp Neurol* 85:597–619, 1984.
77. Freedman LJ and Cassell MD. Thalamic afferents of the rat infralimbic and lateral agranular cortices. *Brain Res Bull* 26:957–964, 1991.
78. Frysinger RC, Marks JD, Trelease RB, Schechtman VL, and Harper RM. Sleep states attenuate the pressor response to central amygdala stimulation. *Exp Neurol* 83:604–617, 1984.
79. Frysztak RJ and Neafsey EJ. The effect of medial frontal cortex lesions on cardiovascular conditioned emotional responses in the rat. *Brain Res* 643:181–193, 1994.
80. Fulwiler CE and Saper CB. Subnuclear organization of the efferent connections of the parabrachial nucleus in the rat. *Brain Res* 319:229–259, 1984.
81. Galeno TM and Brody MB. Hemodynamic responses to amygdaloid stimulation in spontaneously hypertensive rats. *Am J Physiol* 245:R281–R286, 1983.

82. Galeno TM, Van Hoesen GW, and Brody MJ. Central amygdaloid nucleus lesion attenuates exaggerated hemodynamic responses to noise stress in the spontaneously hypertensive rat. *Brain Res* 291:249–259, 1984.
83. Gallagher M, Kapp BS, Frysinger RC, and Rapp PR. β-Adrenergic manipulation in amygdala central n. alters rabbit heart rate conditioning. *Pharmacol Biochem Behav* 12:419–426, 1980.
84. Gallagher M, Kapp BS, McNall CL, and Pascoe JP. Opiate effects in the amygdala central nucleus on heart rate conditioning in rabbits. *Pharmacol Biochem Behav* 14:497–505, 1981.
85. Ganchrow D and Erickson RP. Thalamocortical relations in gustation. *Brain Res* 36:298–305, 1972.
86. Gelsema AJ, McKitrick DJ, and Calaresu FR. Cardiovascular responses to chemical and electrical stimulation of amygdala in rats. *Am J Physiol* 253: R712–R718, 1987.
87. Gilchrist JM. Arrhythmogenic seizures: diagnosis by simultaneous EEG/ECG recording. *Neurology* 35:1503–1506, 1985.
88. Glass RI and Zack MM, Jr. Increase in deaths from ischaemic heart-disease after blizzards. *Lancet* 1:485–487, 1979.
89. Grillot M, Fauvel JP, Cottet-Emard JM, Laville M, Peyrin L, Pozet N, and Zech P. Spectral analysis of stress-induced change in blood pressure and heart rate in normotensive subjects. *J Cardiovasc Pharmacol* 25:448–452, 1995.
90. Hachinski VC, Oppenheimer SM, Wilson JX, Guiraudon C, and Cechetto DF. Asymmetry of sympathetic consequences of experimental stroke. *Arch Neurol* 49:697–702, 1992.
91. Hachinski VC, Smith KE, Silver MD, Gibson CJ, and Ciriello J. Acute myocardial and plasma catecholamine changes in experimental stroke. *Stroke* 17:387–390, 1986.
92. Hachinski VC, Wilson JX, Smith KE, and Cechetto DF. Effect of age on autonomic and cardiac responses in a rat stroke model. *Arch Neurol* 49:690–696, 1992.
93. Hall RE, Livingston RB, and Bloor CM. Orbital cortical influences on cardiovascular dynamics and myocardial structure in conscious monkeys. *J Neurosurg* 46:648–653, 1977.
94. Halsell CB. Organization of parabrachial nucleus efferents to the thalamus and amygdala in the golden hamster. *J Comp Neurol* 317:57–78, 1992.
95. Hamilton RB and Norgren R. Central projections of gustatory nerves in the rat. *J Comp Neurol* 222:560–577, 1984.
96. Hamilton RB, Pritchard TC, and Norgren R. Central distribution of the cervical vagus nerve in Old and New World primates. *J Auton Nerv Syst* 19:153–169, 1987.
97. Hamm TE, Jr, Kaplan JR, Clarkson TB, and Bullock BC. Effects of gender and social behavior on the development of coronary artery atherosclerosis in cynomolgus macaques. *Atherosclerosis* 48:221–233, 1983.
98. Han ZS, Gu GB, Sun CQ, and Ju G. Convergence of somatosensory and baroreceptive inputs onto parabrachio-subfornical organ neurons in the rat: an electrophysiological study. *Brain Res* 566:239–247, 1991.
99. Haynes SG, Feinleib M, and Kannel WB. The relationship of psychosocial factors to coronary heart disease in the Framingham Study. III. Eight-year incidence of coronary heart disease. *Am J Epidemiol* 111:37–58, 1980.

100. Henry JP, Ely DL, Stephens PM, Ratcliffe HL, Santisteban GA, and Shapiro AP. The role of psychosocial factors in the development of arteriosclerosis in CBA mice. Observations on the heart, kidney and aorta. *Atherosclerosis* 14:203–218, 1971.
101. Herbert H, Moga MM, and Saper CB. Connections of the parabrachial nucleus with the nucleus of the solitary tract and the medullary reticular formation in the rat. *J Comp Neurol* 293:540–580, 1990.
102. Hoff EC, Kell JF, Jr., and Carroll MN, Jr. Effects of cortical stimulation and lesions on cardiovascular function. *Physiological Rev* 43:68–114, 1963.
103. Hoffman BL and Ramussen T. Stimulation studies of insular cortex of *Macaca mulatta*. *J Neurophysiol* 16:343–351, 1953.
104. Hopkins DA and Holstege G. Amygdaloid projections to the mesencephalon, pons and medulla oblongata in the cat. *Exp Brain Res* 32:529–547, 1978.
105. Hurley KM, Herbert H, Moga MM, and Saper CB. Efferent projections of the infralimbic cortex of the rat. *J Comp Neurol* 308:249–276, 1991.
106. Hurley-Gius KM and Neafsey EJ. The medial frontal cortex and gastric motility: microstimulation results and their possible significance for the overall pattern of organization of rat frontal and parietal cortex. *Brain Res* 365:241–248, 1986.
107. Iwata J, Chida K, and LeDoux JE. Cardiovascular responses elicited by stimulation of neurons in the central amygdaloid nucleus in awake but not anesthetized rats resemble conditioned emotional responses. *Brain Res* 418:183–188, 1987.
108. Iwata J, LeDoux JE, Meeley MP, Arneric S, and Reis DJ. Intrinsic neurons in the amygdaloid field projected to by the medial geniculate body mediate emotional responses conditioned to acoustic stimuli. *Brain Res* 383:195–214, 1986.
109. Johansson G, Jonsson L, Lannek N, Blomgren L, Lindberg P, and Poupa O. Severe stress-cardiopathy in pigs. *Am Heart J* 87:451–457, 1974.
110. Kaada BR. Somato-motor, autonomic electrocorticographic responses to electrical stimulation of 'rhinencephalic' and other structures in primates, cat and dog. *Acta Physiol Scand* 24:1–285, 1951.
111. Kaada BR. Stimulation and regional ablation of the amygdaloid complex with reference to functional representations. In: Eleftheriou BE, ed. *The Neurobiology of the Amygdala*. New York: Plenum Press, 1972, pp 205–281.
112. Kalia M and Mesulam MM. Brain stem projections of sensory and motor components of the vagus complex in the cat: I. The cervical vagus and nodose ganglion. *J Comp Neurol* 193:435–465, 1980.
113. Kalia M and Mesulam MM. Brain stem projections of sensory and motor components of the vagus complex in the cat: II. Laryngeal, tracheobronchial, pulmonary, cardiac, and gastrointestinal branches. *J Comp Neurol* 193:467–508, 1980.
114. Kalia M and Richter D. Morphology of physiologically identified slowly adapting lung stretch receptor afferents stained with intra-axonal horseradish peroxidase in the nucleus of the tractus solitarius of the cat. I. A light microscopic analysis. *J Comp Neurol* 241:503–520, 1985.
115. Kalia M and Welles RV. Brain stem projections of the aortic nerve in the cat: a study using tetramethyl benzidine as the substrate for horseradish peroxidase. *Brain Res* 188:23–32, 1980.

116. Kaplan JR, Manuck SB, Clarkson TB, Lusso FM, and Taub DM. Social status, environment, and atherosclerosis in cynomolgus monkeys. *Arteriosclerosis* 2:359–368, 1982.
117. Kaplan JR, Manuck SB, Clarkson TB, Lusso FM, Taub DM, and Miller EW. Social stress and atherosclerosis in normocholesterolemic monkeys. *Science* 220:733–735, 1983.
118. Kapp BS, Frysinger RC, Gallagher M, and Haselton JR. Amygdala central nucleus lesions: effect on heart rate conditioning in the rabbit. *Physiol Behav* 23:1109–1117, 1979.
119. Kawachi I, Colditz GA, Ascherio A, Rimm EB, Giovannucci E, Stampfer MJ, and Willett WC. Prospective study of phobic anxiety and risk of coronary heart disease in men. *Circulation* 89:1992–1997, 1994.
120. Kawachi I, Sparrow D, Spiro A, III, Vokonas P, and Weiss ST. A prospective study of anger and coronary heart disease. The Normative Aging Study. *Circulation* 94:2090–2095, 1996.
121. Kawachi I, Sparrow D, Vokonas PS, and Weiss ST. Symptoms of anxiety and risk of coronary heart disease. The Normative Aging Study [see comments]. *Circulation* 90:2225–2229, 1994.
122. Kennard MA. Focal autonomic representation in the cortex and its relation to sham rage. *J Neuropathol Exper Neurol* 4:295–304, 1945.
123. King AB, Menon RS, Gatti JS, Hachinski VC, and Cechetto DF. Cardiovascular reactivity and mental stress: an fMRI study. *Neurosci Abstr* 24:125–125, 1998.
124. King AB, Menon RS, Hachinski V, and Cechetto DF. Human forebrain activation by visceral stimuli. *J Comp Neurol* 413:572–582, 1999.
125. Kiok MC, Terrence CF, Fromm GH, and Lavine S. Sinus arrest in epilepsy. *Neurology* 36:115–116, 1986.
126. Klingelhofer J and Sander D. Cardiovascular consequences of clinical stroke. *Baillieres Clin Neurol* 6:309–335, 1997.
127. Koch M and Ebert U. Enhancement of the acoustic startle response by stimulation of an excitatory pathway from the central amygdala/basal nucleus of Meynert to the pontine reticular formation. *Exp Brain Res* 93:231–241, 1993.
128. Kosar E, Grill HJ, and Norgren R. Gustatory cortex in the rat. I. Physiological properties and cytoarchitecture. *Brain Res* 379:329–341, 1986.
129. Krantz DS, Kop WJ, Santiago HT, and Gottdiener JS. Mental stress as a trigger of myocardial ischemia and infarction. *Cardiol Clin* 14:271–287, 1996.
130. Krettek JE and Price JL. A direct input from the amygdala to the thalamus and the cerebral cortex. *Brain Res* 67:169–174, 1974.
131. Krettek JE and Price JL. The cortical projections of the mediodorsal nucleus and adjacent thalamic nuclei in the rat. *J Comp Neurol* 171:157–191, 1977.
132. Krettek JE and Price JL. Projections from the amygdaloid complex to the cerebral cortex and thalamus in the rat and cat. *J Comp Neurol* 172:687–722, 1977.
133. Krettek JE and Price JL. Projections from the amygdaloid complex and adjacent olfactory structures to the entorhinal cortex and to the subiculum in the rat and cat. *J Comp Neurol* 172:723–752, 1977.
134. Krukoff TL, Morton TL, Harris KH, and Jhamandas JH. Expression of c-fos protein in rat brain elicited by electrical stimulation of the pontine parabrachial nucleus. *J Neurosci* 12:3582–3590, 1992.
135. Lasiter PS. Thalamocortical relations in taste aversion learning: II. Involve-

ment of the medial ventrobasal thalamic complex in taste aversion learning. *Behav Neurosci* 99:477–495, 1985.
136. LeDoux JE, Farb CR, and Romanski LM. Overlapping projections to the amygdala and striatum from auditory processing areas of the thalamus and cortex. *Neurosci Lett* 134:139–144, 1991.
137. LeDoux JE, Iwata J, Cicchetti P, and Reis DJ. Different projections of the central amygdaloid nucleus mediate autonomic and behavioral correlates of conditioned fear. *J Neurosci* 8:2517–2529, 1988.
138. LeDoux JE, Sakaguchi A, Iwata J, and Reis DJ. Interruption of projections from the medial geniculate body to an archi-neostriatal field disrupts the classical conditioning of emotional responses to acoustic stimuli. *Neuroscience* 17:615–627, 1986.
139. Leor J, Poole WK, and Kloner RA. Sudden cardiac death triggered by an earthquake [see comments]. *N Engl J Med* 334:413–419, 1996.
140. Lofving B. Cardiovascular adjustments induced from the rostral cingulate gyrus. *Acta Physiol Scand* 53:1–82, 1961.
141. Lown B, Verrier RL, and Rabinowitz SH. Neural and psychologic mechanisms and the problem of sudden cardiac death. *Am J Cardiol* 39:890–902, 1977.
142. Malmgren R, Warlow C, Bamford J, and Sandercock P. Geographical and secular trends in stroke incidence. *Lancet* 2:1196–1200, 1987.
143. Manuck SB, Kaplan JR, and Clarkson TB. Behaviorally induced heart rate reactivity and atherosclerosis in cynomolgus monkeys. *Psychosom Med* 45:95–108, 1983.
144. Manuck SB, Olsson G, Hjemdahl P, and Rehnqvist N. Does cardiovascular reactivity to mental stress have prognostic value in postinfarction patients? A pilot study. *Psychosom Med* 54:102–108, 1992.
145. McLeod JG. The representation of the splanchnic afferent pathways in the thalamus of the cat. *J Physiol* 140:462–478, 1958.
146. Meisel SR, Kutz I, Dayan KI, Pauzner H, Chetboun I, Arbel T, and David D. Effect of Iraqi missile war on incidence of acute myocardial infarction and sudden death in Israeli civilians [see comments]. *Lancet* 338:660–661, 1991.
147. Mittleman MA, Maclure M, Sherwood JB, Mulry RP, Tofler GH, Jacobs SB, Friedman R, Benson H, and Muller JE. Triggering of acute myocardial infarction onset by episodes of anger. Determinants of Myocardial Infarction Onset Study Investigators [see comments]. *Circulation* 92:1720–1725, 1995.
148. Mizuno N, Takahashi O, Satoda T, and Matsushima R. Amygdalospinal projections in the macaque monkey. *Neurosci Lett* 53:327–330, 1985.
149. Moga MM, Herbert H, Hurley KM, Yasui Y, Gray TS, and Saper SB. Organization of cortical, basal forebrain, and hypothalamic afferents to the parabrachial nucleus in the rat. *J Comp Neurol* 295:624–661, 1990.
150. Moga MM, Weis RP, and Moore RY. Efferent projections of the paraventricular thalamic nucleus in the rat. *J Comp Neurol* 359:221–238, 1995.
151. Morin LP, Blanchard J, and Moore RY. Intergeniculate leaflet and suprachiasmatic nucleus organization and connections in the golden hamster. *Vis Neurosci* 8:219–230, 1992.
152. Myers A and Dewar HA. Circumstances attending 100 sudden deaths from coronary artery disease with coroner's necropsies. *Br Heart J* 37:1133–1143, 1975.

153. Myers MG, Norris JW, Hachinski VC, Weingert ME, and Sole MJ. Cardiac sequelae of acute stroke. *Stroke* 13:838–842, 1982.
154. Natelson BH and Chang Q. Sudden death. A neurocardiologic phenomenon [published erratum appears in Neurol Clin 1993;11(3):ix]. *Neurol Clin* 11:293–308, 1993.
155. Neafsey EJ, Hurley-Gius KM, and Arvanitis D. The topographical organization of neurons in the rat medial frontal, insular and olfactory cortex projecting to the solitary nucleus, olfactory bulb, periaqueductal gray and superior colliculus. *Brain Res* 377:561–570, 1986.
156. Nearing BD, Huang AH, and Verrier RL. Dynamic tracking of cardiac vulnerability by complex demodulation of the T wave. *Science* 252:437–440, 1991.
157. Nearing BD, Oesterle SN, and Verrier RL. Quantification of ischaemia induced vulnerability by precordial T wave alternans analysis in dog and human. *Cardiovasc Res* 28:1440–1449, 1994.
158. Norgren R. Projections from the nucleus of the solitary tract in the rat. *Neuroscience* 3:207–218, 1978.
159. Norgren R. Central neural mechanisms of taste. In: Barian-Simth I, ed. *Handbook of Physiology, Section 1, The Nervous System, Vol. III, Sensory Processes, Part 2*. Bethesda: American Physiology Society 1984, pp 1087–1128.
160. Norgren R and Wolf G. Projections of thalamic gustatory and lingual areas in the rat. *Brain Res* 92:123–129, 1975.
161. Norris JW, Froggatt GM, and Hachinski VC. Cardiac arrhythmias in acute stroke. *Stroke* 9:392–396, 1978.
162. Oakley B and Pfaffman C. Electrophysiologically monitored lesions in the gustatory thalamic relay of the albino rat. *J Comp Physiol Psychol* 55:155–160, 1962.
163. Ogawa H, Ito S, Murayama N, and Hasegawa K. Taste area in granular and dysgranular insular cortices in the rat identified by stimulation of the entire oral cavity. *Neurosci Res (NY)* 9:196–201, 1990.
164. Oppenheimer SM. Neurogenic cardiac effects of cerebrovascular disease. *Curr Opin Neurol* 7:20–24, 1994.
165. Oppenheimer SM and Cechetto DF. Cardiac chronotropic organization of the rat insular cortex. *Brain Res* 533:66–72, 1990.
166. Oppenheimer SM, Cechetto DF, and Hachinski VC. Cerebrogenic cardiac arrhythmias. Cerebral electrocardiographic influences and their role in sudden death. *Arch Neurol* 47:513–519, 1990.
167. Oppenheimer SM, Gelb A, Girvin JP, and Hachinski VC. Cardiovascular effects of human insular cortex stimulation. *Neurology* 42:1727–1732, 1992.
168. Oppenheimer SM, Kedem G, and Martin WM. Left-insular cortex lesions perturb cardiac autonomic tone in humans. *Clin Auton Res* 6:131–140, 1996.
169. Oppenheimer SM, Saleh T, and Cechetto DF. Lateral hypothalamic area neurotransmission and neuromodulation of the specific cardiac effects of insular cortex stimulation. *Brain Res* 581:133–142, 1992.
170. Oppenheimer SM, Wilson JX, Guiraudon C, and Cechetto DF. Insular cortex stimulation produces lethal cardiac arrhythmias: a mechanism of sudden death? *Brain Res* 550:115–121, 1991.
171. Panneton WM and Loewy AD. Projections of the carotid sinus nerve to the nucleus of the solitary tract in the cat. *Brain Res* 191:239–244, 1980.
172. Parkes CM, Benjamin B, and Fitzgerald RG. Broken heart: a statistical study of increased mortality among widowers. *BMJ* 1:740–743, 1969.

173. Patton HD and Amassian VE. Thalamic relay of splanchnic afferent fibers. *Am J Physiol* 167:815–816, 1951.
174. Penfield W and Faulk ME, Jr. The insula: further observations on its function. *Brain* 78:445–470, 1955.
175. Peters ML, Godaert GL, Ballieux RE, van Vliet M, Willemsen JJ, Sweep FC, and Heijnen CJ. Cardiovascular and endocrine responses to experimental stress: effects of mental effort and controllability. *Psychoneuroendocrinology* 23:1–17, 1998.
176. Powell DA, Buchanan S, and Hernandez L. Electrical stimulation of insular cortex elicits cardiac inhibition but insular lesions do not abolish conditioned bradycardia in rabbits. *Behav Brain Res* 17:125–144, 1985.
177. Price JL and Amaral DG. An autoradiographic study of the projections of the central nucleus of the monkey amygdala. *J Neurosci* 1:1242–1259, 1981.
178. Pritchard TC, Hamilton RB, Morse JR, and Norgren R. Projections of thalamic gustatory and lingual areas in the monkey, *Macaca fascicularis*. *J Comp Neurol* 244:213–228, 1986.
179. Ratcliffe HL and Snyder RL. Coronary arterial lesions in chickens: origin and rates of development in relation to sex and social factors. *Circ Res* 17:403–413, 1965.
180. Ratcliffe HL and Snyder RL. Arteriosclerotic stenosis of the intramural coronary arteries of chickens: further evidence of a relation to social factors. *Br J Exp Pathol* 48:357–365, 1967.
181. Ray JP and Price JL. The organization of the thalamocortical connections of the mediodorsal thalamic nucleus in the rat, related to the ventral forebrain–prefrontal cortex topography. *J Comp Neurol* 323:167–197, 1992.
182. Ray JP and Price JL. The organization of projections from the mediodorsal nucleus of the thalamus to orbital and medial prefrontal cortex in macaque monkeys. *J Comp Neurol* 337:1–31, 1993.
183. Ricardo JA and Koh ET. Anatomical evidence of direct projections from the nucleus of the solitary tract to the hypothalamus, amygdala, and other forebrain structures in the rat. *Brain Res* 153:1–26, 1978.
184. Roberts WC, Potkin BN, Solus DE, and Reddy SG. Mode of death, frequency of healed and acute myocardial infarction, number of major epicardial coronary arteries severely narrowed by atherosclerotic plaque, and heart weight in fatal atherosclerotic coronary artery disease: analysis of 889 patients studied at necropsy [see comments]. *J Am Coll Cardiol* 15:196–203, 1990.
185. Room P, Russchen FT, Groenewegen HJ, and Lohman AH. Efferent connections of the prelimbic (area 32) and the infralimbic (area 25) cortices: an anterograde tracing study in the cat. *J Comp Neurol* 242:40–55, 1985.
186. Rosene DL and Van Hoesen GW. Hippocampal efferents reach widespread areas of cerebral cortex and amygdala in the rhesus monkey. *Science* 198:315–317, 1977.
187. Rosenman RH. Modification of the coronary behavior pattern (type A) in the context of cardiac rehabilitation. *Rev Esp Cardiol* 38(Suppl 3):50–55, 1985.
188. Rosenman RH, Brand RJ, Jenkins D, Friedman M, Straus R, and Wurm M. Coronary heart disease in Western Collaborative Group Study. Final follow-up experience of 8 1/2 years. *JAMA* 233:872–877, 1975.
189. Ruggiero DA, Mraovitch S, Granata AR, Anwar M, and Reis DJ. A role of insular cortex in cardiovascular function. *J Comp Neurol* 257:189–207, 1987.
190. Russchen FT. Amygdalopetal projections in the cat. I. Cortical afferent con-

nections. A study with retrograde and anterograde tracing techniques. *J Comp Neurol* 206:159–179, 1982.
191. Russchen FT, Amaral DG, and Price JL. The afferent input to the magnocellular division of the mediodorsal thalamic nucleus in the monkey, *Macaca fascicularis*. *J Comp Neurol* 256:175–210, 1987.
192. Saad MA, Elghozi JL, and Meyer P. Baroreflex sensitivity alteration following transient hemispheric ischaemia in rats: protective effect of alpha-methyldopa and guanfacine. *Clin Exp Pharmacol Physiol* 13:525–534, 1986.
193. Saad MA, Huerta F, Trancard J, and Elghozi JL. Effects of middle cerebral artery occlusion on baroreceptor reflex control of heart rate in the rat. *J Auton Nerv Syst* 27:165–172, 1989.
194. Saleh TM and Cechetto DF. Peptides in the parabrachial nucleus modulate visceral input to the thalamus. *Am J Physiol* 264:R668–R675, 1993.
195. Saleh TM and Cechetto DF. Neurotransmitters in the parabrachial nucleus mediating visceral input to the thalamus in rats. *Am J Physiol* 266:R1287–R1296, 1994.
196. Saleh TM and Cechetto DF. Neurochemical interactions in the parabrachial nucleus mediating visceral inputs to visceral thalamic neurons. *Am J Physiol* 268:R786–R795, 1995.
197. Saleh TM and Cechetto DF. Peptide changes in the parabrachial nucleus following cervical vagal stimulation. *J Comp Neurol* 366:390–405, 1996.
198. Samuels MA. Neurally induced cardiac damage. Definition of the problem. *Neurol Clin* 11:273–292, 1993.
199. Sander D and Klingelhofer J. Changes of circadian blood pressure patterns after hemodynamic and thromboembolic brain infarction. *Stroke* 25:1730–1737, 1994.
200. Sander D and Klingelhofer J. Changes of circadian blood pressure patterns and cardiovascular parameters indicate lateralization of sympathetic activation following hemispheric brain infarction. *J Neurol* 242:313–318, 1995.
201. Sandrew BB, Edwards DL, Poletti CE, and Foote WE. Amygdalospinal projections in the cat. *Brain Res* 373:235 239, 1986.
202. Saper CB. Convergence of autonomic and limbic connections in the insular cortex of the rat. *J Comp Neurol* 210:163–173, 1982.
203. Saper CB. Reciprocal parabrachial-cortical connections in the rat. *Brain Res* 242:33–40, 1982.
204. Saper CB. Organization of cerebral cortical afferent systems in the rat. II. Hypothalamocortical projections. *J Comp Neurol* 237:21–46, 1985.
205. Saper CB and Loewy ad. Efferent connections of the parabrachial nucleus in the rat. *Brain Res* 197:291–317, 1980.
206. Schwaber JS, Kapp BS, Higgins GA, and Rapp PR. Amygdaloid and basal forebrain direct connections with the nucleus of the solitary tract and the dorsal motor nucleus. *J Neurosci* 2:1424–1438, 1982.
207. Scott TR, Plata-Salaman CR, Smith VL, and Giza BK. Gustatory neural coding in the monkey cortex: stimulus intensity. *J Neurophysiol* 65:76–86, 1991.
208. Shekelle RB, Gale M, and Norusis M. Type A score (Jenkins Activity Survey) and risk of recurrent coronary heart disease in the aspirin myocardial infarction study. *Am J Cardiol* 56:221–225, 1985.
209. Shekhar A, Hingtgen JN, and DiMicco JA. Selective enhancement of shock avoidance responding elicited by GABA blockade in the posterior hypothalamus of rats. *Brain Res* 420:118–128, 1987.

210. Shipley MT. Insular cortex projection to the nucleus of the solitary tract and brainstem visceromotor regions in the mouse. *Brain Res Bull* 8:139–148, 1982.
211. Shipley MT and Sanders MS. Special senses are really special: evidence for a reciprocal, bilateral pathway between insular cortex and nucleus parabrachialis. *Brain Res Bull* 8:493–501, 1982.
212. Silver FL, Norris JW, Lewis AJ, and Hachinski VC. Early mortality following stroke: a prospective review. *Stroke* 15:492–496, 1984.
213. Smith KE, Hachinski VC, Gibson CJ, and Ciriello J. Changes in plasma catecholamine levels after insula damage in experimental stroke. *Brain Res* 375:182–185, 1986.
214. Smith-Swintosky VL, Plata-Salaman CR, and Scott TR. Gustatory neural coding in the monkey cortex: stimulus quality. *J Neurophysiol* 66:1156–1165, 1991.
215. Steptoe A and Ross A. Psychophysiological reactivity and the prediction of cardiovascular disorders. *J Psychosom Res* 25:23–31, 1981.
216. Sudakov KV. Effects of acute emotional stress on the brain and autonomic variables. *Baillieres Clin Neurol* 6:261–274, 1997.
217. Swanson LW. A direct projection from Ammon's horn to prefrontal cortex in the rat. *Brain Res* 217:150–154, 1981.
218. Szilagyi JE, Taylor AA, and Skinner JE. Cryoblockade of the ventromedial frontal cortex reverses hypertension in the rat. *Hypertension* 9:576–581, 1987.
219. Taguchi H, Masuda T, and Yokota T. Cardiac sympathetic afferent input onto neurons in nucleus ventralis posterolateralis in cat thalamus. *Brain Res* 436:240–252, 1987.
220. Takagishi M and Chiba T. Efferent projections of the infralimbic (area 25) region of the medial prefrontal cortex in the rat: an anterograde tracer PHA-L study. *Brain Res* 566:26–39, 1991.
221. Talman WT and Kelkar P. Neural control of the heart. Central and peripheral. *Neurol Clin* 11:239–256, 1993.
222. Terreberry RR and Neafsey EJ. Rat medial frontal cortex: a visceral motor region with a direct projection to the solitary nucleus. *Brain Res* 278:245–249, 1983.
223. Tofler GH, Stone PH, Maclure M, Edelman E, Davis VG, Robertson T, Antman EM, and Muller JE. Analysis of possible triggers of acute myocardial infarction (the MILIS study). *Am J Cardiol* 66:22–27, 1990.
224. Tokgozoglu SL, Batur MK, Top uoglu MA, Saribas O, Kes S, and Oto A. Effects of stroke localization on cardiac autonomic balance and sudden death. *Stroke* 30:1307–1311, 1999.
225. Travers JB, Travers SP, and Norgren R. Gustatory neural processing in the hindbrain. *Annu Rev Neurosci* 10:595–632, 1987.
226. Trichopoulos D, Katsouyanni K, Zavitsanos X, Tzonou A, and Dalla-Vorgia P. Psychological stress and fatal heart attack: the Athens (1981) earthquake natural experiment. *Lancet* 1:441–444, 1983.
227. Valeriano J and Elson J. Electrocardiographic changes in central nervous system disease. *Neurol Clin* 11:257–272, 1993.
228. van der Kooy D, Koda LY, McGinty JF, Gerfen CR, and Bloom FE. The organization of projections from the cortex, amygdala, and hypothalamus to the nucleus of the solitary tract in rat. *J Comp Neurol* 224:1–24, 1984.
229. van der Kooy D, McGinty JF, Koda LY, Gerfen CR, and Bloom FE. Visceral cortex: a direct connection from prefrontal cortex to the solitary nucleus in rat. *Neurosci Lett* 33:123–127, 1982.

230. Verberne AJ. Medullary sympathoexcitatory neurons are inhibited by activation of the medial prefrontal cortex in the rat. *Am J Physiol* 270:R713–R719, 1996.
231. Verberne AJ, Lewis SJ, Worland PJ, Beart PM, Jarrott B, Christie MJ, and Louis WJ. Medial prefrontal cortical lesions modulate baroreflex sensitivity in the rat. *Brain Res* 426:243–249, 1987.
232. Verrier RL. Mechanisms of behaviorally induced arrhythmias. *Circulation* 76:I48–I56, 1987.
233. Verrier RL, Calvert A, and Lown B. Effect of posterior hypothalamic stimulation on ventricular fibrillation threshold. *Am J Physiol* 228:923–927, 1975.
234. Verrier RL and Lown B. Behavioral stress and cardiac arrhythmias. *Annu Rev Physiol* 46:155–176, 1984.
235. Von Euler US and Folkow B. The effect of stimulation of autonomic areas in the cerebral cortex upon the adrenaline and noradrenaline secretion from the adrenal gland of the cat. *Acta Physiol Scand* 42:313–320, 1958.
236. Waldrop TG, Bauer RM, and Iwamoto GA. Microinjection of GABA antagonists into the posterior hypothalamus elicits locomotor activity and a cardiorespiratory activation. *Brain Res* 444:84–94, 1988.
237. Wall PD and Davis CD. Three cerebral cortical systems affecting autonomic function. *J Neurophysiol* 14:507–517, 1951.
238. Ward AA. The cingular gyrus: area 24. *J Neurophysiol* 11:13–23, 1948.
239. Warwick-Evans L, Walker J, and Evans J. A comparison of psychologically induced cardiovascular reactivity in laboratory and natural environments. *J Psychosom Res* 32:493–504, 1988.
240. Watts AG and Swanson LW. Efferent projections of the suprachiasmatic nucleus: II. Studies using retrograde transport of fluorescent dyes and simultaneous peptide immunohistochemistry in the rat. *J Comp Neurol* 258:230–252, 1987.
241. Watts AG, Swanson LW, and Sanchez-Watts G. Efferent projections of the suprachiasmatic nucleus: I. Studies using anterograde transport of *Phaseolus vulgaris* leucoagglutinin in the rat. *J Comp Neurol* 258:204–229, 1987.
242. Way M and Cechetto DF. Neurotransmitters in the lateral hypothalamic area (LHA) mediating cardiovascular responses from the infralimbic cortex (ILC). *Neurosci Abstr* 22:391–391, 1996.
243. Whitehead MC and Frank ME. Anatomy of the gustatory system in the hamster: central projections of the chorda tympani and the lingual nerve. *J Comp Neurol* 220:378–395, 1983.
244. Wible JH, Jr, Luft FC, and DiMicco JA. Hypothalamic GABA suppresses sympathetic outflow to the cardiovascular system. *Am J Physiol* 254:R680–R687, 1988.
245. Yamamoto T and Kawamura Y. Gustatory responses from circumvallate and foliate papillae of the rat. *Nippon Seirigaku Zasshi* 34:83–84, 1972.
246. Yamamoto T and Kawamura Y. Cortical responses to electrical and gustatory stimuli in the rabbit. *Brain Res* 94:447–463, 1975.
247. Yamamoto T and Kawamura Y. Gustatory reaction time in human adults. *Physiol Behav* 26:715–719, 1981.
248. Yamamoto T, Matsuo R, and Kawamura Y. Localization of cortical gustatory area in rats and its role in taste discrimination. *J Neurophysiol* 44:440–455, 1980.

249. Yasui Y, Breder CD, Saper CB, and Cechetto DF. Autonomic responses and efferent pathways from the insular cortex in the rat. *J Comp Neurol* 303:355–374, 1991.
250. Zamrini EY, Meador KJ, Loring DW, Nichols FT, Lee GP, Figueroa RE, and Thompson WO. Unilateral cerebral inactivation produces differential left/right heart rate responses [see comments]. *Neurology* 40:1408–1411, 1990.
251. Zhang Z and Oppenheimer SM. Characterization, distribution and lateralization of baroreceptor-related neurons in the rat insular cortex. *Brain Res* 760:243–250, 1997.
252. Zhang ZH, Rashba S, and Oppenheimer SM. Insular cortex lesions alter baroreceptor sensitivity in the urethane-anesthetized rat. *Brain Res* 813:73–81, 1998.

8

Ontogeny of the Cardiac Nervous System

Phyllis M. Gootman

This chapter summarizes the major findings from research on maturation of extrinsic and intrinsic neurons regulating the heart. It includes some speculations on the relevance of this research to clinical issues such as prematurity, heart failure associated with congenital heart disease, and the etiology of sudden infant death syndrome (SIDS). The topics chosen for discussion represent highlights in the field of neurocardiology. Thus, the references cited are selective rather than exhaustive. While there are numerous review articles on cardiac development, few are devoted to the ontogeny of the cardiac neuronal hierarchy.

Perinatal Development of Extrinsic Cardiac Neuronal Control

Localization of Cardiomotor Regulatory Regions

Surprisingly, the number of studies localizing central neuronal vasoactive sites in neonates is limited. Most of these studies have been carried out in piglets.[10,27-29,32,36,37] For instance, there is only one study on colonic blood flow responses to hypothalamic stimulation in puppies.[9] Electrical stimulation of central nervous system vasoactive sites in neonatal swine reveals a postnatal maturation of cardiovascular responses.[29,30] The magnitude of the cardiovascular responses induced in this way and the number of vasoactive sites identified increase during postnatal development.[27] The central nervous system does not begin to integrate multiple inputs from baroreceptor and somatic afferent neurons, as occurs during the Valsalva maneuver,[40,56] until several weeks after birth.[28] Progressive central neuronal maturation is required for this information processing, even though baroreceptor and chemoreceptor reflex mechanisms are functional.[30,34] Furthermore, centrally coordinated respiratory modulation of baroreceptor reflexes is not present in piglets until about 25 days of age.[56] Although perinatal development of the brain stem regions involved in cardiorespiratory rhythm generation has not been examined in detail,[104] peripheral sympathetic efferent postganglionic nerve activity in neonatal swine displays cardiac and respiratory cycle–related periodicities.[31,34,103] The coherence of activities generated by sympathetic efferent neuronal outflows from different spinal cord levels reveals another aspect of postnatal maturation—age-related changes in response to stresses.[42,56] Using c-*fos* as a marker of neuronal activation, nucleus tractus solitarius neurons are activated by alterations in baroreceptor[90] or chemoreceptor[102] sensory inputs in the neonate. Age-related changes in response to hypoxia occur, with 2-week-olds showing greater c-*fos* labeling than newborns. Different age-related changes occur in neurons in the nucleus tractus solitarius and the area postrema.[89,102] This demonstrates the selectivity of such maturation.

Cardiovascular Reflexes

In mammals, cardiovascular reflexes are initiated by afferent neurons associated with mechanosensory neurites located in the carotid arteries and aorta or heart, as well as chemosensory neurites in the carotid and aortic bodies, the myocardium, and pulmonary vasculature (Chapter 3). Cardiovascular reflexes mature during perinatal development.[30,98,104] In neonatal swine, altered baroreceptor activity does not lead to alterations in heart rate until 10 days after birth. Furthermore, hypoxic stimulation of cardiovascular chemosensory afferent neurons does not elicit a heart rate response until more than 2 weeks of postnatal life. Thus, blood pressure regulation becomes discernable soon after birth and increases in sensitivity thereafter.[30] Baroreceptor reflex gain also increases postnatally.[54] A recent study on infants subjected to baroreflex stimulation by tilting their head up[24] showed a biphasic tachycardia/bradycardia response in 3-month-olds; either no change in heart rate or either tachycardia or bradycardia was elicited at 1 month of age.[30]

By birth, cardiopulmonary receptor activation by phenyl biguanide evokes reflex responses in swine.[31,95] Porcine ventricular sensory neurites respond to stimulation by veratrum alkaloids to induce bradycardia at birth.[31,60] Thus, cardiac sensory neurons are functional in the early neonatal period. These sensory neurons are capable of transducing stimuli in a manner similar to that found in adults.[12] Mesenteric and renal vascular responses can also be initiated by 2 weeks of age. Cardiopulmonary J receptors respond to stimulation with phenyl biguanide, inducing atrioventricular conduction block by 1 week of postnatal age.[110] In a study with chronically instrumented fetal, newborn, and 6- to 8-week-old lambs, activation of cardiopulmonary reflexes by expansion of total blood volume evoked heart rate responses in postnatal, not fetal, lambs. This intervention did not affect baroreceptor reflex gain until 6–8 weeks of age.[72] In piglets, fully mature sympathetic efferent neuronal activity and cardiovascular responses to a complex afferent stimulus such as the Valsalva maneuver do not become evident until 7 weeks of age; a progressive maturation of this reflex occurs before that age.[40,54]

Extrinsic Innervation of the Heart

Autonomic innervation of the developing heart has been examined in fetal and neonatal hearts of several mammalian species. Adrenergic neurons and fibers have been detected by spectrofluorometry in term fetal rabbits[22] and by immunocytochemistry in mid-term fetal dogs.[112] Peptidergic innervation has been identified in neonatal[43] but not fetal dog hearts.[113] Cholinergic fibers have been detected in fetal pig hearts throughout gestation, adrenergic axons making their appearance in late gestation.[66] Pharmacological blockade studies in chronically instrumented fetal lambs revealed that the level of cerebral cortical activity is a determinant of sympathetic versus parasympathetic dominance.[116] Denervation of sympathetic efferent neurons that innervate the heart (by bilateral stellectomy) induces no alterations in cardiac responses elicited in 1-week old piglets, indicative of a lack of functional innervation by these neurons at that age. Bilateral stellectomy before 8 weeks of age does affect cardiac control.[111] These and other studies[44] indicate that the cardiac sympathetic efferent nervous system is mature by that age. Thus, studies of autonomic innervation of the heart and vasculature support the view that such innervation may be present before central reflex control mechanisms become functional.[29,30,47,48,66] These data imply that cardiovascular reflexes mature after afferent and efferent neuronal functional innervation.[12,33,46]

In postnatal rat hearts, immunohistochemical fluorescence studies demonstrated that tyrosine hydroxylase reactivity (the rate-limiting enzyme involved in norepinephrine synthesis) is present at birth, especially in nodal and conduction tissues; it increases until the 20th postnatal day.[79,107] The authors of these studies cited earlier literature to suggest that, in the rat, anatomical changes precede functional development of the cardiovascular neuronal hierarchy before the first postnatal week.

Functional studies in swine involving denervation versus stimulation of decentralized vagal efferent postganglionic axons show significant development in the cardiac parasympathetic efferent nervous system shortly after birth.[11,31,44] Physiological studies indicate minimum spontaneous activity generated by neurons in stellate ganglia of neonates.[101] There is a delay in the onset of heart rate and contractile responses elicited by stellate ganglion[33] or vagus nerve[44] stimulation, with parasympathetic efferent neuronal innervation preceding sympathetic innervation.[44] A decrease in resting heart rate and an increase in heart rate variability are characteristic of perinatal cardiac innervation in many mammals,[56,63,119] including humans.[35,70,71,91] These data suggest that the balance of autonomic control of neonatal hearts evolves differentially during early neonatal life.[81,85]

Immunohistochemical studies in dog hearts indicate that adrenergic innervation occurs in the atrium before the ventricle and that the adult pattern of innervation is achieved only by the second postnatal month.[112] These studies support previous functional data indicating the varied time for functional innervation of the heart by parasympathetic versus sympathetic efferent neurons.[44] Studies that compared neonatal and 3-month-old swine found no age-related difference in conduction system innervation;[14] however, there is asymmetry of atrial and ventricular innervation by adrenergic, cholinergic, and peptidergic axons.[15] That functional studies are not in total accord with these anatomical findings[44] suggests that there may be a delay of function after the heart becomes innervated. For example, when sleeping kittens were subjected to adrenergic or cholinergic blockade, a shift from sympathetic to parasympathetic efferent neuronal dominance over resting heart rate occurred during the first 18 days of life.[18] In piglets, cardiac autonomic neurons are also known to be present before functional innervation occurs.[30,47,48] Furthermore, in the youngest piglets, minimal spontaneous activity is generated by neurons in intrathoracic sympathetic ganglia.[101] Age-related delays in the appearance of heart rate and contractile force changes induced during stellate ganglion stimulation have also been reported in developing swine,[33] dogs,[44] and cats.[68] Generally speaking, vagal efferent neurons innervate the hearts of swine,[39] dogs,[44] and rats[74] at an earlier age. Vagus nerve stimulation before and during right stellate ganglion stimulation also reveals an age-related inhibition of the vagally induce bradycardia in maturing dogs.[86] Such interactions are minimal in neonates; by 1 month of age they are similar to those found in adults. In summary, the results of studies carried out on extrinsic cardiac neurons in the neonate reveal asynchronous development of the cardiac nervous system, thus catastrophic responses to stress may occur during the early postnatal period because of different levels of extrinsic cardiac neuronal maturation (see below).

Perinatal Development of Intrinsic Cardiac Neuronal Control

The mammalian embryonic heart has functional properties that enable the fetal heart to undergo progressive changes in myocardial ultrastructure and biochemistry that underlie the electrical and mechanical characteristics of its myocytes.[5,61,79]

Cardiac Rhythmicity and Conduction of Electrical Activity

Ontogenesis of myocardial electrical properties has been studied in chick and rat embryos.[57,108] Cardiac myocyte action potentials are detectable at a very early stage. The precontractile embryonic heart generates spontaneous, rhythmic action potentials that are usually synchronous in nature. Heart rate decreases with lowered body temperature. This effect lessens as the embryo ages, even though the heart is not yet innervated. Cardiomyocyte contraction and excitation–contraction coupling occur before extrinsic innervation of the heart occurs. The ionic currents underlying the myocardial action potential continue to evolve during fetal and neonatal life; cardiomyocyte resting potentials become more negative and action potentials increase in amplitude, as do membrane depolarizations and repolarizations.[108] Ultrastructural alterations supporting these ionic changes have been identified in membranes derived from fetal human ventricles,[59] as well as fetal and neonatal dog hearts.[26] Low resistance gap junctions of the developing human left ventricle change as well.[83] The Ca^{2+} handling sarcolemma and sarcoplasmic reticulum are functional in embryonic rat, chick, and humans hearts.[77] Species differences in cardiac electrophysiological changes have been identified in conjunction with postnatal development, including the ontogeny of electrocardiographic waveforms.[65]

Characteristic pacemaker potentials have been recorded from various sites in early embryonic chick and rat hearts; a specific atrial pacemaker site develops only later in embryonic life.[57] Action potentials are conducted radially at a uniformly slow rate in these hearts. Among the many studies on the ontogenesis of the sinus and atrioventricular nodes and the ventricular conduction system,[75] 10- to 18-day-old gestational rat hearts have been used to reconstruct three-dimensional conduction pathways based on immunohistochemical and electron microscopic evidence. Nodal cells are identifiable at 12 days of age. Right and left bundle branches of the ventricular conduction system are identifiable by 10 days of age. A single bundle of His appears by the 14th day of age, which subsequently communicates with the atrioventricular node by the 16th day.[75] There is wide variation among the types of Purkinje fibers found in neonatal hearts from different species. Groups of non-contracting cardiac myocytes are seen to increase in number from the earliest embryonic stage through the stage of ventricular septation. On the basis of cardiac gene expression, a definitive ventricular conduction system appears to develop from the interventricular myocardium first as a ring on top of the septum. The velocity of conduction through this specialized myocyte system increases during fetal and postnatal life as its number of low-resistance gap junctions increases.

Influx of calcium ions across the myocyte sarcolemma ensures excitation–contraction coupling in the fetal heart[108] so that sarcolemmal sodium–calcium exchange becomes functional during neonatal development.[45] Postnatal maturation of the sarcoplasmic reticulum[77] provides for calcium storage and release during excitation–contraction coupling,[108] although this mechanism is immature in neonates compared to that in adults. Taken together, these observations indicate that during perinatal development, electrical mechanisms coordinating the unidirectional propulsion of output from the heart are available during the precontractile stage of myocardial development.

Myocardial Contractility and Stretch Mechanisms

Perinatal development of contractile function depends on changes in myoarchitecture of the heart,[97] its ultrastructure,[61] and molecular components.[64,76] A review of functional studies on chick, rat, and human embryonic hearts summarizes evidence for the early development of contractility prior to the appearance of extrinsic innervation: atrial filling is passive and followed by atrial contraction that generates increasing peak systolic pressure with embryonic age.[59] The cardiac jelly lining the ventricles of early embryos impedes ventricular filling and thus end-diastolic pressure. Ventricular systolic pressure and stroke volume increase with age, as does the end-systolic pressure–volume relationship reflecting rapid changes in afterload during ejection. The appearance of adult contractile characteristics early in neonatal life indicates that the myocardial contractile apparatus involves biomechanical mechanisms that evolve early during embryonic development.

Results obtained by studying cardiac contraction in fetal and neonatal mammals have been presented in relation to findings in 1- to 17-year-olds undergoing echocardiography.[13] The left ventricle of young children exhibited a faster velocity of myocardial shortening, greater shortening, and a lower afterload than that found in children older than 4 years of age. However, isolated fetal and neonatal myocardial tissue derived from several animal species has a lower capacity for force generation than the adult myocardium.[13] The wide variety of studies that have focused on the role of calcium ion exchange in the development of contractile force has been reviewed in the context of the ontogeny of calcium ion handling by cardiomyocytes.[79] Calcium uptake into and release from the sarcoplasmic reticulum increases while the sensitivity of contractile proteins and ATPase decreases perinatally, paralleling changes in cardiac myocyte ultrastructure and contractile proteins.

The myocardial response to stretch is manifest by increased contractile force and speed of shortening in the atria and ventricles or isolated myocardial segments derived from either chamber. Developmental changes in myocyte structure and function allow maturation of cardiomyocyte responses to stretch, which is necessary for adaptation to the sudden changes in pressure and volume loads that occur at birth. Pre-innervated embryonic hearts of several species respond to stretch with an increase in ventricular systolic pressure (and its rate of development) and stroke volume, without a change in heart rate.[59] This increase in contractile force is initiated by increased influx of calcium ions through stretched sarcolemmal channels.[108] Rapid growth of the left ventricle in early neonatal swine[5] is attributable to stretch-induced increases in contractile function that has been shown to involve increased sensitivity of contractile proteins to calcium,[23] as well as the activation of mechanosensitive ion channels in cardiomyocyte membranes.[8]

The right ventricle exhibits difficulty in contracting against the sudden increase in resistance offered by the pulmonary vasculature during the first postnatal hours as the low-resistance fetal circulatory pathways close. However, progressive experimental occlusion of the pulmonary artery in swine within 24 hours or at 3–5 days of age results in a decrease in right ventricular stroke volume as maturation proceeds; this has been attributed to the greater right ventricular muscle mass identified in neonatal swine.[6] The magnitude of the cardiomyocyte responses elicited by stretch increases postnatally in swine and sheep, both in vivo and in isolated myocardial preparations.[21] A study in chronically instrumented lambs demonstrated that the left ventricle fills faster in the newborn than in 2-month-olds,[115] partly as a result of a faster rate of myocardial relaxation. In contrast, when isolated perfused guinea pig hearts were subjected to increases in filling pressure, the observed increase in rate of ventricular relaxation was found to be similar in neonates and adults.[58]

A role for intrinsic cardiac neurons in altering these stretch mechanisms is suggested by studies on mechanosensory neuronal activity in adult dog hearts.[20] Many ventricular mechanosensory neurites generate action potentials that occur during specific phases of the cardiac cycle, particularly during late diastole. The activity they generate increases when the ventricles become stretched, for instance, during partial outflow tract obstruction or post-extrasystolic filling. Thus one might speculate that intrinsic cardiac neurons provide a supplementary contribution to the intrinsic myocardial response to stretch (Chapter 3).

Ontogeny of the Intrinsic Cardiac Nervous System

Intrinsic cardiac neurons have been identified at an early fetal age, even before ingrowth of nerve fibers extrinsic to the heart.[3,84] This observation is based on immunohistochemical analysis of fetal atria tissue derived from rabbits[87] or humans.[82] Cholinesterase-containing atrial and ventricular neurons have been identified in rabbit fetus hearts at gestation day 15.[88] Atrial, but not ventricular, tissue derived from human fetal hearts contains intrinsic neurons by 14 weeks gestation, as identified by a neuron-specific gene product.[51] Intrinsic cardiac adrenergic cell types have been detected in pre-innervation human fetal hearts at 20 weeks gestation.[46] Human atrial and ventricular epicardial ganglionated plexuses contain acetylcholinesterase staining intrinsic cardiac neurons that decrease in number from fetal and neonatal life to infancy and adulthood.[82] The populations of adrenergic cell types decreases during the early neonatal period as the population of cholinesterase-containing neurons increases.[51] The intrinsic cardiac nervous system of swine aged 1–4 postnatal weeks contains acetycholinesterase- and tyrosine hydroxylase–positive somata and nerves.[15] This is important because adult intrinsic cardiac adrenergic neurons may be involved in the genesis of ventricular arrhythmias.[3,53]

Nonadrenergic and noncholinergic neural control of cardiac function includes purinergic and peptidergic neural mechanisms that are both extrinsic and intrinsic to the neonatal heart.[3,50,88] With respect to fetal intrinsic cardiac neurons, only the reactivity to peptides has been examined extensively. In fetal human hearts, peptidergic intrinsic cardiac nerve fibers and somata are detectable by 7 weeks gestation,[43] a relatively late embryonic stage of development. Immunofluorescence staining revealed neuropeptide Y reactivity by 10 weeks gestation; vasoactive intestinal polypeptide and somatostatin reactivities were observed at 10–12 weeks and substance P reactivity occurred at 18–24 weeks. The pattern of distribution of neurons and axons in atrial and ventricular tissues differs during neonatal development, depending on the peptide studied. Neuropeptide Y immunoreactivity has been detected in intrinsic cardiac ganglia of the fetal rat by 16 gestational days,[100] followed by an age-related increase in the number of neuronal somata and axons associated with that peptide. During postnatal development of the rat heart,[106] neuropeptide

Y immunoreactivity is associated with few atrial axons and neuronal somata by birth. Both increase during subsequent maturation, with cell bodies becoming highly reactive by the 40th postnatal day. Vasoactive intestinal peptide reactivity was observed by 10 days, somata being highly reactive by the 40th postnatal day. However, no intrinsic neurons reactive to substance P were detected in the developing atria of this mammal. Hearts of swine contain axons that are immunoreactive to multiple peptides by 1–4 postnatal weeks of age; only somatostatin-reactive cell bodies have been detected in this species at that age.[15] Adenosine is known to affect the electrophysiological properties of dissociated fetal, neonatal, and adult rat atria myocytes.[109] Adenosine activates muscarinic sensitive-cardiomyocyte potassium ion channels associated with 14-day but not 12-day fetal hearts. The amplitude of current generated by a given dose of adenosine increases through birth and early neonatal life until the 10th postnatal day; it decreases during the subsequent postnatal period.

Many chemicals to which adult intrinsic cardiac neurons respond are known to modulate these neurons during postnatal maturation.[3] The developing heart contains neurons responsive to histamine,[99] angiotensin II,[55] and nitric oxide.[100] Isolated myocytes from guinea pig right and left atria and right ventricular papillary muscle are sensitive to histamine by birth, producing adult-like responses by 5–10 postnatal days.[99] Although H_1 receptor responses are not elicited in the immature myocardium, H_2 receptor–induced responses can be evoked in immature right atrial and ventricular tissue that resemble those induced in adult myocardial tissue. Angiotensin II receptors are detectable in myocardial tissue from fetal and neonatal rats by autoradiography.[55] These cardiomyocyte receptors are distributed diffusely throughout atrial and ventricular tissue by 12 days (mid) gestation, their density increasing thereafter into early postnatal life.[55] The low density of angiotensin II receptor subtypes has precluded their quantification on neonatal cardiomyocytes.

Nitrergic immunoreactivity has been found in intrinsic cardiac ganglia of fetal rat hearts by 19 days gestation,[100] later than many other intrinsic neuron immunoreactivities. During postnatal development, an unexpected decrease in the number of these cell bodies was observed. It is logical to assume that interactions among these chemically sensitive neurons contribute to the complex perinatal development of the intrinsic cardiac nervous system.[55] Taken together, the observations summarized above indicate the complex ontogeny of the intrinsic cardiac nervous system. The functional role of each component during cardiac development requires further investigation if this nervous system is to be targeted therapeutically in the neonatal period. It may be that intrinsic cardiac neurons act as linkages during development of electrophysiological control of cardiac contraction through excitation–contraction coupling, biochemical control of contractile force, and biomechanical control of myocardial responses to stretch.

RELEVANT PATHOLOGIES IN THE PERINATAL PERIOD

Premature Birth

Prematurity of birth can be associated with cardiomyocyte dysfunction due to the immaturity of the autonomic nervous system. Among the measures used in the assessment of autonomic function in infants, determination of heart rate variability (i.e., the beat to beat fluctuations in cardiac cycle duration) is important.[35,70,114] Receptor blockade experiments have provided evidence that high- and low-frequency components of the constructed power spectrum of heart rate variability can differentiate to some degree the sympathetic and parasympathetic efferent neuronal control of heart rate, respectively.[2,16,67,81]

Alterations in the high- and low-frequency patterns of heart rate variability have been identified in the perinatal period of at least three mammalian species. Third-trimester fetal lamb hearts display less heart rate variability and smaller effects of adrenergic or cholinergic blockade on this index[73] than do neonatal hearts.[105] In swine, a study conducted at intervals from 8 to 33 postnatal days revealed a continuing increase in heart rate variability, especially in its low-frequency components, with increasing age.[63] In humans, although the low-frequency component is the largest, the high-frequency component continues to increase postnatally from preterm to full-term infancy.[11,114] Furthermore, it increases more from 3 days to 14 years of age[70] or from 4 months to 4 years of age,[4] depending on the study.

Major contributors to heart rate variability include modulation by respiration[11,41] and the baroreceptor reflex.[118] Respiratory rhythm analysis while heart rate variability is being determined in premature and full-term infants provides evidence that respiration modulates its high-frequency component.[11] Alteration of baroreceptor reflex activity in third-trimester fetal lambs consequent to raising or lowering arterial pressure by phenylephrine or nitroprusside, respectively, produces a steeply rising slope on a graph of heart rate variability versus arterial pressure, chiefly via increases in its low-frequency component.[118] Use of receptor blockade has established that modulation of heart rate variability by the baroreceptor reflex is mediated primarily by cholinergic efferent neurons. Immaturity of the baroreflex, as well as cardiorespiratory integration,[69] is reflected during the early perinatal period in low heart rate variability. From the demonstration that heart rate variability is virtually absent after cardiac transplantation in adult humans[92] and dogs[78] until extrinsic re-innervation develops, one may conclude that heart rate variability is not primarily due to the intrinsic cardiac nervous system but rather to extracardiac neurons.[78]

Congenital Cardiac Malformations and Cardiac Failure

Congenital cardiac malformations may lead to cardiac failure. They can be caused by arrested or aberrant cardiogenesis due to genetic defects.[25] Common types of congenital heart disease relate to the incomplete development of the atrial or ventricular septum. Atrial septal defects have been attributed to impairment of critical interactions occurring between embryonic mesenchymal tissues during the evolution of the atrial myocardium.[117] Ventricular septal defects have been attributed to altered embryonic neural crest development.[62] Biopsies of the right atrium during surgery in children with either of these cardiac malformations reveal depletion of myocardial contractile elements, perineural fibrosis in groups of unmyelinated nerve fibers, and absence of contact between vesiculated axon terminals and myocytes.[17] Septal defects lead to shunting of blood between left and right cardiac chambers and to volume overloading that depends on the size of the septal defect. Although this overload may be tolerated by activating intrinsic myocardial stretch mechanisms and subsequent myocardial thickening, large septal defects lead to heart failure in infancy. Counts of right atrial neurons in postmortem samples derived from children who died in heart failure due to congenital heart disease do not differ from those found in tissues from nondiseased hearts.[1] Nevertheless, given the above findings, functional failure in some types of intrinsic cardiac neurons might be expected.

Some cases of ventricular septal defect are associated with congenital obstruction of the pulmonary valve, leading to inadequate pulmonary blood flow so that normal oxygenation of pulmonary arterial blood does not occur. In a lamb model of congenital heart disease in which atrial septal defects that cause hypoxemia and right ventricular overload were produced surgically, down-regulation of cardiomyocyte β-adrenergic receptors and adenylate cyclase activity occurred during the development of heart failure.[7] The cellular localization of these biochemical changes has not been determined. However, a morphologic study of atrial neurons sampled from adult patients with ischemic hearts at the time of surgery may be relevant.[49] The ultrastructural abnormalities thus detected included laminated cytoplasmic inclusions in the cell bodies and disrupted axoplasm of intrinsic cardiac ganglion axon terminals. It is therefore not unreasonable to speculate that these changes could occur in hypoxemic congenital heart disease.

Neuronal Imbalance in Sudden Infant Death Syndrome

This syndrome is presumed to be of multifactorial etiology. There is growing evidence for the role of defective autonomic neuronal control of the heart in this syndrome.[38,39,104] For the last 10 years we have been exploring the effects of chronic autonomic imbalance on cardiovascular reflexes as a model for SIDS. While neuronal imbalance could occur within the brain stem regulatory system or within effector pathways or at the level of the effectors themselves,[96] we have developed the premise that selective chronic effector denervation would reveal a pattern of imbalance within the cardiac neuronal hierarchy (see Chapter 4). To that end, we explored changes induced in cardiovascular reflex responses and alterations in patterns of these responses. Recently, we have taken two additional approaches: chronic telemetry and c-*fos* activation as markers for changes in neuronal activity in areas of the brain stem known to be vital to autonomic neuronal regulation of cardiovascular function.

Selected cardiac denervation early in postnatal life reveals the maturational role of autonomic innervation in the regulation of cardiac function. Poincare plots were used to differentiate the delay in onset of autonomic efferent neuronal control of regional cardiac function. One week following selected cardiac sympathetic or parasympathetic efferent neuronal denervation, there was little difference in these plots; a right vagotomy or right stellectomy induced demonstrable alterations in this control by 3 weeks of age.[119] The normal trend of decreasing postnatal heart rate was absent following either type of denervation. In chronic vagotomoized animals, the trend of increasing R-R intervals was no longer present 8 weeks after efferent neuronal denervation. Right stellectomized animals, by contrast, revealed increasing R-R intervals. Among reflex responses to blood pressure elevation (induced by phenylephrine) after 8 weeks of chronic denervation, ventricular bigeminy was identified. Upon arousal from sleep, the newborn infant has an elevated arterial blood pressure; if there is a critical delay in the development of the cardiac neuronal hierarchy, SIDS might develop as a consequence. Another possible occurrence is asynchrony in the interplay between extrinsic and intrinsic cardiac neurons, thus inducing cardiac dysrhythmias. Currently, we lack information on how the interplay between these two neuronal systems might play a role in regulating the neonatal heart.

Heart rate variability is depressed in near miss and SIDS victims.[84,93,94] It is also depressed in neonatal swine subjected to right stellate ganglionectomy.[63] Since imbalance between extrinsic adrenergic and cholinergic nerves innervating the heart has been shown to lead to cardiac dysrhythmias,[94] and altered heart rate variability leads to electrical instability of the heart,[19] it is not surprising that arrhythmias occur in SIDS. Recent autopsy material from cases of SIDS provides histological evidence of abnormally high resorption degeneration in the cardiac conduction system.[71] In those cases in which electrocardiograms had been recorded, over half of these patients displayed cardiac dysrhythmias. There is also compelling evidence that ventricular premature contractions and/or tachycardia, along with ventricular fibrillation, can be induced by neurochemical stimulation of intrinsic cardiac neurons in adult dogs.[3,55]

Taken together, these data indicate the potential importance of the role of the cardiac neuronal hierarchy in various cardiac pathologies that develop in the perinatal period. It is apparent that we need much more information about the ontogeny of the entire cardiac nervous system before neurocardiological therapies can be successfully developed to help manage neonatal cardiac disease.

ACKNOWLEDGMENTS

Work toward this chapter was supported by USPHS Grants from the NIH: HL-20864 and HD-28931. The author would like to acknowledge the invaluable assistance of Nancy M. Buckley, M.D., in the preparation of this manuscript and Mrs. Susan Ingenito for library research.

REFERENCES

1. Abdulla AK, Freestaci A, Amorim D, and Olsen EG. Assessment of neurons in congenital heart disease with heart failure. *Am J Cardiovasc Pathol* 3:265–269, 1990.
2. Akselrod S, Gordon D, Ubel FA, Shannon DC, Berger AC, and Cohen RJ. Power spectrum analysis of heart rat fluctuation: a quantitative probe of beat-to-beat cardiovascular control. *Science* 213:220–222, 1981.
3. Armour JA. Anatomy and function of peripheral autonomic neurons involved in cardiac regulation. In: Shepherd JT and Vatner SF, eds. *Nervous Control of the Heart*. Amsterdam: Harwood Academic Press, 1996, pp 29–47.
4. Bar-Haim Y, Marshall PJ, and Fox NA. Developmental changes in heart period and high frequency heart period variability from 4 months to 4 years of age. *Dev Psychobiol* 37:44–56, 2000.
5. Beinlich CJ and Morgan HE. Control of growth in neonatal pig hearts. *Mol Cell Biochem* 119:3–9, 1993.
6. Belik J and Light RB. Effects of increased afterload on right ventricular function in newborn pigs. *J Appl Physiol* 66:863–869, 1989.
7. Bernstein DE, Voss S, Huang R, Doshi R, and Crane C. Differential regula-

tion of right and left beta-adrenergic receptors in newborn lambs with experimental cyanotic heart disease. *J Clin Invest* 85:68–74, 1990.
8. Bett GCL and Sachs F. Cardiac mechanosensitivity and stretch-activated ion channels [review]. *Trends Cardiovasc Med* 7:4–8, 1997.
9. Brodie TA, Devedas M, Rysavy J, Delaney JP, and Leonard AS. The effect of hypoxia and posterior hypothalamic stimulation on colonic blood flow in the weaning puppy. *J Pediatr Surg* 8:747–756, 1973.
10. Buckley NM, Gootman PM, Yellin EL, and Brazeau P. Age-related cardiovascular effects of catecholamines in anesthetized piglets. *Circ Res* 45:282–292, 1979.
11. Chatow U, Davidson S, Reichman BL, and Akselrod S. Development and maturation of the autonomic nervous system in premature and full term infants using spectral analysis of heart rate fluctuation. *Pediatr Res* 37:294–302, 1995.
12. Chen RP-C, Thompson GW, and Armour JA. Transduction capabilities of neonatal ventricular afferent neurons in situ. *Auton Neurosci* 87:1–8, 2001.
13. Colan SD, Parness IA, Spevak PJ, and Sanders SP. Developmental modulation of myocardial mechanics: age and growth related alterations in afterload and contractility. *J Am Coll Cardiol* 19:619–629, 1992.
14. Crick SJ, Anderson RH, Ho SY, and Sheppard MN. Localization and quantitation of autonomic innervation in the porcine heart II: endocardium, myocardium and epicardium. *J Anat* 195:359–373, 1999a.
15. Crick SJ, Sheppard MN, Ho SY, and Anderson RH. Localization and quantitation of autonomic innervation in the porcine heart I: Conduction system. *J Anat* 195:341–357, 1999b.
16. Dalton KJ, Dawes GS, and Patrick JE. The autonomic nervous system and fetal heart rate and blood pressure variability in the fetal lamb. *Am J Obstet Gynecol* 146:456–462, 1983.
17. Dastur DK, Vevaina SC, and Manghani DK. Fine structure of A: autonomic nerve fibers and terminals in human myocardium; and B: myocardial changes in congenital heart disease. *Ultrastruct Pathol* 13:413–431, 1989.
18. Egbert JR and Katona PG. Development of autonomic heart rate control in the kitten during sleep. *Am J Physiol* 238:H829–H835, 1980.
19. Fetsch TH, Reinhardt L, Wichter TH, Borggrefe M, and Breithardt G. Heart rate variability and electrical stability. *Basic Res Cardiol* 93(Suppl 1):117–124, 1998.
20. Foreman RD, Blair RW, Holmes HR, and Armour JA. Correlation of ventricular mechanosensory neurite activity with myocardial sensory field deformation. *Am J Physiol* 276:R979–R989, 1999.
21. Friedman WF. Physiological properties of the developing heart. *Pediatr Cardiol* 6:3–12, 1986.
22. Friedman WF, Pool PE, Jacobowitz D, Seagren SC, and Braunwald E. Sympathetic innervation of the developing rabbit heart. Biochemical and histological comparisons of fetal, neonatal, and adult myocardium. *Circ Res* 23:25–32, 1968.
23. Fuchs F. Mechanical modulation of the Ca^{2+} regulatory protein complex in cardiac muscle. *News Physiol Sci* 10:6–12, 1995.
24. Galland BC, Hayman RM, Taylor BJ, Boltin DPF, Sayers RM, and Williams SM. Factors affecting heart rate variability and heart rate responses to tilting infants aged 1 and 3 months. *Pediatr Res* 48:360–368, 2000.

25. Gelb BD. Recent advances in the understanding of genetic causes of congenital heart defects. *Front Biosci* 5:D321–D333, 2000.
26. Goldstein MA and Traeger L. Ultrastructural changes in postnatal development of the cardiac myocyte. In: Legato MJ, ed. *The Developing Heart*. Boston: Martinus Nijhoff, 1985, pp 1–20.
27. Gootman N, Gootman PM, Buckley NM, Cohen MI, Levine MI, and Spielberg R. Central vasomotor regulation in the newborn piglet (*Sus scrofa*). *Am J Physiol* 222:994–999, 1972.
28. Gootman N, Gootman PM, Crane LA, and Buckley BJ. Integrated cardiovascular to combined somatic and visceral afferent stimulation in newborn piglets. *Biol Neonate* 36:70–77, 1979.
29. Gootman PM. Development of central autonomic regulation of cardiovascular function. In: Gootman PM, ed. *Developmental Neurobiology of the Autonomic Nervous System*. Totowa, NJ: Humana Press, 1986, pp 279–325.
30. Gootman PM. Developmental aspects of reflex control of the circulation. In: Gilmore JP, Zucker IH, eds. *Reflex Control of the Circulation*. Boca Raton, FL: CRC Press. 1991, pp 965–1027.
31. Gootman PM, Buckley BJ, DiRusso SM, Gootman N, Yao AC, Pierce PE, Griswold PG, Epstein MD, Cohen HL, and Nudel DB. Age-related responses to stimulation of cardiopulmonary receptors in swine. *Am J Physiol* 251:H748–H755, 1986.
32. Gootman PM, Buckley BJ, Gootman N, and Salinas-Zeballos T. Localization of vasoactive sites in the thalamus of newborn swine. In: Jones CT and Nathanielsz PW, eds. *Physiological Development of Fetus and Newborn*. London: Academic Press, 1985, pp 599–604.
33. Gootman PM, Gandhi MR, Coren CV, Kaplan NM, Pisana FM, Buckley BJ, Armour JA, and Gootman N. Cardiac responses elicited by stimulation of loci within the stellate ganglion of developing swine. *J Auton Nerv Syst* 38:191–200, 1992.
34. Gootman PM, Gandhi MR, Steele AM, Hundley BW, Cohen HL, Eberle LP, and Sica AL. Respiratory modulation of sympathetic activity in neonatal swine. *Am J Physiol* 261:R1147–R1154, 1991.
35. Gootman PM and Gootman N. The assessment of the autonomic nervous system in newborn babies. In: Eyre JA, ed. *The Neurophysiological Examination of The Newborn Infant. Clinics in Developmental Medicine, No. 120*. London: Mac Keith Press, 1992, pp 168–194.
36. Gootman PM, Gootman N, and Buckley BJ. Maturation of central autonomic control of the circulation. *Fed Proc* 42:1648–1655, 1983.
37. Gootman PM, Gootman N, and Buckley BJ. Localization of central neural vasoactive (VA) sites in developing swine. In: Tumbleson ME, ed. *Swine in Biomedical Research, Vol. III*. New York: Plenum Publishing Corp., 1986, pp 1623–1642.
38. Gootman PM, Gootman N, and Sica AL. A neurocardiac theory for sudden infant death syndrome: role of the autonomic nervous system. *J SIDS Infant Mortal* 1:169–181, 1996.
39. Gootman PM, Hopkins DA, Buckley NM, and Gootman N. Vagal cardiac nerves of the developing swine. In: Ferrans VJ, Rosenquist G, and Weinstein C, eds. *Cardiac Morphogenesis*. New York: Elsevier Science Publishing 1985, pp 267–274.

40. Gootman PM, Hundley BW, Condemi G, and Cohen HL. Postnatal development of cardiovascular and sympathetic responses to stimulated Valsalva maneuvers in neonatal swine. In: Yoshikawa M, Uono M, Tanabe H, and Ishikawa S, eds. *New Trends in Autonomic Nervous System Research, Basic and Clinical Integration.* New York: Elsevier Science Publishing, 1991, pp 349–351.
41. Gootman PM, Hundley BW, and Gootman N. The presence of coherence in sympathetic and phrenic activities in a developing mammal. *Acta Neurobiol Exp* 56:137–145, 1996.
42. Gootman PM, Hundley BW, Sica AL, and Gootman N. Coherence of efferent sympathetic and phrenic activity in a neonatal animal: relation to SIDS? In: Rognum TO, ed. *Sudden Infant Death Syndrome: New Trends in the Nineties.* Oslo: Scandinavian University Press, 1995, pp 246–252.
43. Gordon L, Polak JM, Moscose GI, Smith A, Kuhn DM, and Wharton J. Development of the peptidergic innervation of the human heart. *J Anat* 183:131–140, 1993.
44. Haddad C and Armour JA. Ontogeny of the canine intrathoracic cardiac nervous system. *Am J Physiol* 261:R920–R927, 1991.
45. Haddock PS, Coetzee WA, Nakamura TY, Balaguru D, Boerth SR, and Artman M. Perinatal maturation of myocardial contraction: the role of Na^+-Ca^{2+} exchange. In: Legato MJ, ed. *The Developing Heart.* Philadelphia: Lippincott-Raven, 1997, pp 231–245.
46. Hassall CJ, Penketh R, Rodeck C, and Burnstock G. The intracardiac neurons of the fetal human heart in culture. *Anat Embryol* 182:329–337, 1990.
47. Hopkins DA, Gootman PM, Gootman N, and Armour JA. Anatomy of medullary and peripheral autonomic neurons innervating the neonatal porcine heart. *J Auton Nerv Syst* 64:74–84, 1997.
48. Hopkins DA, Gootman PM, Gootman N, DiRusso SM, and Zeballos ME. Brainstem cells of origin of the cervical vagus and cardiopulmonary nerves in the neonatal pig (*Sus scrofa*). *Brain Res* 306:63–72, 1984.
49. Hopkins DA, Macdonald SE, Murphy DA, and Armour JA. Pathology of intrinsic cardiac neurons from ischemic human hearts. *Anat Rec* 259:424–436, 2000.
50. Horackova M and Armour JA. Role of peripheral autonomic neurons in maintaining adequate cardiac function. *Cardiovasc Res* 30:326–335, 1995.
51. Horackova M, Slavikova J, and Byczko Z. Postnatal development of the rat intrinsic cardiac nervous system: a confocal laser scanning microscopy study in whole-mount atria. *Tissue Cell* 32:377–388, 2000.
52. Huang MH, Smith FM, and Armour JA. Modulation of in situ canine intrinsic cardiac neuronal activity by nicotinic, muscarinic and β-adrenergic agonists. *Am J Physiol* 265:R659–R669, 1993.
53. Huang MH, Wolf SG, and Armour JA. Ventricular arrhythmias induced by chemically modified intrinsic cardiac neurons. *Cardiovasc Res* 28:636–642, 1994.
54. Hundley BW, Sica ASL, and Gootman PM. Rhythmicities in sympathetic discharge: a possible signal of cardiorespiratory integration in developing animals. *Ann NY Acad Sci* 940:416–430, 2001.
55. Hunt RA, Ciuffo GM, Saavedra JM, and Tucker DC. Quantification and localization of angiotensin II receptors and angiotensin converting enzyme in the developing rat heart. *Cardiovasc Res* 29:834–840, 1995.

56. Jarenwattananon M, Buckley BJ, Gootman N, and Kaplan NA. Age-dependent cardiovascular effects of verapamil in newborn swine. *Pediatr Res* 20:428–432, 1986.
57. Kamino K. Optical approaches to ontogeny of electrical activity and related functional organization during early heart development. *Physiol Rev* 71:53–91, 1991.
58. Kaufman TM, Horton JW, White DJ, and Mahony L. Age-related change in myocardial relaxation and sacroplasmic reticulum function. *Am J Physiol* 259:H309–H316, 1990.
59. Keller BB. Overview: functional maturation and coupling of the embryonic cardiovascular system. In: Clark EB, Markwald RR, and Takao A, eds. *Developmental Mechanisms of Heart Disease.* New York: Futura, pp 367–385, 1955.
60. Khan MS, Zhao N, Sica AL, Gootman N, and Gootman PM. Changes in R-R and Q-T intervals following cardiac vagotomy in neonatal swine. *Soc Exp Biol Med* 226:32–36, 2001.
61. Kim H, Kim D, Lee I, Rak B, Sawa Y, and Schaper J. Human fetal heart development after mid-term: morphometry and ultrastructural study. *J Mol Cell Cardiol* 24:949–965, 1992.
62. Kirby ML. Cardiovascular morphogenesis: recent research advances. *Pediatr Res* 21:219–224, 1987.
63. Lipsitz LA, Pincus SM, Morin RJ, Tong SW, Eberle LP, and Gootman PM. Preliminary evidence for the evolution in complexity of heart rate dynamics during autonomic maturation in neonatal swine. *J Auton Nerv Syst* 65:1–9, 1997.
64. Lompre A-M. The sarco(endo)plasmic reticulum Ca^{2+}-ATPase in the cardiovascular system during growth and proliferation. *Trends Cardiovasc Med* 8:75–82, 1998.
65. Lukas A. Electrophysiologic changes in the mammalian heart during postnatal development. In: Ostadal B, Gagano M, Takeda M, and Dhalla NS, eds. *The Developing Heart.* Philadelphia: Lippincott-Raven Press, 1997, pp 173–188.
66. Macdonald AA, Poot P, Colenbrander B, Meyer JC, and Wensing CJ. Development of nervous tissue in the heart of the fetal and neonatal pig and the effect of decapitation in utero. *Anat Embryol* 168:405–417, 1983.
67. Malliani A, Pagani M, Lombardi F, and Cerutti S. Cardiovascular neural regulation explored in the frequency domain. *Circulation* 84:1482–1492, 1991.
68. Masliukov PM, Fateev MM, and Nozdrachev AD. Age-dependent changes of electrophysiologic characteristics of the stellate ganglion conducting pathways in kittens. *Auton Neurosci* 83:12–18, 2000.
69. Massimini M, Porta A, Mariotti A, Malliani A, and Montano M. Heart rate variability is encoded in the spontaneous discharge of thalamic somatosensory neurons in cat. *J Physiol (Lond)* 526:387–396, 2000.
70. Massin M and von Bernuth G. Normal ranges of heart rate variability during infancy and childhood. *Pediatr Cardiol* 18:297–302, 1997.
71. Matturri L, Ottaviani G, Ramos SG, and Rossi L. Sudden infant death syndrome (SIDS): a study of the cardiac conduction system. *Cardiovasc Pathol* 9:137–145, 2000.
72. Merrill DC, Segar JL, McWeeny OJ, Smith BA, and Robillard JE. Cardiopulmonary and arterial baroreflex responses to acute volume expansion during fetal and postnatal development. *Am J Physiol* 267:H1467–H1475, 1994.

73. Metsala T, Siimes A, and Valmaki I. The effects of change in sympathovagal balance on heart rate and blood pressure variability in the fetal lamb. *Acta Physiol Scand* 154:85–92, 1995.
74. Minami N and Head GA. Cardiac vagal responsiveness during development in spontaneously hypertensive rats. *Auton Neurosci* 82:115–122, 2000.
75. Moorman AFM, deJong F, Denyn MMFJ, and Lamers WH. Development of the cardiac conduction system [review] *Circ Res* 82:629–644, 1998.
76. Moorman AFM and Lamers WH. Molecular anatomy of the developing heart. *Trends Cardiovasc Med* 4:257–264, 1994.
77. Moorman AFM, Schumacher CA, deBoer PAT, Hagoort JJ, Bezstarosti K, van den Hoff MJB, Wagenaar GTM, Lamers JMJ, Wuytack F, Christoffel VM, and Fiolet JWT. Presence of functional sarcoplasmic reticulum in the developing heart and its confinement to chamber myocardium. *Dev Biol* 223:279–290, 2000.
78. Murphy DA, Thompson GW, Ardell JL, McCraty R, Stevenson RS, Sangatang VE, Cardinal R, Wilkinson M, Craig S, Smith FM, Kingma JG, and Armour JA. The heart reinnervate after transplantation. *Ann Thorac Surg* 69:1769–1781, 2000.
79. Nijjar MS and Dhalla NS. Biochemical basis of calcium handling in developing myocardium. In: Ostadal B, Gagano M, Takeda M, Dhalla NS, eds. *The Developing Heart*. Philadelphia: Lippincott-Raven, 1997, pp 147–171.
80. Nyquist-Battie C, Cochran PK, Sands SA, and Chronwall BM. Development of neuropeptide Y and tyrosine hydroxylase immunoreactive innervation in postnatal rat heart. *Peptides* 15:1461–1469, 1994.
81. Pagani M, Lombardi F, Guzzetti S, Rimoldi O, Furlan R, Pizzinelli P, Sandrone G, Malfatto G, Dell-Orto S, and Piccaluga E. Power spectral analysis of heart rate and arterial pressure variabilities as a marker of sympatho-vagal interaction in man and conscious dog. *Circ Res* 59:178–193, 1986.
82. Pauza DH, Skripka V, Pauziene N, and Stropus R. Morphology, distribution and variability of the epicardiac neural ganglionated sub-plexes in the human heart. *Anat Rec* 259:353–382, 2000.
83. Peters NS, Severs NJ, Rothberg SM, Lincoln C, Yacoub MH, and Green CR. Spatiotemporal relations between gap junction and fascia adherens junctions during postnatal development and its confinement to chamber myocardium. *Circulation* 90:713–725, 1994.
84. Pincus SM, Cummins TR, and Haddad GG. Heart rate control in normal and aborted-SIDS infants. *Am J Physiol* 264:R638–R646, 1993.
85. Pomeranz B, Macaulay RJ, Caudill MA, Kutz I, Adam D, Gordon D, Kilborn KM, Barger AC, Shannon DC, and Cohen RJ. Assessment of autonomic function in humans by heart rate spectral analysis. *Am J Physiol* 248:H151–H153, 1985.
86. Rios R, Stolfi A, Campbell PH, and Pichoff AS. Postnatal development of the putative neuropeptide-Y-mediated sympathetic-parasympathetic autonomic interaction. *Cardiovasc Res* 31:E96–103, 1996.
87. Roberts LA. Morphological innervation pattern of the developing rabbit heart. *Am J Anat* 190:370–384, 1991.
88. Rubino A, Hassell CJS, and Burnstock G. Autonomic control of the myocardium: non-adrenergic noncholinergic (NANC) mechanisms. Shepherd JT and Vatner SF, eds. *Nervous Control of the Heart*. Amsterdam: Harwood Academic Publishers, 1996, pp 139–171.

89. Ruggiero DA, Gootman PM, Ingenito S, Wong C, Gootman N, and Sica AL. The area postrema of newborn swine is activated by hypercapnia: relevance to sudden infant death syndrome? *J Auton Nerv Syst* 76:167–175, 1999.
90. Ruggiero DA, Tong S, Anwar M, Gootman N, and Gootman PM. Hypotension induced expression of c-*fos* gene transcript in the medulla oblongata of piglets. *Brain Res* 706:199–209, 1996.
91. Sahni R, Schulze KF, Kashyap S, Ohviakist U, Fifer WP, and Myers MM. Maturational changes in heart rate and heart rate variability in low birth weight infants. *Dev Psychobiol* 37:73–81, 2000.
92. Sands KEF, Appel ML, Lilly LS, Schoen FJ, Mudge GH, and Cohen RJ. Power spectrum analysis of heart rate variability in human cardiac transplant recipients. *Circulation* 79:76–82, 1989.
93. Schechtman VL, Harper RM, Kluge KA, Wilson AJ, Hoffman HJ, and Southall DP. Cardiac and respiratory patterns in normal infants and victims of the SIDS. *Sleep* 11:413–424, 1988.
94. Schechtman VL, Harper RM, Kluge KA, Wilson AJ, Hoffman HJ, and Southall DP. Heart rate variability in normal infants and victims of the SIDS. *Early Hum Dev* 19:167–181, 1989.
95. Schleman M, Gootman N, and Gootman PM. Cardiovascular and respiratory responses to right atrial injections of phenyldiguanide in pentobarbital-anesthetized newborn piglets. *Pediatr Res* 13:1271–1274, 1979.
96. Schwartz PJ. Sympathetic imbalance and cardiac arrhythmias. In: Randall DC, ed. *Nervous Control of Cardiovascular Function.* New York: Oxford University Press, 1984, pp 636–642.
97. Sedmara D, Pexieder T, Vuillemin M, Thompson RP, and Anderson RH. Developmental patterning of the myocardium. *Anat Rec* 258:319–337, 2000.
98. Segar JL. Ontogeny of the arterial and cardiopulmonary baroreflex during fetal and postnatal life. *Am J Physiol* 273:R457–R471, 1997.
99. Shigenobu K, Sawada K, and Kasuya Y. Changes in sensitivity to histamine of guinea pig cardiac muscles during postnatal development. *Can J Physiol Pharmcol* 58:1300–1306, 1980.
100. Shoba T and Tay SSW. Nitrergic and peptidergic innervation of the developing rat heart. *Anat Embryol* 201:491–500, 2000.
101. Sica AL, Gootman PM, Gootman N, and Armour JA. Neuronal activity of the stellate ganglia in neonatal swine. *J Auton Nerv Syst* 48:273–277, 1994.
102. Sica AL, Gootman PM, and Ruggiero DA. CO_2-induced expression of c-fos in the nucleus of the solitary tract and the area postrema of developing swine. *Brain Res* 837:106–116, 1999.
103. Sica AL, Hundley BW, Ruggiero DA, and Gootman PM. Emergence of lung-inflation related sympathetic nerve activity in spinal cord transected neonatal swine. *Brain Res* 767:380–383, 1997.
104. Sica AL, Hundley BW, Ruggiero DA, and Gootman PM. The sympathetic nervous system of the developing mammal. In: Scharf SMS, Pinsky SM, and Magder MP, eds. *Respiratory–Circulatory Interactions in Health and Disease.* New York: Marcel Dekker, 2001, pp 145–181.
105. Siimes ASI, Valimaki IAT, Antila KJ, Julkunem MKA, Metsala TH, Halkola LT, and Sarajas HSS. Regulation of heart rate variability by the autonomic nervous system in neonatal lambs. *Pediatr Res* 27:383–391, 1990.
106. Slavikova J. Distribution of peptide containing neurons in the developing rat

right atrium, studied using immunofluorescence and confocal laser scanning. *Neurochem Res* 22:1013–1021, 1997.
107. Slavikova J, Goldstein M, and Dahlström A. The postnatal development of tyrosine hydroxylase immunoreactive nerves in rat atrium, studied with immunofluorescence and confocal laser scanning microscopy. *J Auton Nerv Syst* 43:159–170, 1993.
108. Sperelakis N, Katsube Y, Sada H, and Masudo H. Developmental changes in ionic currents of the heart. In: Ostadal B, Gagano M, Takeda M, Dhalla NS, eds. *The Developing Heart*. Philadelphia: Lippincott-Raven, 1997, pp 147–171.
109. Takano M and Noma A. Development of muscarinic potassium currents in fetal and neonatal rat heart. *Am J Physiol* 272:H1188–H1195, 1997.
110. Tong SW, Frasier ID, Ingenito S, Sica AL, Gootman N, and Gootman PM. Age-related cardiovascular responses to phenylbiguanide in piglets. In: Tumbleson M and Schook L, eds. *Advances in Swine Biomedical Research*. New York: Plenum Press, 1996, pp 123–130.
111. Tong SW, Frasier ID, Ingenito S, Sica AL, Gootman N, and Gootman PM. Age-related effects of cardiac sympathetic denervation on the responses to cardiopulmonary receptor stimulation in piglets. *Pediatr Res* 41:72–77, 1997.
112. Ursell PC, Ren CL, and Danilo P, Jr. Anatomic distribution of autonomic neural tissue in the developing dog heart: I. Sympathetic innervation. *Anat Rec* 226:71–80, 1990.
113. Ursell PC, Ren CL, and Danilo P, Jr. Anatomic distribution of autonomic neural tissue in the developing dog heart: II Non-adrenergic non-cholinergic innervation. *Anat Rec* 230:531–538, 1991.
114. Valimaki I and Rantonen T. Spectral analysis of heart rate and blood pressure variability. *Clin Perinatol* 26:967–980, 1999.
115. Velvis H and Klopfenstein HS. Filling characteristics of the left ventricle in newborn lambs. *Am J Physiol* 269:H2039–H2043, 1995.
116. Wakasuki A, Murata Y, Ninomiya Y, Masaoku N, Tyner JG, and Kutty KK. Autonomic nervous system regulation of baseline heart rate in the fetal lamb. *Am J Obstet Gynecol* 167:519–523, 1992.
117. Wessels A, Anderson RH, Markwald RR, Webb S, Brown NA, Viragh SZ, Moorman AFM, and Lamers WH. Atrial development in the human heart: immunohistochemical study with emphasis on the role of mesenchymal tissues. *Anat Rec* 259:288–300, 2000.
118. Yu Z-Y and Lumbers ER. Measurement of baroreceptor-mediated effects on heart rate variability in fetal sheep. *Pediatr Res* 47:233–239, 2000.
119. Zhao N, Khan M, Ingenito S, Sica AL, Gootman N, and Gootman PM. Electrocardiographic changes during postnatal development in conscious swine with cardiac autonomic imbalance. *Auton Neurosci* 88:167–174, 2001.

9

Aging and Neural Responses in the Heart

JAMES G. DOBSON, JR. AND RICHARD A. FENTON

The nervous system is important in the modulation of the peripheral circulation and cardiac pump to ensure an adequate supply of blood to all mammalian tissues. A major component of the control of heart function derives from arterial baroreflexes that exert their influence via the autonomic parasympathetic and sympathetic outflow to the nodal tissue and myocardium.

As adult mammals age, profound changes occur in the cardiovascular responses to autonomic nerve activity. Generally, there is a depressed responsiveness. For example, one cardiovascular manifestation of aging is the vascular hypotension[148] that results from a reduced heart rate response to an orthostatic challenge.[137] Although baroreflex regulation of sympathetic activity appears to remain unchanged with aging,[22,40,147] an overall decrease in cardiac vagal activity and heightened sympathetic discharge under basal conditions is observed.[40] Furthermore, an age-induced reduction of norepinephrine reuptake as determined by enhanced neurotransmitter overflow would be expected to amplify adrenergic signaling.[44] Yet the arterial baroreflex control of the heart rate is attenuated in the aged heart.[40] As a result, with a fall in sinus pressure the heart rate does not increase commensurate with expectations. Although it has been suggested that orthostatic intolerance can result partly from inadequate increases in released norepinephrine in response to reduced baroreceptor activity,[57] an age-induced change in end-organ sensitivity to neurotransmitters most likely plays a primary role. Since it appears that age-induced morphological changes in neural structures within the heart[1] do not affect their functional activity,[3] the focus of this chapter will be on age-induced changes in neurotransmitter release and myocardial responsiveness to neurotransmitters.

Autonomic Function in the Aging Heart

In the pathologically free heart stress such as exercise elicits an increase in the inotropic state as a result of the sympathetic-mediated release of norepinephrine and epinephrine. These catecholamines subsequently activate β_1 (β_1R), β_2 (β_2R), and α_1 (α_1R) receptors on the myo-cardium, resulting in an activation via a stimulatory guanine nucleotide binding protein (G_s)[114] of adenylyl cyclase (β_1R),[8,90,139] an increase in L-type Ca^{2+} current (β_1R, β_2R),[18] and an increase in protein kinase C (PKC) activity[81] and inositide hydrolysis (α_1R).[11] Upon activation of the cyclase, a cascade of transmembrane and intracellular signaling is initiated with subsequent phosphorylation of various myocardial proteins instrumental to the enhancement of contractile function and metabolism.[4,43,49,54,69,73,151]

Aging and Functional Responses to Adrenergic Catecholamines

It has long been recognized that the augmentation of cardiac contractile performance elicited by adrenergic stimulation is diminished in the aged heart. This observation has been made for humans,[19] monkeys,[125] canines,[161] and rats,[88] the most commonly studied models of aging,[56] with males exhibiting a greater response decline than that in their female counterparts.[154] The increase in contractile function (positive inotropy) elicited by β_1R stimulation is reduced in the aged as compared to the young adult heart.[19,86,89,109,155,157,159,161] Using isolated perfused intraventricular septa from young adult (6- to 8-month) and aged (24-month) rat hearts, Guarnieri et al.[65] reported that the maximum rate of force production elicited by β_1R stimulation was reduced in aged septa. A similar age-related decrement in response to norepinephrine and isoproterenol, a β_1 agonist, has been observed in superfused trabecular muscles by Lakatta et al.[88] and in isolated rat ventricular myocytes by Sakai et al.[123] Because the latter studies used in vitro preparations, the results indicated that the age-induced decrement in responsiveness to β_1R stimulation is essentially a postsynaptic phenomenon.

In addition to effects on contractile responsiveness, aging reduces the augmentation in human heart rate observed with increases in serum catecholamine elicited by stressful stimuli such as static exercise, hypoxia, and hypercapnia.[86,109] Aging also diminishes chronotropic responses to the infusion of isoproterenol in senescent beagles[161] and humans,[155] compared to those of their younger adult counterparts.

Our results obtained with young adult (3- to 4-month) and aged (18- to 20-month) isolated, constant-pressure perfused rat hearts indicate that the aged heart is less mechanically responsive to β_1R stimulation than that of the young adult heart[31,33,34] and clearly substantiate the above-cited classic findings. However, our studies (as discussed in more detail below) indicate that the antiadrenergic action of the nucleoside adenosine is an important factor in the reduced responsiveness of the aged adult heart to β_1R stimulation.[31,33,34,53] Blocking the antiadrenergic manifestations of adenosine in the aged heart returns adrenergic responsiveness toward that observed in the young adult heart.[31]

α_1-Adrenergic receptors modulate the automaticity of Purkinje fibers,[23] mediate vasoconstriction of blood vessels,[66] and enhance the inotropy of the myocardium.[15] The effect of aging on α_1R responsiveness has been investigated in rats, where it was found that methoxamine-induced inotropy was attenuated in right ventricular strips.[84] These observations were confirmed in humans when left ventricular systolic function was assessed with echocardiography.[153] This age-induced attenuation of positive inotropism most likely resulted from a reduced α_1R-mediated phosphoinositide hydrolysis which has been observed in rat hearts with aging.[11] With respect to vascular responsiveness, in the presence of atropine blockade, phenylephrine infusions resulted in a reduction in α_1R-induced vascular constriction in concert with an attenuated cardiac contractile activity in human subjects 60–75 years of age.[153] Changes in left ventricular end-diastolic diameters with phenylephrine were unaffected by aging. A reduction in myocardial α_1R number, but not apparent dissociation constant, has been reported to result from an age-induced reduction in receptor transcription.[60,84] However, others have reported no change in rat vascular α-adrenergic responses[145] and no age-induced changes in α_1R mRNA levels. These findings have led to the conclusion that aging does not affect transcriptional regulation of α_1R.[99]

Presynaptic Regulation of Autonomic Responses

In humans, circulating plasma levels of adrenergic neurotransmitters are elevated with aging.[45] This condition might be expected to result from either enhanced release or depressed reuptake of the released neurotransmitters. Stores of adrenergic neurotransmitter in the heart are reduced with aging,[21,85] a possible result of a diminished number of neurons in the heart.[1,64] Although the release of norepinephrine induced pharmacologically by tyramine is unaffected by aging,[64,85,140] norepinephrine overflow from the isolated aged male rat heart in response to right sympathetic nerve stimulation is reduced compared to that in the young adult.[20] This effect of aging was not observed in hearts from female rats.[152]

Extracellular levels of norepinephrine are influenced by several processes. These include transmitter release in response to neural depolarization, modulation of release by presynaptic activities of α_2R, β_2R, and adenosine A_1 receptors (A_1R), and reuptake (Fig. 9–1). Studies using potassium depolarized cardiac synaptosomes that had been loaded with ^3H-labeled norepinephrine suggest that depolarization-induced transmitter release is reduced in the aged rat heart,[140] perhaps as a result of impaired Ca^{2+} influx into nerve terminals.[141] These observations were made in hearts obtained from male, not female, rats, further suggesting a gender-sensitive mechanism of aging.[160] Modulation of transmitter release is also influenced by aging. The activity of prejunctional β_2R that enhance transmitter release has been reported to be reduced in the aged heart,[37,101] as have the inhibitory actions of prejunctional α_2R[20,37] and A_1R.[142] Clearly, the net impact of aging on norepinephrine release would depend on the relative effect of aging on the activities of the different receptors.

How aging affects transmitter reuptake remains controversial, perhaps because uptake is dependent on nerve terminals available for uptake, a number that is depressed in the aged heart.[37,64] Uptake of norepinephrine released from electrically stimulated rat atria has been reported to be depressed with aging,[37] whereas neuronal uptake was observed to be enhanced in neurally stimulated isolated aged rat hearts.[20,64]

Postsynaptic Regulation of Autonomic Responses

The heart responds to neurotransmitters by mechanisms that involve activation of agonist-specific receptors and transduction of the signal by second messengers such as cyclic adenosine monophosphate (cAMP) and

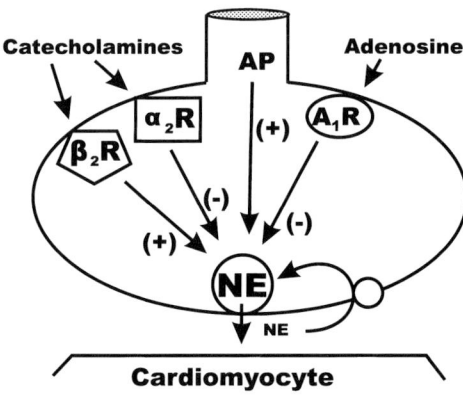

FIGURE 9–1 Depiction of neurohumoral control of norepinephrine (NE) levels at the adrenergic nerve terminal. Action potentials (AP) and stimulation of β_2 receptors (β_2R) enhance [(+)] release, whereas stimulation of α_2 (α_2R) and adenosine A_1 (A_1R) receptors depress [(−)] release.

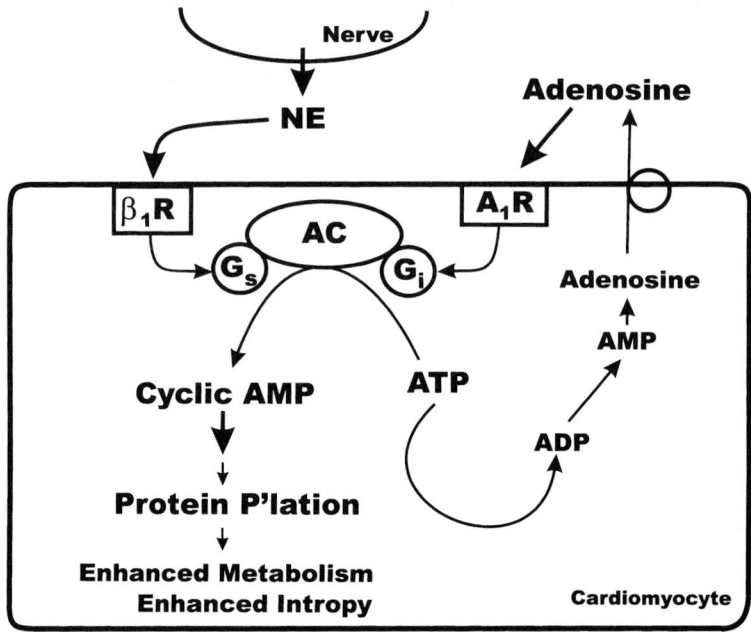

FIGURE 9–2 Schematic of biochemical and transport events depicting the interaction of adrenergic- and adenosinergic-stimulation in the myocardium. Please see text for details. AC, adenylyl cyclase; Gs, Gi, stimulatory and inhibitory guanine nucleotide binding proteins, respectively; NE, norepinephrine; P'lation, phosphorylation.

Ca^{2+}. Catecholamines that interact with β_1R initiate their positive inotropic and glycogenolytic responses by elevating cellular levels of cAMP (Fig. 9–2). This results from the transmembrane coupling of the receptor to adenylyl cyclase via the α subunit of G_s, resulting in the activation of the adenylyl cyclase catalytic subunit.[36,39,114,150] The adenylyl cyclase catalyzes the formation of cAMP, which in turn activates cAMP-dependent protein kinase (PKA), leading to the phosphorylation of a number of myocardial proteins such as the C protein of myosin, glycogen phosphorylase, troponin I, phospholamban, and P-light chain of myosin.[4,25,49,79,123,144] The phosphorylation of these proteins is believed to influence contractile, sarcoplasmic reticulum, sarcolemmal, and enzymatic protein function including Ca^{2+} handling by the myocardial cells.[26]

Although it is recognized that fundamental mechanisms of excitation–contraction (E-C) coupling are also altered with aging,[74,79] considerable attention has been placed on revealing age-induced changes in β_1-adrenergic signal transduction to explain the reduced responsiveness of the myocardium to stimulation by norepinephrine. Although there appears to be some suggestion that β-receptor number and affinity remain unchanged as the myocardium ages,[10,13,65,82,106,121] this conclusion is hardly unanimous.[17,68,130,160] However, for reasons to be discussed in a later section, interpretation of these data requires care because endogenous adenosine presumably present in membrane preparations[90] may modulate adrenergic binding and confound the determination of receptor agonist affinity.[117] Age-induced effects in ventricular $β_1R$ mRNA are conflicting,[67,68] thus a pretranslational effect of aging on $β_1R$ density remains to be conclusively defined. Aging was not found to affect the activities, immunodetectable levels, or expressed mRNA for β-receptor kinase (βARK1) or GRK5,[160] thus minimizing a role for enhanced receptor inactivation in reduced adrenergic responses observed in the aged heart. Similar negative findings have been reported for adrenergic-stimulated substrate phosphorylation. Although aging has been found to depress adrenergic-induced phosphorylation of troponin I and phospholamban,[78,123] isobutylmethylxanthine added to inhibit phosphodiesterase and elevate cAMP levels reversed this depression.[123] In sarcoplasmic reticular-enriched membranes from rat hearts, the incorporation of phosphate into phospholamban in response to exogenous PKA was not altered by aging.[79] In the absence of any apparent enhancement of dephosphorylation,[123] it would appear that aging affects adrenergic signaling processes only prior to targetted protein phosphorylation.

Available evidence suggests that the reduced levels of cAMP attained in the aged heart with adrenergic stimulation[9,31,78,113] result from a reduction in adrenergic-sensitive adenylyl cyclase activity.[104,128,129,160] It has been observed that activation of the catalytic subunit of adenylyl cyclase by forskolin is attenuated with aging,[129,160] as is the forskolin binding site number.[138] This suggests an impairment in the capacity to activate adenylyl cyclase, which is also independent of changes in mRNA expressions for adenylyl cyclase types V and VI.[131]

Age-induced changes in G-protein constituency of the heart may affect the efficacy of adrenergic-induced adenylyl cyclase activation. However, the role of $G_{sα}$ levels in reduced adrenergic responsiveness is at present inconclusive. As assessed by immunoreactivity, aging has been reported to decrease[68,121] or have no effect on[10,13,80,138] the levels of $G_{sα}$ attained in the myocardium. As will be discussed below, enhanced levels of inhibitory G-protein α subunits ($G_{iα}$) would be predicted to attenuate adrenergic stimulation of adenylyl cyclase. However, immunoreactivity to $G_{iα}$ has also been found to increase[10,13,121] or not change[68,80,138,160] with aging.

Aging and Signal Transduction of the Antiadrenergic Modulators Acetylcholine and Adenosine

Parasympathetic innervation provides antiadrenergic modulation of the β_1-adrenergic effectors[12] based on systemic requirements. However, adenosinergic modulation is responsible for local antiadrenergic effects because adenosine is generally released by the tissue in which the antiadrenergic effect is manifest.

Acetylcholine Responses in the Aged Heart

Parasympathetic stimulation of the heart is affected by aging. In a human study in which baroreflex activity was assessed by the bradycardic response to phenylephrine, it was concluded that muscarinic receptor activity in the heart is attenuated with advanced age.[110] A similar conclusion was reached in a study using pirenzepine, a presynaptic muscarinic M_1 receptor antagonist.[12] In human atrial myocardium, carbachol-induced inhibition of forskolin-stimulated inotropy was found to be attenuated with age.[63] Cholinergic-induced inhibition of adrenergic- and forskolin-stimulated adenylyl cyclase activity in cardiac membranes was strongly reduced by aging.[12,103] An interesting dichotomy has been reported for atrial and ventricular myocardium of the rat. Right atrial M_2R mRNA levels, found to be highest in the sinus node, were significantly depressed by aging.[67] However, despite an unchanged M_2R density in the ventricle, mRNA levels for this receptor type were found to be significantly elevated in the aged ventricular myocardium when compared to that of the young adult.[68]

Adenosine in the Aged Heart

While β_1R stimulation of the heart is capable of markedly enhancing myocardial contractility and glycogenolysis, adenosine, a naturally occurring nucleoside, is known to attenuate these evoked responses via the inhibitory G protein, G_i (Fig. 9-2). Adenosine reduces the catecholamine-induced increases in calcium membrane current[7,135] and intracellular Ca^{2+} transient magnitude[54] as well as cAMP accumulation[24,134] by diminishing β_1R coupling and reducing adenylyl cyclase activity.[90,118] Also reduced are the adrenergic-stimulated activation of PKA,[29] phosphorylation of myocardial proteins,[49,61,120] augmentation of phosphorylase activity,[24,29] and the elevation of atrial[27,28,115] and ventricular[29,30,41,42,91,105,134] contractility. These antiadrenergic effects of adenosine are prevented by theophylline,[29,105] a methylxanthine known to block the actions of adenosine at concentrations that do not inhibit phosphodiesterase activity.[29] The inhibitory action of adenosine in ventricular myocardium occurs at low concentrations (0.1–10 μM) which have no direct effects on the above parameters that are detectable when the nucleoside is administered in the absence of catecholamines.[24,27,29,30,115] At concentrations as low as 10 nM, phenylisopropyladenosine (PIA), a nonmetabolized adenosine analog, has been found to decrease the isoproterenol-induced activation of adenylyl cyclase activity in adenosine deaminase–treated cardiac membranes.[90,118] These results have substantiated the notion that adenosine acts extracellularly[32,50,93,156] via an inhibitory A_1R activity.[90,93–95,118] This effect is sensitive to pertussis toxin, indicating the involvement of an inhibitory G_i protein.[14,76,87] Of considerable interest is the observation that the administration of adenosine deaminase to both oxygenated isolated atria[27,30] and perfused hearts[35] causes isoproterenol-elicited contractile responses greater than those normally observed in the absence of the enzyme. These results suggest that endogenous adenosine normally dampens the contractile response of the oxygenated heart to β_1R stimulation. Adenosine also antagonizes the positive chronotropic effect of norepinephrine in spontaneously beating right atria.[122,124] However, adenosine does not reduce the positive inotropic response in rat atria caused by α-adrenergic receptor stimulation with phenylephrine.[27]

In addition to the antiadrenergic action, adenosine has other actions in the heart that are known to affect neural modulation of heart function. Adenosine A_1 and/or A_2 receptors on cardiopulmonary afferents play a primary role in transducing myocardial ischemia to central neurons.[149] Adenosine, acting upon intracardiac neuronal A_1 receptors, stabilizes the intrinsic cardiac nervous system during reperfusion following transient myocardial ischemia.[2] Adenosine inhibits cardiac norepinephrine release,[71,83,112] depresses sinoatrial (SA) node activity,[72,122] and has been observed to shift pacemaker activity from the SA node to the crista terminalis[158] and prolong the atrial-ventricular (AV) conduction time.[5,6,143]

Available evidence indicates that adenosine receptor activation plays an important role in the altered responsiveness of the aged heart to enhanced sympathetic neural activity.[31,33,34,96,146] However, it is unclear, whether this effect is a result of an age-induced change in A_1R function[58,70,75,82,116,127] or elevated levels of interstitial adenosine found in the myocardium[31,33,53,70,96] or both.

Adenosine A_1R in the aged myocardium
The responsiveness of the myocardium to elevated levels of norepinephrine is reduced with aging. To explore whether the antiadrenergic effect

of adenosine plays a role in this attenuation, experiments were conducted in which the action of endogenous adenosine was blocked with the adenosine receptor antagonist theophylline.[33] In these experiments, the age-induced loss of contractile responsiveness to adrenergic stimulation in the rat heart was reversed so that the enhanced contractilities of the two age groups were equivalent (Fig. 9–3). Contractile and metabolic responses (Fig. 9–4) to adrenergic stimulation were similarly restored in aged hearts treated with the adenosine antagonist 8-sulphophenyltheophylline (8-SPT)[31] or the enzyme adenosine deaminase.[31] These data suggest that much of the age-induced depression in adrenergic responsiveness can be attributed to the antiadrenergic action of adenosine. A similar conclusion was reached with humans in the investigation of aging and isoproterenol-induced changes in heart rate.[146]

A heightened antiadrenergic action in the aged heart would result from either enhanced A_1R binding affinities or receptor density. Results to date have been complex and conflicting. Experiments investigating A_1R characteristics have indicated that the sensitivity of the antiadrenergic action of adenosine in the heart increases with age, as evidenced by a reduction in the IC_{50} for the adenosine analog PIA (Fig. 9–5).[116] Furthermore, the density of ventricular A_1R was found to become elevated as the heart ages (Fig. 9–5).[116] A greater A_1R-induced negative chronotropy also

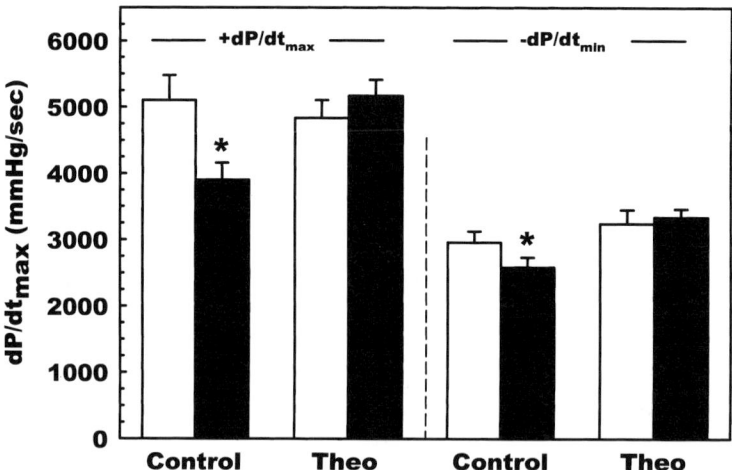

FIGURE 9–3 Effect of aging on isoproterenol-induced increases in maximal rates of left ventricular pressure development ($+dP/dt_{max}$) and relaxation ($-dP/dt_{max}$) of isolated rat hearts in the absence (Control) or presence (Theo) of 50 μM theophylline. Open bars represent young animals (4 months). Cross-hatched bars indicate aged animals (19 months). Values are the mean ± SE for 23 (control) or 9 (Theo) hearts. *, significance from the corresponding young adult value.

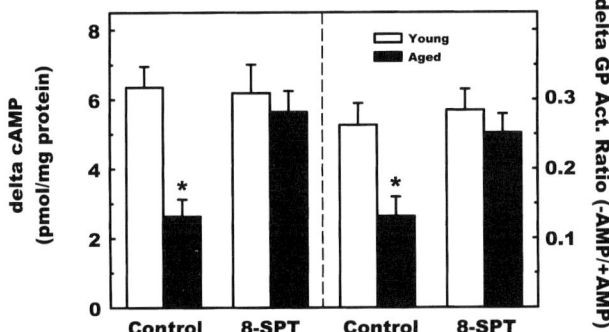

FIGURE 9–4 Effect of aging on isoproterenol-induced increases in cAMP and glycogen phosphorylase activity ratio (GP Act. Ratio) of isolated rat hearts in the absence (Control) or presence (8-SPT) of 50 μM 8-sulphophenyltheophylline. An increase in the GP Act. Ratio reflects an activation of the enzyme. Values are the mean ± SE for 12 (control) or 6 (8-SPT) hearts. *, significance from the corresponding young adult value.

has been reported for isolated hearts,[70,75] further suggesting an enhanced sensitivity with age. However, it would appear, that conclusions about A_1R receptors are tissue- and species-specific. In rat atria, the A_1R density has been found to increase with age with no change observed for the K_d.[77,82] This may explain the reduction in EC_{50} for PIA-induced negative

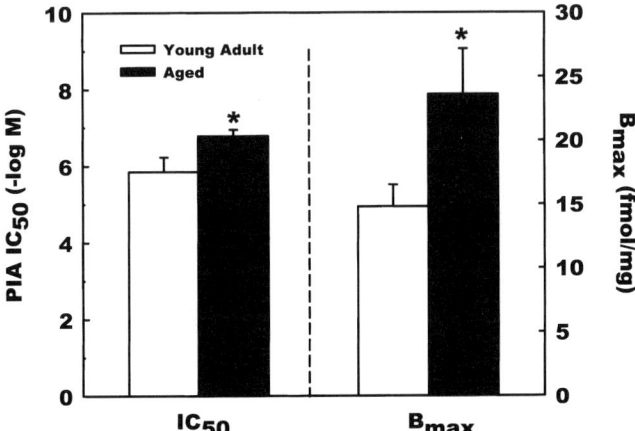

FIGURE 9–5 Effect of aging on the IC_{50} of phenylisopropyladenosine (PIA) and adenosine A_1 receptor density (B_{max}) for isolated young adult (mean 4 months) or aged (mean 19 months) rat hearts. The IC_{50} (antiadrenergic action) was determined in hearts stimulated with 100 nM isoproterenol. Values are the mean ± SE for five to six hearts. *, significance from the corresponding young adult value.

chronotropy in the aged rat heart.[77] However, in rabbit atria, aging does not affect this receptor density.[102] In the ventricular myocardium, the A_1R density has been reported to be increased with aging (unchanged K_d) in the rabbit.[102] In the aged rat ventricle, by contrast, the A_1R density has been reported to be increased (Fig. 9–5),[116] reduced,[82] or not changed[16] with an age-induced reduction in the percentage of high-affinity binding sites reported.[16,59]

Others have suggested that the enhanced efficacy of adenosine in the aged heart to induce bradycardia results not only from changes in receptor function but also from a reduced myocardial uptake of adenosine with aging.[75] Thus, the latter would lead to an increase in interstitial adenosine levels in aged hearts and therefore a greater antiadrenergic effect, as will be discussed below.

It has also been reported that the antiadrenergic action of adenosine is lost with aging.[16] In membrane preparations from 24-month Fischer 344 rats, unlike with 6-month rats, isoproterenol- and forskolin-stimulated adenylyl cyclase was resistant to attenuation by cyclopentyladenosine (CPA) or sulphophenyladenosine (SPA).[58] The antiadrenergic function of carbachol remained strong, suggesting an aging effect on adenosine-specific signaling. The decrease in adenosine sensitivity was attributed to an age-related decrease in A_1R/G_i coupling.[16] It is clear that considerable work remains to clarify the effects of aging on the signaling mechanisms by which adenosine manifests an antiadrenergic action.

Adenosine levels in the aged myocardium
As with an enhancement of A_1R function, elevated levels of interstitial adenosine in the aged heart would increase the manifestation of the antiadrenergic action. To investigate this possibility, adenosine concentrations in coronary effluent[33] and epicardial transudates[31] were determined with young adult and aged rat hearts. Transudates have been found to accurately represent interstitial fluid[50,55] and contain adenosine in levels exceeding those of the coronary effluent by greater than four- to six-fold[31,51] (Fig. 9–6). Basal adenosine release as determined from coronary effluents and transudate adenosine concentrations were both found to be significantly greater in aged than in young adult hearts. These elevations resulted from a reduced reuptake of adenosine by the myocardium.[96] Nitrobenzylthioinosine saturation-binding studies indicated a reduced number of adenosine transporter sites in the aged heart despite an increased affinity for adenosine.[53,96] The depressive effect of aging on myocardial adenosine transport has been reported by others.[70,75]

Since aging causes an increased net release of adenosine from the aged rat and guinea pig myocardium,[31,33,75,96] the universality of aging to fa-

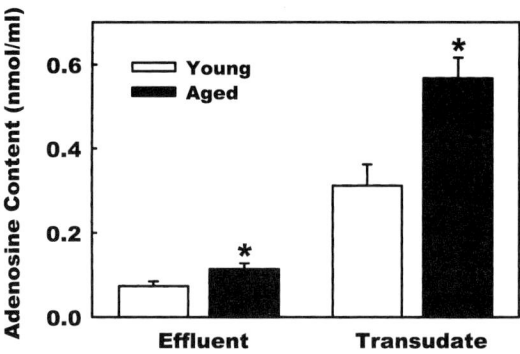

FIGURE 9-6 Effect of aging on adenosine release into the coronary effluent and adenosine content of epicardial transudates obtained from young adult (mean 4 months) and aged (mean 18 months) rat hearts. Values are the mean ± SE for 31 (effluent) and 12 (transudate) hearts. *, significance from the corresponding young adult value.

cilitate adenosine release from other cell types was explored.[46] Adenosine release was determined from confluent cultures of low- (population doubling level 23–25, designated "young") and high- (population doubling level 43–45, designated "aged") passage human lung fibroblasts (IMR-90). The release of adenosine was found to be greater from the aged fibroblasts (Fig. 9–7). Thus, in vitro aging of human lung fibroblasts caused an increase in the amount of adenosine released into the medium.

Additional experiments were conducted with confluent cultures of human skin fibroblasts obtained from fetal and 66-year-old donors. Both groups of cells were cultured to five population doublings. The aged skin

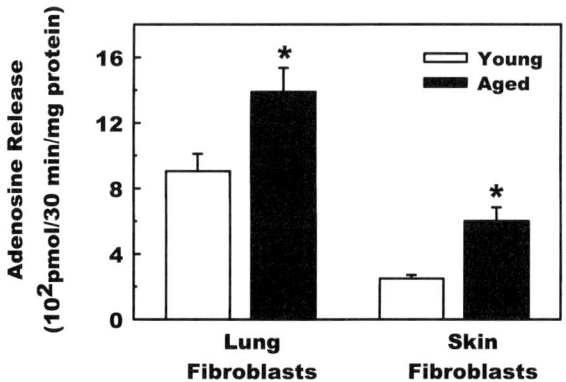

FIGURE 9-7 Effect of in vitro and in vivo aging on adenosine release from cultured fibroblasts. Adenosine release into the bathing medium from young human lung fibroblasts (IMR-90) having a population doubling level (PDL) of 23–25 (young) was compared to in vitro aged IMR-90 fibroblasts having a PDL of 43–45 (aged). Adenosine release into the bathing medium was also determined for human skin fibroblasts from fetal (young) and 66-year-old (aged) donors both cultured to a PDL of 5. Values are the mean ± SE for 10 lung and 6 skin fibroblast cultures. *, significance from the corresponding young value.

fibroblasts released more adenosine than the younger fibroblasts (Fig. 9–7). Therefore, regardless of whether the fibroblasts were aged in vitro or in vivo, the release of adenosine from the aged cells was always greater. These findings suggest that aging is associated with an enhanced release of adenosine from many cell types, including those comprising the heart. Thus, the enhanced release of adenosine may be a general feature of aging.

AGING MODULATES β RECEPTOR–INDUCED ACTIONS FROM JUVENILE THROUGHOUT AGED ADULTHOOD

Adult heart aging causes a reduction of β receptor–induced cardiac contractile and metabolic responsiveness from young adult to aged adulthood. More recently, studies have been performed to determine whether this aging process is actually initiated in the immature or juvenile heart, only to be continued throughout adulthood. Since we had already reported on the enhanced antiadrenergic action of adenosine that occurs in

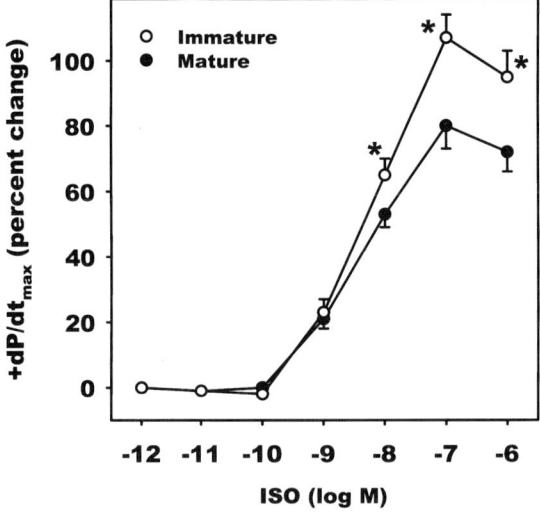

FIGURE 9–8 The effect of β_1-adrenergic stimulation with isoproterenol (ISO) on the contractile response (+dP/dt$_{max}$ in percent increase above basal) of isolated perfused (12 ml/min/g) immature (24 ± 2 days) and mature (90 ± 4 days) rat hearts stimulated to contract at 300 contractions per minute. Basal +dP/dt$_{max}$ was 2840 ± 430 mmHg per second. Values are mean ± SE for 15–16 hearts. All values ≥10^{-9} ISO are significant above the absence of ISO. *, significance from the corresponding mature value.

the aged heart, compared to that in the young adult heart, these studies were undertaken using juvenile and mature (young adult) rats that were 24 and 90 days of age, respectfully.

The contractile response to $\beta_1 R$ stimulation elicited by isoproterenol was greater in the juvenile than in the mature heart (Fig. 9–8). The juvenile heart also showed an enhanced antiadrenergic activity to the $A_1 R$ agonist chlorocyclopentyladenosine (CCPA). This was demonstrated as a greater reduction by CCPA of the isoproterenol-elicited contractile response in the juvenile hearts (Fig. 9–9). In addition, CCPA caused a greater inhibition of the isoproterenol-induced activation of adenylyl cyclase in cardiac membranes obtained from juvenile hearts than that observed with mature hearts (Fig. 9–10). Compared to the mature heart, these findings indicate that the juvenile heart was more responsive to $\beta_1 R$ stimulation and that the younger heart demonstrated a greater antiadrenergic manifestation upon $A_1 R$ stimulation.[126,127]

Because the contractile and metabolic responsiveness of the mammalian heart to $\beta_1 R$ stimulation is clearly depressed with aging, a comparison of a more complete aging spectrum from the juvenile stage throughout adulthood was considered. A third group of aged (19-month) rats was compared to the juvenile and young adult (mature) hearts. As expected, $\beta_1 R$ stimulation with isoproterenol showed a progressively greater depression with aging (Fig. 9–11). The adenosine release, as determined in the coronary effluent of the perfused hearts, increased with aging. The release of adenosine was inversely related to the isoproterenol-elicited contractile response over the three age groups. This suggests that

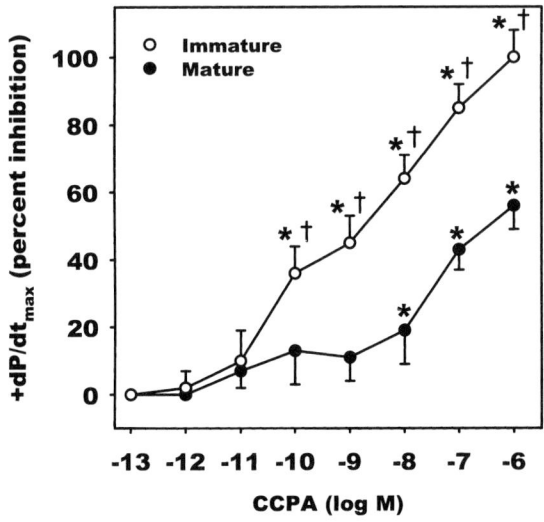

FIGURE 9–9 Effect of chlorocyclopentyladenosine (CCPA) inhibition on the 10 nM isoproterenol-induced increase in contractility ($+dP/dt_{max}$) in immature and mature perfused rat hearts. See legend of Figure 9–8 for more details. Values are the mean $\pm$ SE for six hearts. *, significance from zero. †, significance from the corresponding mature value.

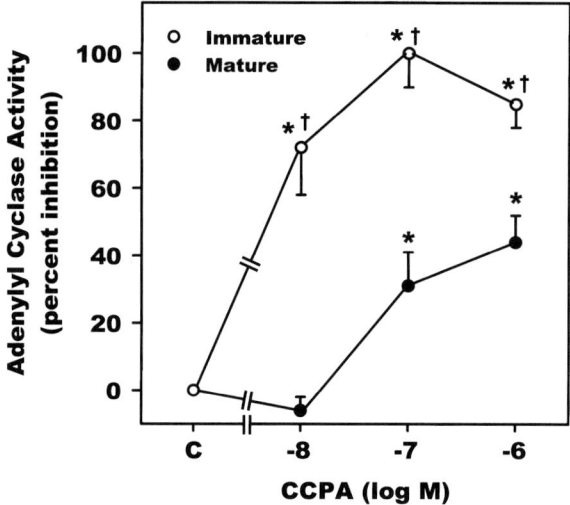

FIGURE 9–10 Effect of CCPA on β-adrenergic (100 nM isoproterenol)-elicited activation of adenylyl cyclase activity of myocardial membranes obtained from immature and mature rat hearts. Values are the mean ± SE for five hearts. See legend of Figure 9–8 for further details.

higher endogenous adenosine levels cause a greater antiadrenergic action in the catecholamine-stimulated heart as it ages. It is also interesting that the inhibition of adenylyl cyclase activity by an adenosine-mediated mechanism displayed a biphasic pattern (Fig. 9–11). The antiadrenergic

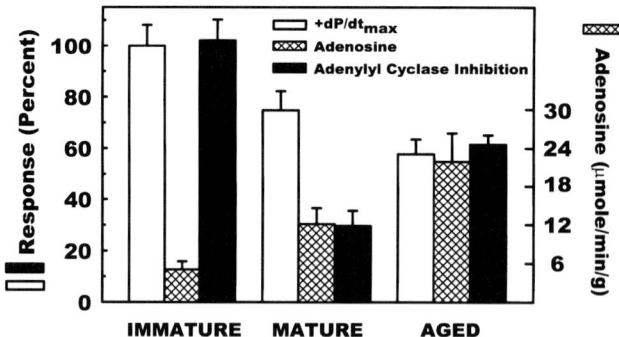

FIGURE 9–11 Effect of aging from immaturity to aged adulthood on the isoproterenol contractile ($+dP/dt_{max}$) responsiveness (open bar), coronary effluent adenosine release (hatched bar), and adenosine A_1 receptor inhibition of isoproterenol-activated adenylyl cyclase activity with CCPA (striped bar) for juvenile (immature), adult (mature), and aged adult (aged) hearts. Values are the mean ± SE for five hearts. The values are all significantly different between the age groups.

action appears to be greatest with membranes from immature hearts, least with mature heart membranes, and moderate with membranes from the aged heart. Thus the potential for the antiadrenergic action to be expressed is greatest in the juvenile heart. However, the adenosine levels in these hearts are minimal when compared to those of mature and aged hearts. It is also of interest that the antiadrenergic action is greater in the aged adult heart than in the mature or young adult heart. This feature may be beneficial to the aged adult heart in that it can be protected from an overresponse to $\beta_1 R$ stimulation resulting from physical or mental stress.

CLINICAL IMPLICATIONS OF AGE-INDUCED CHANGES IN MYOCARDIAL NEUROHUMORAL RESPONSIVENESS

While it is known that aging clearly has profound effects on the neural regulation of the cardiovascular system, much remains to be determined regarding the processes of development and maturation through adulthood. Aging affects not only the nerves that modulate the heart but also the local processes within the myocardium that modulate responses of the heart to neural activity.[97] Investigators interested in aging have only just begun to scratch the surface of the clinical ramifications of the aging process on heart function.

Consideration of adenosine and the antiadrenergic actions of this nucleoside has been found to be of particular clinical importance. Aging of the adult myocardium leads to elevated levels of interstitial adenosine and an enhanced efficacy of adenosine receptor activity. These two factors foster a greater mediation of the antiadrenergic-induced attenuation of $\beta_1 R$ stimulation in the aged than in the young adult heart. It is believed that a magnified antiadrenergic effect in the aged heart protects the aged heart from overresponding to the β_1-adrenergic stimulation associated with stress and exercise. Thus, in the aged heart, adenosine manifests a heightened ability to reduce myocardial injury and the arrhythmogenesis that may accompany strong adrenergic stimulation.[47] Clinically, it would be imperative to understand these processes and limit any therapies in the aged heart that would diminish the naturally facilitated manifestation of the antiadrenergic action of adenosine.[98]

Adenosine is also reported to be cardioprotective in the ischemic heart.[62,92] Increased levels of this nucleoside in the aged adult myocardium may be protective[52] by limiting functional and morphological damage elicited by endogenous norepinephrine[97,119] released into the myocardium during ischemia.[132,133] Protection may also continue into the reperfusion period following the ischemic insult.[2,108] Clinically, this may be important during surgical procedures in which coronary blood flow to the aged heart is diminished or terminated for an extended period of time. Furthermore, enhanced adenosine actions may be important to the survival of the aged heart during ischemic insults resulting from coronary vessel obstruction.[100] Thus, a naturally occurring augmentation with aging of an innate cardioprotective mechanism ensures the improved probability that aged myocardium will survive a reduction of perfusion. Further understanding of enhanced adenosine cardioprotection may provide insight into methods by which this property of adenosine could be imparted to young adult hearts.

In a manner probably independent of adrenergic stimulation, adenosine via receptor-mediated mechanisms plays an important role in the manifestation of preconditioning, whereby multiple short ischemic episodes initiate mechanisms that protect the myocardium against the deleterious effects of a longer-duration ischemia.[107,136] This phenomenon reduces the contractile stunning and necrosis that become apparent with reperfusion of the flow-deprived myocardium.[38,111] However, despite an enhanced antiadrenergic action of adenosine in the aged heart, it is paradoxical that the mechanism of preconditioning in the rat is markedly attenuated with aging.[48] More study is required to determine both the robustness of adenosine-induced preconditioning in the human heart and the signaling pathways shared with the antiadrenergic action. Perhaps with pharmacological intervention, preconditioning mediated by adenosine could be enhanced artificially in the aged heart.

REFERENCES

1. Akamatsu FE, De-Souza RR, and Liberti EA. Fall in the number of intracardiac neurons in aging rats. *Mech Ageing Dev* 109:153–161, 1999.
2. Arora RC and Armour JA. Adenosine A_1 receptor activation reduces myocardial reperfusion effects on intrinsic cardiac nervous system. *Am J Physiol (Regul Integr Comp Physiol)* 284:R1314–R1321, 2003.
3. Atkinson CJ and Santer RM. Quantitative studies on myelinated and unmyelinated nerve fibres in the interatrial septal region of aged rat hearts. *J Auton Nerv Syst* 77:172–176, 1999.
4. Barany M and Barany K. Protein phosphorylation in cardiac and vascular smooth muscle. *Am J Physiol* 241:H117–H128, 1981.
5. Belardinelli L, Belloni FL, Rubio R, and Berne RM. Atrioventricular conduction disturbances during hypoxia. Possible role of adenosine in rabbit and guinea-pig heart. *Circ Res* 47:684–691, 1980.
6. Belardinelli L, Fenton RA, West A, Linden J, Althaus JS, and Berne RM. Extracellular action of adenosine and the antagonism by aminophylline on the atrioventricular conduction of isolated perfused guinea pig and rat hearts. *Circ Res* 51:569–579, 1982.

7. Belardinelli L and Isenberg G. Actions of adenosine and isoproterenol on isolated mammalian ventricular myocytes. *Circ Res* 53:287–297, 1983.
8. Birnbaumer L, Codina J, Mattera R, Cerione RA, Hildebrandt JD, Sunyer T, Rojas FJ, Caron MG, Lefkowitz RJ, and Iyengar R. Regulation of hormone receptors and adenylyl cyclases by guanine nucleotide binding N proteins. *Rec Prog Hormone Res* 41:41–99, 1985.
9. Blumenthal EJ and Malkinson AM. Age-dependent changes in murine protein kinase and protease enzymes. *Mech Ageing Dev* 46:201–217, 1988.
10. Bohm M, Dorner H, Htun P, Lensche H, Platt D, and Erdmann E. Effects of exercise on myocardial adenylate cyclase and $G_i\alpha$ expression in senescence. *Am J Physiol* 264:H805–H814, 1993.
11. Borst SE, Narang N, Crews FT, and Scarpace PJ. Reduced α_1-adrenergic receptor–mediated inositide hydrolysis in cardiac atria of senescent rats. *J Cardiovasc Pharmacol* 16:444–448, 1990.
12. Brodde OE, Konschak U, Becker K, Ruter F, Poller U, Jakubetz J, Radke J, and Zerkowski HR. Cardiac muscarinic receptors decrease with age—in vitro and in vivo studies. *J Clin Invest* 101:471–478, 1998.
13. Brodde OE, Zerkowski HR, Schranz D, Broedesitz A, Michelreher M, Schaferbeisenbusch E, Piotrowski JA, and Oelert H. Age-dependent changes in the β-adrenoceptor-G-protein(s)-adenylyl cyclase system in human right atrium. *J Cardiovasc Pharmacol* 26:20–26, 1995.
14. Brown LA, Humphrey SM, and Harding SE. The anti-adrenergic effect of adenosine and its blockade by pertussus toxin: a comparative study in myocytes isolated from guinea-pig, rat and failing human hearts. *Br J Pharmacol* 101:484–488, 1990.
15. Bruckner R, Mugge A, and Scholz H. Existence and functional role of alpha$_1$-adrenoceptors in the mammalian heart. *J Mol Cell Cardiol* 17:639–645, 1985.
16. Cai G, Wang H-Y, Gao E, Horwitz J, Snyder DL, Pelleg A, Roberts J, and Friedman E. Reduced adenosine A$_1$ receptor and Gα protein coupling in rat ventricular myocardium during aging. *Circ Res* 81:1065–1071, 1997.
17. Cerbai E, Guerra L, Varani K, Barbieri M, Borea PA, and Mugelli A. β-Adrenoceptor subtypes in young and old rat ventricular myocytes: a combined patch-clamp and binding study. *Br J Pharmacol* 116:1835–1842, 1995.
18. Chen-Izu Y, Xiao RP, Izu LT, Chen H, Kuschel M, Spurgeon H, and Lakatta EG. G$_i$-dependent localization of β_2-adrenergic receptor signaling to L-type Ca^{2+} channels. *Biophys J* 79:2547–2556, 2000.
19. Conway J, Wheeler R, and Sannerstedt R. Sympathetic nervous activity during exercise in relation to age. *Cardiovasc Res* 5:577–581, 1971.
20. Daly RN, Goldberg PB, and Roberts J. The effect of age on presynaptic α_2 adrenoceptor autoregulation of norepinephrine release. *J Gerontol* 44:B59–B66, 1989.
21. Dawson R, Jr. and Meldrum MJ. Norepinephrine content in cardiovascular tissues from the aged Fischer 344 rat. *Gerontology* 38:185–191, 1992.
22. Dawson SL, Robinson TG, Youde JH, Martin A, James MA, Weston PJ, Panerai RB, and Potter JF. Older subjects show no age-related decrease in cardiac baroreceptor sensitivity. *Age Ageing* 28:347–353, 1999.
23. del Balzo U, Rosen MR, Malfatto G, Kaplan LM, and Steinberg SF. Specific α_1-adrenergic receptor subtypes modulate catecholamine-induced increases and decreases in ventricular automaticity. *Circ Res* 67:1535–1551, 1990.

24. Dobson JG, Jr. Reduction by adenosine of the isoproterenol-induced increase in cyclic adenosine 3',5'-monophosphate formation and glycogen phosphorylase activity in rat heart muscle. *Circ Res* 43:785–792, 1978.
25. Dobson JG, Jr. Catecholamine-induced phosphorylation of cardiac muscle proteins. *Biochim Biophys Acta* 675:123–131, 1981.
26. Dobson JG, Jr. Cyclic AMP-dependent activation of protein kinases in the myocardium. In: Delius W, Gerlach E, Grobecker H, and Kubler W, eds. *Catecholamines and the Heart*. New York: Springer-Verlag, 1981, pp 128–141.
27. Dobson JG, Jr. Adenosine reduces catecholamine contractile responses in oxygenated and hypoxic atria. *Am J Physiol* 245:H468–H474, 1983.
28. Dobson JG, Jr. Interaction between adenosine and inotropic interventions in guinea pig atria. *Am J Physiol* 245:H475–H480, 1983.
29. Dobson JG, Jr. Mechanism of adenosine inhibition of catecholamine-induced elicited responses in heart. *Circ Res* 52:151–160, 1983.
30. Dobson JG, Jr. and Fenton RA. Antiadrenergic effects of adenosine in the heart. In: Berne RM, Rall TW, and Rubio R, eds. *Regulatory Function of Adenosine*. Boston: Nijhoff, MA, 1983, pp 363–376.
31. Dobson JG, Jr. and Fenton RA. Adenosine inhibition of β-adrenergic induced responses in aged hearts. *Am J Physiol* 265:H494–H503, 1993.
32. Dobson JG, Jr., Fenton RA, and Romano FD. The antiadrenergic actions of adenosine in the heart. In: Gerlach E and Becker BF, eds. *Topics and Perspectives in Adenosine Research*. Berlin: Springer-Verlag, 1987, pp 356–368.
33. Dobson JG, Jr., Fenton RA, and Romano FD. Increased myocardial adenosine production and reduction of β-adrenergic contractile response in aged hearts. *Circ Res* 66:1381–1390, 1990.
34. Dobson JG, Jr., Fenton RA, and Romano FD. Adenosine and the reduced responsiveness of the aged heart to adrenergic stimulation. In: Imai S and Nakazawa M, eds. *Role of Adenosine and Adenine Nucleotides in Biological Systems*. Amsterdam, Elsevier, 1991, pp 377–386.
35. Dobson JG, Jr., Ordway RW, and Fenton RA. Endogenous adenosine inhibits catecholamine contractile responses in normoxic hearts. *Am J Physiol* 251:H455–H462, 1986.
36. Dobson JG, Jr., Ross J, Jr., and Mayer SE. The role of cyclic adenosine 3',5'-monophosphate and calcium in the regulation of contractility and glycogen phosphorylase activity in guinea pig papillary muscle. *Circ Res* 39:388–395, 1976.
37. Docherty JR. Effects of aging on prejunctional control of neurotransmission in the rat. *Ann NY Acad Sci* 786:264–273, 1996.
38. Downey JM and Cohen MV. Signal transduction in ischemic preconditioning. *Adv Exp Med Biol* 430:39–55, 1997.
39. Drummond GI and Duncan L. Adenyl cyclase in cardiac tissue. *J Biol Chem* 245:976–983, 1970.
40. Ebert TJ, Morgan BJ, Barney JA, Denahan T, and Smith JJ. Effects of aging on baroreflex regulation of sympathetic activity in humans. *Am J Physiol* 263:H798–H803, 1992.
41. Endoh M, Kushida H, Norota I, and Takanashi M. Pharmacological characteristics of adenosine-induced inhibition of dog ventricular activity. Dependence on the pre-existing level of β-adrenoceptor activation. *Naunyn Schmiedebergs Arch Pharmacol* 344:70–78, 1991.

42. Endoh M and Yamashita S. Adenosine antagonizes the positive inotropic action mediated via β-, but not α-adrenoceptors in the rabbit papillary muscle. *Eur J Pharmacol* 65:445–448, 1980.
43. Epstein SE, Levey GS, and Skelton CL. Adenylate cyclase and cyclic AMP. Biochemical links in the regulation of myocardial contractility. *Circulation* 43:437–448, 1971.
44. Esler MD, Thompson JM, Kaye DM, Turner AG, Jennings GL, Cox HS, Lambert GW, and Seals DR. Effects of aging on the responsiveness of the human cardiac sympathetic nerves to stressors. *Circulation* 91:351–358, 1995.
45. Esler MD, Turner AG, Kaye DM, Thompson JM, Kingwell BA, Morris M, Lambert GW, Jennings GL, Cox HS, and Seals DR. Aging effects on human sympathetic neuronal function. *Am J Physiol* 268:R278–R285, 1995.
46. Ethier MF, Hickler RB, and Dobson JG, Jr. Aging increases adenosine and inosine release by human fibroblast cultures. *Mech Ageing Dev* 50:159–168, 1989.
47. Fenton RA. Purines and ventricular arrhythmias. In: Abd-Elfattah AS and Wechsler AS, eds. *Purines and Myocardial Protection*. Boston: Kluwer, 1996, pp 383–394.
48. Fenton RA, Dickson EW, Meyer TE, and Dobson JG, Jr. Aging reduces the cardioprotective effect of ischemic preconditioning in rat heart. *J Mol Cell Cardiol* 32:1371–1375, 2000.
49. Fenton RA and Dobson JG, Jr. Adenosine and calcium alter adrenergic-induced intact heart protein phosphorylation. *Am J Physiol* 246:H559–H565, 1984.
50. Fenton RA and Dobson JG, Jr. Measurement by fluorescence of interstitial adenosine levels in normoxic, hypoxic and ischemic perfused rat hearts. *Circ Res* 60:177–184, 1987.
51. Fenton RA and Dobson JG, Jr. Hypoxia enhances isoproterenol-induced increase in heart interstitial adenosine depressing β-adrenergic contractile responses. *Circ Res* 72:571–578, 1993.
52. Fenton RA, Galeckas KJ, and Dobson JG, Jr. Endogenous adenosine reduces depression of cardiac function induced by β-adrenergic stimulation during low flow perfusion. *J Mol Cell Cardiol* 27:2373–2383, 1995.
53. Fenton RA, Lorbar M, and Dobson JG, Jr. Adenosine and cardiac aging. In: Burnstock G, Dobson JG, Jr, Liang BT, and Linden J, eds. *Cardiovascular Biology of Purines*. Boston: Kluwer, 1998, pp 143–158.
54. Fenton RA, Moore EDW, Fay FS, and Dobson JG, Jr. Adenosine reduces the Ca^{2+} transients of isoproterenol-stimulated rat ventricular myocytes. *Am J Physiol* 261:C1107–C1114, 1991.
55. Fenton RA, Tsimikas S, and Dobson JG, Jr. Influence of β-adrenergic stimulation and contraction frequency on heart interstitial adenosine. *Circ Res* 66:457–468, 1990.
56. Folkow B and Svanborg A. Physiology of cardiovascular aging. *Physiol Rev* 73:725–764, 1993.
57. Gabbett T, Gass G, Gass E, Morris N, Bennett G, and Thalib L. Norepinephrine and epinephrine responses during orthostatic intolerance in healthy elderly men. *Jpn J Physiol* 50:59–66, 2000.
58. Gao E, Snyder DL, Johnson MD, Friedman E, Roberts J, and Horwitz J. The effect of age on adenosine A_1 receptor function in the rat heart. *J Mol Cell Cardiol* 29:593–602, 1997.

59. Gao E, Snyder DL, Roberts J, Friedman E, Cai G, Pelleg A, and Horwitz J. Age-related decline in β adrenergic and adenosine A_1 receptor function in the heart are attenuated by dietary restriction. *J Pharmacol Exp Ther* 285: 186–192, 1998.
60. Gascon S, Dierssen M, Marmol F, Vivas NM, and Badia A. Effects of age on α_1-adrenoceptor subtypes in the heart ventricular muscle of the rat. *J Pharm Pharmacol* 45:907–909, 1993.
61. George EE, Romano FD, and Dobson JG, Jr. Adenosine and acetylcholine reduce isoproterenol-induced protein phosphorylation of rat myocytes. *J Mol Cell Cardiol* 23:749–764, 1991.
62. Gerlock T, Bentsen D, and Weiss HR. Local adenosine infusion and myocardial oxygen supply and consumption in reperfused canine myocardium. *Cardiovasc Res* 25:630–636, 1991.
63. Gliessler C, Wangemann T, Zerkowski HR, and Brodde OE. Age-dependent decrease in the negative inotropic effect of carbachol on isolated human right atrium. *Eur J Pharmacol* 357:199–202, 1998.
64. Goldberg PB, Kreider MS, McLean MR, and Roberts J. Effects of aging at the adrenergic cardiac neuroeffector junction. *Fed Proc* 45:45–47, 1986.
65. Guarnieri T, Filburn CR, Zitnik G, Roth GS, and Lakatta EG. Contractile and biochemical correlates of β-adrenergic stimulation of the aged heart. *Am J Physiol* 239:H501–H508, 1980.
66. Han C, Li J, and Minneman KP. Subtypes of α_1-adrenoceptors in rat blood vessels. *Eur J Pharmacol* 190:97–104, 1990.
67. Hardouin S, Bourgeois F, Toraasson M, Oubenaissa A, Elalouf JM, Fellmann D, Dakhli T, Swynghedauw B, and Moalic JM. β-Adrenergic and muscarinic receptor mRNA accumulation in the sinoatrial node area of adult and senescent rat hearts. *Mech Ageing Dev* 100:277–297, 1998.
68. Hardouin S, Mansier P, Bertin B, Dakhly T, Swynghedauw B, and Moalic JM. β-Adrenergic and muscarinic receptor expression are regulated in opposite ways during senescence in rat left ventricle. *J Mol Cell Cardiol* 29:309–319, 1997.
69. Hayes JS, Bowling N, and Boder GB. Contractility and protein phosphorylation in cardiomyocytes: effects of isoproterenol and AR-L57. *Am J Physiol* 247:H157–H169, 1984.
70. Headrick JP. Impact of aging on adenosine levels, A_1/A_2 responses, arrhythmogenesis, and energy metabolism in rat heart. *Am J Physiol* 270:H897–H906, 1996.
71. Hedqvist P and Fredholm BB. Inhibitory effect of adenosine on adrenergic neuroeffector transmission in the rabbit heart. *Acta Physiol Scand* 105:120–122, 1979.
72. Heller LJ and Olsson RA. Inhibition of rat ventricular automaticity by adenosine. *Am J Physiol* 248:H907–H913, 1985.
73. Hescheler J, Nawrath H, Tang M, and Trautwein W. Adrenoceptor-mediated changes of excitation and contraction in ventricular heart muscle from guinea-pigs and rabbits. *J Physiol (Lond)* 397:657–670, 1988.
74. Heyliger AR and McNeil JH. Effects of aging on phospholamban phosphorylation and calcium transport. *Mol Cell Biochem* 85:75–79, 1989.
75. Hinschen AK, Rose'meyer RB, and Headrick JP. Age-related changes in A_1-adenosine receptor-mediated bradycardia. *Am J Physiol* 278:H789–H795, 2000.

76. Hopwood AM, Harding SE, and Harris P. Pertussis toxin reduces the antiadrenergic effect of 2-chloroadenosine on papillary muscle and the direct negative inotropic effect of 2-chloroadenosine on atrium. *Eur J Pharmacol* 141:423–428, 1987.
77. Janczewski AM and Lakatta EG. Thapsigargin inhibits Ca^{2+} uptake, and Ca^{2+} depletes sarcoplasmic reticulum in intact cardiac myocytes. *Am J Physiol* 265:H517–H522, 1993.
78. Jiang MT, Moffat MP, and Narayanan N. Age-related alterations in the phosphorylation of sarcoplasmic reticulum and myofibrillar proteins and diminished contractile response to isoproterenol in intact rat ventricle. *Circ Res* 72:102–111, 1993.
79. Jiang, M-T and Narayanan N. Effects of aging on phospholamban phosphorylation and calcium transport. *Mech Ageing Dev* 54:87–101, 1990.
80. Johnson MD, Zhou Y, Friedman E, and Roberts J. Expression of G protein α subunits in the aging cardiovascular system. *J Gerontol A Biol Sci Med Sci* 50A:B14–B19, 1995.
81. Kaku T, Lakatta E, and Filburn C. α-Adrenergic regulation of phosphoinositide metabolism and protein kinase C in isolated cardiac myocytes. *Am J Physiol* 260:C635–C642, 1991.
82. Kapicka CL, Montamat SC, Mudumbi RV, Jacks SM, Olson RD, and Vestal RE. Effects of cyclopentyladenosine on isoproterenol response in adult and senescent cardiac tissue from Fischer 344 rats. *J Pharmacol Exper Ther* 293:599–606, 2000.
83. Khan MT and Malik KU. Inhibitory effect of adenosine and adenine nucleotides on potassium-evoked efflux of [^{3}H]-noradrenaline from the rat isolated heart: lack of relationship to prostaglandins. *Br J Pharmacol* 68:551–561, 1980.
84. Kimball KA, Cornett LE, Seifen E, and Kennedy RH. Aging: changes in cardiac α_1-adrenoceptor responsiveness and expression. *Eur J Pharmacol* 208:231–238, 1991.
85. Kreider MS, Goldberg PB, and Roberts J. The effect of age on release of norepinephrine by tyramine from rat heart. *Mech Ageing Dev* 36:281–285, 1986.
86. Kronenberg RS and Drage CW. Attenuation of the ventilatory and heart rate responses to hypoxia and hypercapnia with aging in normal men. *J Clin Invest* 52:1812–1819, 1973.
87. Kubalak SW, Newman WH, and Webb JG. Differential effect of pertussis toxin on adenosine and muscarinic inhibition of cyclic AMP accumulation in canine ventricular myocytes. *J Mol Cell Cardiol* 23:199–205, 1991.
88. Lakatta EG, Gerstenblith G, Angell CS, Shock NW, and Weisfeldt ML. Diminished inotropic response of aged myocardium to catecholamines. *Circ Res* 36:262–269, 1975.
89. Lakatta EG and Yin FCP. Myocardial aging: functional alterations and related cellular mechanisms. *Am J Physiol* 242:H927–H941, 1982.
90. LaMonica DA, Frohloff N, and Dobson JG, Jr. Adenosine inhibition of catecholamine-stimulated cardiac membrane adenylate cyclase. *Am J Physiol* 248:H737–H744, 1985.
91. Law WR, Carney PJ, and McLane MP. Influence of adenosine on the stimulatory effect of isoprenaline and insulin on myocardial contractility in vivo. *Cardiovasc Res* 25:151–157, 1991.

92. Ledingham S, Katayama O, Lachno D, Patel N, and Yacoub M. Beneficial effect of adenosine during reperfusion following prolonged cardioplegic arrest. *Cardiovasc Res* 24:247–253, 1990.
93. Liang BT and Donovan LA. Differential desensitization of A_1 adenosine receptor–mediated inhibition of cardiac myocyte contractility and adenylate cyclase activity. *Circ Res* 67:406–414, 1990.
94. Linden J. Structure and function of A_1 adenosine receptors. *FASEB J* 5:2668–2676, 1991.
95. Londos C, Cooper DMF, and Wolff J. Subclasses of external adenosine receptors. *Proc Natl Acad Sci USA* 77:2551–2554, 1980.
96. Lorbar M, Fenton RA, Duffy AJ, Graybill CA, and Dobson JG, Jr. Effect of aging on myocardial adenosine production, adenosine uptake and adenosine kinase activity in rats. *J Mol Cell Cardiol* 31:401–412, 1999.
97. Lorbar M, Skalova K, Nabi A, Chung ES, Fenton RA, Dobson JG, Jr., and Meyer TE. Norepinephrine concentrations in the epicardial transudate reflect early changes in adrenergic activity in the isolated perfused heart. *J Mol Cell Cardiol* 32:1695–1701, 2000.
98. Meyer TE, Chung ES, Perlini S, Norton GR, Woodiwiss AJ, Lorbar M, Fenton RA, and Dobson JG, Jr. Antiadrenergic effects of adenosine in pressure overload hypertrophy. *Hypertension* 37:862–868, 2001.
99. Miller JW, Hu ZW, Okazaki M, Fujinaga M, and Hoffman BB. Expression of alpha 1 adrenergic receptor subtype mRNAs in the rat cardiovascular system with aging. *Mech Ageing Dev* 87:75–89, 1996.
100. Monahan TS, Sawmiller DR, Fenton RA, and Dobson JG, Jr. Adenosine A_2 receptor activation increases contractility in the isolated perfused heart. *Am J Physiol* 279:H1472–H1481, 2000.
101. Mortimer ML, Tumer N, Johnson MD, and Roberts J. Effect of age on presynaptic β_2 receptor mediated responses in the rat. *Mech Ageing Dev* 59:17–25, 1991.
102. Mudumbi RV, Olson RD, Hubler BE, Montamat SC, and Vestal RE. Age-related effects in rabbit hearts of N^6-R-phenylisopropyladenosine, an adenosine A_1 receptor agonist. *J Gerontol* 50A:B351–B357, 1995.
103. Narayanan N and Derby JA. Alterations in the properties of β-adrenergic receptors of myocardial membranes in aging: impairments in agonist–receptor interactions and guanine nucleotide regulation accompany diminished catecholamine-responsiveness of adenylate cyclase. *Mech Aging Dev* 19:127–139, 1982.
104. Narayanan N and Tucker L. Autonomic interactions in the raging heart: age-associated decrease in muscarinic cholinergic receptor mediated inhibition of β-adrenergic activation of adenylate cyclase. *Mech Ageing Dev* 34:249–259, 1986.
105. Newman WH, Lee JT, and Webb JG. Persistent desensitization of the heart to the inotropic action of isoproterenol by adenosine. *Res Commun Chem Pathol Pharmacol* 66:233–254, 1989.
106. O'Connor SW, Scarpace PJ, and Abrass IB. Age-associated decrease in the catalytic unit activity of rat myocardial adenylate cyclase. *Mech Ageing Dev* 21:357–363, 1983.
107. Oldenburg O, Cohen MV, Yellon DM, and Downey JM. Mitochondrial K_{ATP} channels: role in cardioprotection. *Cardiovasc Res* 55:429–437, 2002.
108. Perlini S, Khoury E, Norton GR, Chung ES, Fenton RA, Dobson JG, Jr., and

Meyer TE. Adenosine mediates sustained antiadrenergic depression via activation of protein kinase C in the rat heart. *Circ Res* 83:761–771, 1998.
109. Petrofsky JS and Lind AR. Isometric strength, endurance, and the blood pressure and heart rate responses during isometric exercise in healthy men and women, with special reference to age and body fat content. *Pflugers Arch* 360:49–61, 1975.
110. Poller U, Nedelka G, Radke J, Ponicke K, and Brodde OE. Age-dependent changes in cardiac muscarinic receptor function in healthy volunteers. *J Am Coll Cardiol* 29:187–193, 1997.
111. Reisert PS, Dobson JG, Jr., and Fenton RA. Anoxia-induced changes in purine nucleotide metabolism of in vitro aged human fibroblasts. *Life Sci* 70:1369–1382, 2002.
112. Richardt G, Waas W, Kranzhofer R, Cheng B, Lohse MJ, and Schomig A. Interaction between the release of adenosine and noradrenaline during sympathetic stimulation. A feed-back mechanism in rat heart. *J Mol Cell Cardiol* 21:269–277, 1989.
113. Robberecht P, Gillard M, Waelbroek M, Camus JC, and Neef P. Alterations of rat cardiac adenylate cyclase activity with age. *Eur J Pharmacol* 126:91–95, 1986.
114. Robishaw JD and Foster KA. Role of G-proteins in the regulation of the cardiovascular system. *Annu Rev Physiol* 51:229–244, 1989.
115. Rockoff JB and Dobson JG, Jr. Inhibition by adenosine of catecholamine-induced increase in rat atrial contractility. *Am J Physiol* 239:H365–H370, 1980.
116. Romano FD and Dobson JG, Jr. Adenosine attenuation of isoproterenol-stimulated adenylyl cyclase activity is enhanced with aging in the adult heart. *Life Sci* 58:493–502, 1996.
117. Romano FD, Fenton RA, and Dobson JG, Jr. The adenosine R_i agonist, phenylisopropyladenosine, reduces high affinity isoproterenol binding to the β-adrenergic receptor of rat myocardial membranes. *Sec Mess Phosphoproteins* 12:29–43, 1988.
118. Romano FD, Macdonald SG, and Dobson JG, Jr. Adenosine receptor coupling to adenylate cyclase of rat ventricular myocyte membranes. *Am J Physiol* 257:H1088–H1095, 1989.
119. Rona G. Catecholamine cardiotoxicity. *J Mol Cell Cardiol* 17:291–306, 1985.
120. Rosenthal RA and Lowenstein JM. Inhibition of phosphorylation of troponin I in rat heart by adenosine and 5'-chloro-5'-deoxyadenosine. *Biochem Pharmacol* 42:685–692, 1991.
121. Roth DA, White CD, Podoli DA, and Mazzeo RS. Alterations in myocardial signal transduction due to aging and chronic dynamic exercise. *J Appl Physiol* 84:177–184, 1998.
122. Sadavongvivad C, Satayavivad J, Prachayasittikul V, and Mo-Suwun L. Modification of relative potencies of beta-adrenoceptor agonists by negative chronotropic agents in rat atrium. *Gen Pharmacol* 8:263–267, 1977.
123. Sakai M, Danziger RS, Staddon JM, Lakatta EG, and Hansford RG. Decrease with senescence in the norepinephrine-induced phosphorylation of myofilament proteins in isolated rat cardiac myocytes. *J Mol Cell Cardiol* 21:1327–1336, 1989.
124. Samet MK and Rutledge CO. Antagonism of the positive chronotropic effect of norepinephrine by purine nucleoside in rat atria. *J Pharmacol Exper Ther* 232:106–110, 1985.
125. Sato N, Kiuchi K, Shen Y-T, Vatner SF, and Vatner DE. Adrenergic respon-

siveness is reduced, while baseline cardiac function is preserved in old adult conscious monkeys. *Am J Physiol* 269:H1664–H1671, 1995.
126. Sawmiller DR, Fenton RA, and Dobson JG, Jr. Myocardial adenosine A_1 and A_2 receptor activities between juvenile and adult stages of development. *Am J Physiol* 271:H235–H243, 1996.
127. Sawmiller DR, Fenton RA, and Dobson JG, Jr. Myocardial adenosine A_1 receptor sensitivity during juvenile and adult stages of maturation. *Am J Physiol* 274:H627–H635, 1998.
128. Scarpace PJ. Decreased β-adrenergic responsiveness during senescence. *Fed Proc* 45:51–54, 1986.
129. Scarpace PJ. Forskolin activation of adenylate cyclase in rat myocardium with age: effects of guanine nucleotide analogs. *Mech Ageing Dev* 52:169–178, 1990.
130. Scarpace PJ and Abrass IB. Beta-adrenergic agonist-mediated desensitization in senescent rats. *Mech Ageing Dev* 35:255–264, 1986.
131. Scarpace PJ, Matheny M, and Tumer N. Myocardial adenylyl cyclase type V and VI mRNA: differential regulation with age. *J Cardiovasc Pharmacol* 27:86–90, 1996.
132. Schomig A. Catecholamines in myocardial ischemia: systemic and cardiac release. *Circulation* 82(Suppl II):II-13–II-22, 1990.
133. Schomig A, Haass M, and Richardt G. Catecholamine release and arrhythmias in acute myocardial ischemia. *Eur Heart J* 124:F38–F47, 1991.
134. Schrader J, Baumann G, and Gerlach E. Adenosine as inhibitor of myocardial effects of catecholamines. *Pflugers Arch* 372:29–35, 1977.
135. Schrader J, Rubio R, and Berne RM. Inhibition of slow action potentials of guinea pig atrial muscle by adenosine: a possible effect of Ca^{2+} influx. *J Mol Cell Cardiol* 7:427–433, 1975.
136. Schulz R, Cohen MV, Behrends M, Downey JM, and Heusch G. Signal transduction of ischemic preconditioning. *Cardiovasc Res* 52:181–198, 2001.
137. Shi X, Wray DW, Formes KJ, Wang H-W, Hayes PM, O-Yurvati AH, Weiss MS, and Reese IP. Orthostatic hypotension in aging humans. *Am J Physiol* 279:H1548–H1554, 2000.
138. Shu Y and Scarpace PJ. Forskolin binding sites and G-protein immunoreactivity in rat hearts during aging. *J Cardiovasc Pharmacol* 23:188–193, 1994.
139. Smit MJ and Iyengar R. Mammalian adenylyl cyclase. In: Cooper DMF, ed. *Advances in Second Messenger and Phosphorylation Research.* Philadelphia: Lippincott-Ravin, 1998, pp 1–21.
140. Snyder DL, Aloyo VJ, McIlvain HB, Johnson MD, and Roberts J. Effect of age on potassium- and tyramine-induced release of norepinephrine from cardiac synaptosomes in male F344 rats. *J Gerontol* 47:B190–B197, 1992.
141. Snyder DL, Johnson MD, Aloyo V, Eskin B, and Roberts J. Age-related changes in cardiac norepinephrine release: role of calcium movement. *J Gerontol* 50:B358–B367, 1995.
142. Snyder DL, Wang W, Pelleg A, Friedman E, Horwitz J, and Roberts J. Effect of aging on A_1-adenosine receptor–mediated inhibition of norepinephrine release in the rat heart. *J Cardiovasc Pharmacol* 31:352–358, 1998.
143. Stafford A. Potentiation of adenosine and the adenine nucleotides by dipyridamole. *Br J Pharmacol Chemother* 28:218–227, 1966.
144. Stull JT. Phosphorylation of contractile proteins in relation to muscle function. *Adv Cyclic Nucl Res* 13:39–93, 1980.

145. Su N and Narayanan N. Age-related alteration in cholinergic but not alpha-adrenergic response of rat coronary vasculature. *Cardiovasc Res* 27:284–290, 1993.
146. Suteparuk S, Nies AS, Andros E, and Gerber JG. The role of adenosine in promoting cardiac β-adrenergic subsensitivity in aging humans. *J Gerontol* 50:B128–B134, 1995.
147. Tanaka H, Davy KP, and Seals DR. Cardiopulmonary baroreflex inhibition of sympathetic nerve activity is preserved with age in healthy humans. *J Physiol* 515:249–254, 1999.
148. Taylor JA, Hand GA, Johnson DG, and Seals DR. Sympathoadrenal–circulatory regulation of arterial pressure during orthostatic stress in young and older men. *Am J Physiol* 263:R1147–R1155, 1992.
149. Thompson GW, Horackova M, and Armour JA. Role of P_1 purinergic receptors in myocardial ischemia sensory transduction. *Cardiovasc Res* 53:888–901, 2002.
150. Tolkovsky AM and Levitzki A. Coupling of a single adenylate cyclase to two receptors: adenosine and catecholamine. *Biochemistry* 17:3811–3817, 1978.
151. Tsien RW, Bean BP, Hess P, Lansman JB, Nilius B, and Nowycky MC. Mechanisms of calcium channel modulation by β-adrenergic agents and dihydropyridine calcium agonists. *J Mol Cell Cardiol* 18:691–710, 1986.
152. Tumer N, Mortimer ML, and Roberts J. Gender differences in the effect of age on adrenergic neurotransmission in the heart. *Exp Gerontol* 27:301–307, 1992.
153. Turner MJ, Mier CM, Spina RJ, and Ehsani AA. Effects of age and gender on cardiovascular responses to phenylephrine. *J Gerontol A Biol Sci Med Sci* 54:M17–M24, 1999.
154. Turner MJ, Mier CM, Spina RJ, Schechtman KB, and Ehsani AA. Effects of age and gender on the cardiovascular responses to isoproterenol. *J Gerontol A Biol Sci Med Sci* 54:B393–B400, 1999.
155. Vestal RE, Wood AJJ, and Shand DG. Reduced β-adrenoceptor sensitivity in the elderly. *Clin Pharmacol Ther* 26:181–186, 1979.
156. Wei HW, Friedrichs GS, and Merrill GF. Endogenous adenosine inhibits catecholamine contractile responses in normoxic hearts. *Cardiovasc Res* 25:529–536, 1991.
157. Weisfeldt ML. Left ventricular function. In: Weisfeldt ML, ed. *Aging*. New York: Raven Press, 1980, pp 297–316.
158. West GA and Belardinelli L. Sinus slowing and pacemaker shift caused by adenosine in rabbit SA node. *Pflugers Arch* 403:66–74, 1985.
159. White M, Roden R, Minobe W, Khan F, Larrabee P, Wollmering M, Port JD, Anderson F, Campbell D, Feldman AM, and Bristow MR. Age-related changes in β-adrenergic neuroeffector systems in the human heart. *Circulation* 90:1225–1238, 1994.
160. Xiao RP, Tomhave ED, Wang DJ, Ji X, Boluyt MO, Cheng H, Lakatta EG, and Koch WJ. Age-associated reductions in cardiac beta1- and beta2-adrenergic responses without changes in inhibitory G proteins or receptor kinases. *J Clin Invest* 101:1273–1282, 1998.
161. Yin FCP, Raizes GS, Guarnieri T, Spurgeon HA, Lakatta EG, Fortuin NJ, and Weisfeldt ML. Age-associated decrease in ventricular response to haemodynamic stress during beta-adrenergic blockade. *Br Heart J* 40:1349–1355, 1978.

10

The Genesis of Pain during Myocardial Ischemia and Infarction

CHRISTER SYLVÉN

Heberdeen first described angina pectoris in 1772.[20] At the time it was not possible to differentiate between reversible ischemia and acute myocardial infarction. Keefer and Resnik made that distinction in 1932 through electrocardiographic analysis.[26] They were the first to describe reversible myocardial ischemia with transient ST changes, as opposed to acute myocardial infarction with definitive changes of the QRS complex. A few years later, Lewis formulated the idea that angina pectoris might be due to an imbalance in the oxygen supply/demand ratio of the myo-cardium.[32] He applied the concept of ischemia put forward by Virchow in 1858 to the heart. This term was derived from the two Greek words, *ischo*, to keep back, and *haima*, blood. In Virchow's own words: "So habe Ich den neuen Ausdruck der ischaemie vorgeschlagen, um damit die Hemmung der Blutzüfuhr, die Vermehrung des Einströmens zu bezeichnen." "Thereby, I have suggested the new concept of ischemia in order to describe obstruction of the arterial blood supply." Lewis advanced the hypothesis that the pain thus produced was due to the local release of a substance with the following characteristics: *(1)* substantial release during ischemia, *(2)* capacity to excite sensory neurites, and *(3)* capacity to provoke painful sensations. A number of candidate substances have been proposed for such a role, including potassium, acetylcholine, bradykinin, serotonin, substance *P*, and adenosine. So far only adenosine fulfils all of the criteria proposed by Lewis, and this has led to hypotheses about the molecular basis for the etiology of angina pectoris.[42]

CARDIAC SYMPTOMS

Typically, angina pectoris is described as central chest pain that radiates into the left arm and the fourth and fifth fingers of the left hand. This suggests that the pain of angina pectoris is manifested in a manner similar to that of somatic pain. However, many investigators have demonstrated that specific symptomatology is seldom associated with cardiac pathology.[21,31] A frequent characteristic of the symptoms that patients with isolated left or right main coronary artery stenosis report is the central substernal localization of their pain.[10] The pain associated with left or right coronary artery–derived myocardial ischemia radiates in any direction from there.[42,43] Central chest pain may be viewed as visceral in origin, while radiating pain represents its referred component. When patients admitted to the coronary care unit are asked about the character of their ischemic pain, generally they report two or three specific traits associated with it (Fig. 10–1). Each is expressed with varied intensity, according to the Borg CR-10 scale.[13] No symptomatic differences were reported among patients with respect to whether they had acute myocardial infarction, unstable angina pectoris, or even a lack of myocardial ischemia. Patients who report extension of pain over their chest wall have a greater probability of having acute myocardial infarction (Fig. 10–2).

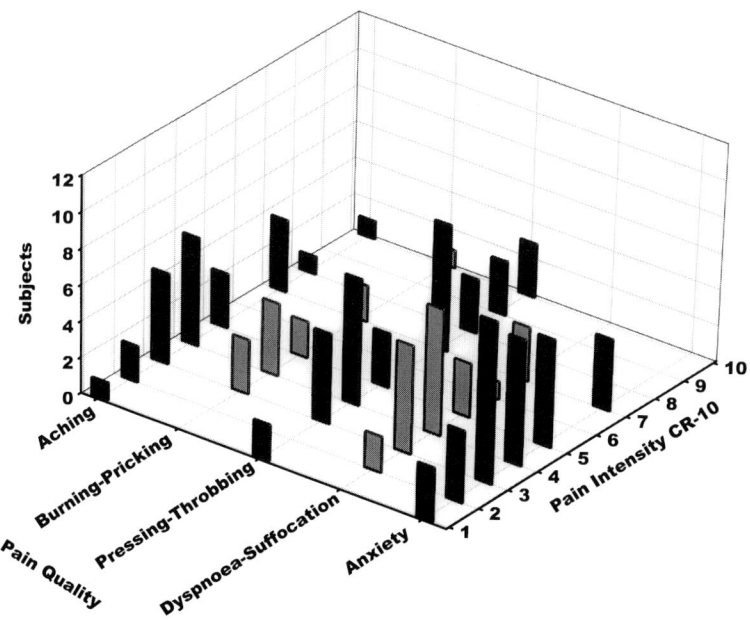

FIGURE 10–1 Pain quality and intensity reported by patients treated for acute myocardial infarction in a coronary care unit. The quality of pain described by patients was rated according to its intensity, according to the Borg CR-10 scale. (Reproduced with permission, from Eriksson et al.[13])

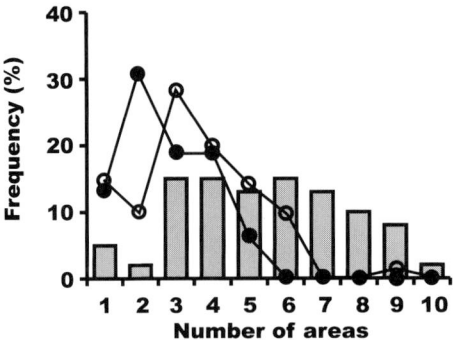

FIGURE 10–2 Extension of pain over the surface of the thorax in coronary care patients with acute myocardial infarction (as represented by heights of columns) and unstable angina pectoris (●) versus nonischemic chest pain (○). Each patient was shown a figure of the thorax and asked to draw the area where pain was experienced. Pain extension was analysed on the basis of a preset anterior chest wall grid consisting of 10 grid areas. (Reproduced with permission, from Eriksson et al.[13])

Thus pain elicited during acute myocardial infarction or reversible myocardial ischemia is usually multimodal in nature and diffuse in character. Furthermore, its visceral component is usually located substernally and related to the central thorax. With increasingly severe ischemia, the area over which pain is referred increases in size. Although fairly constant in location among individual patients, it should be recalled that pain can be referred to various loci independent of the site of the myocardial ischemia.

THE SUBSTRATE

The myocardium is made up of highly specialized tissues. One of its unique characteristics is that it supplies its own nutrients that convert chemical energy into mechanical force to cope with the circulatory demands of the body on a beat-to-beat basis. The oxygen and energy supply to the myocardium is thus a critical factor, as, even during rest, almost all of the available oxygen in coronary arterial blood is extracted by the myocardium.[34] The major compensatory mechanism for increasing demand is therefore very dependent on coronary arterial vasodilatation. If this vasodilation cannot compensate for increasing demand, an unfavorable oxygen supply/demand ratio arises that leads to myocardial ischemia. This is reflected in decreased local creatine phosphate concentrations and decreasing energy substrates associated with decreasing levels of locally released ATP, accompanied at the same time by increases in locally released adenosine (Fig. 10–3).

Creatine phosphate reduced by 10% ⟶ Adenosine increases by 100%

Myocardial ischemia ⟶ 1000x increase in adenosine

FIGURE 10–3 Adenosine is a messenger during ischemia. Depicted here are the dynamics of adenosine formation during ischemia.

Myocardial Adenosine

Adenosine is recognized as a messenger that reflects the myocardial energy state.[43] Endothelial cells and red blood cells take up most of the adenosine released locally within the myocardium. Consequently, circulating adenosine has a half-life of less than 10 seconds.[35] Adenosine release can increase 1000-fold during severe myocardial ischemia.[11] ATP and adenosine, two substances that reflect the energy state of the myocardium, act as primary messengers.[2,37] Creatine phosphate, ATP, and adenosine concentrations in coronary sinus blood normally oscillate during each cardiac cycle, presumably reflective of their levels released during systole as opposed to diastole. The concentration of adenosine within normal myocardial tissue oscillates at around 1 μM. Thus the normal myocardium continuously releases small amounts of adenosine that effect local vasomotor tone and regional neuronal tissue. Concentrations of adenosine as low as 1 μM can affect adjacent cardiac sensory neurites associated with different populations of cardiac afferent neurons.[52] Adenosine is involved in sympathetic efferent neuronally mediated vasomotion[38] and can potentiate the effects that nicotine exerts on autonomic neurons.[17] Adenosine also activates intrinsic cardiac neurons to influence cardiodynamics.[23]

Adenosine Acts Via Three Membrane-bound Receptor Subtypes

Locally produced adenosine modifies not only cardiomyocytes but also intrinsic cardiac neuronal tissues. Presumably, that is why adenosine may exert varied and even opposing effects on end-organ function, depending on whether affected purinoceptors are associated with local neurons or cardiomyocytes (Fig. 10–4). From a theoretical perspective, adenosine may exert both algesic and analgesic effects, depending on the neuromodulatory or cardiomyocyte effects it induces. The first evidence that adenosine might be a pain messenger in myocardial ischemia was presented in 1986.[45] When adenosine is administered intravenously to healthy volunteers, angina pectoris–like pain is provoked in a dose-

CARDIAC AFFERENT NEURONS

Modify (excites or inhibits) A_1 or A_2 adenosine receptors associated with cardiac sensory neurites

CARDIAC EFFERENT NEURONS

Prejunctional: A_1 inhibition of cholinergic and adrenergic neurons
                    A_2 excitation of cholinergic neurons

Postjunctional: A_1 enhancement of vascular smooth muscle contraction
                     A_2 inhibition of smooth muscle contraction

FIGURE 10–4 The spectrum of neuromodulation associated with intravenous administration of adenosine.

dependent manner. These effects can be counteracted by adenosine receptor blockade via systemic vascular administration of theophylline (Fig. 10–5). These findings indicate that pain of cardiac origin can involve membrane-bound adenosine receptors. Subsequently, adenosine has been shown to exert psychophysical effects as well.[47]

The same quality of pain is initiated by intravenous administration of adenosine in patients with angiographically proven coronary artery disease as occurs during effort angina.[44] Upon provocation of symptoms by intravenous doses of adenosine, no electrocardiographic changes occur. According to the patients tested, the pain provoked by adenosine did not differ in quality or body referral site from anginal symptoms provoked by daily routine. When adenosine is administered into a diseased coronary artery, it provokes the same kind of pain as that which occurs during exercise—doing so in a dose-dependent manner.[7,28] Likewise, when adenosine is administered intraarterially in other vascular beds, pain is provoked from the corresponding vascular bed region in a dose-dependent manner.[29,43,51] These findings indicate that the sensory neurites of cardiac afferent neurons respond to exogenously applied adenosine to generate symptoms, as well as enhancing sympathetic efferent neuronal dependent vasomotor activity.[38]

Too Much or Too Little Pain

Not all patients with ischemic heart disease experience symptoms of angina pectoris. Many have silent ischemic episodes, which represents a considerable clinical problem. Silent ischemia has two main facets. One

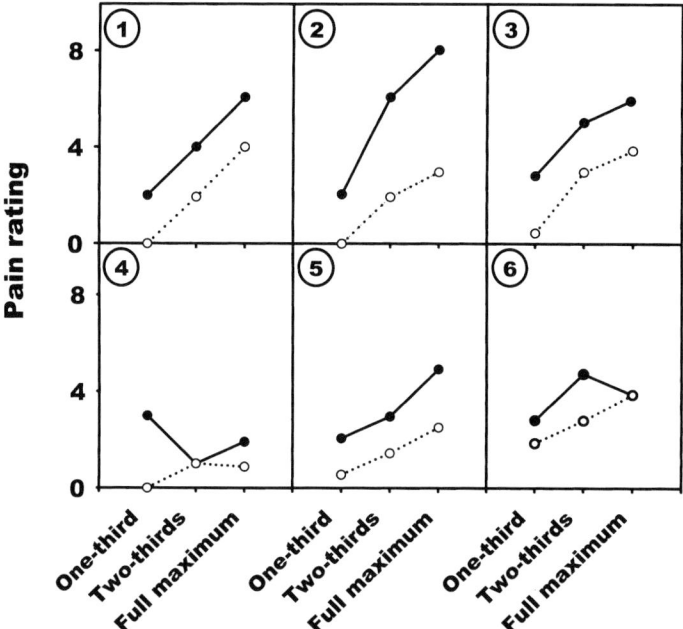

FIGURE 10–5 Dose–response relationships of adenosine given as intravenous bolus and chest pain elicited before (●) and after (○) theophylline administration. The intensity of pain was rated using the Borg CR-10 scale. (Reproduced with permission, from Sylvén et al.[44])

is that about half of the patients suffering from acute myocardial infarction do not have a history of angina pectoris. Thus they do not experience pain during episodes of myocardial ischemia or during myocardial infarction. This may relate to the fact that they experience uncharacteristic symptoms.[25] The other aspect of this problem is that many patients with angina pectoris have episodes of silent myocardial ischemia; these occur with a frequency as high as 80%–90% in these patients.[5] While episodes of modest myocardial ischemia seldom provoke symptoms, about 50% of the longer duration and more severe ischemic episodes are accompanied by symptoms.[34] A considerable number of patients who suffer from incapacitating chest pain (angina pectoris) have no evidence of coronary disease, the so-called syndrome X. Thus there is a spectrum of responsiveness from silent myocardial ischemia to incapacitating angina pectoris, even in patients without signs of ischemic heart disease. These two extremes of the spectrum, silent ischemia and syndrome X, differ in a number of personality traits as well as sensory and pain characteristics.[43] The latter include scores for nervousness, excitability, masculinity, and a tendency to complain, as well as varied thresholds and tolerance of pain elicited by forearm ischemia, for instance. These characteristics also include different responses to the cold pressor test, skin electrical stimulation, intravenous adenosine infusion, or dental pulp stimulation.

Syndrome X Patients

Pain elicited by adenosine in patients with syndrome X or ischemic heart disease differs from that elicited in healthy controls (Fig. 10–6).[30] Patients with syndrome X have a reduced threshold for maximal painful stimuli; at the same time they report the highest intensity of provoked pain for a given stimulus. Healthy volunteers, by contrast, endure higher doses of painful stimuli but report the lowest intensity for provocation of anginal pain. Patients with ischemic heart disease lie between these two extremes with respect to their pain tolerance. It could be that patients with ischemic heart disease represent a subgroup of the general population. For instance, healthy controls may include individuals with symptomatic or silent ischemic heart disease.

The pain that adenosine provokes in these individuals is not counteracted by the administration of metoprolol, naloxone, ibuprofen, clonidine, atropin, or nitroglycerin.[50] Individuals who do not smoke but received nicotine from chewing gum, for instance, experienced greater intensity of

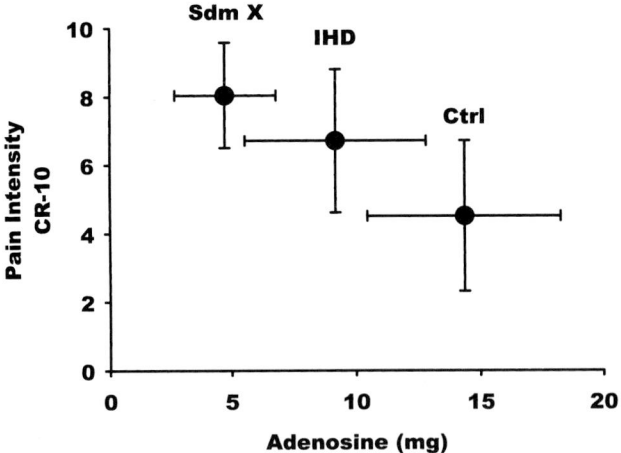

FIGURE 10–6 Provocation of angina pectoris–like chest pain in patients with syndrome X (Sdm X) compared with that in patients with ischemic heart disease (IHD; verified by coronary angiography) and controls (Ctrl). The x-axis represents dose of adenosine administered intravenously; the y-axis represents pain intensity experienced, according to the Borg CR-10 scale. Values are given as mean ± standard deviation. (Reproduced with permission, from Lagerquist et al.[30])

adenosine-provoked angina pectoris–like chest pain.[46] Substance P, however, did not induce such pain; rather, it accentuated adenosine-provoked anginal pain.[8] These findings indicate that neuromodulator effects of adenosine involve the sensitization of afferent neurons so that pain is perceived. Other substances may participate in modifying adenosine-induced cardiac symptoms, since many chemicals in addition to adensoine activate individual cardiac afferent neurons that project to neurons in the medulla and spinal cord (Chapter 3). Adenosine also activates sympathetic efferent neurons,[3,9] including those on the heart.[1]

For all of these reasons, exogenously administered adenosine may modify a number of components within the cardiac neuronal hierarchy to provoke angina pectoris–like symptoms. Does that mean that endogenously released adenosine can provoke symptoms? This question has been examined in three ways. First, adenosine receptor blocking agents such as theophylline or bamiphylline, the latter being considered a selective adenosine A_1 receptor antagonist, can counteract exercise-induced angina pectoris.[6,18] Second, because the coronary steal phenomenon may be involved in the genesis of these symptoms, the ischemic forearm modle was used to compare the results, since vascular steal does not exist in the latter model. In the forearm model, theophylline obtunds the pain of local ischemia (Fig. 10–7).[24] Thus it appears that endogenously released adenosine can provoke pain in various vascular beds.

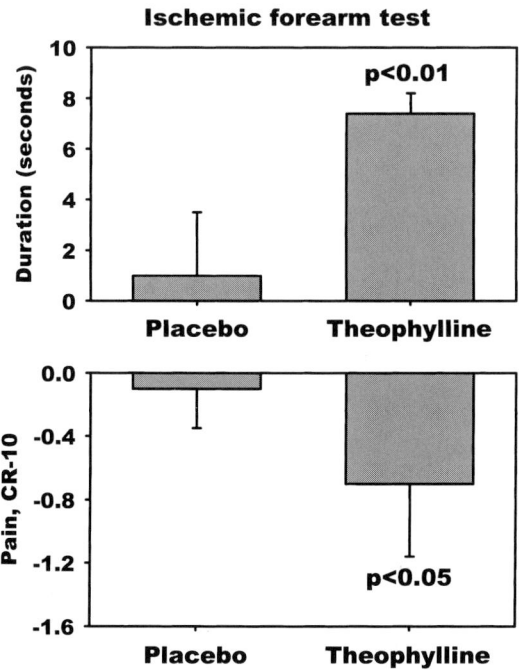

FIGURE 10–7 Average pain provoked in the ischemic forearm model by adenosine infused into the brachial artery on two separate occasions while saline (placebo) or theophylline were administered intravenously in a double-blind manner. The duration of the forearm work and the maximal pain intensity elicited are presented according to the Borg CR-10 scale. (Reproduced with permission, from Jonzen et al.[24])

Syndrome X is characterized by the genesis of incapacitating angina pectoris and ST depression during exercise in the presence of normal coronary arteries, as determined by angiography. Even though no definite evidence of myocardial ischemia has been identified in this clinical constellation,[43] it has been called "microvascular angina pectoris."[27,36] These patients experience pain during physical exercise, a state in which sympathetic efferent neuronal "tone" to the heart increases (Chapter 4). Epinephrine has been infused intravenously to mimic this increased sympathetic efferent neuronal tone.[12] Epinephrine infusion provokes the habitual chest pain in patients suffering from syndrome X; it fails to do so in normal individuals (Fig. 10–8). Echocardiographic evidence demonstrates that individuals suffering from syndrome X have normal or even improved ejection fractions in this state, suggesting that the epinephrine infusion does not cause myocardial ischemia even when symptoms are provoked.

Exercise and Anxiety States

Patients with life styles limited by the severity of their exercise-induced chest pain are thought to be physically deconditioned.[14] Therefore, a group of these patients was subjected to physical training, 3 days a week, over an 8-week period of time.[16] Before physical training, their exercise capacity was below the reference average for their age; after training it was found to equal that of healthy volunteers (Fig. 10–9). These patients nonetheless still experienced exercise-induced chest pain, although the curve had shifted to the right. Even though these patients were able to

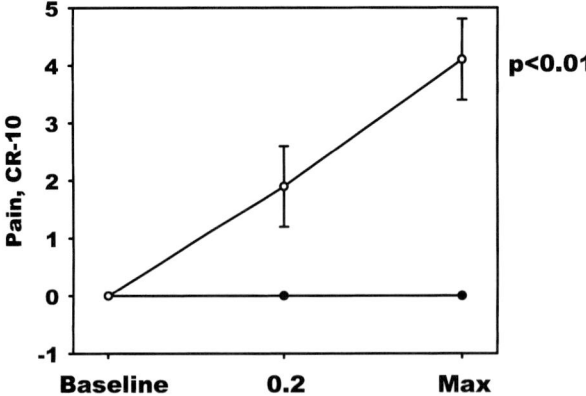

FIGURE 10–8 Provocation of chest pain by intravenous infusion of epinephrine into patients with syndrome X (○) as compared to that in age- and sex-matched controls (●). (Reproduced with permission, from Eriksson et al.[12])

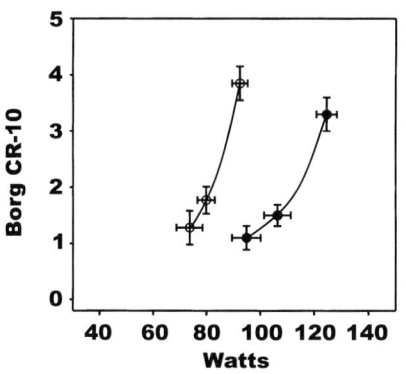

FIGURE 10–9 Angina pectoris provoked in patients with syndrome X during bicycle ergometric testing before (○) and after (●) 8 weeks of physical training. Pain intensity was rated by the Borg CR-10 scale. Values are given as mean ± standard error of the mean. (Reproduced with permission, from Eriksson et al.[16])

attain an increased workload, the degree of ST segment depression was similar in both groups. These data suggest that such ST depression is not related to exercise-induced myocardial ischemia. In these patients, the dose–response curves obtained during adenosine-provoked chest pain were similar, regardless of whether tests were performed before or following the training period. Thus, after 8 weeks of physical training, physical deconditioning had been reduced despite the fact that patients' pain response to enhanced sympathetic tone remained unchanged. Accordingly, patients with syndrome X appear to be conditioned to enhanced sympathetic efferent neuronal tone in response to stress (Fig. 10–10), pre-

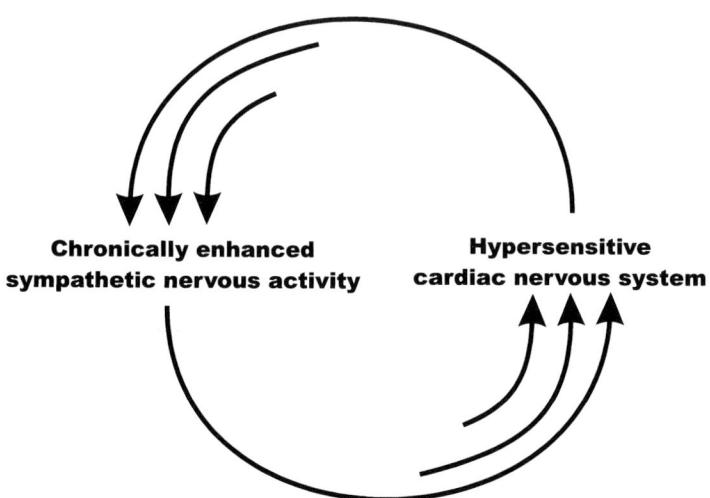

FIGURE 10–10 Proposed mechanisms whereby sympathetic efferent neurons are involved in the genesis of pain in patients with syndrome X. (Reproduced with permission, from Jonzon et al.[24])

sumably via a hyperactive cardiac sympathetic nervous system.[4,39,53] This syndrome may be viewed as one member of the group of chronic hypersensitive neuronal disorders that includes fibromyalgia, irritable colon, nonspecific vertigo, back pain, headache, and insomia. In other words, syndrome X might be viewed as a burnout syndrome with the heart as its locus minoris resistentie. This view is supported by the fact that experiencing central chest pain in situations of anxiety is a frequent occurrence in this population.[53] We found that 30%–40% of medical students experience similar symptoms during anxiety states. As anxiety increases with age and with repeated development of such symptoms, hypersensitivity of the cardiac afferent nervous system may develop.

As reported by Marchland and co-workers,[33] one interesting finding is that coffee counteracts the algesic effects of transcutaneous electrical stimulation (Fig. 10–11). Because the active substance in coffee is caffeine and caffeine is related to theophylline, it may act as an adenosine receptor–blocking agent. Thus caffeine may act to not only modulate cardiac neuronal function but also exert an analgesic effect on the cardiac nervous system. This hypothesis was tested in patients with symptomatic ischemic heart disease associated with verified coronary artery disease.[48] In a double-blind, placebo-controlled crossover study, these patients received low-dose adenosine infused intravenously before and during exercise (Fig. 10–12). While no differences were observed in hemodynamic and ST segment alterations during exercise stress testing, exercise-induced angina pectoris was reduced by the presence of adenosine. To elaborate on this observation, the effects of adenosine were tested in the forearm ischemia

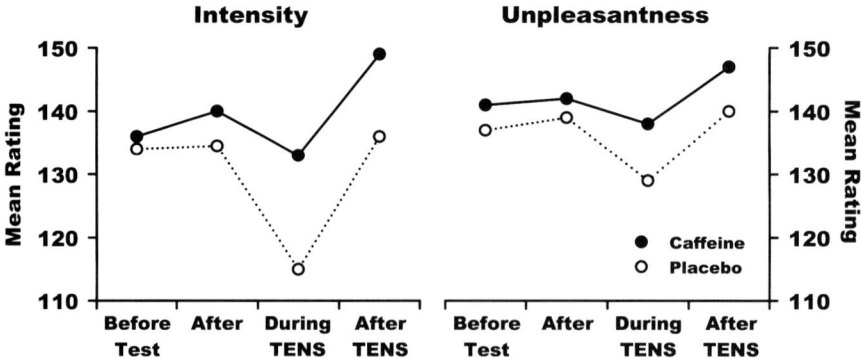

FIGURE 10–11 Effects of caffeine on the intensity (left panel) and unpleasantness (right panel) of symptoms elicited before and after stress testing, as well as during and after transcutaneous electrical nerve stimulation (TENS) application. (Reproduced with permission, from Marchand et al.[33])

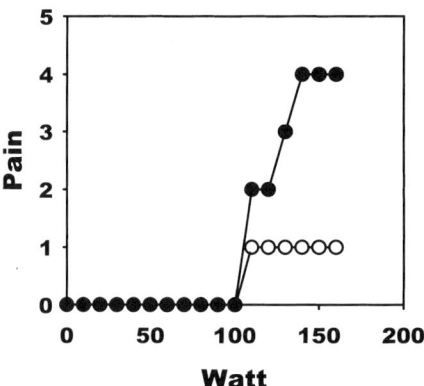

FIGURE 10–12 Effect of administering a low dose of adenosine (35 $\mu g/kg^{-1}/min^{-1}$, i.v.) on pain sensed before and during exercise. Exercise-induced chest pain was quantified with the Borg CR-10 scale. This study was performed in a double-blind crossover fashion (placebo: ●; adenosine: ○). (Reproduced with permission, from Sylvén et al.[47])

model. In a double-blind, placebo-controlled crossover study, adenosine was infused into the brachial artery of patients with syndrome X and matched healthy controls before and during ischemic forearm work.[15] In this study, the effects of adenosine were confined primarily to the forearm vasculature, thereby precluding any direct effects on central neurons or other blood vessels that would occur if adenosine were administered into the systemic circulation. In these subjects, adenosine induced analgesic effects in control subjects as well as in patients with syndrome X. Because the effects induced by adenosine were no longer elicited in the presence of theophyllamine, it was concluded that membrane-bound extracellular adenosine receptors were involved in the genesis of these symptoms.

Opioid Receptors

Adenosine and opioids modify not only intrathoracic cardiac afferent neurons but also intrathoracic local circuit neurons.[1,22] Opioidergic receptors also play an important role in the genesis of angina pectoris.[40,41] Interactions between adenosine and opioidergic receptors have clinical relevance, especially since activation of μ-opioid receptors counteracts the adenosine receptor 2_A intracellular signaling pathway.[19] We therefore determined whether adenosine-induced pain could be counteracted by systemic administration of the opioid agonists metenkephalin or β-endorphin.[49] While metenkephalin did not affect adenosine-provoked pain, β-endorphin was found to be capable of modifying adenosine-induced cardiac symptoms (Fig. 10–13). Although intravenously administered β-endorphin probably does not pass the blood–brain barrier, it may act to counteract adenosine-provoked pain via adenosine receptors associated with various populations of cardiac afferent neurons (Chapter 3) or intrinsic cardiac neurons involved in regulating regional cardiac function.[23]

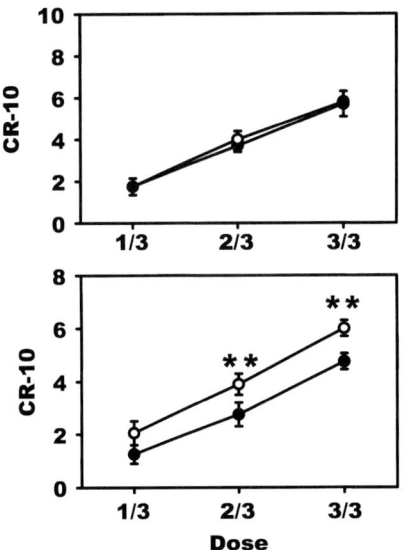

FIGURE 10–13 Effects of metenkaphalin (above) and β-endorphin (below) administered double-blind (●) versus saline as a placebo (○) on the effects of intravenous bolus doses of adenosine in inducing angina pectoris–like chest pain (pain intensity on vertical axes rated according to the Borg CR-10 scale). (Reproduced with permission, from Sylvén et al.[48])

PERSPECTIVES

The discovery that adenosine is an important modulator of afferent neuronal transduction has implications for the manifestation of cardiac symptoms.[43] This has opened up the possibility of investigating the mechanisms of pain genesis at the molecular level. The complexity of adenosine physiology is reflected in its role as a pain modulator (Fig. 10–14). Its mode of release during myocardial ischemia accounts in part for the varied duration, intensity, and localization of associated symptoms. The varied spatiotemporal summation of effects thus elicited presumably also re-

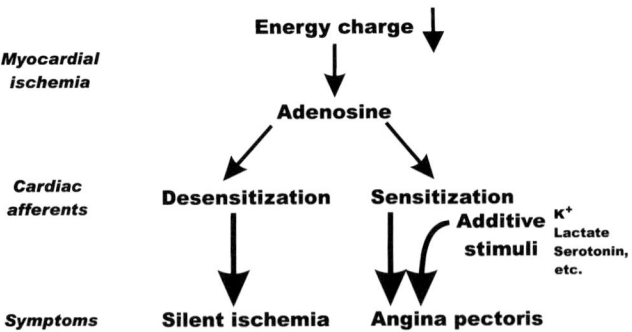

FIGURE 10–14 Flow diagram illustrating current views concerning the role that adenosine plays in peripheral algesic/analgesic neuromodulation during myocardial ischemia. (Reproduced with permission, from Sylvén.[42])

sults in the varied algogenic or analgesic responses that are reported. With respect to the genesis of pain, the message arising from local myocardial events involves the processing of sensory information by peripheral and central neurons (Chapters 4, 6, and 7). Although the specific mechanisms involved remain unexplored, the varied neuronal responses elicited presumably reflect the divergent populations of cardiac afferent and efferent neurons involved. That may be why one cannot reasonably predict whether a particular bout of myocardial ischemia will provoke symptoms or even the type and character of the symptoms produced. It may be that no direct relation necessarily exists between the site of myocardial ischemia and the pattern and type of attending referred pain. Thus, the functional complexity of the entire cardiac nervous system is reflected in the complex symptomatology attending cardiac ischemia.

REFERENCES

1. Armour JA, Huang MH, Pelleg A, and Sylvén C. Responsiveness of in situ canine nodose ganglion cardiac afferent neurons to epicardial mechanoreceptor and/or chemoreceptor stimuli. *Cardiovasc Res* 28:1218–1225, 1994.
2. Azam F and Hudson RE. Dissolved ATP in the sea and its utilisation by marine bacteria. *Nature* 267:696–698, 1977.
3. Biaggioni I, Killian TJ, Mosqueda-Garcia R, Robertson RM, and Robertson D. Adenosine increases sympathetic nerve traffic in humans. *Circulation* 83:1668–1675, 1991.
4. Cannon RO, Quyyumi A, Schenke WH, Fananapazia L, Tucker SE, Ganghan AM, Graeely RH, Cattau EL, and Epstein SE. Abnormal cardiac sensitivity in patients with chest pain and normal coronary arteries. *J Am Coll Cardiol* 16:1359–1366, 1990.
5. Collins P and Fox KM. Pathophysiology of angina. *Lancet* 335:94–96, 1990.
6. Crea F, Galassi AR, Kaski JC, El-Tamini H, Kaski JC, Davies G, and Maseri A. Effect of theophylline on exercise-induced myocardial ischaemia. *Lancet* 8640:683–686, 1989.
7. Crea F, Pupita G, Galassi AR, El-Tamini H, Kaski JC, Davies G, and Maseri A. Role of adenosine in pathogenesis of anginal pain. *Circulation* 81: 164–172, 1990.
8. Crea F, Tomai F, Iamele M, Crossman DC, Pappagallo M, Versaci F, Chiariello L, and Gioffré PA. Substance P potentiates the algogenic effects of intraarterial infusion of adenosine. *J Am Coll Cardiol* 24:477–482, 1994.
9. Dibner-Dunlap ME, Kinugawa T, and Thames MD. Activation of cardiac sympathetic afferents: effects of exogenous adenosine and adenosine analogues. *Am J Physiol* 265:H395–400, 1993.
10. Droste C. Schmerzperzeption und periphere Schmerzlokalisation bei Angina Pectoris. *Z Kardiol* 77(Suppl 5):15–33, 1988.
11. Edlund A, Fredholm BB, Patrignani P, Patrono D, Wennmalm Å, and Wennmalm M. Release of two vasodilators—adenosine and prostacyclin—from isolated rabbit heart during controlled hypoxia. *J Physiol* 340:487–501, 1983.

12. Eriksson B, Svedenhag J, Martinsson A, and Sylvén C. Effect of epinephrine infusion on chest pain in syndrome X in the absence of signs of myocardial ischemia. *Am J Cardiol* 75:241–245, 1995.
13. Eriksson B, Vourisalo D, and Sylvén C. Diagnostic potential of chest pain characteristics in coronary care. *J Intern Med* 235:473–478, 1994.
14. Eriksson BE, Jansson E, Kaijser L, and Sylvén C. Exercise performance, autonomic control and skeletal muscle function in female Syndrome X patients. *Am J Cardiol* 84:176–180, 1999.
15. Eriksson BE, Sadig B, Svedenhag J, and Sylvén C. Intraarterially administered adenosine has analgesic effects in the ischemic forearm test in controls but not syndrome X patients. *Clin Sci* 98:15–20, 2000.
16. Eriksson BE, Tyni-Lenné R, Svedenhag J, Hallin R, Jensen-Urstad K, Jensen-Urstad M, Bergman K, and Sylvén C. Physical training in syndrome X. *J Am Coll Cardiol* 36:1619–1625, 2000.
17. Evoniuk GE, von Borstel RW, and Wurtman RJ. Adenosine affects sympathetic neurotransmission at multiple sites in vivo. *J Pharmacol Exp Ther* 236:350–355, 1986.
18. Gaspardone A, Crea F, Iamele M, Tomai F, Versaci F, Pellegrino A, Chiariello L, and Gioffré PA. Bamiphylline improves exercise-induced myocardial ischemia through a novel mechanism of action. *Circulation* 88:502–508, 1993.
19. Greengard P, Allen PB, and Nairn AC. Beyond the dopamine receptor: the DARPP-32/protein phosphatase-1 cascade. *Neuron* 23:435–447, 1999.
20. Heberdeen W. Some account of a disorder of the breast. *Med Trans* 2:59–67, 1772.
21. Herlitz J, Hjalmarsson Å, Holmberg S, Rydén L, Svedberg K, and Waagstein F. Variability, prediction and prognostic significance of chest pain in acute myocardial infarction. *Cardiology* 73:13–21, 1986.
22. Huang MH, Sylvén C, Horackova M, and Armour JA. Ventricular sensory neurons in canine dorsal root ganglia: effects of adenosine and substance P. *Am J Physiol* 269:R318–R324, 1995.
23. Huang MH, Sylvén C, Pelleg A, Smith FM, and Armour JA. Modulation of in situ canine intrinsic cardiac neurons by locally applied adenosine, ATP or their analogs. *Am J Physiol* 265:R914–R922, 1993.
24. Jonzon B, Sylvén C, and Kaijser L. Theophylline during pain in the ischemic forearm test. *Cardiovasc Res* 23:807–809, 1989.
25. Kannel WB and Abbott RD. Incidence and prognosis of unrecognized myocardial infarction. An up-date on the Framingham study. *N Engl J Med* 311:1144–1147, 1984.
26. Keefer S and Resnik W. Angina pectoris: a syndrome caused by anoxemia of the myocardium. *Arch Intern Med* 41:769–807, 1928.
27. Kemp H, Vokonas P, Cohn P, and Gorlin R. The anginal syndrome associated with normal coronary angiograms: report of a six-year experience. *Am J Med* 54:735–742, 1973.
28. Lagerqvist B, Sylvén C, Beermann B, Helmius G, and Waldenström A. Intracoronary adenosine causes angina pectoris like pain—an inquiry into the nature of visceral pain. *Cardiovasc Res* 24:609–613, 1990.
29. Lagerqvist B, Sylvén C, Theodorsen E, Kaijser L, Helmius G, and Waldenström A. Adenosine induced chest pain—a comparison between intracoronary bolus injection and steady state infusion. *Cardiovasc Res* 26:810–814, 1992.

30. Lagerqvuist B, Sylvén C, and Waldenström A. Low threshold for adenosine induced chest pain in patients with angina pectoris and normal coronary angiogram. *Br Heart J* 68:282–283, 1992.
31. Ledwich JR. Chest pain in the early recognition of large infarcts. *Can Med Assoc J* 116:38–43, 1977.
32. Lewis T. Pain in muscular ischemia—its relation to anginal pain. *Arch Intern Med* 49:713–727, 1932.
33. Marchand S, Li J, and Charest J. Effects of caffeine on analgesia from transcutaneous electrical nerve stimulation. *N Engl J Med* 333:325–326, 1995.
34. Maseri A, Crea F, Kaski JC, and Davies G. Mechanisms and significance of cardiac ischemic pain. *Prog Cardiovasc Dis* 35:1–18, 1992.
35. Olsson RA and Pearson ID. Cardiovascular purinoceptors. *Physiol Rev* 70:761–845, 1990.
36. Opherk D, Schuler G, Wettaur K, Manthey J, Schwarz F, and Kubler W. Four-year follow-up in patients with angina pectoris and normal coronary angiograms (syndrome X). *Circulation* 80:1610–1616, 1989.
37. Pothier F, Couillard P, and Forget J. ATP and the autonomy of the contractile vacuole in *Amoeba proteus*. *J Exp Zool* 230:211–218, 1984.
38. Sadigh-Lindell B, Sylvén C, Hagerman I, Bergland M, Terenius L, Franzen O, and Eriksson BE. Oscillation of pain intensity during adenosine infusion. Relation to beta-endorphin and sympathetic tone. *Neuroreport* 12:1571–1575, 2001.
39. Shapiro LM, Crake T, and Poole-Wilson PA. Is altered cardiac sensation responsible for chest pain in patients with normal coronary arteries? *BMJ* 296: 170–171, 1988.
40. Sheps DS, Adams KF, and Hinderliter A. Endorphins are related to pain perception in coronary artery disease. *Am J Cardiol* 59:523–527, 1987.
41. Sheps DS, Ballenger MN, De Gent GE, Krittayaphong R, Dittman E, Maixner W, McCartney W, Golden RN, Koch G, and Light KC. Psychophysical responses to a speech stressor: correlation of plasma beta-endorphin levels at rest and after psychological stress with thermally measured pain threshold in patients with coronary artery disease. *J Am Coll Cardiol* 25:1504–1506, 1995.
42. Sylvén C. Angina pectoris. Clinical characteristics, neurophysiological and molecular mechanisms. *Pain* 36:145–167, 1989.
43. Sylvén C. Neurophysiological aspects of angina pectoris. *Z Kardiol* 86(Suppl 1):95–105, 1997.
44. Sylvén C, Beermann B, Edlund A, Lewander R, Jonzon B, and Mogensen L. Provocation of chest pain in patients with coronary insufficiency using the vasodilator adenosine. *Eur Heart J* 9(Suppl N):6–10, 1988.
45. Sylvén C, Beermann B, Jonzon B, and Brandt R. Angina pectoris–like pain provoked by IV adenosine in healthy volunteers. *BMJ* 293:227–230, 1986.
46. Sylvén C, Beermann B, Kaijser L, and Jonzon B. Nicotine enhances angina pectoris–like chest pain and atrioventricular blockade provoked by i.v. bolus of adenosine in healthy volunteers. *J Cardiovasc Pharmacol* 16:962–965, 1990.
47. Sylvén C, Borg G, Brandt R, Beermann B, and Jonzon B. Dose–effect relationship of adenosine provoked angina pectoris–like pain—a study of the phychophysical power function. *Eur Heart J* 9:86–91, 1988.
48. Sylvén C, Eriksson B, Jensen J, Geigant E, and Hallin R. Analgesic effects of adenosine during exercise-provoked myocardial ischemia. A double-blind placebo-controlled crossover study. *Neuroreport* 7:1521–1525, 1996.

49. Sylvén C, Eriksson B, Sheps D, and Maixner W. Intravenous infusion of β-endorphin but not of metenkephalin counteracts angina pectoris–like pain provoked by intravenous bolus injection of adenosine. *Neuroreport* 7:1982–1984, 1996.
50. Sylvén C, Jonzon B, Brandt R, and Beermann B. Adenosine provoked angina pectoris–like pain—time characteristics, influence of autonomic blockade and naloxone. *Eur Heart J* 8:738–743, 1987.
51. Sylvén C, Kaijser L, Jonzon B, and Fredholm BB. Effect of close intraarterial adenosine on forearm ischemic-like pain. *Cardiovasc Res* 22:674–678, 1988.
52. Thompson GW, Horackova M, and Armour JA. Role of P_1 purinergic receptors in myocardial ischemia sensory transduction. *Cardiovasc Res* 53:888–901, 2002.
53. Tyni-Lenné R, Stryjan S, Ericksson B, Berglund M, and Sylvén C. Beneficial therapeutic effects of physical training and relaxation therapy in women with coronary syndrome X. *Physiother Res Int* 7:35–43, 2002.

11

Neuronal Modulation of Atrial and Ventricular Electrical Properties

RENÉ CARDINAL AND PIERRE L. PAGÉ

As reviewed in Chapter 4, anatomically and functionally complex neuronal aggregates that are involved in coordinating regional cardiac function exist in intrathoracic extracardiac as well as intrinsic cardiac ganglia. It has been proposed that the intrinsic cardiac nervous system represents the final common pathway for the control of regional cardiac function.[5] This system integrates afferent neuronal information arising from the heart to exert spatial and temporal control over cardiac efferent neurons regulating different cardiac regions. As such, it forms part of a hierarchy of intrathoracic and central neuronal feedback loops involved in regulating regional cardiac dynamics.[6] In this scheme, neurons located in the various intrinsic cardiac ganglionated plexuses play a major role in beat-to-beat regulation of regional cardiac function, a role that has traditionally been minimized to the benefit of local mechanical interactions (the Frank-Starling hypothesis).

One outstanding issue in the field of neurocardiology concerns the patterns of efferent neuronal projections to various cardiac regions arising from the different ganglionated plexuses located in divergent atrial and ventricular regions. At present, this is a subject of considerable controversy. Some authors believe that neurons in the right atrial ganglionated plexus, for instance, subserve solely sinus nodal function whereas those in the inferior vena caval–inferior left ventricular ganglionated plexus exert predominant control over the atrioventricular node. In contrast, it has been our contention that the multiple neurons existing within a given ganglionated plexus modulate divergent cardiac regions while displaying preferential control over regional cardiac function.

Functional Anatomy of Intrinsic Cardiac Neurons Modulating Sinus and Atrioventricular Nodal Function

It is classical knowledge that electrical stimulation of the right vagus nerve in experimental animals, such as canines, exerts predominant effects on heart rate, whereas electrical stimulation of the left vagus nerve exerts relatively greater effects on atrioventricular (AV) conduction.[21] In 1973 Lazzara et al.[40] reported that exploration of the epicardial surface of the canine atria with bipolar electrodes used for selective stimulation of intrinsic cardiac nerves

> uncovered two epicardial loci (SA site and AV site) where it was possible to specifically alter vagal tone on the SA or the AV node. The SA site was located in the intercaval region of the right atrium just posterior to the sulcus terminalis and near the pericardial reflection. It was at the anterior, superior border of a triangular accumulation of fat. . . . The AV site was located in a pocket formed between the terminations of the inferior vena cava and the coronary sinus on the posterior inferior right atrium.

They added that "within the limits of the methods used, no effects on ordinary atrial muscle were detected." The effects on atrial muscle were estimated by measuring changes in intraatrial conduction between two distant sites and changes in refractory periods determined using the extrastimulus technique.

Similar conclusions emerged from experiments in which the right or left cervical vagus nerve was stimulated electrically in conjunction with selective intrapericardial denervation. Randall and Ardell[3,57] thus demonstrated in anesthetized canines that projections exist from both the right and left vagus nerves to the sinus node region via fatty tissues located in the region of the right pulmonary venous–right atrial (RPV-RA) junction. Right and left vagal inputs to the AV node, by contrast, occur via tissues located at the inferior vena caval–inferior left atrial (IVC-ILA) junction. Thus, in the canine heart, parasympathetic efferent postganglionic neuronal aggregates associated with fatty tissues in the so-called ventral right atrial (VRA) and IVC-ILA ganglionated plexuses are described as major sites of convergence for preferential parasympathetic efferent neuronal inputs to the sinus node and AV node, respectively. Chiou et al.[20] have provided physiological evidence that some vagal efferent preganglionic axons that project to the VRA and IVC-ILA ganglionated plexuses course through fat located between the medial superior vena cava and aortic root. These findings may have produced confusion, however, as this area is the location of the cranial medial ventricular ganglionated plexus that contains parasympathetic efferent postganglionic neurons that project axons to diverse atrial and ventricular regions, including the sinoatrial (SA) and AV nodes.[67]

Histological analyses have revealed the existence of collections of cholinergic neurons embedded in the epicardial fat (Chapter 2), supporting the notion that these loci contain synapses between classical pre- and postganglionic efferent parasympathetic neurons.[58,59] It remains to be determined whether the association of neurons with fatty tissues is of any biological significance, or whether their fatty locations should merely be considered anatomic landmarks. Collections of intrinsic cardiac ganglia associated with interconnecting nerves are designated *ganglionated plexuses* (a more accurate terminology than *fat pad*). The right atrial and inferior vena cava–inferior atrial ganglionated plexuses are among the seven major atrial and ventricular ganglionated plexuses that have been identified in the canine heart.[67,68] These include the following:

1. The right atrial ganglionated plexus (with ventral and dorsal components)
2. The inferior vena cava–inferior atrial ganglionated plexus
3. The ventral left atrial ganglionated plexus (cranial, intermediate, and caudal components)
4. The dorsal atrial ganglionated plexus (right and left components)
5. The cranial medial ganglionated plexus
6. The cranial lateral right ventricular ganglionated plexus,
7. The cranial lateral left ventricular ganglionated plexus.

It is important to realize that this nomenclature is of limited functional significance and thus serves the purpose of anatomical localization of these different populations of neurons, since *(1)* there is substantial variability in size and extension of neuronal structures among such ganglionated plexuses in different cardiac preparations, and *(2)* each intrinsic cardiac ganglionated plexus consists of neuronal clusters of relatively greater density within the more widely distributed intrinsic cardiac neuronal network.[14,54] In fact, the relatively more extended ganglionated plexuses can be subdivided into several components (cranial, intermediate, and caudal components, or right and left components). Moreover, a nomenclature that is useful in the canine heart may not necessarily be entirely applicable to hearts of other mammals. Thus a modified nomenclature for the porcine[11] and the human[9] intrinsic cardiac nervous systems has been proposed to account for differences in morphology between canine, porcine, and human hearts observed postmortem. Pauza et al.[55] proposed a slightly different nomenclature for the human epicardial ganglionated plexuses. Despite the differences in nomenclature presented to date, on the basis of our own experience and that of others with intraoperative stimulation of intrinsic cardiac neuronal elements,[18,52] we believe that there are analogies between the neuronal structures existing in the human, porcine, and canine hearts. In particular, an anatomically and functionally analogue to the canine right atrial ganglionated plexus (RAGP) exists in the human heart within the epicardial fat pad overlying an area encompassing the right superior pulmonary vein, the superior vena cava, the interatrial sulcus, and the ventral right atrium.[9] Selective electrical stimuli applied in the canine RAGP induce prolongation of the sinus cycle length without affecting AV nodal conduction.[18,52] Also, the structure designated the *posteromedial left atrial ganglionated plexus* in the human heart[9] bears some anatomical analogy to the canine inferior vena caval–inferior atrial ganglionated plexus.

Attention has also been directed to the intrapericardial course of sympathetic efferent postganglionic nerves. Ardell et al.[4] reported that ablation of the right atrial or IVC-ILA ganglionated plexuses induces selective parasympathectomy of the SA and AV nodes, respectively. Ablation of either or both of these ganglionated plexuses, however, produces little or no attenuation of the chronotropic and dromotropic responses elicited by right or left stellate ganglion stimulation. Rather, chronotropic responses elicited by right stellate ganglion stimulation are abolished when the medial aspect of the superior vena cava at the right atrial junction is ablated, as well as the region adjacent to the right pulmonary artery between the superior vena cava and ascending aorta. Left stellate ganglion stimulation effects are abolished after transecting the ventrolateral cardiac nerve and dissecting tissue around the left pulmonary artery and left pulmonary veins. From the results of experiments using selective intrapericardial denervation (in conjunction with extrapericardial nerve stimulation), these authors described the intrapericardial projections of axons derived from intrathoracic extrapericardial parasympathetic and sympathetic efferent nerves. They concluded that there was a clear divergence of sympathetic and parasympathetic efferent nerve projections onto different regions of the canine heart.

Ganglionated plexuses do not contain exclusively parasympathetic efferent postganglionic neurons. Brief electrical stimuli delivered to loci in the RAGP of canine hearts in situ induce an abrupt bradycardia followed by tachycardia that develops after cessation of stimulation.[15] When these electrical stimuli are performed in the presence of atropine, the bradycardia response stops while the tachycardia response is maintained. However, focal electrical stimulation of loci within the intrinsic cardiac ganglionated plexuses can activate both cell bodies and axons of passage. It is therefore important to demonstrate that similar biphasic chronotropic responses can be induced following local injection of nicotine into loci within a ganglionated plexus.[67]

Such effects can be elicited when nicotine is administered in small doses into the sinus node artery that perfuses the canine right atrial ganglionated plexus, either in situ[49] or in vitro.[61,66] In these preparations, the initial bradycardia response (stopped by atropine) and the delayed positive chronotropic response (stopped by β-adrenergic receptor blockade) are both suppressed by autonomic ganglionic blockade (hexamethonium) or excision of the ganglionated plexus (Fig. 11–1). These findings indicate that the negative chronotropic responses elicited by local nicotine administration are mediated via nicotinic receptors expressed on the cell bodies of cholinergic efferent neurons and that the positive chronotropic responses are mediated via nicotinic receptors expressed on the cell bodies of adrenergic efferent neurons.[36,67] These data are in accord with the fact that adrenergic and cholinergic efferent postganglionic neurons are both present in the mammalian intrinsic cardiac nervous system (Chapter 2).

Different peptides, such as bradykinin, calcitonin gene–related peptide (CGRP), D-Ala^2 D-Leu^5-enkephalin, oxytocin, substance P, or vasoactive intestinal peptide (VIP), when injected in microliter quantities in the vicinity of spontaneously active canine intrinsic cardiac neurons in situ, either decrease or, more frequently, increase the activity generated by these neurons.[10] Administration of C-type natriuetic peptide,[12] VIP,[56] angiotensin II,[39] oxytocin,[37] substance P, or bradykinin into the regional arterial blood supply of specific populations of intrinsic cardiac neurons in microliter quantities also induces alterations in their activity. Neuronal responses, if robust enough, can be accompanied by alterations in cardiac rate and force in situ.[10,37] In isolated right atrial preparations, local administration of oxytocin induces negative chronotropic and inotropic responses that are mediated in part via cholinergic efferent neurons.[48] In isolated atrial preparations, responses elicited by low doses of angiotensin II (10^{-11} M) are blocked by β-adrenoceptor blockade; those elicited by high concentrations of angiotensin II (10^{-6} M) are blocked by losartan, not by β-adrenergic receptor blockade.[66] Thus, the positive chronotropic responses elicited by low doses of angiotensin II are presumably mediated via angiotensin II receptors expressed on adrenergic neuronal cell bodies[42,60] and terminals,[37] while those elicited by higher doses involve non-adrenergic, possibly cardiomyocytic mechanisms.[7] These findings are consistent with the notion of a complex neurochemical organization within mammalian intrinsic cardiac ganglionated plexuses. Neuronal and cardiovascular responses occurred less frequently following acute decentralization of the intrinsic cardiac nervous system. This finding suggests that these responses depend in part on intrathoracic extracardiac and central reflex mechanisms.[7]

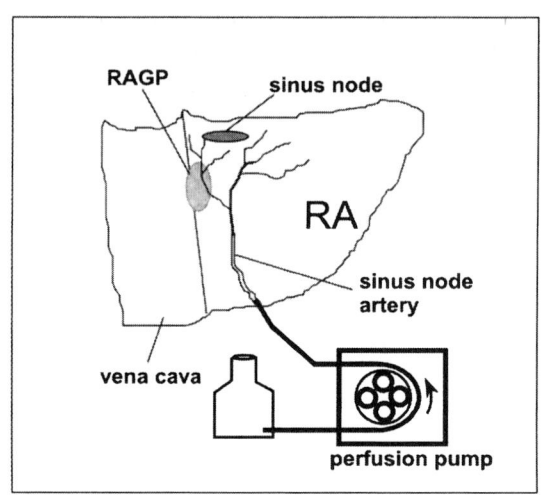
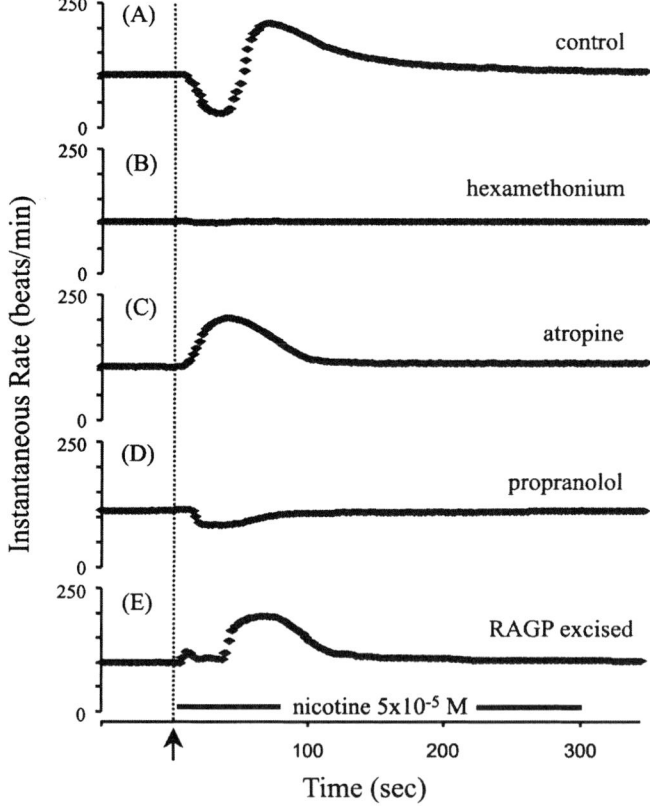

Although the ventral RAGP has been the most frequent target for electrical or pharmacological activation of its components, heart rate effects can also be induced in response to pharmacological modification of neurons in other intrinsic cardiac ganglionated plexuses. Yuan et al.[67] reported that tachycardia or bradycardia, as well as positive or negative atrial and ventricular contractile responses, can be elicited when nicotine is administered in low doses to selective populations of ventral left atrial, dorsal atrial, or cranial medial ventricular neurons. Some, but not all, of the responses elicited are abolished after acute decentralization of the intrinsic cardiac nervous system. Bradycardia and atrial force suppression induced by local nicotine administration are abolished by atropine, whereas the tachycardic and contractile augmentor responses elicited are suppressed by β-adrenergic receptor blockade. These findings indicate that cholinergic and adrenergic efferent neurons are distributed among the various mammalian intrinsic cardiac ganglionated plexuses.

An alternative to naming the ganglionated plexuses after their anatomical location (e.g., the RAGP and IVC-ILA plexus) would be to name them after their presumed myocardial target structures—i.e., the sinus node and AV node. This proposition has been made on the basis of anatomical and physiological data suggesting that separate groups of functionally selective cardioinhibitory neurons project from the brain stem to the feline heart.[13,31] However, experimental data indicate that neurons of canine RAGP ganglionated plexus, for instance, project axons to atrial muscle outside the sinus node region,[53] whereas some in the IVC-ILA ganglionated plexus project to the SA node and ventricles.[67] In addition, some of the neurons in ventricular ganglionated plexuses control SA nodal function.[67] Thus current data paint a much richer picture of control by efferent neurons in various regions of the heart than had been considered previously. Some of these findings are reviewed in the next section.

FIGURE 11–1 Time course of the chronotropic responses to nicotine perfusion into sinus node artery alone (control: **A**) and concomitantly with hexamethonium 10^{-6}M (**B**), atropine 10^{-6} M (**C**), or propranolol 10^{-6} M (**D**), or after ablation of the right atrial ganglionated plexus (RAGP; **E**). The upper panel shows a diagramatic representation of the isolated right atrial preparation superfused in a tissue bath and perfused via the sinus node artery. The control response to nicotine (A) presented a biphasic course with an initial decrease in instantaneous rate (expressed on a per-minute basis) followed by an increase in rate. Both effects were abolished by the ganglionic nicotinic receptor blockade (B), whereas the bradycardia component was abolished by muscarinic receptor blockade (C) or RAGP ablation (E), and the tachycardic component was abolished by β-adrenergic receptor blockade (D). Modified from Yin et al.[66]

Autonomic Efferent Neuronal Projections to Cardiac Tissues

Atrial Projections

The ease with which heart rate and AV conduction time can be measured has probably been a factor explaining the emphasis devoted to modulation of sinus nodal chronotropic function and AV nodal dromotropic function by neurons within various intrinsic cardiac ganglionated plexuses. It has been proposed that neurons in the RAGP exert exclusive control over adjacent tissues, including the SA node.[31] On closer inspection, activation of neurons in various loci throughout the right atrial ganglionated plexuses exerts widely distributed effects over electrical and mechanical events in both atria.[15,53,67]

The repolarization phase of the atrial action potential is shortened markedly in response to parasympathetic efferent neuronal stimulation.[34,35] Because of the difficulty in measuring intracellular action potentials in situ, the extra-stimulus technique has been used to determine refractory periods to study regional atrial effects induced in response to stimulation of intrathoracic autonomic efferent neuronal elements.[2,69] By measuring the effective refractory periods (ERP) at multiple atrial sites in anesthetized canines, Zipes et al.[69] showed that ERP shortens significantly more at right atrial sites than at left atrial ones in response to stimulating the right as compared to left vagus nerve, whereas effects of a similar magnitude are induced at left atrial sites in response to right or left vagal nerve stimulation; maximal effects were induced in the region of the sinus node in either case. However, the spatial and temporal resolution of electrical changes induced using the extra-stimulus technique is limited by the fact that only one site can be sampled at a time and that each determination requires minutes to complete.

An alternative approach is to analyze changes induced in the configuration of simultaneously recorded multiple atrial extracellular unipolar electrograms.[51,53,64] Figure 11–2 illustrates the fact that electrical changes can be induced in various regions of both atrial surfaces when neuronal elements in a locus of the RAGP are stimulated. These changes occur primarily during the repolarization phase (atrial T wave) of individual epicardial electrograms, with little or no change in the activation complex (RS deflection). In contrast to recordings made in the ventricles (see below), atrial unipolar electrograms do not display clear ST segments because the plateau phase of the intracellular action potential of atrial myocytes is very short and thus merges with the rapid repolarization phase.[34,35] The difference between the areas subtended by individual car-

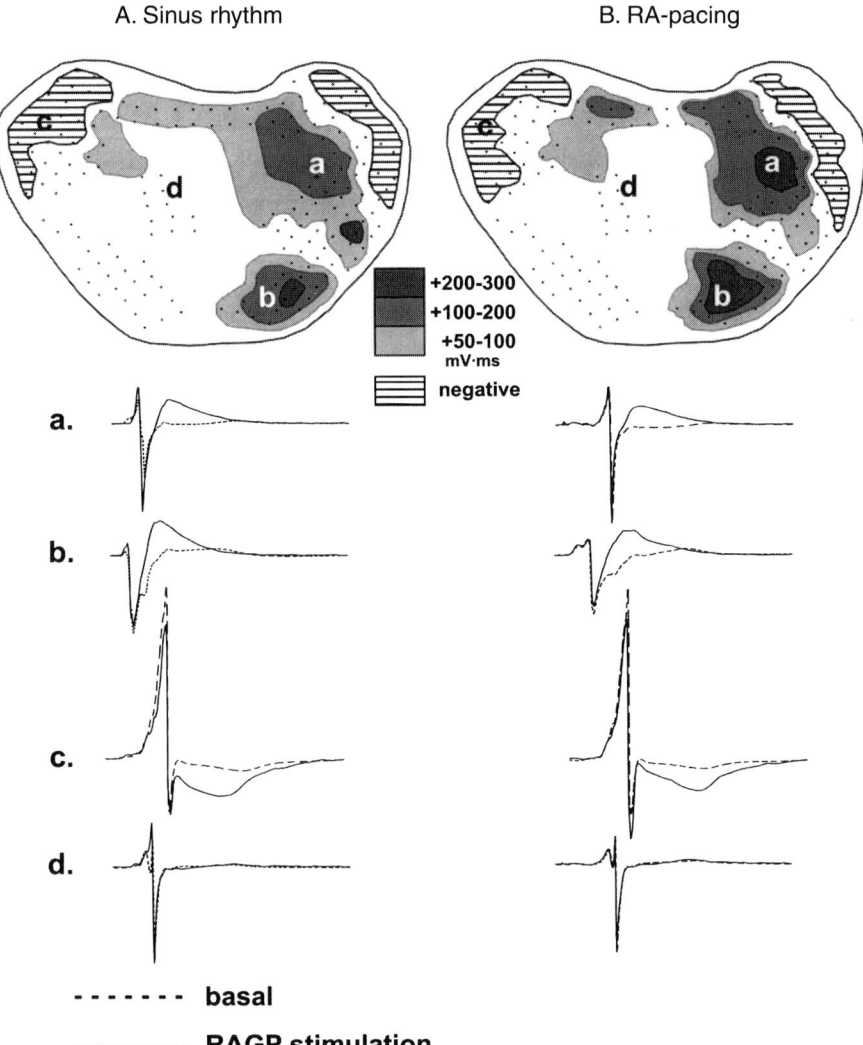

FIGURE 11–2 Changes in atrial unipolar electrogram configuration induced in response to electrical stimulation of the right atrial ganglionated plexus (RAGP) in an anesthetized canine. Lower traces show unipolar electrograms recorded from the atrial surface at selected sites *(a–d)* under basal conditions (broken line) and RAGP stimulation (solid line). Upper maps show the spatial distribution of changes in the area subtended by the unipolar electrograms (area measured at each site under RAGP stimulation minus the area measured at the same site under basal condition, in mV · ms). Positive changes occurred at most recording sites (as in a and b), whereas negative changes occurred at some sites (as in c). The atrial surface is represented as though unfolded and viewed from a posterior projection.

diac unipolar electrograms recorded before versus during neuronal activation (i.e., RAGP stimulation) can be used as a measure of the locally induced alterations by efferent neuronal elements. In the example illustrated in Figure 11–2, unipolar electrograms were recorded simultaneously from multiple atrial epicardial sites via 128 recording contacts derived from flexible silicone templates sutured to the epicardial surfaces of the atria.[53]

In order to analyze multiple atrial unipolar electrograms without interference from ventricular QRS complexes in canine preparations, complete AV block was first induced by the injection of formaldehyde into the His bundle region. The maps thus derived (Fig. 11–2, upper diagrams) indicate the localized changes induced in response to electrical stimulation of a discrete site in the RAGP in control states (sinus rhythm) and during fixed atrial pacing. Changes identified between basal and stimulation states were considered physiologically significant if they were ≥50 mv · ms (corresponding to twice the standard deviation of measurements repeated under basal conditions). Similar alterations in atrial electrical activity were induced by activating a selected population of right atrial neurons either during sinus rhythm (Fig. 11–2A) or when the atrial rate was fixed at 150 beats per minute by right atrial pacing (Fig. 11–2B). Marked positive changes occurred in the superior (which includes the sinus node region) and inferior parts of the right atrial wall. Positive changes were detected in the interatrial band and superior left ventricular areas, whereas negative changes were detected in the right and left atrial appendages.

Similar changes in regional atrial electrical events can be induced by electrically activating the right vagosympathetic complex (Fig. 11–3A). Positive deflection changes were induced in the electrograms obtained from the right atrial free wall in all preparations; positive deflection changes were also elicited in the interatrial band and left atrial free wall in 50% of these preparations. When the left vagosympathetic complex was activated electrically, electrical changes were limited spatially to the right atrial sinus node region of the right atrium, with more widespread changes occurring in the left atrium (Fig. 11–3B). These findings indicate that the atrial projections of right- or left-sided parasympathetic efferent preganglionic axons are distributed bilaterally. Parasympathetic efferent postganglionic neurons innervating the right atrium are located within the right atrial ganglionated plexus. Variability of such innervation patterns occurs among preparations in response to electrical stimulation of the right or left vagosympathetic complexes, or even discrete loci within the right atrial ganglionated plexus.

As discussed above, a widely distributed intrinsic cardiac nervous system associated with the human heart has been demonstrated by gross and microscopic examination of human hearts postmortem. In intraoperative studies,[52] we have found that electrical stimuli applied to selective foci

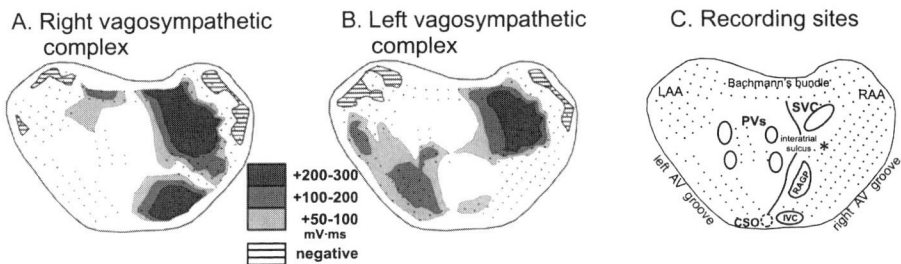

FIGURE 11–3 Atrial distribution of changes in unipolar electrogram configuration in response to electrical stimulation of the right (**A**) or left (**B**) vagosympathetic complex in an anesthetized canine. Changes were determined as described in Figure 11–2. In A, changes occurred mainly in the right atrial free wall, whereas they extended to the left atrial wall in B. **C**. Recording site locations and anatomic landmarks on a representation of the atrial surface. CSO, orifice of the coronary sinus; LAA, left atrial appendage; PVs, pulmonary veins; RAA, right atrial appendage; SVC, superior vena cava. The asterisk indicates the approximate sinus node location in the basal state.

within the human ventral RAGP induces changes in atrial unipolar electrograms that extend over the right atrial free wall to the medial aspect of the right atrial appendage (Fig. 11–4). These effects are similar to those induced in canine preparations when loci in the RAGP are stimulated (see above). These data suggest that the distributive processing of information

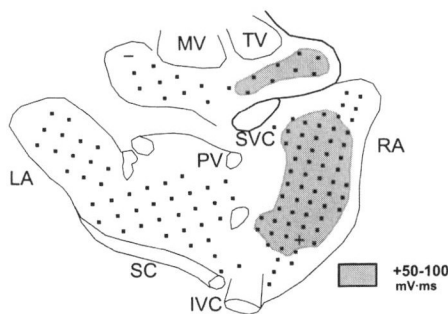

RAGP stimulation (human)

FIGURE 11–4 Atrial distribution of changes in unipolar electrogram configuration in response to electrical stimulation of the right atrial ganglionated plexus (RAGP) in a patient undergoing coronary artery bypass surgery. Changes (determined as described in Figure 11–2) occurred in the right atrial (RA) free wall and extended to the right-hand portion of Bachmann's bundle. IVC, inferior vena cava; LA, left atrial; MV, mitral valve; PV, pulmonary veins; SC, sinus coronarius; SVC, superior vena cava; TV, tricuspid valve.

within the intrinsic cardiac nervous system affects atrial electrical events in humans in a manner similar to that identified in the canine model.

Ventricular Projections

In the past, we have depicted the effects that activated intrathoracic extracardiac efferent neurons exert on the area subtended by unipolar electrograms recorded throughout the ventricular epicardial surface (QRST area changes).[64] Differential local ventricular innervation patterns are displayed by efferent axons coursing in the different mediastinal cardiopulmonary nerves.[1,17] This index allows one to study atrial innervation patterns as well (see Fig. 11–2). With respect to ventricular unipolar electrograms, the activation complex (QRS or RS) derived from epicardial unipolar electrocardiograms can be readily separated from the T wave, reflecting the fact that the ventricular action potential displays a clear plateau (or phase of slow repolarization) before rapid repolarization begins. Therefore, ventricular responses to neuronal activation can be readily determined from alterations in local activation–recovery intervals so induced, as measured from the steepest negative slope of the activation complex to the maximum positive slope of the T wave (Fig. 11–5). This variable is an excellent one with which to monitor both temporal alterations in local repolarization intervals induced by different neuronal elements within the cardiac neuroaxis and the regionality of such effects.[47]

Preliminary data indicate that the activation–recovery intervals in multiple regions of the ventricular epicardium shorten in response to the excitation of nicotine-sensitive neurons in major intrinsic cardiac ganglionated plexuses in the anesthetized canine preparation. For instance, the magnitude of shortening induced by nicotine-sensitive neurons in the caudal region of the RAGP is especially pronounced in the basal regions of the right ventricular sinus (Fig. 11–5A; data obtained when heart rate was fixed by atrial pacing). In contrast, nicotine-sensitive neurons in the cranial ventricular ganglionated plexus exert maximum influence on electrical changes in the apical region of the left ventricle (Fig. 11–5B). Thus neurons in one region of an intrinsic cardiac ganglionated plexus can influence widespread regions of the ventricles while at the same time affecting the sinus node to induce bradycardia or tachycardia. These findings support the concept that adrenergic and cholinergic neurons present in each major atrial or ventricular ganglionated plexus modulate various regions of the heart, while displaying preferential control over specific cardiac regions—some of which may be distant from each neuronal population. Taken together, it appears that neurons in atrial and ventricular

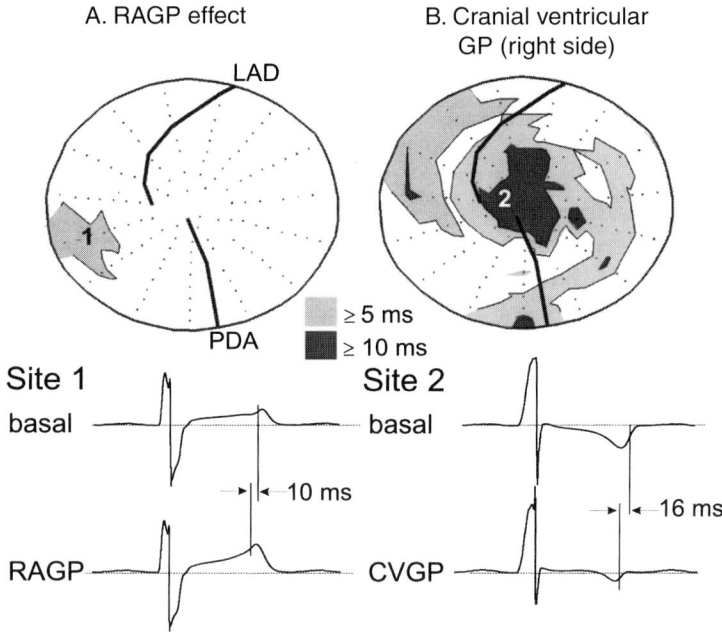

FIGURE 11–5 Shortening of ventricular repolarization intervals by chemical stimulation of the RAGP (**A**) or the cranial ventricular GP (**B**) in a healthy canine preparation. Polar representation of the ventricular surface in which the apex is at the center and the base parallel to the circumflex coronary artery. Activation-recovery intervals were measured from the point of steepest negative sloped the activation complex to the point of steepest positive slope in the T wave, as illustrated in unipolar electrograms recorded from two selected sites. Shortening occurred in response to nicotine (10 μg) administered into a locus of the right atrial ganglionated plexus (RAGP) or the cranial ventricular ganglionated plexus (CVGP). LAD, left anterior descending coronary artery; PDA, posterior descending artery.

ganglionated plexus control the electrical behavior of atrial and ventricular tissues, even modulating tissues remote from their location.

EFFERENT NEURONAL CONTROL OF ATRIAL ELECTRICAL EVENTS

Investigating the autonomic neuronal effects of surgical procedures used to treat atrial fibrillation has enabled us to determine the contribution of atrial denervation to sinus node function by assessing the intracardiac course of autonomic efferent axons that arise from more centrally located somata. The Maze procedure is used in patients with chronic atrial fibrillation to restore sinus node rhythm.[22,23] The rationale underlying the efficacy of the Maze operation is that incisions performed in both atria create fragments of atrial myocardium that should be small enough to prevent sustained wavelet formation (the cause of fibrillation) while at the same time retaining sufficiently connected atrial tissues to ensure adequate mechanical contraction. The pattern of the incisions used in this procedure is designed to spare vascularization as much as possible. The procedure is known to produce temporary chronotropic incompetence that has been presumed to be related to denervation of the sinus node region.

We have employed a canine model of the Maze procedure to investigate the functional anatomy of the atrial nervous system. In nine normal canine preparations, Maze incisions were performed according to the technique described by Cox et al.,[22,23] excluding cryolesions. The pattern of Maze lesions employed is displayed on the right-hand maps shown in Figure 11–6. Prior to the Maze procedure, electrical stimulation of a right- or left-sided vagosympathetic trunk induced bradycardia (-67 ± 20 and -35 ± 10 beats per minute, respectively) in all nine preparations. These interventions induced marked changes in the unipolar electrograms recorded throughout the right atrium and in some areas of the left atrium (Fig. 11–6A,B, left-hand maps). After the Maze procedure, the bradycardia responses induced by electrical stimulation of either vagosympathetic complex were no longer elicited. Vagally induced alterations in atrial unipolar electrograms were completely suppressed in five preparations following the surgical procedure (see Fig. 11–6A, right-hand map), whereas regional electrocardiographic effects induced persisted in the four remaining preparations (Fig. 11–6B: right-hand map). In about one-third of the preparations in which these regional effects persisted, responses to right-sided vagus nerve stimulation was retained in the cranial right atrium; they also persisted in the inferior septum in another third of the animals. Responses to left-sided vagal stimulation were preserved in the superior and inferior parts of the right atrium, in Bachmann's bundle, and the superior septum following this surgical intervention.

These findings support the concept that the atrial free wall and interatrial septum are richly innervated by parasympathetic efferent preganglionic neurons whose axons course in either vagosympathetic complex.[24,26,27,51] The axons associated with parasympathetic efferent preganglionic neurons course along the superior vena cava and pulmonary vein complex to converge on parasympathetic efferent postganglionic neurons in the dorsal right atrial ganglionated plexus, adjacent to the ori-

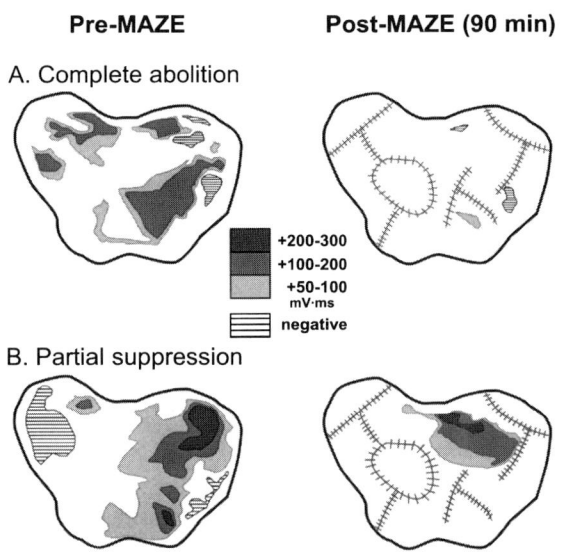

FIGURE 11–6 Complete (A) or partial (B) abolition, by the atrial incisions of the Maze III procedure, of the changes in unipolar electrogram configuration induced in response to electrical stimulation of the right atrial ganglionated plexus in two anesthetized canines. Changes were determined at each electrode site (as described in Figure 11–2) prior to (left-hand maps) and after (right-hand maps) performing the Maze III procedure (right hand maps) in two canine preparations. The locations of the incisions are indicated in the right-hand maps. Responses to right atrial ganglionated plexus stimulation were completely abolished in case 1 (A), whereas changes persisted in the upper right atrial wall in case 2 (B).

gins of the right-sided pulmonary veins. These parasympathetic efferent postganglionic neurons project their axons to tissue in the superior atrial septum, the mid- and lower right atrium, and to most of the left atrium. The persistent control of the inferior right atrium by these neurons after dissecting the superior vena cava, along with the suppression of their function after RAGP ablation, indicates that the inferior right atrium is innervated predominantly by parasympathetic efferent postganglionic neurons located in the dorsal RAGP.[24,27]

Thus, the sinus node area and the superior right atrium are innervated by parasympathetic efferent preganglionic axons coursing in either vagosympathetic complex that project axons to neurons in the RAGP as well as other cephalic ganglionated plexuses (Fig. 11–3). This finding is in direct contrast to data derived from reports suggesting that neurons in the RAGP subserve an exclusive role in parasympathetic efferent control of sinus node function.[3,14,59] Furthermore, the persistence of vagal efferent neuronal effects after a sequential dissection protocol that includes the superior left atrium[24,27] demonstrates that this control derives mainly from nerves coursing in the left-sided vagus. These data suggest that parasympathetic efferent preganglionic axons coursing through the mediastinum to the superior atrial septum also target the cranial left atrium. Furthermore, right- and left-sided vagal efferent postganglionic neurons innervate Bachmann's bundle, the superior portion of the atrial septum, and the superior right atrium, regions not necessarily affected by the Maze procedure (see Fig. 11–6).

Efferent Neuronal Control of Ventricular Electrical Events

The intrinsic cardiac nervous system controls not only the contractile performance of ventricular muscle but also its electrical behavior. Ventricular contractility responds to electrical or chemical activation of neurons in the various intrinsic cardiac ganglionated plexuses, including those in the right atrium.[67] To date, the ventricular patterns of projection arising from efferent neurons in different intrinsic cardiac ganglionated plexuses remain unknown. It is possible that such cardiac innervation patterns display less interindividual variability than that displayed during activation of intrathoracic ganglia or different extrinsic cardiopulmonary nerves,[64] as reviewed in the previous edition of this book.[16] A greater consistency in the spatial distribution of responses to electrical or chemical activation of neurons in individual loci within each intrinsic cardiac ganglionated plexus would be in keeping with the notion that the intrinsic cardiac nervous system represents the final common pathway for neuronal control of regional cardiac function (Chapter 4). In agreement with that notion is the concept that efferent neurons in one intrinsic cardiac ganglionated plexus project exclusively to adjacent tissues so that neurons, for instance, in the RAGP exert exclusive control over SA nodal function.[31]

In previous studies, we monitored the effects that specific populations of intrathoracic extracardiac efferent neurons exert on the area subtended by unipolar electrograms recorded throughout the ventricular epicardial surface (QRST area changes) to determine local innervation patterns displayed by various populations of intrathoracic extracardiac efferent neurons.[1,17,64] This approach is similar to the one used to study patterns of atrial innervation (see Fig. 11–2). With respect to ventricular unipolar electrograms, the activation complex (QRS or RS) derived from epicardial unipolar electrocardiograms can be readily separated from the T wave, reflecting the fact that the ventricular action potential displays a clear plateau (or phase of slow repolarization) before rapid repolarization begins. Therefore, ventricular responses to neuronal activation can be readily determined from alterations induced in local activation–recovery intervals, as measured from the steepest negative slope of the activation complex to the maximum positive slope of the T wave (Fig. 11–5). This variable represents an excellent one with which to monitor transient alterations in regional repolarization intervals induced by different neuronal elements within the cardiac neuroaxis.[47]

Preliminary data indicate that activation–recovery intervals shorten in various epicardial regions of the ventricle in response to activating nicotine-sensitive neurons in selective regions of the major intrinsic cardiac ganglionated plexuses of anesthetized canine preparations. For instance, the magnitude of shortening induced by nicotine-sensitive neurons in the caudal region of the RAGP is especially pronounced in the basal regions of the right ventricular sinus (Fig. 11–5A; data obtained when heart rate was fixed by atrial pacing). In contrast, neurons in the cranial ventricular ganglionated plexus activated by local application of minute doses of nicotine affect electrical changes primarily, but not exclusively, in the apical region of the left ventricle (Fig. 11–5B). At the same time, these neurons exert less influence over widespread ventricular regions and the sinus node region, as indicated by bradycardia followed by tachycardia. These findings support the concept that adrenergic and cholinergic neurons located in each major atrial or ventricular ganglionated plexus modulate multiple atrial and ventricular sites, while displaying preferential control over specific cardiac regions—some of which may be distant from the neurons so activated. Taken together, these data indicate that atrial and ventricular neurons control the electrical behavior of tissues throughout the atria and ventricles, frequently modulating tissues remote from their location.

Shortened activation recovery intervals at ventricular sites can also be induced when angiotensin II is administered to populations of intrinsic cardiac neurons via their local coronary artery blood supply. Angiotensin II, when administered into the regional arterial blood supply of right atrial neurons, not only increases the activity generated by such neurons but also induces concomitant positive cardiac inotropic effects.[39,41] The concentration of catecholamines liberated into ventricular interstitial fluid (ISF), as determined by regional microdialysis, can increase as much as fivefold when right atrial neurons are exposed to angiotensin II.[29] As this may occur without any change in catecholamine concentration in coronary sinus plasma, it appears that measurement of ISF content provides a much more accurate index of efferent neuronal responses elicited than conventional coronary blood AV difference measurements. That angiotensin II–sensitive intrinsic cardiac neurons modulate cardiac electrical events supports the contention that various populations of neurons located throughout the mammalian intrinsic cardiac nervous system exert control over regional cardiac electrical events. The electrical changes induced depend on the population of neurons involved as well as the neurotransmitter or neuromodulator to which they are exposed.

Clinical Relevance

The involvement of intrinsic cardiac neurons in regulating cardiac electrical and mechanical events raises questions about their role during the evolution of specific cardiac pathological syndromes. In chronic obstructive coronary artery disease (whether or not associated with prior myocardial infarction), conditions precipitating myocardial ischemia and angina (e.g., increased physical activity) can be associated with increased sympathetic efferent neuronal activity. Accordingly, β-adrenoceptor–blocking agents remain a cornerstone of therapy in such a state. These agents are presumed to exert their primary effects via cardiac myocyte β-adrenoceptors to reduce myocardial O_2 demand.[50] It has been proposed that the intrinsic cardiac nervous system might be a target for anti-ischemic interventions with drugs that affect cardiomyocytes and/or vascular smooth muscle.[6] Such agents include angiotensin II receptor and β-adrenoceptor blockers known to influence the intrathoracic cardiac nervous system.[5]

Activation of the dorsal aspect of the cranial thoracic spinal cord with high-frequency electrical stimuli (50 Hz) of short duration (0.2 ms) has been proposed as an alternative therapeutic modality in patients with chronic angina pectoris refractory to standard medical and surgical therapy.[45,63] The mechanisms of its anti-anginal action remain unclear. One possibility is that its anti-anginal effects result from suppression of pain perception, a mechanism that has received support from experiments conducted in primates.[19] This has raised concern for patients' safety if they were deprived of an important warning signal of myocardial ischemic insult. Whereas inhibition of transmission in the spinal cord appears to be a relevant mechanism of action of spinal cord stimulation with regard to neurogenic pain, clinical studies suggest that the relationship between anginal pain and myocardial ischemia is not affected significantly by spinal cord stimulation (as reviewed in Mannheimer et al.[43]). It is therefore necessary to consider the possibility that spinal cord stimulation induces its anti-ischemic effects through improved perfusion and/or a decrease in myocardial O_2 consumption at a given level of exercise (for instance, induced by rapid cardiac pacing). Clinical investigations have provided evidence supporting the anti-ischemic effects of this therapy in the form of a decreased magnitude of ECG ST-segment depression during exercise (at comparable workload) or in response to rapid cardiac pacing.[33,44,62] Favorable responses to these tests occur in association with clinical improvement (decreased frequency of spontaneous anginal attacks and reduced sublingual nitrate consumption).

In two clinical studies, myocardial blood flow appeared to be globally unaffected by spinal cord stimulation therapy.[25,32] However, homogenization of blood flow during this therapy was demonstrated by positron-emission tomography (PET) in one study,[32] which suggests that redistribution of coronary flow from nonischemic to ischemic areas occurred. The occurrence of anti-ischemic effects independent of improved perfusion could be due to a reduction in energy expenditure or an increase in mechanical efficiency (ratio between useful work performed and oxygen consumed). Such neuronally mediated effects might conceivably also occur via suppression of adrenergic influences on the ischemic myocardium or through neuronal release of cardioprotective substances.

Recently, it has been reported that dorsal spinal cord stimulation performed in anesthetized canines suppresses the activity generated by intrinsic cardiac neurons.[30] Spinal cord stimulation also suppressed the excitatory effects induced by regional ventricular ischemia on the intrinsic cardiac nervous system.[8] However, this procedure did not influence the distribution of blood flow in either the nonischemic or the ischemic myocardium following occlusions of the left anterior descending coronary artery of 4 minutes duration in canines.[38] In a recent series of experiments, we showed that metabolic stress induced by either rapid cardiac pacing at 240 per minute or intracoronary angiotensin II administration induced ST segment changes in the unipolar ventricular electrograms recorded from the chronically ischemic myocardium of canines in which the blood flow in the left circumflex coronary artery (LCx) was gradually obliterated over a 3-week period via an ameroid constrictor (Fig. 11–7). In such a chronic preparation, intracoronary administration of angiotensin II induces an increase in ventricular ischemic regions that display ST segment displacement (compare shaded areas in Fig. 11–7A,B). The magnitude of this effect, one presumably related to activation of intrinsic cardiac neurons by the locally administered angiotensin II,[41] was reduced when spinal cord stimulation was performed concomitantly with the intracoronary administration of angiotensin II (Fig. 11–7C). This anti-ischemic effect occurred concomitant with inhibition of intrinsic cardiac neuronal activity enhancement secondary to regional ventricular ischemia. These responses might account in part for the effect that spinal cord stimulation exerts on ventricular electrical events (Fig. 11–7C).

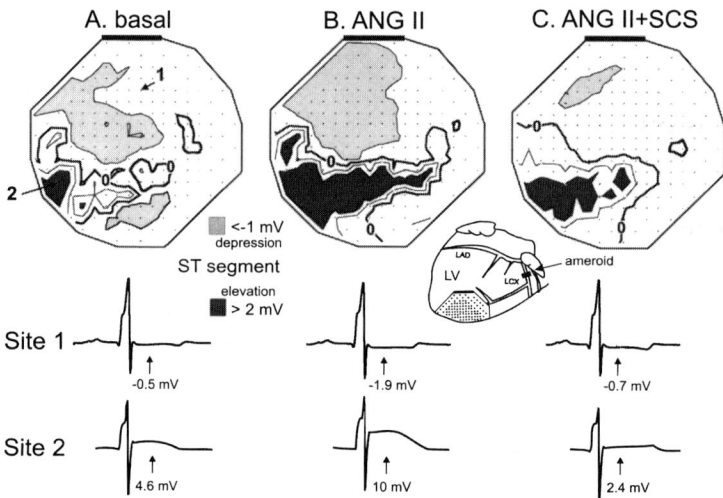

FIGURE 11–7 ST segment changes elicited in a canine preparation of chronic myocardial ischemia (**A**) that were exacerbated by intracoronary administration of angiotensin II (ANG II) (**B**). These effects were improved by concomitant spinal cord stimulation (SCS) (**C**). Hypoperfusion of the left circumflex coronary artery (LCX) was induced by gradual occlusion over several weeks of an ameroid constrictor implanted around the LCX. Unipolar electrograms recorded in the LCX territory displayed ST segment depression in some areas (site 1 and maps, light shading) and ST segment elevation in other areas (site 2 and maps, dark shading). The magnitude and spatial extent of ST segment displacements were augmented by angiotensin II perfused into the right coronary artery proximal to the arterial supply of the right atrial ganglionated plexus (B: ANG II, total dose of 40 μg over 1 minute). Exacerbation of ST segment changes was partially suppressed by spinal cord stimulation (C: SCS at 50 Hz, 0.2 ms, 90% motor threshold intensity) via an epidural electrode extending over the lower cervical and upper thoracic spinal segments. LAD, left anterior descending coronary artery; LV, left ventricle.

Improvements in the myocardial metabolic status might be associated with yet other modifications of the heart's neurohumoral environment. It is noteworthy that spinal cord stimulation augments the release of opioids into the coronary venous effluent in patients subjected to pacing-induced angina pectoris[28] since opioid agonists have been found to exert cardioprotective effects in several experimental paradigms, including ischemic preconditioning (for review, see Schultz and Gross[65]). Thus, neuronal release of vasodilator substances is yet another possibility to be considered by analogy with peripheral vascular disease in which the pain-relieving effect of spinal cord stimulation is thought to be due, at least in part, to the vasodilator action of calcitonin gene–related peptide and other vasoactive substances liberated locally as a consequence of the therapy.[46]

PERSPECTIVES

The findings reviewed in this chapter support the view that the intrinsic cardiac nervous system exerts tonic control over the electrical properties of cardiac muscle. Furthermore, they indicate that therapeutic interventions aimed at the intrinsic cardiac nervous system might have salutary effects on pathological cardiac electrical events. In chronic, obstructive coronary artery disease without prior myocardial infarction, conditions precipitating myocardial ischemia and angina (e.g., increased physical activity) are associated with increased sympathetic efferent neuronal activity.[50] Accordingly, β-adrenoceptor blocking agents remain a cornerstone of therapy devised to manage obstructive coronary artery disease, exerting their effects ultimately by reducing myocardial O_2 demand. The considerations discussed in this chapter raise the possibility that the intrinsic cardiac nervous system might not only be involved in such pathological processes, but also be a target for anti-ischemic therapy. Several drugs that affect cardiomyocytes or vascular smooth muscle also influence the intrinsic cardiac nervous system. These include angiotensin-converting enzyme inhibitors, angiotensin II receptor blockers, and β-adrenoceptor blockers. Likewise, stimulation of the dorsal aspect of the upper thoracic spinal cord reduces deleterious cardiac events associated with chronic regional myocardial ischemia primarily via the intrinsic cardiac nervous system. Spinal cord stimulation provides a unique experimental paradigm with which to explore the relationship between the intrinsic cardiac nervous system, spinal cord neurons, and cardiac electrical events. The ideas discussed in this chapter not only challenge our current concepts about the regulation of cardiac electrical events but also present an opportunity to devise new therapeutic approaches to the problem of cardiac arrhythmia management.

ACKNOWLEDGMENTS
The Canadian Institutes of Health Research and the Canadian Heart and Stroke Foundation provided financial support for this work.

REFERENCES

1. Abildskov JA, Evans AK, Lux RL, and Burgess MJ. Ventricular recovery properties and QRST deflection area in cardiac electrograms. *Am J Physiol* 239: H227–H231, 1980.
2. Alessi R, Nasynowitz M, Abildskov JA, and Moe GK. Nonuniform vagal effects on the atrial refractory period. *Am J Physiol* 194:406–411, 1958.

3. Ardell JL and Randall WC. Selective vagal innervation of sinoatrial and atrioventricular nodes in the canine heart. *Am J Physiol* 251:H764–H773, 1986.
4. Ardell JL, Randall WC, Cannon WJ, Schmacht DC, and Tasdemiroglu E. Differential sympathetic regulation of automatic, conductile, and contractile tissue in dog heart. *Am J Physiol* 255:H1050–H1059, 1988.
5. Armour JA. Anatomy and function of the intrathoracic neurons regulating the mammalian heart. In: Zucker IH and Gilmore JP, ed. *Reflex Control of the Circulation*. Boca Raton, FL: CRC Press, 1991, pp. 1–37.
6. Armour JA. Myocardial ischemia and the cardiac nervous system. *Cardiovasc Res* 41:41–54, 1999.
7. Armour JA, Huang MH, and Smith FM. Peptidergic modulation of in situ canine cardiac neurons. *Peptides* 14:191–202, 1993.
8. Armour JA, Linderoth B, Arora RC, DeJongste MJ, Ardell JL, Kingma GJ, Hill M, and Foreman RD. Long-term modulation of the intrinsic cardiac nervous system by spinal cord neurons in normal and ischaemic hearts. *Auton Neurosci* 95:71–79, 2002.
9. Armour JA, Murphy DA, Yuan BX, Macdonald S, and Hopkins DA. Gross and microscopic anatomy of the human intrinsic cardiac nervous system. *Anat Rec* 247:289–298, 1997.
10. Armour JA, Yuan BX, and Butler CK. Cardiac responses elicited by peptides administered to canine intrinsic cardiac neurons. *Peptides* 11:753–761, 1990.
11. Arora RC, Waldmann M, Hopkins DA, and Armour JA. Porcine intrinsic cardiac ganglia. *Anat Rec* 271:249–258, 2003.
12. Beaulieu P, Cardinal R, Pagé P, Francoeur F, Tremblay J, and Lambert C. Positive chronotropic and inotropic effects of C-type natriuretic peptide in dogs. *Am J Physiol* 273:H1933–H1940, 1997.
13. Blinder KJ, Johnson TA, and Massari VJ. Negative inotropic vagal preganglionic neurons in the nucleus ambiguus of the cat: neuroanatomical comparison with negative chronotropic neurons utilizing dual retrograde tracers. *Brain Res* 804:325–330, 1998.
14. Bluemel KM, Wurster RD, Randall WC, Duff MJ, and O'Toole MF. Parasympathetic postganglionic pathways to the sinoatrial node. *Am J Physiol* 259: H1504–H1510, 1990.
15. Butler CK, Smith FM, Cardinal R, Murphy DA, Hopkins DA, and Armour JA. Cardiac responses to electrical stimulation of discrete loci in canine atrial and ventricular ganglionated plexi. *Am J Physiol* 259:H1365–H1373, 1990.
16. Cardinal R. Autonomic modulation of myocardial electrical properties and cardiac rhythm. In: Armour JA and Ardell JL, eds. *Neurocardiology*. New York: Oxford University Press, 1994, pp 165–191.
17. Cardinal R, Savard P, Armour JA, Scherlag BJ, Vermeulen M, Pagé P, and Nadeau R. Ventricular patterns of efferent sympathetic innervation and origins of sympathetically induced ventricular tachycardias. In: *Cardiac Mapping*. Shenasa M, Borggrefe M, Breithardt G, eds. Mount Kisco, NY: Futura Publishing Co., 1993, pp 263–273.
18. Carlson MD, Geha AS, Hsu J, Martin PJ, Levy MN, Jacobs G, and Waldo AL. Selective stimulation of parasympathetic nerve fibers to the human sinoatrial node. *Circulation* 85:1311–1317, 1992.
19. Chandler MJ, Brennan TJ, Garrison DW, Kim KS, Schwartz PJ, and Foreman RD. A mechanism of cardiac pain suppression by spinal cord stimulation: implications for patients with angina pectoris. *Eur Heart J* 14:96–105, 1993.

20. Chiou CW, Eble JN, and Zipes DP. Efferent vagal innervation of the canine atria, sinus and atrioventricular nodes: the third fat pad. *Circulation* 95:2573–2584, 1997.
21. Cohn AE. On the difference in the effects of stimulation of the two vagus nerves on rate and conduction of the dog's heart. *J Exp Med* 16:732–747, 1912.
22. Cox JL, Boineau JP, Schuessler RB, Jaquiss DB, and Lappas DG. Modification of the Maze procedure for atrial flutter and atrial fibrillation. I. Rationale and surgical results. *J Thorac Cardiovasc Surg* 110:473–484, 1995.
23. Cox JL, Jaquiss RD, Schuessler RB, and Boineau JP. Modification of the MAZE procedure for atrial flutter and atrial fibrillation. II. Surgical technique of the MAZE III procedure. *J Thorac Cardiovasc Surg* 110:485–495, 1995.
24. Davis Z, Jacobs HK, Bonilla J, Anderson RR, Thomas C, and Forst W. Retaining the aortic fat pad during surgery decreases postoperative atrial fibrillation. *Heart Surg Forum* 3(2):108–112, 2000.
25. De Landsheere C, Mannheimer C, Habets A, Guillaume M, Bourgeois I, Augustinsson LE, Eliasson T, Lamotte D, Kulbertus H, and Rigo P. Effect of spinal cord stimulation on regional myocardial perfusion assessed by positron emission tomography. *Am J Cardiol* 69:1143–1149, 1992.
26. Do QB, Dandan N, Cardinal R, and Pagé P. Étude de l'innervation autonomique du septum inter-auriculaire par cartographie iso-intégrale chez le chien. *Ann Chir* 50:659–666, 1996.
27. Do QB, Pagé P, Dandan N, and Cardinal R. Effect of intrapericardial dissections on atrial innervation: assessment by integral distribution mapping. *Can J Cardiol* 11(Suppl E): 95E, 1995.
28. Eliasson T, Mannheimer C, Waagstein F, Andersson B, Bergh CH, Augustinsson LE, Hedner T, and Larson G. Myocardial turnover of endogenous opioids and calcitonin-gene-related peptide in the human heart and the effects of spinal cord stimulation on pacing-induced angina pectoris. *Cardiology* 89:170–177, 1998.
29. Farrell DM, Wei CC, Tallaj J, Ardell JL, Armour JA, Hageman GR, Bradley WE, and Dell'Italia LJ. Angiotensin II modulates catecholamine release into interstitial fluid of canine myocardium in vivo. *Am J Physiol* 281:H813–H822, 2001.
30. Foreman RD, Linderoth B, Ardell JL, Barron KW, Chandler MJ, Hull SS, Jr, TerHorst GJ, DeJongste MJL, and Armour JA. Modulation of intrinsic cardiac neurons by spinal cord stimulation: implications for its therapeutic use in angina pectoris. *Cardiovasc Res* 47:367–375, 2000.
31. Gatti PJ, Johson TA, and Massari VJ. Can neurons in the nucleus ambiguus selectively regulate cardiac rate and atrio-ventricular conduction? *J Auton Nerv Syst* 57:123–127, 1996.
32. Hautvast RW, Blanksma PK, DeJongste MJ, Pruim J, van der Wall EE, Vaalburg W, and Lie KI. Effect of spinal cord stimulation on myocardial blood flow assessed by positron emission tomography in patients with refractory angina pectoris. *Am J Cardiol* 77:462–467, 1996.
33. Hautvast RW, DeJongste MJ, Staal MJ, van Gilst WH, and Lie KI. Spinal cord stimulation in chronic intractable angina pectoris: a randomized controlled efficacy study. *Am Heart J* 136:943–944, 1998.
34. Hoffman BF and Cranefield PF. *Electrophysiology of the Heart*. Mount Kisco, NY: Futura Publishing Company, 1976, pp 53–57.
35. Hoffman BF and Suckling EE. Cardiac cellular potentials: effect of vagal stimulation and acetylcholine. *Am J Physiol* 173:312–320, 1953.

36. Huang MH, Friend DS, Sunday ME, Singh K, Haley K, Austen KF, Kelly RA, and Smith TW. An intrinsic adrenergic system in mammalian heart. *J Clin Invest* 98:1298–1303, 1996.
37. Hughes J and Roth RH. Evidence that angiotensin enhances transmitter release during sympathetic nerve stimulation. *Br J Pharmacol* 41:239–255, 1971.
38. Kingma JG, Linderoth B, Ardell JL, Armour JA, DeJongste MJ, and Foreman RD. Neuromodulation therapy does not influence blood flow distribution of left-ventricular dynamics during acute myocardial ischemia. *Auton Neurosci* 91:47–54, 2001.
39. Lambert C, Godin D, Fortier P, and Nadau R. Direct effects in vivo of angiotensin I and II on the canine sinus node. *Can J Physiol Pharmacol* 69:389–392, 1991.
40. Lazzara R, Scherlag BJ, Robinson MJ, and Samet P. Selective in situ parasympathetic control of the canine sinoatrial and atrioventricular nodes. *Circ Res* 32:393–401, 1973.
41. Levett JM, Murphy MD, McGuirt AS, Ardell JL, and Armour JA. Cardiac augmentation can be maintained by continuous exposure of intrinsic cardiac neurons to a β-adrenergic agonist or angiotensin II. *J Surg Res* 66:167–173, 1996.
42. Lindmar R, Loffelholz K, and Muscholl E. A muscarinic mechanism inhibiting the release of noradrenaline from peripheral adrenergic nerve fibers by nicotinic agents. *Br J Pharmacol* 32:280–294, 1968.
43. Mannheimer C, Camici P, Chester MR, Collins A, DeJongste M, Eliasson T, Follath F, Hellemans I, Herlitz J, Lüscher T, Paisc M, and Thelle D. The problem of chronic refractory angina. Report from the ESC Joint Study Group on the treatment of refractory angina. *Eur Heart J* 23:355–370, 2002.
44. Mannheimer C, Eliasson T, Andersson B, Bergh CH, Augustinsson LE, Emanuelsson H, and Waagstein F. Effects of spinal cord stimulation in angina pectoris induced by pacing and possible mechanism of action. *BMJ* 307:477–480, 1993.
45. Mannheimer C, Eliasson T, Augustinsson LE, Blomstrand C, Emanuelsson H, Larsson S, Norssell H, and Hjalmarsson A. Electrical stimulation versus coronary artery bypass surgery in severe angina pectoris. The ESBY study. *Circulation* 97:1157–1163, 1998.
46. Meyerson BA and Linderoth B. Spinal cord stimulation. In: Loeser JD, ed. *Bonica's Management of Pain*. Philadelphia: Lippincott-Raven, 2000, pp 1857–1876.
47. Millar CK, Kralios FA, and Lux RL. Correlation between refractory periods and activation-recovery intervals from electrograms: effects of rate and adrenergic interventions. *Circulation* 72:1372–1379, 1985.
48. Mukkadam-Daher S, Yin YL, Roy J, Gutkowska J, and Cardinal R. Negative inotropic and chronotropic effects of oxytocin. *Hypertension* 38:292–296, 2001.
49. Nadeau RA and James TN. Effect of nicotine on heart rate studied by direct perfusion of sinus node. *Am J Physiol* 212:911–916, 1967.
50. Opie LH. *Drugs for the Heart*, 4th ed. Philadelphia: WB Saunders, 1995, p 1.
51. Pagé P, Dandan N, Cardinal R, and Nadeau R. Repolarization changes induced in left atrial regions by parasympathetic neurons located within the right atrial wall. *PACE* 18(Part II): 904, 1995.
52. Pagé P, Yin Y, and Cardinal R. Parasympathetic innervation of the human heart: an intraoperative mapping study. *PACE* 22(Part II):716, 1999.
53. Pagé PL, Dandan N, Savard P, Nadeau R, Armour JA, and Cardinal R. Regional distribution of atrial electrical changes induced by stimulation of ex-

tracardiac and intracardiac neural elements. *J Thorac Cardiovasc Surg* 109:377–388, 1995.
54. Pauza DH, Skripka V, Pauziene N, and Stropus R. Anatomical study of the neural ganglionated plexus in the canine right atrium: implications for selective denervation and electrophysiology of the sinoatrial node in dog. *Anat Rec* 255:271–294, 1999.
55. Pauza DH, Skripka V, Pauziene N, and Stropus R. Morphology, distribution, and variability of the epicardiac neural ganglionated subplexuses in the human heart. *Anat Rec* 259:353–382, 2000.
56. Pinter A, Nadeau R, Dandan N, and Pagé PL. Effect of vasoactive intestinal peptide on pacemaker location and heart rate in the dog atrium. *Can J Physiol Pharmacol* 76:457–462, 1998.
57. Randall WC and Ardell JL. Selective parasympathectomy of automatic and conductile tissues of the canine heart. *Am J Physiol* 248:H61–H68, 1985.
58. Randall WC, Ardell JL, Calderwood D, Milosavljevic M, and Goyal SC. Parasympathetic ganglia innervating the canine atrioventricular node region. *J Auton Nerv Syst* 16:311–323, 1986.
59. Randall WC, Ardell JL, Wurster RD, and Milosavljevic M. Vagal postganglionic innervation of the canine sinoatrial node. *J Auton Nerv Syst* 20:13–23, 1987.
60. Reit E. Actions of angiotensin on the adrenal medulla and autonomic ganglia. *Fed Proc* 31:1338–1343, 1972.
61. Ren LM, Furukawa Y, Karasawa Y, Murakami M, Takei M, Narita M, and Chiba S. Effects of tetrodotoxin and imipramine on the cardiac responses to nicotine in isolated, blood-perfused canine heart preparations. *J Cardiovasc Pharmacol* 18:77–84, 1990.
62. Sanderson JE, Brooksby P, Waterhouse D, Palmer RPG, and Neubauer K. Epidural spinal electrical stimulation for severe angina: a study of its effects on symptoms, exercise tolerance and degree of ischaemia. *Eur Heart J* 13:628–633, 1992.
63. Sanderson JE, Ibrahim B, Waterhouse D, and Palmer RB. Spinal electrical stimulation for intractable angina—long-term clinical outcome and safety. *Eur Heart J* 15:810–804, 1994.
64. Savard P, Cardinal R, Nadeau RA, and Armour JA. Epicardial distribution of ST segment and T wave changes produced by stimulation of intrathoracic ganglia or cardiopulmonary nerves in dogs. *J Auton Nerv Syst* 34:47, 1991.
65. Schultz JEJ and Gross GJ. Opioids and cardioprotection. *Pharmacol Ther* 89:123–137, 2001.
66. Yin Y, Pagé P, and Cardinal R. Concentration-dependent effects of angiotensin II on sinus rate in canine isolated right atrial preparations. *Can J Physiol Pharmacol* 77:36–41, 1999.
67. Yuan BX, Ardell JL, Hopkins DA, and Armour JA. Differential cardiac responses induced by nicotine sensitive canine atrial and ventricular neurones. *Cardiovasc Res* 27:760–769, 1993.
68. Yuan BX, Ardell JL, Hopkins DA, Losier AM, and Armour JA. Gross and microscopic anatomy of the canine intrinsic cardiac nervous system. *Anat Rec* 239:75–87, 1994.
69. Zipes DP, Mihalick MJ, and Robbins GT. Effects of selective vagal and stellate ganglion stimulation of atrial refractoriness. *Cardiovasc Res* 8:647–655, 1974.

12

Sympathetic Nervous System in the Evolution of Heart Failure

Louis J. Dell'Italia and Jeffrey L. Ardell

In response to a variety of stresses, including exercise, traumatic injury, and blood loss, the need for increased cardiac output is met by a commensurate increase in adrenergic drive. As a result, norepinephrine (NE), the primary neurotransmitter of the adrenergic system, is released from sympathetic nerve endings in the heart. Myocardial adrenergic receptor signaling pathways are activated, resulting in increases in heart rate, rate of electrical conduction, and force of contraction. Early sympathetic neuronal activation in cardiac injury and/or hemodynamic overload increases ventricular inotropy and systemic resistance, thereby maintaining cardiac output and blood pressure. Sustained activation of sympathetic efferent neurons, however, can have several adverse consequences, including increased ventricular wall stress, direct myocyte toxicity, myocardial fibrosis, and lowering of the ventricular fibrillation threshold. Furthermore, there is mounting evidence that multiple intracardiac neurohormonal systems and the adrenergic system are activated simultaneously and cross-regulate each other, even in the absence of elevations in plasma neurohormonal levels as heart failure progresses. The purpose of this chapter is to not only underscore the central role of sympathetic overdrive in early left ventricular dysfunction but also to emphasize its interaction with key neurohormonal systems, in particular the renin–angiotensin system, kallikrein–kinin system, and inflammatory cytokines, in the progression of adverse structural and functional left ventricular remodeling associated with the cardiac pathology.

Left Ventricular Remodeling and the Progression to Heart Failure

Whether myocardial damage is secondary to myocardial infarction, chronic ischemia, inflammation, pressure overload, or volume overload, there is a complex sequence of compensatory events that ultimately result in an adversely remodeled myocardium and a dilated, thin-walled, spherical ventricle. The morphological changes to the heart associated with these pathophysiological events and compensatory mechanisms can be categorized into three stages, as shown in Figure 12–1. First, during acute load, there is an increase in diastolic pressure and/or systolic pressure with some compensatory myocyte hypertrophy. Second, during compensatory hypertrophy, myocyte growth leads to an increase in ventricular wall thickness and chamber diameter. During this stage, there is a complex sequence of dynamic compensatory events involving myocyte morphology, intracellular calcium homeostasis, the extracellular matrix (ECM), and the neurohormonal systems that modulate the heart. Untreated, this results in a progressive dilatation characterized by a disproportionate decrease in the ratio of left ventricular (LV) wall thickness to diameter (weight/diameter) ratio, increase in myocardial wall stress, development of congestive heart failure (CHF), arrhythmias, and sudden death.

It is now well accepted that myocardial remodeling is determined not only by hemodynamic factors but also by local production of neurohormones (e.g., angiotensin II [ANG II], aldosterone, NE, and bradykinin [BK]), growth factors (transforming growth factor β [TGF-β] insulin-like growth factor [IGF]) and reactive inflammatory species (RIS) (Fig. 12–2). Therapeutic approaches to date have been largely directed at these neurohormonal targets, in particular, the noradrenergic system and renin–angiotensin system. Classically, these were considered only in the context of their effects on myocyte function. But as a result of the many clinical trials and animal studies, there is now a general appreciation of the many effects of increased sympathetic drive on other important targets in heart failure, including RIS and ECM, and an understanding that many current therapies act in part by directly modulating the cardiac nervous system. There is increasing evidence that oxidative stress is increased in

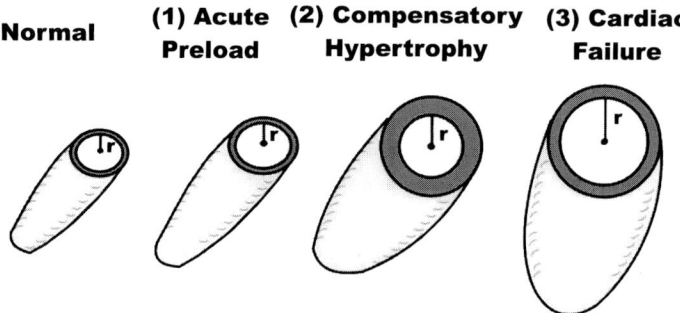

FIGURE 12–1 Schematic representation of the gross morphological changes in the heart from acute preload to the progression to heart failure.

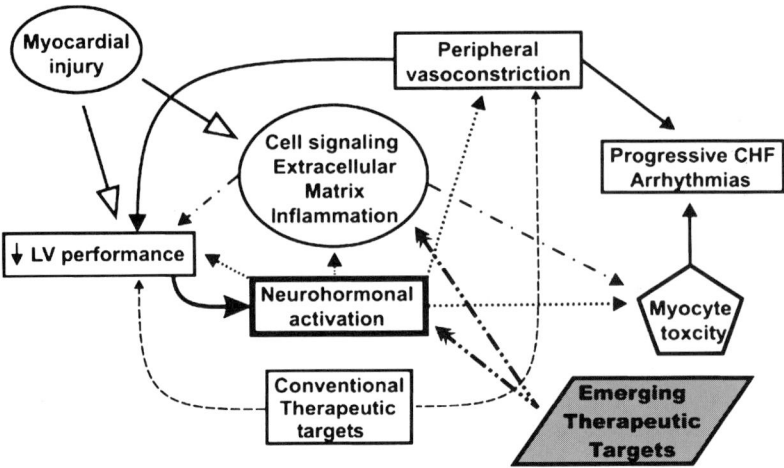

FIGURE 12–2 Schema demonstrating that myocardial remodeling is determined not only by hemodynamic factors but also by local production of neurohormones (e.g., angiotensin II, aldosterone, norepinephrine, bradykinin), growth factors (transforming growth factor-β, insulin-like growth factor), and other targets, including reactive inflammatory species and extracellular matrix. CHF, congestive heart failure; LV, left ventricular.

myocardial failure and may play an important role in the structural and functional changes that lead to the progression of heart failure.[19,30,59] The dynamic plasticity of the ECM is maintained not only by changes in collagen structure and accumulation but also by two functional classes of molecules: matrix metalloproteinases (MMPs) that degrade collagen, and matrix components that inhibit MMPs (TIMPs) or prevent their activation.[78] The balance between MMPs and TIMPs has also been shown to play an important role in animal models of heart failure and in human dilated cardiomyopathy. In this chapter, evidence is presented for the importance of increased sympathetic drive on these interdependent mechanisms in the pathophysiology and progression of cardiomyocyte, ECM, and neurohumoral remodeling in heart failure.

INCREASED ADRENERGIC DRIVE IN HEART FAILURE

There is ample evidence of increased sympathetic efferent neuronal activity in severe CHF.[27,40,58,62,105] However, we now know that the sympathetic efferent nervous system activity is increased in mild heart failure in the absence of increased plasma catecholamine levels.[37,46,91] In the heart, NE and epinephrine (EPI) are released into the myoneural junction from sympathetic efferent postganglionic nerve terminals to interact with β_1 and β_2 receptors on cardiomyocytes, fibroblasts, and other cells in the cardiac tissue to produce their biologic effects. Norepinephrine is a β_1-selective agonist that is about 20-fold more selective for human cardiomyocyte β_1 than β_2 receptors and 10-fold more selective for β_1 receptors than human myocardial α_1 receptors; EPI has a higher selectivity for cardiomyocyte β_2 receptors.[13] For the most part, EPI is extracted by the heart from the blood and stored in sympathetic efferent postganglionic nerve terminals to be released as a cotransmitter with NE.[39,40,84] However, there is now evidence of NE and EPI production by intrinsic cardiac adrenergic cell types that appears to be independent of sympathetic innervation.[55] Nevertheless, the amount of EPI within the canine LV myocardium is approximately 40-fold lower than that of NE.[5] Thus, since EPI content is a small fraction of NE content in intracardiac adrenergic nerves, its recycling is also critical for its continued release. After synaptic release, NE undergoes metabolism. There are two mechanisms involved: (1) the clearance of NE from the myoneural junction (uptake 1) and (2) uptake by adjacent non-neuronal tissues (uptake 2).[39] The remainder of locally released NE that escapes these uptake processes enters the general circulation and is referred to as " NE spillover."

In the early stages of heart failure, decreased myocardial function activates cardiac sympathetic nerves via complex cardiovascular reflexes (Chapter 4) to increase the local release of catecholamines. Using the NE spillover method in established heart failure, investigators found that cardiac sympathetic activity increased, largely due to increased NE release and decreased NE reuptake.[37] In patients with mild congestive heart failure, cardiac NE spillover is increased threefold over that of healthy controls, even before renal and total body NE spillover increases.[91] Studies of NE kinetics in humans using the triple isotope technique have demonstrated a significant reduction in NE release and reuptake in patients with LV failure due to valvular heart disease[90] and in patients with idiopathic dilated cardiomyopathy.[1] Another study showed that cardiac membrane preparations taken from patients with functional class II–IV heart failure exhibited significantly less (30%) NE uptake-carrier density than in individuals with normal heart function.[9] Using another method to assess sympathetic nervous system activity, Grassi and co-workers applied microneurographic techniques to patients with mild heart failure and found increased muscle sympathetic nerve activity.[46] Taken together, these and other studies[35,57] suggest that the cardiac noradrenergic system is activated early in heart failure, resulting in increased local NE into the myocardial interstitium; this exerts deleterious effects on the myocardium prior to elevation of plasma catecholamines.

The long-term exposure to high levels of NE has profound effects on cardiomyocyte and β-adrenergic signal transduction systems. Increased local NE levels could account for the observed decrease in β_1-receptor density, as demonstrated, for example, by Delehanty and co-workers, who used a triple-isotope intracoronary tracer technique in dogs with pacing tachycardia–induced heart failure.[28] The relationship between local NE levels and the β receptor is complex because NE levels are related to local synthesis as well as to extraction from the circulation, release from nerve terminals, reuptake into nerve terminals, and local metabolism (Fig. 12–3). Since transmitter levels are conserved by the reuptake system, it is conceivable that over time a deficiency of uptake could lead to a depletion of NE in the nerve terminal. In support of this mechanism, Armstrong and co-workers reported that intracardiac NE content was de-

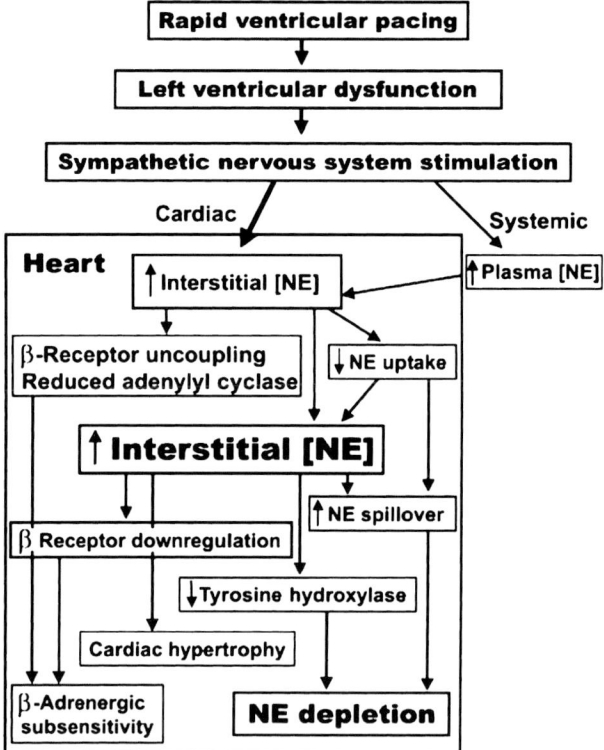

FIGURE 12–3 Hypothetical cause-and-effect relationship regarding temporal changes in left ventricular function, sympathetic stimulation, norepinephrine (NE) uptake activity, tyrosine hydroxylase, β-adrenergic sensitivity, β-adrenoceptor density, and NE content in the heart after rapid ventricular pacing. (From Kawai et al.[61])

creased 50% in dogs with rapid pacing–induced heart failure.[5] Furthermore, Cardinal and Armour have demonstrated that coronary sinus NE levels and the positive inotropic response to stellate ganglion stimulation are markedly decreased in dogs with rapid pacing–induced heart failure.[17] These animal studies suggest a decrease in synaptic NE with heart failure and are consistent with early studies that report depletion of intracardiac NE levels in dog preparations of heart failure and those found in human hearts.

Previous studies in animal models of end-stage heart failure have demonstrated decreased NE tissue stores[17,21–23,28,29,54,72,73] in association with a decrease in NE reuptake protein and kinetics,[54,72,73] a decrease in NE synthesis,[85] and an increase in NE spillover.[72] Neuronal reuptake is the major mechanism of NE clearance from the interstitial fluid (ISF) space and for modulating ISF NE levels in heart failure. Previous studies have demonstrated decreased NE uptake activity and NE uptake-1 carrier protein in end-stage heart failure that correlated with down-regulation of β_1-adrenoreceptor density.[54,72,73] Yet overall, the depletion of cardiac NE in heart failure does not correlate with LV function[85] and is difficult to reconcile with the reported down-regulation of β_1-adrenoreceptor density.[14,15] Importantly, none of these studies directly evaluated whether NE release from sympathetic efferent nerves is elevated or depressed. Moreover, little attention has been given to the potential role of EPI in the cardiac interstitium and its effects on LV function, especially in the context of progressive cardiac disease.

Cardiac microdialysis offers insight into the dynamic neuromyocardial interaction occurring within the heart by providing a direct measurement of interstitial NE and EPI concentrations that can be related to LV function at rest and during sympathetic activation in normal states and in various stages of heart failure. Accordingly, using the cardiac microdialysis technique, Akiyama and co-workers demonstrated a twofold increase in ISF NE concentration with stellate ganglion stimulation[2] and marked regional accumulation of ISF NE concentrations during 40 minutes of ischemia in the dog.[98] Further, they demonstrated that ISF NE levels correlated with ventricular contractility during graded cardiac sympathetic nerve stimulation in the in vivo.[60] Using the cardiac microdialysis technique in open-chest dogs, we have shown that maximal electrical stimulation of intrathoracic adrenergic efferent neurons results in a massive release of NE and EPI into the cardiac ISF space and that transcardiac plasma NE and EPI gradients substantially underestimate sympathetic efferent neuronal NE and EPI release into myoneural tissue[41] (Fig. 12–4). Interstitial fluid NE concentration is determined by the following factors: *(1)* circulating levels of NE that can diffuse into the interstitium—

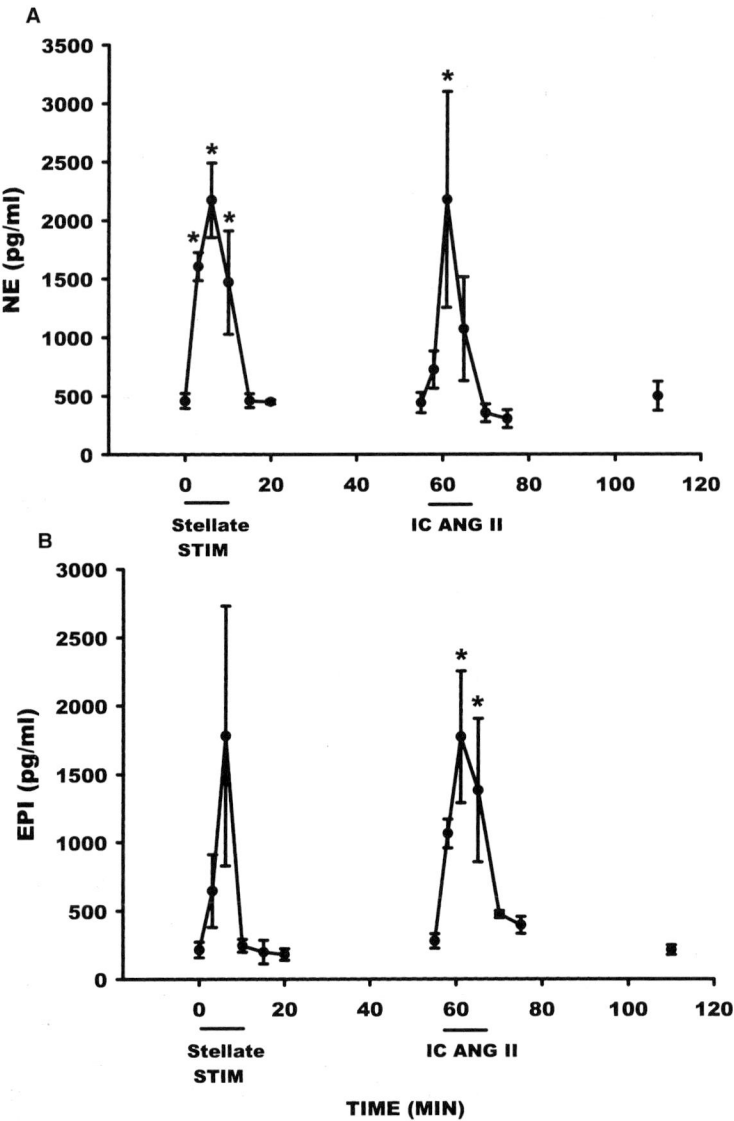

FIGURE 12–4 Interstitial fluid norepinephrine (NE) (**A**) and epinephrine (EPI) (**B**) levels during a 10-minute stellate ganglia stimulation (STIM) (left) and during 10-minute infusion of angiotensin II (ANG II) into a branch of the right coronary artery in dogs with adrenals intact. *$P < 0.05$ versus baseline value of stellate stimulation and ANG II infusion. (From Farrell et al.[41])

the heart is known for an exceptionally avid NE reuptake mechanism that is capable of removing approximately 70% of delivered NE across the coronary circulation in the normal human heart; (2) the rate of reuptake of NE into the neuronal terminals; and (3) the rate of release of NE into the interstitium by cardiac sympathetic efferent nerves. Indeed, from the previous discussion, all of the above mechanisms have been identified as deficient in heart failure.

Most NE in the tissue is stored in the adrenergic neuronal terminal vesicles. As mentioned above, cardiac NE content is determined by the rates of NE release, turnover, and synthesis. As outlined above, NE release and turnover are influenced by cardiac sympathetic tone and NE uptake capacity. The rate of NE synthesis is affected largely by tyrosine hydroxylation, which is the rate-limiting step involved in the catecholamine biosynthesis. An early animal study demonstrated that reduced tyrosine hydroxylase activity played a role in the depletion of cardiac NE stores in heart failure. Eisenhofer et al. showed, however, that the decreased cardiac NE stores in patients with heart failure was caused by chronically increased NE turnover and reduced efficiency of NE reuptake and storage rather than by insufficient tyrosine hydroxylation.[37] Moreover, in a recent study in a rabbit pacing model of heart failure, parallel changes occurred in NE uptake activity and myocardial β-adrenoceptor function, suggesting the pivotal role of NE uptake activity in myocardial β-adrenoceptor down-regulation identified in pacing-induced cardiomyopathy.[61] In summary, the relative contributions of the various factors to cardiac NE depletion in heart failure may vary depending on both the stage and type of hemodynamic overload encountered.

B_1- AND B_2-ADRENORECEPTORS IN HEART FAILURE

As discussed in the previous section, in the early stages of heart failure, an intrinsic decrease in myocardial function ultimately stimulates cardiac sympathetic efferent nerves to release NE. Through this activation of β-adrenergic receptors (β-ARs), heart rate and myocardial contractility are subsequently increased to compensate for the acute myocardial injury. As heart failure worsens, adrenergic neuronal drive continues to increase in reflex response to progressive loss of cardiac function. Long-term exposure to high levels of NE can exert profoundly adverse effects on myocardial and cardiac myocyte biology, including the β-AR signal transduction systems, which results in progressive myocardial dysfunction and worsening heart failure (Fig. 12–2). Thus, in human heart failure, it is generally believed that most of the adverse biological effects of increased cardiac adrenergic efferent neuronal drive are mediated by cardiac tissue β_1-AR.

Treatment of isolated cardiac myocytes with concentrations of NE present in the failing human heart can cause dramatic changes in cell morphology and up to a 60% loss of myocyte viability in a matter of days.[77] This effect can be mimicked by exposing myocytes to varying concentrations of the nonselective β-agonist, isoproterenol. As this cardiomyocyte effect is inhibited pharmacologically by propranolol, it appears that the acute toxic effects of NE are mediated primarily through β-ARs rather than through α-ARs.[77] Recent studies suggest that a major underlying mechanism of NE toxicity involves cAMP-mediated increases in intracellular calcium. Activation of the β_1-AR subtype appears to promote increased calcium influx via cAMP-independent mechanisms as well, including a reported direct interaction of calcium channels with the stimulatory G protein, $G_{\alpha s}$.[25,69,93] In either case, excessive β-AR stimulation eventually results in calcium overload, a condition promoting cell death through a number of mechanisms, including necrosis and apoptosis.

There is mounting evidence that the consequences of β_1- versus β_2-AR stimulation are quite different.[70,100] Although both receptors classically activate adenylate cyclase via stimulation of G_s, β_2 receptors can also stimulate G_i (the myocardial concentrations of which are elevated in CHF). Cardiac β_1-ARs and β_2-ARs have also been shown to differ in their effects on contraction, cytosolic Ca^{2+} concentrations, and Ca^{2+} currents in isolated rat ventricular cells. β_2-ARs are present not only on cardiomyocytes and fibroblasts but also on postganglionic cardiac sympathetic neurons whose nerve terminals, when activated, release NE.[4] It is hypothesized that β_2-AR activation may improve cardiac function in the setting of down-regulation of the β_1-AR in heart failure.[14] In the human and dog heart in vivo, administration of a β_2-AR agonist results in significant increase in LV contractility and increased NE spillover from the heart.[67,83] Furthermore, activation of β_2-ARs of failing human or canine cardiomyocytes increases their calcium transients and thus contractility in vitro.[3]

Transgenic mice overexpressing the β_2-AR at levels of approximately 10-fold above normal show marked potentiation of catecholamine-stimulated inotropy, with no pathological consequences.[108] In fact, up to 100-fold overexpression of β_2-ARs in the mouse heart causes significantly increased cardiac contractile force without any cardiomyopathic consequences for over 1 year.[74] This is in striking contrast to the early cardiomyopathy that results from low-level transgenic overexpression (fivefold) of β_1-ARs in the heart.[38] Thus, although both β_1- and β_2-ARs are present on cardiomyocytes, it appears that the toxic effect of excess catecholamines appears largely mediated by the β_1-AR, while β_2-AR has no adverse effect or may even be protective, especially against apoptosis.[20,25]

Down-regulation of myocardial β_1-AR in heart failure and the resulting increase in relative cardiac β_2-AR expression suggest that cardiac β_2-AR expression and function are of particular importance in this condition. As has been described in a number of investigations, β_2-ARs, although desensitized, do not undergo down-regulation in the failing human heart.[14,76] The reason for this finding is not completely understood. Prior studies in heart failure have demonstrated that genetic variability of β_2-ARs is one determinant of disease progression.[75] The β_2-AR receptor exists in multiple polymorphic forms with different characteristics.[75,110] Of particular interest is the finding that three polymorphic β_2-ARs exhibit altered receptor function in in vitro expression assays. Patients with Ile164 progress more rapidly to death or transplantation than those with Thr164.[75] Strong trends were also seen with Gly16 or Gln27 (both of which have increased down-regulation compared with their counterparts). In addition, patients with the hypofunctional β_2-ARs caused by the fourth transmembrane domain Ile164 polymorphism have a significantly lower peak $\dot{V}O_2$ during treadmill exercise testing—i.e., diminished exercise capacity, than that of patients with Thr164.[110] This is consistent with a recent report showing decreased survival in patients with Ile164. The importance of the β_2-AR in heart failure is currently a topic of intense research that impacts on clinical treatment with a selective β_1-AR blocker or a nonselective β-AR blocker.[12,13]

INTERACTION OF THE RENIN–ANGIOTENSIN SYSTEM AND NORADRENERGIC SYSTEMS

In addition to sympathetic activation mediated via cardiovascular–cardiac reflexes, there is also evidence that ANG II activates intrathoracic cardiac adrenergic efferent postganglionic neurons, thereby resulting in the liberation of catecholamines from their postganglionic nerve terminals.[7,10,41] Recent autoradiographic data from rabbits have demonstrated that AT_1 receptor density in intrinsic cardiac ganglia is ninefold higher than that in the ventricular myocardium.[11] AT_1 receptors are associated with peripheral sympathetic neurons, located within the cardiac conduction system, and have a greater density within intrinsic cardiac neural elements than cardiomyocytes in the rat.[18,32,92] Moreover, a recent study by Kushiku and co-workers demonstrated that high-frequency preganglionic stimulation results in ANG II release from canine sympathetic ganglia that can be blocked by angiotensin-converting enzyme (ACE) inhibitor.[68] In addition, ganglionic cells in culture and in vivo demonstrated an increase in angiotensinogen mRNA after 1 hour of electrical stimulation.[68] These results suggest an intact renin–angiotensin system in ganglionic cells that is up-regulated by high levels of sympathetic activation.

Within the intrathoracic nervous system there are both extracardiac and intrinsic cardiac ganglia which are principally involved in control of regional cardiac function (see Chapter 4). Intrathoracic extracardiac ganglia include the stellate, middle cervical, and mediastinal ganglia. Intrinsic cardiac ganglia include aggregates of neurons located in both atrial and ventricular tissues associated principally with control of specific cardiac function. Angiotensin II induced positive chronotropic effects in adult guinea pig ventricular cardiomyocytes that were cocultured with intrinsic cardiac or extracardiac sympathetic neurons, but not in non-innervated cultured cardiomyocytes.[56] These findings support an ANG II–mediated functional relationship between cardiomyocytes and cardiac neurons. Further, direct ANG II infusion into intrathoracic ganglia containing adrenergic neurons produced augmentation of heart rate as well as right and left ventricular inotropism that was blocked by pretreatment with either a β-AR blocker or an AT_1-receptor blocker.[56,71] These studies indicate that ANG II enhances cardiac contractile function by stimulating intrinsic cardiac adrenergic neurons to release NE into the cardiac interstitium.

In a study using the cardiac microdialysis technique in the dog in vivo, exogenous administration of ANG II to a population of intrinsic cardiac neurons led to an increase in release of NE and EPI into the cardiac ISF space, independent of peripheral systemic effects mediated by adrenal glands (Fig. 12–4).[41] Further, the level of NE in the ISF during exogenous ANG II infusion was equivalent to ISF NE levels achieved during high-level electrical stimulation of the stellate ganglia (i.e., all sympathetic efferent neurons). In contrast to the response to stellate stimulation, activation of adrenergic neurons with ANG II was not associated with spillover of catecholamines from the heart.[41] These findings indicate that different subpopulations of adrenergic neurons can be activated, depending on the stress induced. In another study, direct infusion of ANG II into the cardiac interstitium of the rat heart via microdialysis probes resulted in a dose-dependent increase in interstitial NE that was blocked by the co-administration of an AT_1-receptor blocker.[102]

The anatomical relationship of AT_1 receptors with cardiac neurons may account in part for the fact that ANG II–induced hypertension[34,43] and myocyte necrosis and fibrosis[52,53] are prevented by β-adrenergic blockade. Furthermore, the myocyte necrosis and coronary vascular damage that occur within the first 3 days following elevation of circulating ANG II are prevented by AT_1-receptor blockade and significantly attenuated by $β_1$-receptor blockade. Yet, in this animal model, the ANG II–induced increase in plasma NE did not occur until day 4, and it was prevented by AT_1 receptor blockade. Furthermore, continuous ANG II infusion caused a progressive decrease in $β_1$-AR density in these rat hearts. These studies suggest that the deleterious effects of exogenously infused ANG II are mediated by enhanced local catecholamine release via activation of AT_1 receptors on cardiac adrenergic neurons. Asano and coworkers[5a] found a significant positive correlation between AT_1- and β_1-receptor densities in human failing and unfailing left ventricles, suggesting a possibility that down-regulation of two receptor systems is pathophysiologically related and modulated by local concentrations of ANG II and NE, respectively.

A clinical trial (ELITE) demonstrated that AT_1-antagonist (losartan) was superior to ACE inhibitor therapy (captopril) in lowering mortality (specifically, mortality from sudden death) and in preventing hospitalizations in older patients with heart failure.[86] Recent studies in mice devoid of the AT_{1a} receptor, in which myocardial infarction was evoked by coronary artery ligation, demonstrated that ventricular arrhythmias during reperfusion were significantly less in the knockout than in the wild type, despite no difference in infarct size.[48] Further, pretreatment with a selective AT_1 antagonist in the wild-type mice blocked reperfusion arrhythmias but had no effect on infarct size. Taken together, these findings suggest that ANG II activation of the AT_1 receptor may be critically involved in the induction of ventricular arrhythmias in ischemia and heart failure, in part by enhanced NE release via activation of AT_1 receptors on cardiac neurons.

During progression into CHF, evidence indicates that there is reorganization (or remodeling) of the interactions between tissue ANG II and the intrathoracic noradrenergic system. Himura et al. have shown that chronic NE infusion leads to a reduction of cardiac noradrenergic efferent nerves, as is found in the failing myocardium.[54] This occurred at much higher plasma NE levels in NE-infused animals than in heart failure animals, suggesting a local NE release into cardiac interstitium in the failing heart due to increased sympathetic drive that may also be related to an increase in wall stress or local ANG II mechanisms. In addition, a recent study demonstrated a marked reduction in the transcardiac venoarterial plasma nerve growth factor (NGF) in patients with heart failure compared to levels in normals.[63] The plasma arterial concentration of NGF was also substantially lower in CHF patients. In a rat model of CHF, a 40% reduction ($P < 0.05$) in NGF mRNA expression was apparent in association with a 24% reduction in tissue NGF content ($P < 0.05$). Evidence of reduced sympathetic innervation in the failing heart was apparent, as measured histologically by catecholamine fluorescence and by expression of the neuronal NGF receptor trkA. Norepinephrine (10 μmol/L) exposure reduced both NGF mRNA and protein expression in isolated cardiomyocytes, a result suggesting that myocardial NGF down-regulation may represent an adaptive response to sympathetic overactivity. Chronic myocardial infarction has also been associated with alterations in the innervation of the affected ventricle, and the resultant heterogeneous remodeling of the adrenergic innervation has been associated with induction of spontaneous ventricular tachycardia, ventricular fibrillation, and sudden cardiac death.[16] Taken together, these findings indicate that NGF expression in the heart is dynamic and may be altered in cardiovascular disease states. In CHF, reduced NGF expression may account in part for alterations in sympathetic neuronal function and neuroanatomy.

Data in other animal models suggest that increased local NE release into the interstitium of the failing heart due to increased sympathetic drive may also involve local ANG II mechanisms. Senzaki et al.[95] showed that ANG II infusion for 4 days followed by 48-hour pacing (during continued ANG II infusion) produced a marked exacerbation of LV dysfunction and MMP activation when compared to pacing alone, an effect that was prevented by pretreatment with a high dose of a selective β_1-AR blocker. Further, high-dose β_1-receptor blockade during ANG II infusions prevented MMP activation as well as myocardial tissue damage and inflammation. The mechanism for this synergistic effect remains speculative; however, there is evidence supporting the hypothesis that NE and ANG II may act directly or indirectly to activate MMPs via interactions with inflammatory cytokines or reactive oxygen species.[95]

In the volume overload model of experimentally induced mitral regurgitation (MR) in the dog, neurohumoral interactions between ANG II and the sympathetic nervous system are augmented, with important consequences for the ECM and maintenance of basal cardiac function. The canine model of MR is characterized by an absence of fibrosis and by dissolution of the fine collagen weave.[101] Loss of the fine collagen weave destroys the structural support of the ECM that is necessary for maintenance of normal LV chamber geometry and for the translation of forces from individual cardiomyocytes to the LV chamber.[78] β_1-Receptor blockade decreased renin–angiotensin system sympathoactivation by attenuating the ANG II–mediated NE and EPI release into the cardiac ISF (Figs. 12–5 and 12–6) and circulation and by decreasing LV ACE expression in the early phases of volume overload.[101] β_1-Receptor blockade also attenuates increases in ISF ANG II in MR dogs, most likely because of direct local suppression as well as the suppression of kidney renin production and release. It is now appreciated that cardiac renin receptors and uptake of renin represent an important regulatory mechanism in the formation of cardiac ANG II.[94] Importantly, treatment with β_1-receptor blockade was also associated with prevention of ECM degradation, which is an early key component of the pathological LV remodeling in this volume overload model of heart failure. It is of great interest that treatment of dogs with β-adrenergic blockade for 3 months after 3 months of experimen-

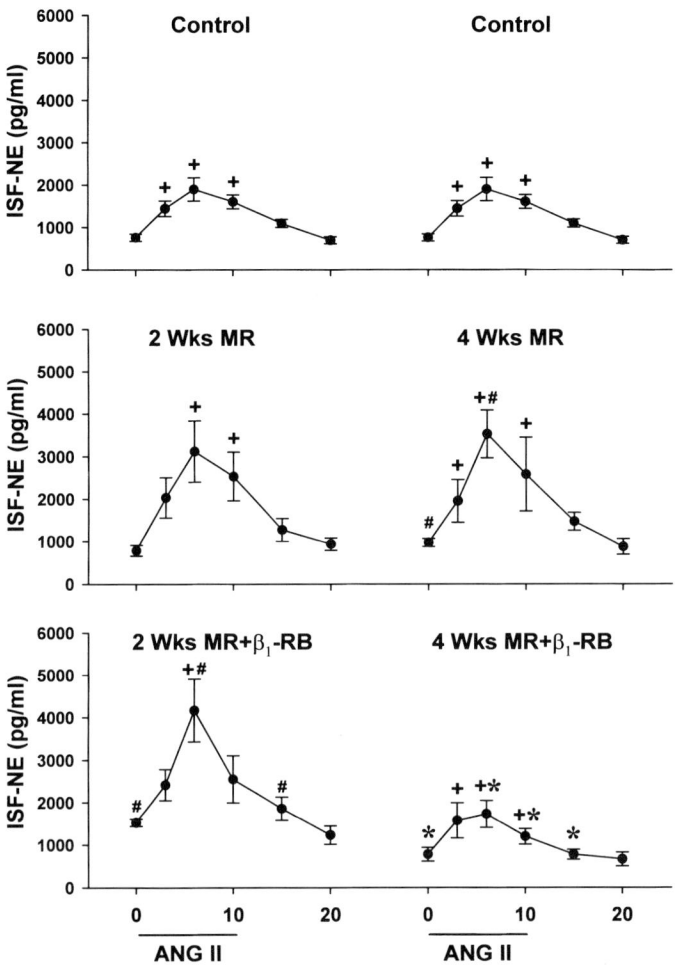

FIGURE 12-5 Interstitial fluid (ISF) norepinephrine (NE) responses to angiotensin II (ANG II) infusion in control, 2- and 4-week mitral regurgitation (MR), and 2- and 4-week MR + β_1-receptor blockade (RB) dogs. $+P < 0.05$ versus baseline; $^\#P < 0.05$ vs. control; $^*P < 0.05$ versus 2-week MR + β_1-RB. (Adapted from Tallaj et al.[101])

tally induced MR resulted in improved LV chamber and isolated cardiomyocyte contractile function, which in turn was associated with an increase in the number of contractile elements within cardiomyocytes.[107]

The suggestion that β_1-receptor blockade impacts the rate of transcardiac collagen degradation is particularly intriguing, and could explain the impressive beneficial effects of β-receptor blockade on LV remodeling in heart failure. With regard to the synergistic effects of the nora-

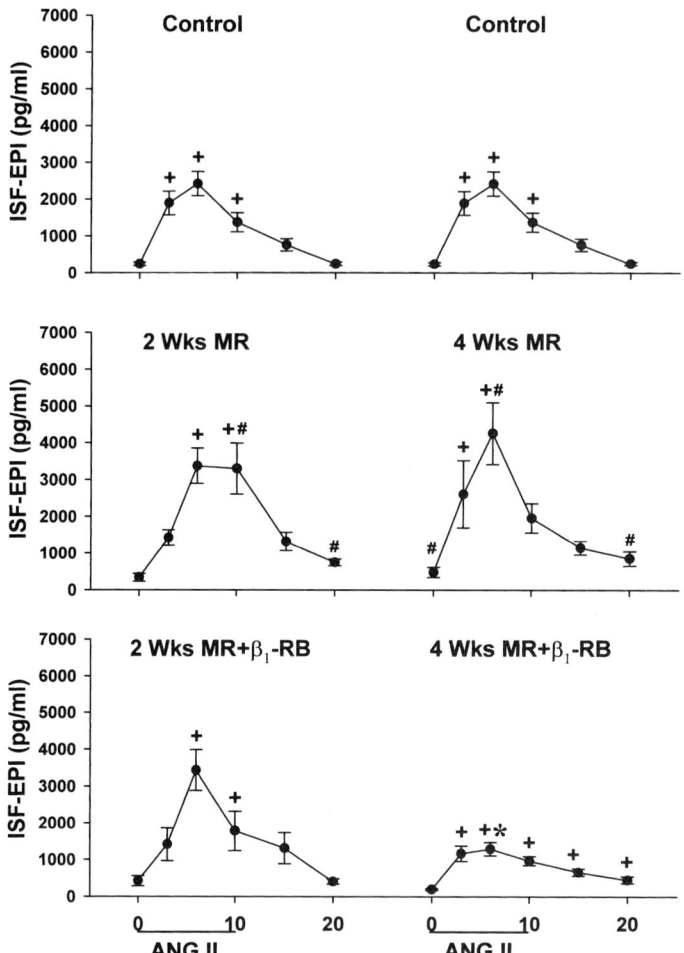

FIGURE 12-6 Interstitial fluid (ISF) epinephrine (EPI) responses to angiotensin II (ANG II) in control, 2- and 4-week mitral regurgitation (MR), and 2- and 4-week MR + β_1-receptor blockade (RB) dogs. $^+P < 0.05$ versus baseline, $^\#P < 0.05$ versus control; $^*P < 0.05$ versus 2-week MR + β_1-RB. (Adapted from Tallaj et al.[101])

drenergic and renin–angiotensin systems, NE and ANG II may act directly or indirectly to activate MMPs via interactions with inflammatory cytokines or reactive oxygen species.[99] Taken together, these animal models demonstrate that β_1-blockade exerts important effects on MMP and renin–angiotensin system activation, as well as on the progression of LV and cardiomyocyte remodeling. That such therapy acts in part by mitigating adverse remodeling of the cardiac nervous system represents a novel model for understanding the complexity of this pathology.

CARDIAC REMODELING IN CLINICAL TRIALS WITH β-RECEPTOR BLOCKADE

In clinical trials of patients with heart failure, improved LV function is defined as an increase in LV ejection fraction (EF) of at least five EF units and a reversal of cardiac remodeling assessed in terms of ejection fraction, ventricular volume or dimension, or LV mass and chamber shape.[8,33,36,43a,45,47,89] According to this definition of a response, favorable changes occur in 50% to 70% of β-AR blocker–treated patients.[31,76] But, it is not intuitively obvious how blocking a pathway that increases contractility in normal hearts should be therapeutic in patients with decreased cardiac function. The mechanism for the improved function with β-AR blocker–treated patients has gained some insight from recent studies in patients with various forms dilated cardiomyopathy.

In a recent study, 53 patients with idiopathic dilated cardiomyopathy were randomly assigned to treatment with a β-AR blocking agent (metoprolol or carvedilol) or placebo and subsequently had RV endomyocardial biopsy 6 months later.[76] Twenty-six of 32 β-blocker–treated patients had an improvement in LV EF of at least 5 EF units (mean [±SE] increase, 18.8 ± 1.8). Compared with the six β-AR blocker–treated patients who did not have a response (mean change, a decrease of 2.5 ± 1.8 EF units), those who did have a response had an increase in sarcoplasmic-reticulum calcium ATPase mRNA and α-myosin heavy-chain mRNA and a decrease in β-myosin heavy-chain mRNA. There were no differences between those who had a response and those who did not in terms of the change in mRNA or protein expression of β-AR. In another study, sarcoplasmic reticulum Ca^{2+} ATPase in the β-AR blocker–treated patients with ischemic and nonischemic cardiomyopathies was greater than that in non–β-AR blocker CHF patients and was not different from that in nonfailing human hearts.[66] Ca^{2+} transients in non–β-AR blocker CHF myocytes had significantly smaller peaks and were prolonged, compared to myocytes from nonfailing hearts. Taken together, β-receptor blockade treatment in CHF patients can normalize the abundance of myocyte Ca^{2+} regulatory proteins and improve Ca^{2+} handling.

In a very elegant study of hearts taken from patients undergoing transplantation, passive ventricular pressure–volume relationships were measured by placing compliant balloons in the extirpated right and left ventricles.[88] In hearts from patients receiving β-AR blocker therapy, there was reduced LV volume (reverse remodeling) (Fig. 12–7) and a restored β-agonist response in cardiac muscle, compared with hearts taken from patients with CHF who did not receive β-AR blockers. The hyperadrenergic state of heart failure results in leaky ryanodine receptor (RyR2)

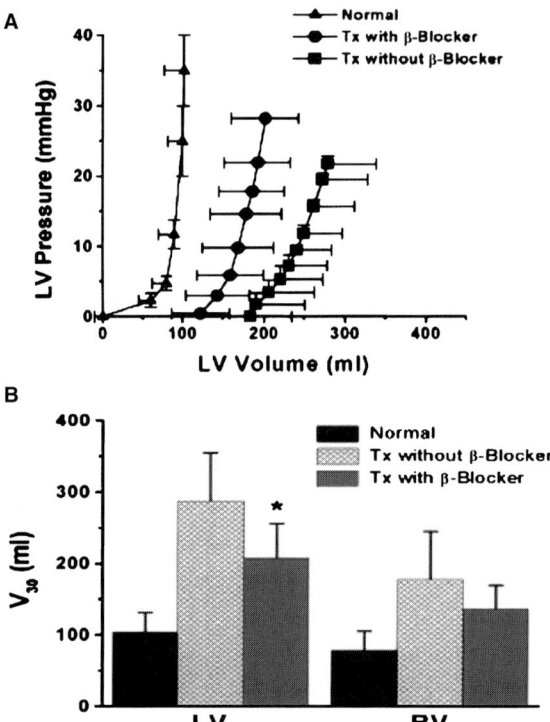

FIGURE 12–7 Ex vivo, passive pressure–volume relationships measured from hearts of transplant patients receiving β-blockers (circles: treatment [Tx] with β-blockers, $n = 6$) were shifted toward significantly lower volumes with steeper slope compared with those measured from transplant patients not receiving β-blockers (squares: treatment without β-blockers, $n = 5$). These curves were shifted toward larger volumes with lower slopes than those of normal hearts not suitable for transplant (triangles: normal, $n = 5$). B. Volume at which ex vivo passive pressure is 30 mmHg (V_{30}) for the left (LV) and right (RV) ventricles of hearts from the three different groups of hearts (normal, $n = 5$; treatment without β-blocker, $n = 7$; treatment with β-blocker, $n = 6$). *$P < 0.05$ for therapy with β-AR blocker (Tx with β-blocker) versus therapy without β-AR blocker (Tx without β-blocker). (From Reiken et al.[88])

channels attributable to protein kinase (PKA) hyperphosphorylation and depletion of the stabilizing FK506 binding protein, FKBP12.6. The improvement in chamber function was associated with restoration of normal FKBP12.6 levels in the cardiac RyR2 receptor macromolecular complex and RyR2 channel function. A similar improvement in LV remodeling was found in patients with idiopathic dilated cardiomyopathy who received a β_1-AR blocking agent (metoprolol) for 6 months, manifested by significant improvement in chamber stiffness, systolic elastance, and isovolumic relaxation index.[64] Taken together with the studies mentioned above, these changes in RyR2 function and the up-regulation of SERCA2a and α-myosin heavy chain likely contribute to improved cardiac contractility observed in patients treated with β-AR blockers.

INTERACTION OF INFLAMMATORY CYTOKINES AND THE NORADRENERGIC SYSTEM

There is increasing evidence that oxidative stress is increased in myocardial failure and may play an important role in the structural and functional changes that lead to the progression of heart failure. The cardiovascular system is continuously exposed to both reactive oxygen species (ROS) and reactive nitrogen species (RNS), collectively termed reactive inflammatory species (RIS). Indeed, ROS are increased and antioxidant capacity is decreased in models of heart failure. In particular, increased iNOS expression and activity has been reported in heart failure of various origins in animal models and in patients.[51,64,114] Furthermore, some reports support the notion that excessive nitric oxide (NO) production contributes to β-adrenergic hyporesponsiveness in patients with heart failure.[44,49,51,111,114] Recent studies in vivo[87] and in vitro[26] provide evidence that β-receptor blockade reduces RIS production in heart failure models and in isolated cardiomyocytes.

Elevated circulating and myocardial levels of TNF-α, IL-1β, and IL-6 have been reported in patients, with plasma levels correlating with severity of disease.[103,106] Inflammatory cytokines induce biological effects similar to the phenotypic changes of heart failure, including contractile depression, myocyte growth and induction of a fetal gene program, myocyte apoptosis, and ECM alterations.[65,99,113] Mechanisms of cytokine-induced contractile depression proposed include altered β-receptor coupling to adenylyl cyclase, increased NO and peroxynitrite formation, and alterations in intracellular Ca^{2+} handling.[24,65,105,109,112]

A recent study demonstrated that LV dysfunction after myocardial infarction in the rat is associated with marked increases in myocardial gene expression and protein production of TNF-α, IL-1β, and IL-6 in the non-infarcted zone without increased expression of myocardial inducible (iNOS) or endothelial (ecNOS). Although there is marked associated β-adrenergic hyporesponsiveness, this is not related to ongoing increased myocardial NO production. Selective β_1-AR blockade with metoprolol in this setting improves LV remodeling and systolic function, restores isoproterenol sensitivity via NO-independent mechanisms, and selectively decreases myocardial gene expression and protein production of TNF-α

and IL-1β but not IL-6. In addition, a nonselective β-AR blocker, carvedilol, significantly inhibited ROS generation and oxidative capacity by leukocytes in vitro.[87] In summary, these results suggest that activation of the adrenergic nervous system during development of heart failure contributes to increased ROS and myocardial expression of TNF-α and IL-1β and that one mechanism underlying the salutary effects of β-blockade in heart failure may relate to attenuation of myocardial expression of ROS and TNF-α and IL-1β.

INTERACTION OF THE KALLIKREIN KININ SYSTEM AND THE NORADRENERGIC SYSTEM

There is mounting evidence that BK, acting at the BK_2 receptor, enhances NE release and exacerbates arrhythmias and ventricular fibrillation in myocardial ischemia/reperfusion.[79–81] Seyedi and co-workers (96,97) demonstrated an active kallikrein/kinin system in a preparation of sympathetic nerve endings from the guinea pig heart that produced NE exocytosis when BK synthesis was increased or when its breakdown was retarded by ACE inhibitor treatment. This observation is consistent with

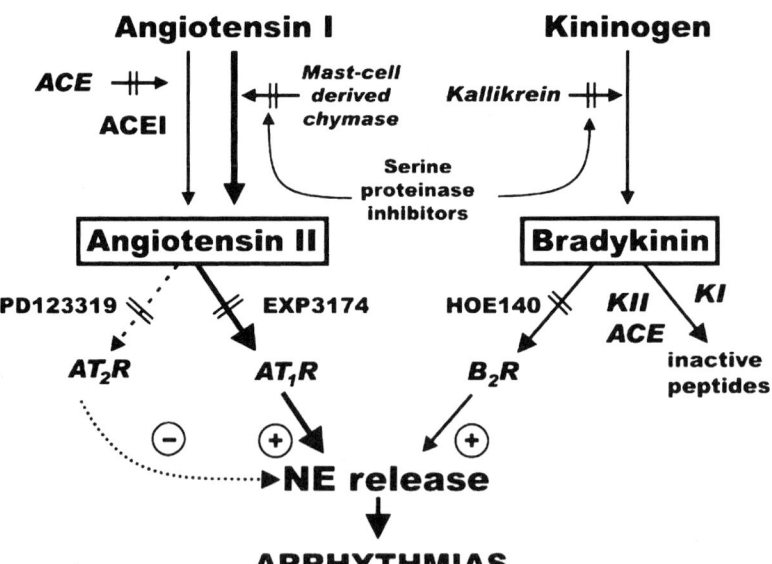

FIGURE 12–8 Schema defining the interaction of the renin–angiotensin system and kallikrein–kinin system in the mechanism of norepinephrine (NE) release from nerve terminals in the heart during myocardial ischemia. (From Maruyama et al.[80])

the finding of diminished NE release from isolated atria of $BK_2r^{-/-}$ mice. Bradykinin facilitates NE release from cardiac sympathetic nerve endings,[96,97] and its production increases in myocardial ischemia.[79,81] Furthermore, B_2R stimulation by exogenous BK markedly enhances carrier-mediated NE in a human model of myocardial ischemia.[50]

A proposed summary, which includes the renin–angiotensin system and kallikein–kinin system in the heart, is outlined in Figure 12–8. In protracted human myocardial ischemia, ANG II is formed locally from ANG I predominantly by ACE and mast cell–derived chymase, a highly efficient ANG II–forming mechanism. Angiotensin II promotes NE release by acting at AT_1 receptors on sympathetic neurons,[56] including their nerve terminals.[82] Although the AT_1 receptor–mediated enhancement of NE release is likely to prevail, ANG II may also exert an AT_2 receptor–mediated inhibitory effect, which is unmasked when AT_1 receptors are blocked.[6,80] Bradykinin production in myocardial ischemia,[81] in part, by protease activation of kallikrein, contributes ischemic NE release.[50] However, some studies report that its effect is probably less important than that of ANG II.[79] Taken together, BK accumulates in the cardiac interstitium where it interacts directly with sympathetic nerve terminals to promote a deleterious effect by excessive NE release.

CONCLUSIONS

Remodeling of the cardiac nervous system directly affects the remodeling of myocytes and of the cardiac extracellular matrix, as underscored by the remarkable effects of β-adrenergic receptor blockade in clinical trials and animal models of heart failure. The central role of a hyperactive sympathetic nervous system in cardiac disease is even more impressive because it is not intuitively obvious how blocking a pathway that increases contractility and has little to no effect on systemic afterload of normal hearts should be of therapeutic benefit to patients with decreased cardiac function. The many beneficial effects of β-AR blockade certainly start at the β-adrenergic receptors, but there are also indirect effects mediated by regulation of other neurohormonal systems and inflammation.

REFERENCES

1. Abraham WT, Lowes BD, Roden RL, Gilbert MR, Havranek EP, Whit M, Zisman LS, Rose CP, and Bristow MR. Mechanism of increased cardiac adrenergic activity in heart failure; evidence for decreased cardiac neuronal norepinephrine reuptake [abstract]. *Circulation* (Suppl) 96(8):I92, 1997.

2. Akiyama T, Yamazaki T, and Ninomiya I. In vivo monitoring of myocardial interstitial norepinephrine by dialysis technique. *Am J Physiol (Heart Circ Physiol)* 261(30):H1643–H1647, 1991.
3. Altschuld RA, Starling RC, Hamin RL, et al. Response of the failing canine and human heart cells to β_2-adrenergic stimulation. *Circulation* 92:1612–1618, 1995.
4. Armour JA. Canine intrinsic cardiac neurons involved in cardiac regulation possess α_1-, α_2, β_1- and β_2-ARs. *Can J Cardiol* 13:277–284, 1997.
5. Armstrong PQ, Stopps TP, Ford SE, and deBold AJ. Rapid ventricular pacing in the dog: pathophysiologic studies of heart failure. *Circulation* 74:1075–1084, 1986.
5a. Asano K, Dutcher DL, Port JD, Minobe WA, Tremmel KD, Roden RL, Bohlmeyer TJ, Bush EW, Jenkin MJ, Abraham WT, Raynolds MV, Zisman LS, Perryman MB, and Bristow MR. Selective downregulation of the AT_1-receptor subtype in failing human ventricular myocardium. *Circulation* 95:1193–1200, 1997.
6. Balt JC, Mathy MJ, Nap A, Pfaffendorf M, and van Zwieten PA. Involvement of the AT(2)-receptor in angiotensin II-induced facilitation of sympathetic neurotransmission. *J Renin Angiotensin Aldosterone Syst* 3:181–187, 2002.
7. Blumberg AL, Ackerly JA, and Peach MJ. Differentiation of neurogenic and myocardial angiotensin II receptors in isolated rabbit atria. *Circ Res* 36:719–726, 1975.
8. Bohm M, Deutsch HJ, Hartmann D, Rosee KL, and Stablein A. Improvement of postreceptor events by metoprolol treatment in patients with chronic heart failure. *J Am Coll Cardiol* 30:992–996, 1997.
9. Bohm M, Rosee KL, Schwinger RHG, and Erdmann E. Evidence for reduction of norepinephrine uptake sites in the failing human heart. *J Am Coll Cardiol* 25:146–153, 1985.
10. Brasch H, Sieroslawski L, and Dominiak P. Angiotensin II increases norepinephrine release from atria by acting on angiotensin subtype 1 receptors. *Hypertension* 22(5):699–704, 1993.
11. Brink M, de Gasparo M, Rogg H, et al. Localization of angiotensin II receptor subtypes in the rabbit heart. *J Mol Cell Cardiol* 27:459–470, 1995.
12. Bristow MR. β-adrenergic receptor blockade in chronic heart failure. *Circulation* 101:558–569, 2001.
13. Bristow MR. What type of β-blocker should be used to treat chronic heart failure? *Circulation* 102:484, 2000.
14. Bristow MR, Ginsburg R, Umans V, Fowler M, Minobe W, Rasmussen R, Zera P, Menlove R, Shah P, Jamieson S, and Stinson EB. β_1- and β_2-adrenergic-receptor subpopulations in nonfailing and failing human ventricular myocardium: coupling of both receptor subtypes to muscle contraction and selective β_1-receptor down-regulation in heart failure. *Circ Res* 59:297–309, 1986.
15. Bristow MR, Minobe W, Raynolds MV, et al. Reduced β_1 receptor mRNA abundance in the failing human heart. *J Clin Invest* 92:2737–2745, 1993.
16. Cao J-M, Chen LS, KenKnight BH, Ohara T, Lee M-H, Tsai J, Lai WW, Karagueuzian HS, Wolf PL, Fishbein MC, and Chen P-S. Nerve sprouting and sudden cardiac death. *Circ Res* 86:816, 2000.

17. Cardinal R, Nadeau R, Laurent C, Boudreau G, and Armour JA. Reduced capacity of cardiac efferent sympathetic neurons to release noradrenaline and modify cardiac function in tachycardia-induced canine heart failure. *Can J Physiol Pharmacol* 74:1070–1078, 1996.
18. Castran E, Kurihara M, Gutkind JS, and Saavendra JM. Specific angiotensin II binding sites in rat stellate and superior cervical ganglia. *Brain Res* 422: 347–351, 1987.
19. Castro L and Freeman BA. Reactive oxygen species in human health and disease. *Nutrition* 17:161, 163–165, 2001.
20. Chesley A, Lundberg MS, Asai T, et al. The β_2-adrenergic receptor delivers an antiapoptotic signal to cardiac myocytes through G_i-dependent coupling to phosphatidylinositol 3'-kinase. *Circ Res* 87:1172–1179, 2000.
21. Chidsey CA, Braunwald E, and Morrow AG. Catecholamine excretion and cardiac stores of norepinephrine in congestive heart failure. *Am J Med* 39:442, 1965.
22. Chidsey CA, Kaiser GA, Sonnenblick EH, et al. Cardiac norepinephrine stores in experimental heart failure in the dog. *J Clin Invest* 43:2386–2393, 1964.
23. Chidsey CA, Sonneblick EH, Morrow AG, and Braunwald E. Norepinephrine stores and contractile force of papillary muscle from the failing human heart. *Circulation* 33:43, 1966.
24. Chung MK, Gulick TS, Rotondo RE, Schreiner GF, and Lange LG. Mechanism of cytokine inhibition of β-adrenergic agonist stimulation of cyclic AMP in rat cardiac myocytes: impairment of signal transduction. *Circ Res* 67:753–763, 1990.
25. Communal C, Singh K, Sawyer DB, and Colucci WS. Opposing effects of β_1- and β_2-adrenergic receptors on cardiac myocyte apoptosis: role of pertussis toxin-sensitive G protein. *Circulation* 100:2210–2212, 1999.
26. Dandona P, Karne R, Ghanim H, Hamouda W, Aljada A, Magsino CH. Carvedilol inhibits reactive oxygen species generation by leukocytes and oxidative damage to amino acids. *Circulation* 101:122–124, 2000.
27. Davis D, Baily R, and Zelis RJ. Abnormalities in systemic norepinephrine kinetics in human congestive heart failure. *Am J Physiol* 254:E760–E766, 1988.
28. Delehanty JM, Himura Y, Elam H, Hood WB, Jr, and Liang C. β-Adrenoceptor downregulation in pacing-induced heart failure is associated with an increased interstitial NE content. *Am J Physiol (Heart Circ Physiol)* 266(35): H930–H935, 1994.
29. DeQuattro V, Nagatsu T, Mendez A, and Verska J. Determinants of cardiac noradrenaline depletion in human congestive heart failure. *Cardiovasc Res* 7:344, 1973.
30. Dhalla AK and Singal PK. Antioxidant changes in hypertrophied and failing guinea pig hearts. *Am J Physiol* 266:H1280–H1285, 1994.
31. Di Lenarda A, Sabbadini G, Salvatore L, Sinagra G, Mestroni L, Pinamonti B, Gregori D, Ciani F, Muzzi A, Klugmann S, Camerini F, and The Heart-Muscle Disease Study. Long-term effects of carvedilol in idiopathic dilated cardiomyopathy with persistent left ventricular dysfunction despite chronic metoprolol. *J Am Coll Cardiol* 33:1926–1934, 1999.
32. Dostal DE and Baker KM. Evidence for a role of an intracardiac renin-angiotensin system in normal and failing hearts. *Trends Cardiovasc Med* 3:67–74, 1993.

33. Doughty RN, Whalley GA, Gamble G, MacMahon S, Sharpe N, on behalf of the Australia-New Zealand Heart Failure Research Collaborative Group. Left ventricular remodeling with carvedilol in patients with congestive heart failure due to ischemic heart disease. *J Am Coll Cardiol* 29:1060–1066, 1997.
34. Doursout MF, Chelley JE, Hartley CJ, Szilagyi J, Montastruc JL, and Buckley JP. Regional blood flows and cardiac function changes induced by angiotensin II in conscious dogs. *J Pharmacol Exp Ther* 246:591–596, 1988.
35. Eaton GM, Cody RJ, Nunziata E, and Binkley PF. Early left ventricular dysfunction elicits activation of sympathetic drive and attenuation of parasympathetic tone in the paced canine model of congestive heart failure. *Circulation* 92:555–561, 1995.
36. Eichhorn EJ and Bristow MR. Medical therapy can improve the biological properties of the chronically failing heart. A new era in the treatment of heart failure. *Circulation* 94:2285–2296, 1996.
37. Eisenhofer G, Friberg P, Rundqvist B, Quyyumi AA, Lambert G, Kaye DM, Kopin IJ, Goldstein DS, and Esler MD. Cardiac sympathetic nerve function in congestive heart failure. *Circulation* 93:1667–1676, 1996.
38. Engelhardt S, Hein L, Wiesmann F, and Lohse MJ. Progressive hypertrophy and heart failure in β_1-adrenergic receptor transgenic mice. *Proc Natl Acad Sci USA* 96:7059–7064, 1999.
39. Esler M, Jennings G, Lambert G, Meredith I, Horne M, and Eisenhofer G. Overflow of catecholamine neurotransmitters to the circulation: source, fate and function. *Physiol Rev* 70(4):963–985, 1990.
40. Esler M, Kaye D, Lambert G, Esler D, and Jennings G. Adrenergic nervous system in heart failure. *Am J Cardiol* 80:7L–14L, 1997.
41. Farrell DM, Wei CC, Tallaj J, et al. Angiotensin II modulates catecholamine release into the interstitial fluid of the canine myocardium in vivo. *Am J Physiol* 281:H813–H822, 2001.
42. Finkel MS, Oddis CV, Jacob TD, Watkins SC, Hattler BG, and Simmons RL. Negative inotropic effects of cytokines on the heart mediated by nitric oxide. *Science* 257:387–389, 1992.
43. Foucart S, Patrick SK, Oster L, and de Champlain J. Effects of chronic treatment with losartan and enalaprilat on [^{3}H]-norepinephrine release from isolated atria of Wistar-Kyoto and spontaneously hypertensive rats. *Am J Hypertens* 9:61–9, 1996.
43a. Fowler MB, Vera-Llonch M, Oster G, Bristow MR, Cohn JN, Colucci WS, Gilbert EM, Lukas MA, Lacey MJ, Richner R, Young ST, and Packer M for the U.S. Carvedilol Heart Failure Study Group. Influence of carvedilol on hospitalizations in heart failure: incidence, resource utilization and costs. *J Am Coll Cardiol* 37:1692–1699, 2001.
43. Fujii AM and Vatner SF. Direct versus indirect pressor and vasoconstrictor actions of angiotensin in conscious dogs. *Hypertension* 7:253–261, 1985.
44. Gealekman O, Abassi Z, Rubinstein I, Winaver J, and Binah O. Role of myocardial inducible nitric oxide synthase in contractile dysfunction and β-adrenergic hyporesponsiveness in rats with experimental volume-overload heart failure. *Circulation* 105:236–243, 2002.
45. Gilbert EM, Abraham WT, Olsen S, Hattler B, White M, Mealy P, Larrabee P, and Bristow MR. Comparative hemodynamic, left ventricular functional,

and antiadrenergic effects of chronic treatment with metoprolol versus carvedilol in the failing heart. *Circulation* 94:2817–2825, 1996.

46. Grassi G, Seravalle G, Cattaneo BM, Lanfranchi A, Vailati S, Giannattasio C, Del Bo A, Sala C, Bolla GB, Pozzi M, and Mancia G. Sympathetic activation and loss of reflex sympathetic control in mild congestive heart failure. *Circulation* 92:3206–3211, 1995.

47. Hall SA, Cigarroa CG, Marcoux L, Risser RC, Grayburn PA, and Eichhorn EJ. Time course of improvement in left ventricular function, mass and geometry in patients with congestive heart failure treated with beta-adrenergic blockade. *J Am Coll Cardiol* 25:1154–1161, 1995.

48. Harada K, Komuro I, Hayashi D, Sugaya T, Murakami, and Yazaki Y. Angiotensin II type 1a receptor is involved in the occurrence of reperfusion arrhythmias. *Circulation* 97:315–317, 1998.

49. Hare JM, Loh E, Creager MA, and Colucci WS. Nitric oxide inhibits the positive inotropic response to β-adrenergic stimulation in humans with left ventricular dysfunction. *Circulation* 92:2198–2203, 1995.

50. Hatta E, Maruyama R, Marshall SJ, Imamura M, and Levi R. Bradykinin promotes ischemic norepinephrine release in guinea pig and human hearts. *J Pharmacol Exp Ther* 288:919–927, 1999.

51. Haywood GA, Tsao PS, von der Leyen HE, Mann MJ, Keeling PJ, Trinidade PT, Lewis NP, Byrne CD, Rickenbacher PR, Bishopric NH, Cooke JP, McKenna WJ, and Fowler MB. Expression of inducible nitric oxide synthase in human heart failure. *Circulation* 93:1087–1094, 1996.

52. Henegar JR, Brower GL, Kabour A, et al. Catecholamine response to chronic ANG II infusion and its role in myocyte and coronary vascular damage. *Am J Physiol* 269:H1564–H1569, 1995.

53. Henegar JR, Schwartz DD, and Janicki JS. ANG II-related myocardial damage: role of cardiac sympathetic catecholamines and β-receptor regulation. *Am J Physiol* 275:H534–H541, 1998.

54. Himura Y, Felton SY, Kashiki M, Lewandowski TJ, Delehanty JM, and Liang C-S. Cardiac noradrenergic nerve terminal abnormalities in dogs with experimental congestive heart failure. *Circulation* 88:1299–1309, 1998.

55. Huang M-H, Friend DS, Sunday ME, Singh K, Haley K, Austen F, Kelly RA, and Smith TW. An intrinsic adrenergic system in mammalian heart. *J Clin Invest* 98:1298–1303, 1996.

56. Horackova M and Armour JA. ANG II modifies cardiomyocyte function via extracardiac and intracardiac neurons: in situ and in vitro studies. *Am J Physiol* 272:R766–R755, 1997.

57. Imamura Y, Ando H, Ashihara T, and Fukuyama T. Myocardial adrenergic nervous activity is intensified in patients without left ventricular volume or pressure overload. *J Am Coll Cardiol* 28:371–375, 1996.

58. Joseph J and Gilbert EM. The sympathetic nervous system in chronic heart failure. *Prog Cardiovasc Dis* 41:9–16, 1998.

59. Kaul N, Siveski-Iliskovic N, Hill M, Slezak J, and Singal PK. Free radicals and the heart. *J Pharmacol Toxicol Methods* 30:55–67, 1993.

60. Kawada T, Yamazaki T, Akiyama T, Shishido T, Miyano H, Sato T, Sugimachi M, Alexander J, Jr, and Sugnagawa K. Interstitial norepinephrine level by cardiac microdialysis correlates with ventricular contractility. *Am J Physiol (Heart Circ Physiol)* 273(42):H1107–H1112, 1997.

61. Kawai H, Mohan A, Hagen J, Dong E, Armstrong J, Stevens SY, and Liang C-S. Alterations in cardiac adrenergic terminal function and β-adrenoreceptor density in pacing-induced heart failure. *Am J Physiol* 278:H1708–H1716, 2000.
62. Kaye DM, Lefkovits J, Jennings GL, Bergin P, Broughton A, and Esler MD. Adverse consequences of high sympathetic nervous activity in the failing human heart. *J Am Coll Cardiol* 26:1257–1263, 1993.
63. Kaye DM, Vaddadi G, Gruskin SL, Du X-J, and Esler MD. Reduced myocardial nerve growth factor expression in human and experimental heart failure. *Circ Res* 86:e80, 2000.
64. Kim MH, Devlin WH, Das SK, Petrusha J, Montgomery D, and Starling MR. Effects of β-adrenergic blocking therapy on left ventricular diastolic relaxation properties in patients with dilated cardiomyopathy. *Circulation* 100:729–735, 1999.
65. Krown KA, Page MT, Nguyen C, Zechner D, Gutierrez V, Comstock KL, Glembotski CC, Quintana PJE, and Sabbadini RA. Tumor necrosis factor alpha-induced apoptosis in cardiac myocytes: involvement of the sphingolipid signaling cascade in cardiac cell death. *J Clin Invest* 98:2854–2865, 1996.
66. Kubo H, Margulies KB, Piacentino V, Gaughan JP, and Houser SR. Patients with end-stage congestive heart failure treated with β-adrenergic receptor antagonists have improved ventricular myocyte calcium regulatory abundance. *Circulation* 104:1012–1018, 2001.
67. Kuschel M, Zhou YY, Spurgeon HA, et al. β_2-adrenergic cAMP signaling is uncoupled from phosphorylation of cytoplasmic proteins in canine heart. *Circulation* 99:2458–2465, 1999.
68. Kushiku K, Yamada H, Shibata K, Tokunaga R, Katsuragi T, and Furukawa T. Upregulation of immunoreactive angiotensin II release and angiotensinogen mRNA expression by high-frequency preganglionic stimulation at the canine cardiac sympathetic ganglia. *Circ Res* 88:110–116, 2001.
69. Lader AS, Xiao YF, Ishikawa Y, Cui Y, Vatner DE, Vatner SF, Homcy CJ, and Cantiello HF. Cardiac Gsα overexpression enhances L-type calcium channels through an adenylyl cyclase independent pathway. *Proc Natl Acad Sci USA* 95:9669–9674, 1998.
70. Lefkowitz RJ, Rockman HA, and Koch WJ. Catecholamines, cardiac β-ARs, and heart failure. *Circulation* 101:1634–1637, 2000.
71. Levett JM, Murphy DA, McGuirt, Ardell AS, and Armour JA. Cardiac augmentation can be maintained by continuous exposure of intrinsic cardiac neurons to a beta-adrenergic agonist or angiotensin II *Surg Res* 66:167–173, 1996.
72. Liang C-S, Fan THM, Sullebarger JT, and Sakamoto S. Decreased adrenergic neuronal uptake activity in experimental right heart failure: A chamber specific contributor to beta-adrenoreceptor downregulation. *J Clin Invest* 84:1267–1275, 1989.
73. Liang C-S, Frantz RP, Suematsu M, et al. Chronic β-adrenoreceptor blockade prevents the development of β-adrenergic subsensitivity in experimental right-sided congestive heart failure in dogs. *Circulation* 84:254–266, 1991.
74. Liggett SB, Tepe NM, Lorenz JN, et al. Early and delayed consequences of

β_2-adrenergic receptor overexpression in mouse hearts: critical role for expression level. *Circulation* 101:1701–1714, 2000.
75. Liggett SB, Wagoner LE, Craft LL, Hornung RW, Hoit BD, McIntosh TC, and Walsh RA. The Ile164 β_2-adrenergic receptor polymorphisms adversely affects the outcome of congestive heart failure. *J Clin Invest* 102:1534–1539, 1998.
76. Lowes BD, Gilbert EM, Abraham WT, Minobe WA, Larrabee P, Ferguson D, Wolfel EE, Lindenfeld J, Tsvetkova T, Robertson AD, Quaife RA, and Bristow MR. Myocardial gene expression in dilated cardiomyopathy treated with beta-blocking agents. *N Engl J Med* 346:1357–1365, 2002.
77. Mann DL, Kent RL, Parsons B, et al. Adrenergic effects on the biology of the adult mammalian cardiocyte. *Circulation* 85:790–804, 1992.
78. Mann DL and Spinale FG. Activation of matrix metalloproteinases in the failing human heart: breaking the tie that binds. *Circulation* 98:1699–1702, 1998.
79. Maruyama R, Hatta E, and Levi R. Norepinephrine release and ventricular fibrillation in myocardial ischemia/reperfusion: roles of angiotensin and bradykinin. *J Cardiovasc Pharmacol* 34:913–915, 1999.
80. Maruyama R, Hatta E, Yasuda K, Smith NCE, and Levi R. Angiotensin-converting enzyme-independent angiotensin formation in a human model of myocardial ischemia: modulation of norepinephrine release by angiotensin type 1 and angiotensin type 2 receptors. *J Pharmacol Exp Ther* 294: 248–254, 2000.
81. Matsuki T, Shoji T, Yoshida S, Kudoh Y, Motoe M, Inoue M, Nakata T, Hosoda S, Shimamoto K, Yellon D, and Iimura O. Sympathetically induced myocardial ischaemia causes the heart to release plasma kinin. *Cardiovasc Res* 21:428–432, 1987.
82. Moura D, Pinheiro H, Paiva MQ, and Guimaraes S. Prejunctional effects of angiotensin II and bradykinin in the heart and blood vessels. *J Auton Pharmacol* 19:321–325, 1999.
83. Newton GE, Azevedo ER, and Parker JD. Inotropic and sympathetic responses to the intracoronary infusion of a β_2-receptor agonist. A human in vivo study. *Circulation* 99:2402–2407, 1999.
84. Peronnet F, Boudreau G, De Champlain J, and Nadeau RA. Effect of increases in myocardial epinephrine content on epinephrine release from the dog heart. *Can J Physiol Pharmacol* 71:884–888, 1993.
85. Pierpont GL, Francis GS, Demaster EG, et al. Heterogeneous myocardial catecholamine concentrations in patients with congestive heart failure. *Am J Cardiol* 60:316–321, 1987.
86. Pitt B, Segal T, Martinez FA, Meurers G, Cowley AJ, Thomas I, Deedwania PC, Ney DE, Snavely DB, and Chang PI, on behalf of the ELITE STUDY Investigators. Randomized trial of losartan versus captopril in patients over 65 with heart failure (Evaluation of Losartan in the Elderly Study, ELITE). *Lancet* 349:747–752, 1997.
87. Prabhu SD, Chandrasekar B, Murray DR, and Freeman GL. β-adrenergic blockade in developing heart failure: effects on myocardial inflammatory cytokines, nitric oxide, and remodeling. *Circulation* 101:2103–2109, 2000.
88. Reiken S, Wehrens XHT, Vest JA, Barbone A, Klotz S, Mancini D, Burkhoff D, and Marks AR. β-Blockers restore calcium release channel function and

improve cardiac muscle performance in human heart failure. *Circulation* 107:2459–2466, 2003.
89. Richards AM, Doughty R, Nicholls MG, Macmahon S, Ikram H, Sharpe N, Espiner EA, Frampton C, and Yandle TG for the Australia-New Zealand Heart Failure Group. Neurohumoral prediction of benefit from carvedilol in ischemic left ventricular dysfunction. *Circulation* 99:786–792, 1999.
90. Rose CP, Burgess JH, and Cousineau D. Tracer norepinephrine kinetics in coronary circulation of patients with heart failure secondary to chronic pressure and volume overload. *J Clin Invest* 76:1740–1747, 1985.
91. Rundqvist B, Elam M, Bergmann-Sverrisdottir Y, Eisenhofer G, and Friberg P. Increased cardiac adrenergic drive precedes generalized sympathetic activation in human heart failure. *Circulation* 95:169–175, 1997.
92. Saavedra J, Viswanathan M, and Shigematsu K. Localization of angiotensin AT1 receptors in the rat heart conduction system. *Eur J Pharmacol* 235:301–303, 1993.
93. Saito S, Hiroi Y, Zou Y, Aikawa R, Toko H, Shibasaki F, Yazaki Y, Nagai R, and Komuro I. Beta-adrenergic pathway induces apoptosis through calcineurin activation in cardiac myocytes. *J Biol Chem* 275:34528–34533, 2000.
94. Saris JJ, Derkx FHM, Lamers JMJ, et al. Cardiomyocytes bind and activate native human prorenin. Role of soluble mannose 6-phospahte receptors. *Hypertension* 37:710–715, 2001.
95. Senzaki H, Paolocci N, Gluzband YA, et al. β-blockade prevents sustained metalloproteinase activation and diastolic stiffening induced by angiotensin II combined with evolving cardiac dysfunction. *Circ Res* 86:807–815, 2000.
96. Seyedi N, Maruyama R, and Levi R. Bradykinin activates a cross-signaling pathway between sensory and adrenergic nerve endings in the heart: a novel mechanism of ischemic norepinephrine release? *J Pharmacol Exp Ther* 290:656–663, 1999.
97. Seyedi N, Win T, Lander HM, and Levi R. Bradykinin B_2-receptor activation augments norepinephrine exocytosis from cardiac sympathetic nerve endings. Mediation by autocrine/paracrine mechanisms. *Circ Res* 81:774–784, 1997.
98. Shindo T, Akiyama T, Yamazaki T, and Ninomiya I. Regional myocardial interstitial norepinephrine kinetics during coronary occlusion and reperfusion. *Am J Physiol (Heart Circ Physiol)* 270(39):H245–H251, 1996.
99. Siwik DA, Pagano PJ, and Colucci WS. Oxidative stress regulates collagen synthesis and matrix metalloproteinase activity in cardiac fibroblasts. *Am J Physiol* 280:C53–C60, 2001.
100. Steinberg SF. The cellular actions of β-adrenergic receptor agonists. Looking beyond cAMP. *Circ Res* 87:1079–1082, 2000.
101. Tallaj J, Wei CC, Hankes GH, Holland M, Rynders P, Dillon AR, Ardell JL, Armour JA, Lucchesi PA, and Dell'Italia LJ. β_1-adrenergic receptor blockade attenuates angiotensin II–mediated catecholamine release into the cardiac interstitium in mitral regurgitation. *Circulation*, 108:225–230, 2003.
102. Teisman AC, Westeink BH, van Veldhuisen DJ, Scholtens E, de Zeeuw D, and van Gilst WH. Direct interaction beween the sympathetic and renin-angiotensin system in myocardial tissue: a microdialysis study in anesthestized rats. *J Auton Nerv Syst* 78:117–121, 2000.
103. Testa M, Yeh M, Lee P, Fanelli R, Loperfido F, Berman JW, and LeJemtel T.

Circulating levels of cytokines and their endogenous modulators in patients with mild to severe congestive heart failure due to coronary artery disease or hypertension. *J Am Coll Cardiol* 28:964–971, 1996.
104. Thaik CM, Calderone A, Takahashi N, and Colucci WS. Interleukin-1β modulates the growth and phenotype of neonatal rat cardiac myocytes. *J Clin Invest* 96:1093–1099, 1995.
105. Thomas JA and Marks BH. Plasma norepinephrine in congestive heart failure. *Am J Cardiol* 41:233–243, 1978.
106. Torre-Amione G, Kapadia S, Lee J, Durand J-B, Bies RD, Young JB, and Mann DL. Tumor necrosis factor-α and tumor necrosis factor receptors in the failing human heart. *Circulation* 93:704–711, 1996.
107. Tsutsui H, Spinale FG, Nagatsu M, et al. Effects of chronic β-adrenergic blockade on the left ventricular and cardiocyte abnormalities of chronic canine mitral regurgitation. *J Clin Invest* 93:2639–2648, 1994.
108. Turki J, Lorenz JN, Green SA, Donnelly ET, Jacento M, and Liggett SB. Myocardial signaling defects and impaired cardiac function of a human β_2-adrenergic receptor polymorphism expressed in transgenic mice. *Proc Natl Acad Sci USA* 93:10483–10488, 1996.
109. Wagner DR, Kubota T, Sanders VJ, McTiernan CF, and Feldman AM. Differential regulation of cardiac expression of IL-6 and TNF-α by A_2- and A_3-adenosine receptors. *Am J Physiol* 276:H2141–H2147, 1999.
110. Wagoner LE, Craft LL, Singh B, Suresh DP, Zengel PW, McGuire N, Abraham WT, Chenier TC, Dorn GW II, and Liggett SB. Polymorphisms of the β_2-adrenergic receptor determine exercise capacity in patients with heart failure. *Circ Res* 86:834, 2000.
111. Yamamoto S, Tsutui H, Tagawa H, Saito K, Takahashi M, Tada H, Yamamoto M, Katoh M, Egashira K, and Takeshita A. Role of myocyte nitric oxide in β-adrenergic hyporesponsiveness in heart failure. *Circulation* 95:1111–1114, 1997.
112. Yokoyama T, Vaca L, Rossen RD, Durante W, Hazarika P, and Mann DL. Cellular basis for the negative inotropic effects of tumor necrosis factor-α in the adult mammalian heart. *J Clin Invest* 92:2303–2312, 1993.
113. Yue P, Massie BM, Simpson PC, and Long CS. Cytokine expression increases in nonmyocytes from rats with postinfarction heart failure. *Am J Physiol* 275:H250–H258, 1998.
114. Ziolo MT, Katoh H, and Bers DM. Expression of inducible nitric oxide synthase depresses β-adrenergic-stimulated calcium release from the sarcoplasmic reticulum in intact ventricular myocytes. *Circulation* 2001;104: 2961–2966.

13

The Pathogenesis of Hypertension

J. MICHAEL WYSS, SCOTT H. CARLSON, AND SUZANNE OPARIL

The nervous system is known to play an important role in the minute-to-minute setting of arterial pressure, but its contribution to chronic blood pressure regulation is less clear. For instance, the activation of baroreflex receptors can acutely reduce vascular resistance, plasma volume, and cardiac function, thereby decreasing arterial pressure, but these receptors reset quickly to a new baseline pressure, and thus their ability to chronically modify arterial pressure is limited under normal conditions. In contrast to this "normal" situation, baroreflex mechanisms appear to be maladaptive in some forms of hypertension and thus may contribute importantly to the blood pressure elevation.[87] Further, primary disturbances in the brain may underlie several forms of hypertension. This chapter reviews available evidence for a role of the nervous system in hypertension and considers newer work suggesting that an examination of circadian rhythms of nervous and cardiovascular system function may clarify the contribution of the nervous system to blood pressure regulation and the pathophysiology of hypertension.

THE PERIPHERAL AUTONOMIC NERVOUS SYSTEM

The autonomic nervous system consists of two separate motor pathways (sympathetic and parasympathetic systems) and two associated sensory feedback systems. The sympathetic and parasympathetic nervous systems are similar in that both are regulated by preganglionic neurons that have neuronal cell bodies in the central nervous system, and by peripherally located postganglionic motor neurons that directly innervate target organs. There are also significant differences between the two systems. For instance, preganglionic sympathetic axons originate in the thoracic region of the spinal cord (T1–L2) and project to ganglia that lie either immediately lateral to the spinal cord (paravertebral) or anterior to the vertebral column (prevertebral). The paravertebral postganglionic neurons project primarily to blood vessels throughout the body, whereas the prevertebral postganglionic neurons primarily innervate visceral organs, including the heart and kidney. Parasympathetic preganglionic neurons originate in the brain stem, primarily dorsal motor nucleus of the vagus and nucleus ambiguus, and in sacral spinal cord segments S2–S4. The dorsal motor nucleus of the vagus and nucleus ambiguus are the origin of the preganglionic parasympathetic innervation of the body rostral to the transverse colon, whereas the sacral spinal cord provides the parasympathetic preganglionic innervation of the organs caudal to the transverse colon. Another difference between the two branches of the autonomic nervous system is that in the sympathetic system, the postganglionic neurons are distant from the target organ that is innervated, while in the parasympathetic nervous system, the postganglionic neurons are located in or near the target organ.

Sensory afferent feedback from the innervated tissue projects through the ganglia from which the organ's motor innervation originates and then gains access to the spinal cord and brain. Sympathetic afferents terminate in the spinal cord at the level that correlates with the ganglia through which they course. For instance, the kidney is innervated by the lower thoracic and upper lumbar sympathetic ganglia and the sensory feedback terminates in those segments of the spinal cord. Parasympathetic sensory innervation follows the projection pattern of the parasympathetic motor axons and terminates in the brain stem and sacral spinal cord.

The major final pathway by which the brain regulates arterial pressure includes the sympathetic and the parasympathetic nervous systems and neurohumoral regulation, largely by the hypothalamus. Activation of the sympathetic nervous system causes tachycardia and increased cardiac contractility, stroke volume, and peripheral resistance. Further, the sympathetic nervous system promotes NaCl and water retention by the kidney, leading to an increase in circulating plasma volume, thereby elevating arterial pressure. The parasympathetic nervous system opposes the actions of the sympathetic nervous system primarily by reducing heart rate and contractility, thereby lowering cardiac output and decreasing arterial pressure. The parasympathetic nervous system has little or no direct control of the vasculature and only secondarily modifies regional blood flow by altering the metabolic demands of organs which it controls. The parasympathetic nervous system has negligible control of renal function, and therefore has little direct affect on fluid and NaCl homeostasis.

Overall, the autonomic nervous system acts primarily as a short-term regulator of blood pressure, adjusting arterial pressure to acute challenges (e.g., standing, running, stress). Long-term control of arterial pressure has traditionally been attributed to the kidney, and the etiology of hypertension has been ascribed almost entirely to deficits in renal function. Considerable evidence suggests that activation of the sympathetic nervous system is the major etiological factor in some forms of hypertension and contributes, at least partially, to all forms of the disease.

Several forms of sensory feedback to the central nervous system (CNS) are important for the chronic regulation of arterial pressure. These include baroreceptor, chemoreceptor, and osmoreceptor pathways. Baroreceptors in the aortic arch and carotid bifurcation primarily monitor arterial pressure and are referred to as high-pressure receptors, while baroreceptors in the atria and pulmonary circulation primarily monitor blood volume, and are therefore termed the low-pressure receptors. High-pressure baroreceptors in the aortic arch project via the vagus to the medulla, while those located in the carotid bifurcation travel to the medulla through Hering's nerve and the glossopharyngeal nerve. Low-pressure receptors pro-ject via the vagus to the brain stem. Baroreceptors in other parts of the body (e.g., the kidney) serve similar functions. Chemoreceptors in the carotid bodies and adjacent to the aorta are sensitive to increased plasma H^+ ion concentrations and thereby indirectly monitor O_2 deficiency and excess CO_2. These receptors normally affect respiration rate and play a role in arterial pressure regulation during extreme hypoxia/ischemia. Osmoreceptors in the hypothalamus respond to increased plasma sodium levels and/or osmolality by directly increasing sympathetic activity.[59,60] Other hypothalamic and brainstem neurons monitor circulating angiotensin II (ANG II) concentration and signal the brain to adjust arterial pressure and plasma volume appropriately. Thus the brain is supplied with a rich sensory feedback that is used to modify the brain's regulation of the cardiovascular system.

THE CONTRIBUTION OF THE SYMPATHETIC NERVOUS SYSTEM TO HYPERTENSION

Essential hypertension is a chronic elevation of arterial pressure that has no identified, proximate cause. Several lines of evidence from animal models of hypertension and human subjects suggest that the sympathetic nervous system may be a primary contributor to the development and the maintenance of hypertension.[29,38] The search for a primary role of the sympathetic nervous system in hypertension has been hampered by the inability to measure levels of sympathetic nervous system activity. Early studies depended on plasma norepinephrine concentration as a surrogate for sympathetic nervous system activity. These data were often dismissed because of the insensitivity of the technique and its inability to differentiate between generalized sympathetic nervous system activity and activity directed to specific organs or vascular beds. Newer techniques that measure norepinephrine spillover from specific target organs[29] provide a much more reliable estimate of norepinephrine release by the sympathetic nerves in a target organ of interest. Similarly, microneurography provides a method for measuring sympathetic nervous system activity that is directed to a specific organ. In humans, microneurography is generally limited to percutaneous investigation of the sympathetic innervation of skeletal muscle and skin. Because of their precision and selectivity, these new techniques offer the potential for providing important insights into the role of the nervous system in hypertension.

Hypertensive patients often display elevated plasma norepinephrine and norepinephrine spillover in target organs, increased muscle sympathetic nerve activity, and sympathetically driven tachycardia.[1,27,29,44,75] These and other findings suggest that sympathetic nervous system overactivity may contribute to the development and maintenance of human essential hypertension.[10,28,42] Several other conditions facilitate blood pressure elevation and the development of hypertension at least in part by increasing sympathetic nervous system activity.[75] For instance, tobacco smoking causes peripheral release of norepinephrine and epinephrine, primarily mediated by nicotine,[46] obesity increases sympathetic nervous system activity by blunting baroreceptors,[43] and type 2 diabetes is associated with both increased sympathetic nervous system activity and hypertension.[2,55] Thus several lines of evidence suggest that essential hypertension is associated with activation of the sympathetic nervous system and that this increased activity contributes to the maintenance of hypertension to target organ damage (especially in the kidney, heart, and blood vessels). Together these effects create a feed-forward system that can greatly amplify hypertension.

The relationship between the sympathetic nervous system and hypertension has been extensively studied using animal models. Employing renal denervation as a primary tool, many studies have indicated that the renal nerves contribute to the development of hypertension but that they are less influential in the maintenance phase of the disorder.[134] Efferent renal sympathetic innervation is necessary for the full and rapid development of hypertension in the spontaneously hypertensive rat of the Okomoto strain (SHR), in the two-kidney, one-clip renovascular hypertensive rat, in the deoxycorticosterone acetate-NaCl (DOCA-NaCl)-treated hypertensive rat, and in the rat made hypertensive by chronic infusion of ANG II. In contrast, one-kidney, one-clip renovascular hypertension in rats and aortic coarctation hypertension in dogs are mediated at least in part by the renal sensory nerves but not by renal motor nerves. Few of these effects are related to defects in peripheral sympathetic mechanisms. Instead they are associated primarily with neurotransmitter and neuropeptide dysfunction(s) in the brain and spinal cord.

NEUROTRANSMITTERS AND NEUROPEPTIDES

The primary final neurotransmitter involved in sympathetic synaptic transmission is norepinephrine, which activates α- and β-adrenergic receptors. Peripheral α_1-adrenergic receptors are primarily responsible for constriction of the vasculature, while most peripheral α_2 receptors are primarily presynaptic and thereby modulate norepinephrine release. Peripheral β_1 receptors are responsible for elevating heart rate and increasing cardiac contractility, while β_2 receptors cause vasodilation of skeletal muscle vasculature during exercise.

Several circulating neuropeptides are able to modify sympathetic nervous system activity and/or effectiveness. Angiotensin II and atrial natriuretic peptide (ANP) are the most extensively studied in this regard. Angiotensin II directly enhances release of norepinephrine in the periphery and blunts baroreflex feedback to the brain.[101,102,108] Active metabolites of ANG II have similar (e.g., angiotensin III) or opposite (angiotensin 1–7) effects. Atrial natriuretic peptide and type C natriuretic peptide (CNP) increase sympathoinhibition and decrease the release of norepinephrine from nerve terminals.[90,103,120,121] Further, both ANG II and ANP/CNP have central effects that regulate sympathetic tone.[13]

Several neuropeptides that are colocalized and released with norepinephrine or other neurotransmitters in peripheral axons can modulate arterial pressure independently or in concert with norepinephrine. Neuropeptide Y (NPY) is released along with norepinephrine by sympathetic nerve terminals. Neuropeptide by itself has little if any effect on sympathetic nervous system target tissues, but it dramatically enhances the responses of peripheral targets to adrenergic/noradrenergic stimulation.[49,130] In both DOCA-NaCl hypertension and in pulmonary hypertension induced by veratrine stimulation of the sympathetic nervous system, increases in plasma concentration of NPY parallel the increases in plasma norepinephrine concentration.[128–130] Further, NPY potentiates the vasoconstrictor effects of adenosine triphosphate (ATP), which is colocalized synaptically with norepinephrine and is released in response to sympathetic activation.[80,81,84,114–116,127] In contrast to NPY, the neuropeptide galanin inhibits norepinephrine release.[16,17]

Other, less well-understood forms of synaptic transmission may be important to the sympathetic nervous system's control of arterial pressure. Several studies suggest that peripheral interplay occurs between afferent and efferent neurons. In the kidney, neurotransmitters released from efferent nerve terminals can affect conduction of information in afferent axons and thereby indirectly modify sympathetic nervous system activity.[20,65] Similarly, peripheral afferent nerves appear to directly innervate neurons in some sympathetic ganglia.[14] Thus, peripheral feedback mechanisms should be considered potential contributors to arterial pressure control. The peripheral (receptive) ends of sympathetic sensory neurons also release neurotransmitters and neuromodulators that can affect peripheral target tissue. The best known example of this is calcitonin gene–related peptide (CGRP), which is released by the peripheral ends of afferent neurons onto blood vessels, causing profound vasodilation.[61–64,83] In the rat, the release of CGRP is inhibited by α_2-adrenoreceptor activation.[110]

Ouabain is a putative endogenous inhibitor of Na^+/K^+ ATPase that has been proposed as a key hypothalamic mediator of sympathoexcitatory responses to dietary NaCl.[9,50,125] Several studies suggest that an increase in brain "ouabain" contributes to salt-sensitive hypertension in SHR and Dahl-S rats as well as the sympathetic hyperactivity observed in congestive heart failure. While several experiments by one group have reported these effects of brain "ouabain," the lack of information on the structure, metabolism, and regulation of this substance have complicated the interpretation of these data.

The brain adrenergic system has also been suggested to play a role in hypertension. Adrenergic receptors in the brain are the target of several effective antihypertensive drugs. In the hypothalamus and cerebral cortex, the action of α_2-adrenergic receptor agonists is mediated by α_2-adrenergic receptors, but in the brain stem, their target is less clear. Both α_2-adrenergic receptors and putative imidazoline receptors reside in many areas of the brain stem, and imidazoline receptor agonists, like clonidine, bind to both receptors with high affinity.[24–26,56] Selective imidazoline agonists have effects similar to those of α_2-adrenergic receptor agonists. They bind to α_2-adrenergic receptor sites, but their affinity is much greater for the imidazoline receptor binding sites, which are primarily in the brain stem. The existence of imidazoline receptors has been hotly debated, largely because of their close similarity to α_2-adrenergic receptors and questions about their endogenous ligand.[22,47] Although the therapeutic benefit of I_1 receptor therapy for the general hypertensive population is unclear,[79] it may have distinct benefits for some hypertensive patients.[96]

THE MEDULLA AND ARTERIAL PRESSURE

The final common pathway for CNS regulation of the sympathetic nervous system is composed of thoracic preganglionic neurons that are regulated directly by descending projections from the cardiovascular centers in the brain stem and diencephalon (Fig. 13–1).[74,77,100] The medulla contains several nuclei that play an important role in cardiovascular control, including the rostral ventrolateral medulla (RVLM), nucleus tractus solitarius (NTS), and area postrema. The RVLM is the nodal point for the regulation of sympathetic tone.[100] Neurons of the RVLM exhibit an intrinsic firing pattern, indicative of their postulated role as the "pacemakers" of the sympathetic nervous system.[48] Both descending and ascending cardiovascular information converges to regulate the activity of RVLM neurons. Descending projections to the RVLM originate in the lateral parabrachial nucleus, periaqueductal gray, paraventricular hypothalamic nucleus, and other parts of the forebrain.[6,48,51,78] Activation of most of these inputs to RVLM increases sympathetic tone and elevates arterial pressure. In addition, the RVLM receives direct inhibitory (GABAergic) input from the caudal ventrolateral medulla (CVLM). Thus, the net RVLM output to the sympathetic preganglionic neurons is a summation of direct descending innervation to RVLM and indirect projections that are relayed by CVLM.

Most excitatory input into the RVLM is mediated by glutamate and AMPA receptors, but several higher centers (e.g., lateral parabrachial nucleus, posterior hypothalamus, and lateral septal area) excite RVLM neurons by the release of acetylcholine (ACh) onto muscarinic receptors (mACh).[70] Acetylcholine content of RVLM is elevated in two models of hypertension (SHR and DOCA-NaCl rats), and inhibition of acetylcholine esterase in the RVLM produces an exaggerated increase in arterial pressure in these models.[71] Together, these findings indicate that the RVLM may contribute to CNS-driven hypertension.[52,113]

The RVLM contains angiotensin receptors (AT_1) which tonically elevate RVLM neuronal activity. AII injections into the cerebral ventricles produce an increase in arterial pressure that is blocked by microinjection of losartan (an AT_1 antagonist) into the RVLM. Further, microinjection of an AT_1 antagonist into the RVLM decreases arterial pressure.[53] The depressor effect of AT1 antagonist microinjections into the RVLM is greater in SHR than in normotensive control rats, a result suggesting an enhanced sensitivity to endogenous ANG II in the RVLM of SHR.[4,35] Angiotensin II in the RVLM also appears to modulate sympathetic responses to baroreceptor input.[105]

The early demonstration that lesions of the NTS result in fulminating hypertension in rats and less severe hypertension in other species led to the conjecture that the NTS was involved in the development of hypertension. Supporting this opinion was the fact that the NTS was the primary nucleus responsible for the intake and initial modification of sensory information from the atrial, aortic, and carotid baroreceptors and chemoreceptors and from cardiovascular-relevant receptors located in the

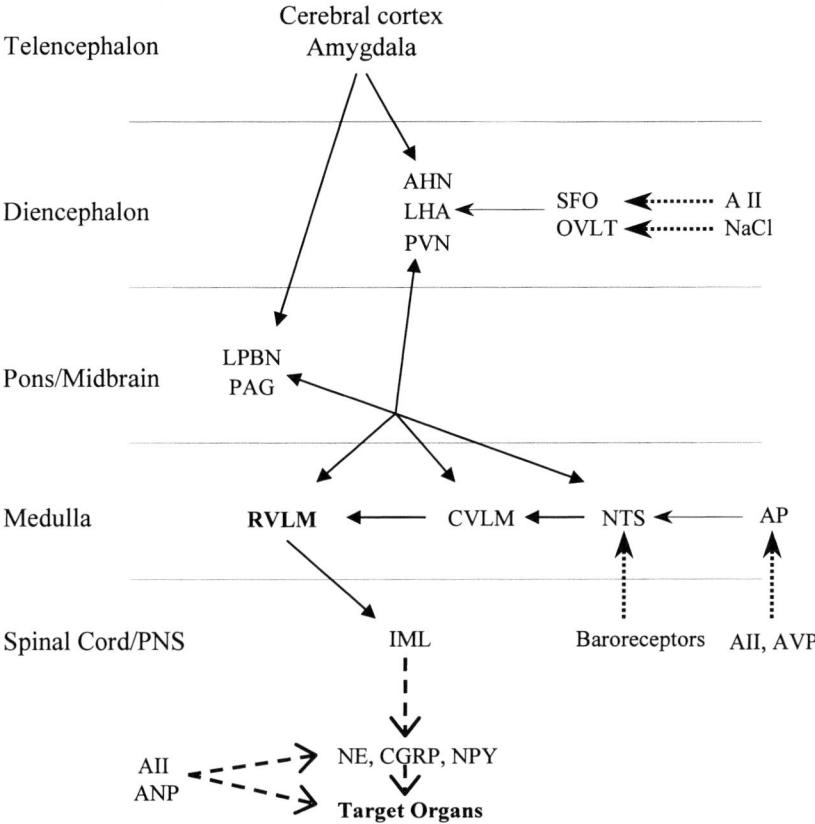

FIGURE 13–1 Line diagram depicting the flow of neuronal information that modifies arterial pressure. Arrows on dotted lines indicate peripheral inputs to the central nervous system (CNS), the arrows on dashed lines indicate the neural output to the target organ, including the presence of the peripheral modulators of that output (e.g., angiotensin II [A II] and atrial natriuretic peptide [ANP]), and the solid arrows indicate CNS pathways. Note that the organum vasculosum of the lamina terminalis (OVLT) is most sensitive to changes in peripheral NaCl, while the subfornical organ (SFO) is more sensitive to circulating A II. AHN, anterior hypothalamic nucleus; AP, area postrema; AVP, arginine vasopressin; CGRP, locally released calcitonin gene–related peptide; CVLM, caudal ventrolateral medulla; IML, intermediolateral preganglionic sympathetic neurons in the spinal cord; LHA, lateral hypothalamic area; LPBN, lateral parabrachial nucleus; NE, locally released noradrenaline; NPY, neuropeptide Y; NTS, nucleus of the solitary tract; PAG, periaqueductal gray; PNS, peripheral nervous system; PVN, posterior hypothalamic nucleus; RVLM, rostral ventrolateral medulla.

kidney, liver, and other peripheral organs. The NTS receives significant descending projections from many regions of the CNS, including the cerebral cortex, and NTS projections indirectly modify sympathetic and parasympathetic nervous system activity and alter the release of vasopressin and other hormone factors from the hypothalamus. The NTS is tonically inhibited by GABA, and baroreflex inputs to the NTS release the neurons from this inhibition.[54] While experimental evidence for a general role of the NTS in the pathogenesis of hypertension remains equivocal, data do suggest that abnormalities in the NTS contribute to hypertension by increasing sympathetic nervous system activity in SHR and some other experimental models of hypertension.[21,99]

In the rat, the area postrema is dorsal to the NTS, and the lack of a blood–brain barrier allows its neurons to monitor plasma concentrations of peptide hormones. Stimulation of these neurons by ANG II decreases baroreflex sensitivity and increases sympathetic activity. Conversely, vasopressin (AVP) binds to V_1 receptors in the area postrema, inhibiting sympathetic nervous system activity and increasing baroreflex sensitivity. Interestingly, lesions of area postrema normalize arterial pressure in some hypertensive animal models. While the area postrema is critical for the development of hypertension in high-renin models such as the mRen rat,[3] it does not appear to modulate salt-sensitive hypertension in rats fed a high-salt diet.[15]

The Hypothalamus and Hypertension

Numerous lesion, stimulation, and neuronal transplantation experiments have suggested that the hypothalamus modifies arterial pressure and is involved in rodent models of hypertension.[85] Transplantation of a hypothalamus from a genetically hypertensive SHR induces hypertension in genetically normotensive recipient Wistar Kyoto rats (WKY).[23] Conversely, transplantation of hypothalamic tissue from WKY rats has no significant effect on arterial pressure in SHR.

Lesion and stimulation experiments indicate that the lateral and posterior hypothalamic areas are generally sympathoexcitatory. Stimulation of either area increases arterial pressure and heart rate, while lesions of the posterior hypothalamic area reduce arterial pressure in DOCA-NaCl rats. Further, imbalances in norepinephrine, ACh, and GABA in the posterior hypothalamic nucleus may contribute to hypertension in SHR rats.[8]

The paraventricular nucleus (PVN) also contributes to arterial pressure regulation (Fig. 13–1). The magnocellular neurons of the PVN and the associated supraoptic nucleus produce vasopressin and release it into the circulation. The parvocellular neurons in the PVN project to several CNS cardiovascular control nuclei, including the RVLM, area postrema, NTS, and intermediolateral nucleus of the spinal cord, and appear to alter cardiovascular function via these connections.[21,39] The SHR display abnormal regulation of neurons in the PVN and the interaction between ANG II and the PVN appears to be altered in several forms of hypertension.[34,68,69,108] Leptin also modifies PVN neuronal activity, potentially contributing to its ability to chronically elevate arterial pressure.[95,107]

The anterior hypothalamus contains several areas that are important in cardiovascular control, and some of these appear to contribute to hypertension. The anteroventral third ventricle (AV3V) is important in several forms of hypertension in the rat. The median preoptic nucleus is the most important cardiovascular nucleus in AV3V. Selective lesions of this nucleus prevent the development of hypertension and/or significantly decrease established hypertension in several animal models. The median preoptic nucleus receives a significant number of cardiovascular/volume inputs from both circumventricular organs and several brain stem nuclei. Other preoptic nuclei regulate water balance, contributing to plasma volume control and modifying arterial pressure. The anterior hypothalamic nucleus, along with the preoptic area, provides important sympathoinhibitory influences, most of which are mediated by projections to sympathoexcitatory nuclei in the diencephalon and brain stem. Stimulation of these nuclei elicits a decrease in arterial pressure and heart rate, whereas lesions in the anterior hypothalamic nucleus increase arterial pressure.

CORTICAL CONTROL OF THE CARDIOVASCULAR SYSTEM

Descending cortical input regulates arterial pressure, and both experimental and clinical evidence indicates that the cardiovascular functions of several cortical regions are lateralized. In the rat, 70% of insular cortex neurons display significant responses to baroreceptor manipulations, while less than 35% of neurons in the surrounding cortex show similar activity. Most of the insular cortex neurons that respond to baroreceptor changes are in the right and not the left posterior insular cortex.[136] In the monkey, cardiovascular information also converges on insular cortex neurons, and approximately twice as many of these baroreceptor-sensitive neurons are found in the right compared to the left hemisphere.[137] In humans, the left (compared to the right) insular cortex appears to dominate parasympathetic control of the cardiovascular system. Strokes that significantly involve the left insular cortex are associated with an increase in sympathetic tone and a decreased phase relationship between heart rate and blood pressure.[86] These data point to the potential importance of the insular cortex in both chronic and acute regulation of cardiovascular function, and suggest that right–left asymmetries in the brain may be important to cardiovascular control.

In addition to the insular cortex, other areas of the cerebral cortex contribute to cardiovascular control. Stimulation of infralimbic cortex (and to a lesser extent the prefrontal cortex) alters arterial pressure,[36,37,122] and many neurons in these areas and in the amygdala send projections to the lateral hypothalamus, the periaqueductal gray, and the medulla. Through these nuclei, the cortical afferents are able to adjust arterial pressure, heart rate, and baroreflex gain.

Salt Sensitivity and the Brain

Excess dietary sodium chloride intake is a significant contributor to hypertension in "salt-sensitive" individuals,[104] and several studies have begun to elucidate the mechanism(s) by which plasma sodium and chloride can alter the activity of neurons in cardiovascular control nuclei. Information about plasma sodium concentration is conveyed to the brain by several different routes. Blood pressure and plasma volume signals (indirect indicies of plasma sodium concentration) are sent to the hypothalamus primarily via neurons in the NTS. The hepatic, renal, mesenteric, and other nerves monitor plasma sodium concentration and/or osmolality in the viscera and transmit this information to the brain stem and from there to the hypothalamus.[58] For instance, local changes in the plasma osmolality of the liver alter neuronal activity in the PVN.[12] Sodium can cross through the blood–brain barrier, thereby gaining direct access to the hypothalamus and potentially affecting the firing rate of neurons in the PVN and other hypothalamic nuclei. Further, the circumventricular organs in the rostral hypothalamus monitor plasma sodium directly.[58] The subfornical organ (SFO) and organum vasculosum of the lamina terminalis (OVLT) are in the rostral edge of the hypothalamus but are outside the blood–brain barrier and are therefore capable of rapid monitoring of circulating substances. The rat SFO neurons are very responsive to changes in plasma ANG II concentration, and they transmit this information to the hypothalamus, indirectly monitoring plasma sodium concentration.[58,60] In the rat, dog, and, presumably, in humans, most of the forebrain effects of plasma ANG II can be blocked by local SFO administration of AT_1 antagonists.[58]

Direct monitoring of plasma sodium concentration in the rat is more dependent on OVLT than on SFO. Bourque and Oliet demonstrated that osmotic challenge to OVLT induces changes in the firing rate of neurons in the hypothalamic supraoptic nucleus.[7] Selective lesions of OVLT eliminate drinking responses to increased plasma osmolarity. The contribution of OVLT and SFO to long-term arterial pressure regulation has not been studied extensively, but several recent findings suggest that these nuclei can influence chronic changes in blood pressure. Kovács and Sawchenko have demonstrated that lesions of the projection from OVLT to the hypothalamus abolish the decrease in corticotrophin-releasing factor that is normally observed in the parvocellular PVN in response to a hyperosmotic challenge.[67]

Studies by Peng et al. indicate that the OVLT pathway to the anterior hypothalamic nucleus is a major contributor to the NaCl-sensitive hypertension in SHR.[92] When SHR are fed a high-NaCl diet, their arterial pressure rapidly increases and is maintained about 30 mmHg higher than that of SHR on a basal NaCl diet. The rise in arterial pressure is associated with a selective decrease in norepinephrine release in the anterior hypothalamic nucleus (AHN), resulting in increased sympathetic nervous system activity, peripheral vasoconstriction, and arterial pressure. Administration of an α_2-adrenergic receptor agonist in this area blocks the NaCl-sensitive rise in arterial pressure in the SHR but has no significant effect on arterial pressure in normotensive controls. We have identified three intermediary steps by which dietary NaCl reduces AHN norepinephrine release. First, dietary NaCl causes an increase in plasma NaCl and a blunting of the plasma NaCl circadian rhythm.[31] Second, alterations in plasma NaCl activate osmosensitive neurons in the OVLT.[92] Third, OVLT input to the AHN appears to increase the release of ANP, with a resultant decrease in the local release of norepinephrine.[57,89] These factors lead to an increased rise in sympathetic nervous system activity during the early-wake phase in SHR on a high-NaCl diet, contributing to NaCl-sensitive hypertension (Fig. 13–2).

CIRCADIAN RHYTHM AND HYPERTENSION

Assessment of the circadian rhythm of arterial pressure has provided a new window into the neural mechanism(s) that underlie hypertension. In patients with established hypertension, the normal-phase relationship between blood pressure, heart rate, and the release of vasoactive hormones is often altered.[97] Hypertensive patients display a reduced amplitude of arterial pressure rhythm with age, largely due to a failure of their arterial pressure to decrease during the nighttime. Normotensive individuals display no similar age-related alteration in the amplitude of their circadian regulation of arterial pressure.[97] Importantly, hypertensive patients who have little if any decrease in arterial pressure during the nighttime and therefore have a significantly blunted circadian rhythm are at increased risk of target organ damage, especially damage to the heart

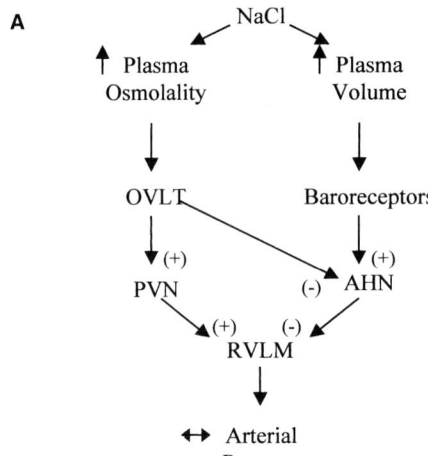
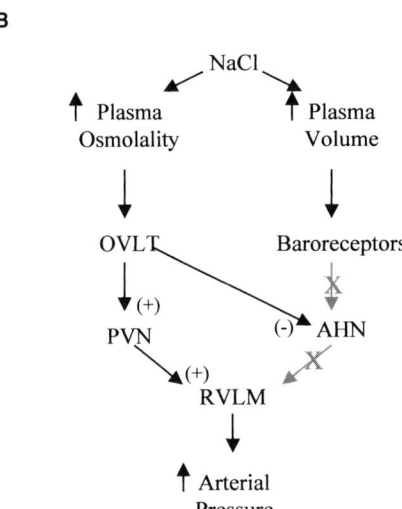

FIGURE 13–2 Diagram demonstrating neural regulation of arterial pressure in response to an increase in plasma NaCl in a normal, NaCl-resistant rat (**A**), and a NaCl-sensitive spontaneously hypertensive rat (SHR) (**B**). Note that in the SHR, inhibition of the anterior hypothalamic nucleus (AHN) leads to a loss of AHN-mediated sympathoinhibition. OVLT, organum vasculosum of the lamina terminals; PVN, posterior hypothalamic nucleus; RVLM, rostral ventrolateral medulla.

and kidney.[72,88,123,124] Thus, consideration of circadian rhythms of arterial pressure is critical to an understanding of the mechanisms that underlie hypertension and hypertension-related target organ damage in humans.

Our laboratories have investigated the relationship of several circadian rhythms to the pathogenesis of NaCl-sensitive hypertension. Our initial focus was on circadian control of arterial pressure (Fig. 13–3). We found that in SHR, as in human subjects, a high-NaCl diet initially causes a marked increase in nighttime arterial pressure (when rats are awake),

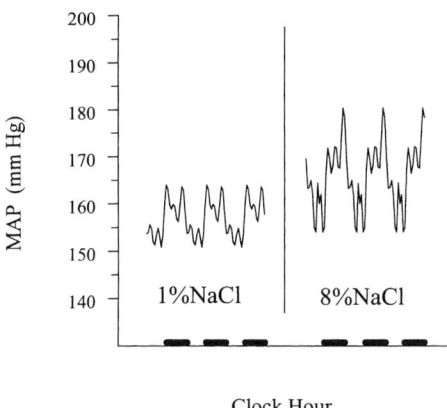

FIGURE 13-3 Demonstration of the circadian mean arterial pressure (MAP) rhythm monitored by radiotelemetry and assessed by PHARMFIT in a male SHR on a basal NaCl diet and 1 week after being placed on a high-NaCl diet. Note that both the rhythm amplitude (height of the wave) and the absolute mean arterial pressure are increased by the high-NaCl diet. The black lines above the x-axis indicate nighttime (lights out).

and a lesser rise in daytime arterial pressure.[11,32] In contrast, later phases of NaCl-sensitive hypertension are marked by a large increase in daytime arterial pressure and a leveling off of nighttime pressure, resulting in a significantly blunted circadian arterial pressure rhythm. In WKY rats, a high-NaCl diet causes only a slight increase in the nighttime arterial pressure that is compensated for by a decrease in daytime arterial pressure.[11]

ESTROGEN REPLACEMENT THERAPY AND HYPERTENSION

The prevalence of hypertension in the United States displays a gender dimorphism. Hypertension in men is more common than in similarly aged women until the age of menopause, after which arterial pressure in women increases rapidly and eventually equals that in men.[66] Compared to age-matched men, premenopausal women are resistant to the hypertensive effects of a high-NaCl diet, but following menopause women and men display a similar incidence of salt-sensitive hypertension.[82] There is evidence that estrogen can blunt the development of hypertension because of its actions on the peripheral vasculature. Estrogen decreases circulating catecholamine levels,[109] attenuates vasoconstrictor responses to norepinephrine by reducing intracellular free calcium,[5,18,73] and enhances vasodilation by increasing nitric oxide release.[19,132] Estrogen may reduce sympathetic nervous system–mediated vasoconstriction at the peripheral vascular level, and may also reduce sympathetic nervous system outflow by modulating baroreflex function.[106,112] Together, these factors[109] contribute to the ability of estrogen to protect females from NaCl-sensitive hypertension. Without estrogen present, the response of female SHR to a high-NaCl diet takes on a "male" phenotype—i.e., the high-NaCl diet elevates sympathetic nervous system activity, thereby chronically elevating arterial pressure (Fig. 13–4).[30,133,135]

We recently carried out a series of experiments demonstrating that both endogenous and dietary estrogens (phytoestrogens) are able to blunt NaCl-sensitive hypertension in female SHR.[33] In female SHR on the basal NaCl diet, arterial pressure was relatively unaffected by the removal of either or both estrogens. Furthermore, in SHR with intact ovaries, the high-NaCl diet did not significantly raise arterial pressure. In contrast, in SHR that had both endogenous (ovariectomy) and exogenous (removal from the diet) sources of estrogen removed, a high-NaCl diet rapidly raised arterial pressure by about 70 mmHg. Depletion of either source of estrogen alone resulted in only about a 20–25 mmHg rise in mean arterial pressure in response to the high-NaCl diet. Blockade of the sympathetic nervous system eliminated the pro-hypertensive effects of the loss of estrogen. Taken together, these findings indicate that estrogens protect female SHR from dietary NaCl-sensitive hypertension and that the sympathetic nervous system plays an important role in this effect.[91] Also, these results demonstrate that dietary phytoestrogens can have a major impact on the interpretation of studies into the physiological role of estrogen in females.

Further complicating the interpretation of studies examining a cardioprotective effect of estrogen is that menopause is often associated with an increase in obesity, which is in itself a major risk factor for hyperten-

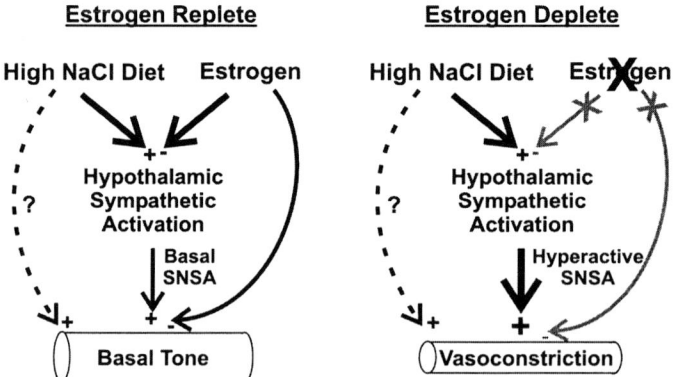

FIGURE 13–4 Two loci where estrogen appears to blunt NaCl-sensitive hypertension in female SHR—i.e., the hypothalamus and the blood vessel. In the estrogen depleted SHR female, there is an increase in sympathetic nervous system activity (SNSA) and a potentiated vasoconstrictor response to each release of neurotransmitter.

sion and cardiovascular disease.[117–119] Studies in humans that have attempted to determine whether hypertension is directly related to loss of estrogen, or only indirectly related via obesity, indicate that the loss of estrogen is an independent risk factor for hypertension in postmenopausal woman.[41,45,111] The effectiveness of estrogen in blunting cardiovascular disease in post-menopausal women remains to be fully elucidated.

FUTURE THERAPY FOR HYPERTENSION

Much current antihypertensive therapy is designed to decrease sympathetic synaptic transmission at the effector organs (e.g., β-blockers, calcium channel antagonists, α_1-antagonists). The antihypertensive effects of angiotensin-converting enzyme inhibitors and ANG II receptor blockers are also mediated by the nervous system, in that they block the ability of ANG II to presynaptically release norepinephrine. Other pharmacologic agents inhibit central activation of the sympathetic nervous system via α_2-adrenergic receptor agonism, by blockade of imidazoline receptors in the brain stem, and by altering the brain's renin–angiotensin system. While all of these therapies are temporary, future therapy to reduce sympathetic outflow from the brain may focus on longer-term treatments that employ antisense gene therapy. Studies involving antisense gene therapy for hypertension in animal models have demonstrated the proof of principle.[98] Injection of antisense oligodeoxynucleotides to either angio-tensinogen mRNA or AT_1-receptor mRNA into the cerebroventricular system caused a profound decrease in arterial pressure that can last several days.[13] In contrast, peripheral injection of the antisense had no antihypertensive effect, which suggests that the antisense therapy was CNS-specific. However, the therapeutic usefulness of antisense strategies has been limited by the relatively short-term effects of oligodeoxynucleotide-delivered antisense DNA. More recent experiments have found that injection of the antisense DNA for the angiotensin AT_1 receptor, coupled to a nonpathogenic adenoassociated virus,[93,94] decreases arterial pressure for up to 9 weeks in SHR. Systemic retroviral delivery of antisense to AT_1 receptors had a longer-lasting[76] or permanent[126] effect, and this therapy also prevented hypertension-associated target organ damage in SHR. Similar retroviral antisense therapy using genes directed against angiotensin-converting enzyme prevented renal vascular damage in SHR, without major reduction in arterial pressure.[40] These findings highlight the potential of antisense gene therapy in future treatment of hypertension.

Conclusions

The central nervous system contributes importantly to essential hypertension in humans and to the development of hypertension in a variety of animal models. The RVLM, NTS, hypothalamus, and cerebral cortex all appear to be involved in the pathogenesis of hypertension. New molecular techniques like antisense technology, in concert with integrative physiological approaches, offer insights into the pathogenesis of hypertension and potential therapies for the disease.

References

1. Aggarwal A, Esler MD, Lambert GW, Hastings J, Johnston L, and Kaye DM. Norepinephrine turnover is increased in suprabulbar subcortical brain regions and is related to whole-body sympathetic activity in human heart failure. *Circulation* 105:1031–1033, 2002.
2. Anderson EA, Hoffman RP, and Balon TW. Hyperinsulinemia produces both sympathetic neural activation and vasodilation in normal humans. *J Clin Invest* 87:2246–2252, 1991.
3. Averill DB, Matsumura K, Ganten D, and Ferrario CM. Role of area postrema in transgene hypertension. *Hypertension* 27:591–297, 1996.
4. Averill DB, Tsuchihashi T, Khosla MC, and Ferrario CM. Losartan, nonpeptide angiotensin II-type 1 (AT1) receptor antagonist, attenuates pressor and sympathoexcitatory responses evoked by angiotensin II and L-glutamate in rostral ventrolateral medulla. *Brain Res* 665:245–252, 1994.
5. Bairey MCN, Kop W, Krantz DS, Helmers KF, Berman DS, and Rozanski A. Cardiovascular stress response and coronary artery disease: evidence of an adverse postmenopausal effect in women. *Am Heart J* 135:881–887, 1998.
6. Barman SM. Descending projections of hypothalamic neurons with sympathetic nerve-related activity. *J Neurophysiol* 64:1019–1032, 1990.
7. Bourque CW and Oliet SH. Osmoreceptors in the central nervous system. *Annu Rev Physiol* 59:601–619, 1997.
8. Brexenoff HE and Xiao YF. Acetylcholine in the posterior hypothalamic nucleus is involved in the elevated blood pressure in the spontaneously hypertensive rat. *Life Sci* 45:1163–1170, 1989.
9. Budzikowski AS, Huang BS, and Leenen FH. Brain "ouabain", a neurosteroid, mediates sympathetic hyperactivity in salt-sensitive hypertension. *Clin Exp Hypertens* 20:119–140, 1998.
10. Calhoun DA and Mutinga ML. Race, family history of hypertension, and sympathetic response to cold pressor testing. *Blood Press* 6:209–213, 1997.
11. Calhoun DA, Zhu S, Wyss JM, and Oparil S. Diurnal blood pressure variation and dietary salt in spontaneously hypertensive rats. *Hypertension* 24:1–7, 1994.
12. Carlson SH, Beitz A, and Osborn JW. Intragastric hypertonic saline increases vasopressin and central fos immunoreactivity in conscious rats. *Am J Physiol (Regul Integr Comp Physiol)* 272:R750–R758, 1997.

13. Carlson SH, Oparil S, Chen YF, and Wyss JM. Blood pressure and NaCl-sensitive hypertension are influenced by angiotensin-converting enzyme gene expression in transgenic mice. *Hypertension* 39:214–218, 2002.
14. Coggan JS, Gruener R, and Kruelen DL. Electrophysiological properties and cholinergic responses in guinea-pig celiac ganglion neurons in primary culture. *J Auton Nerv Syst* 34:147–155, 1991.
15. Collister JP and Osborn JW. The area postrema does not modulate the long-term salt sensitivity of arterial pressure. *Am J Physiol* 275:R1209–R1217, 1998.
16. Degli Uberti EC, Ambrosio MR, Bondanelli M, Trasforini G, Margutti A, Valentini A, Rossi R, and Franceschetti P. Human galanin reduces plasma norepinephrine levels in man. *J Clin Endocrinol Metab* 80:1894–1898, 1995.
17. Degli Uberti EC, Bondanelli M, Margutti A, Ambrosio MR, Valentini A, Campo M, Franceschetti P, Zatelli MC, Pansini R, and Trasforini G. Acute administration of human galanin in normal subjects reduces the potentiating effect of pyridostigmine-induced cholinergic enhancement on release of norepinephrine and pancreatic polypeptide. *Neuroendocrinology* 64:398–404, 1996.
18. Del Rio G, Velardo A, Menozzi R, Zizzo GTV, Venneri MG, Marrama P, and Petraglia F. Acute estradiol and progesterone administration reduced cardiovascular and catecholamine responses to mental stress in menopausal women. *Neuroendocrinology* 67:269–274, 1998.
19. De Meersman RE, Zion AS, Giardina EG, Weir JP, Lieberman JS, and Downey JA. Estrogen replacement, vascular distensibility, and blood pressures in postmenopausal women. *Am J Physiol* 274:H1539–H1544, 1998.
20. Dibona GF and Kopp UC. Neural control of renal function. *Physiol Rev* 77:75–197, 1997.
21. Durgam VR, Vitela M, and Mifflin SW. Enhanced gamma-aminobutyric acid-B receptor agonist responses and mRNA within the nucleus of the solitary tract in hypertension. *Hypertension* 33:530–536, 1999.
22. Eglen RM, Hudson AL, Kendall DA, et al. Seeing through a glass darkly: casting light on imidazoline "I" sites. *Trends Pharmacol Sci* 19:381–390, 1998.
23. Eilam R, Malach R, Bergmann F, and Segal M. Hypertension induced by hypothalamic transplantation from genetically hypertensive to normotensive rats. *J Neurosci* 11:401–411, 1991.
24. Ernsberger P, Friedman JE, and Koletsky RJ. The I1-imidazoline receptor: from binding site to therapeutic target in cardiovascular disease. *J Hypertens Suppl* 15:S9–23, 1997.
25. Ernsberger P, Giuliano R, Willette RN, and Reis DJ. Role of imidazole receptors in the vasodepressor response to clonidine analogs in the rostral ventrolateral medulla. *J Pharmacol Exp Ther* 253:408–418, 1990.
26. Ernsberger P and Haxhiu MA. The I1-imidazoline-binding site is a functional receptor mediating vasodepression via the ventral medulla. *Am J Physiol* 273:R1572–R1579, 1997.
27. Esler M. Differentiation in the effects of the angiotensin II receptor blocker class on autonomic function. *J Hypertens* 20(Suppl 5):S13–S19, 2002.
28. Esler M, Lambert G, Kaye D, Rumantir M, Hastings J, and Seals DR. Influence of ageing on the sympathetic nervous system and adrenal medulla at rest and during stress. *Biogerontology* 3:45–49, 2002.
29. Esler MD. Sympathetic nervous system: contribution to human hypertension and related cardiovascular diseases. *J Cardiovasc Pharmacol* 26:S24–S28, 1995.

30. Ezimokhai M and Osman N. The effect of sodium based hypo-osmolality on arterial smooth muscle reactivity in vitro. *Res Exp Med* 197:269–279, 1998.
31. Fang Z, Carlson SH, Peng N, and Wyss JM. Circadian rhythm of plasma sodium is disrupted in spontaneously hypertensive rats fed a high-NaCl diet. *Am J Physiol (Regul Integr Comp Physiol)* 278:R1490–R1495, 2000.
32. Fang Z, Sripairojthikoon W, Calhoun DA, Zhu S, Berecek KH, and Wyss JM. Interaction between lifetime captopril treatment and NaCl-sensitive hypertension in spontaneously hypertensive rats and Wistar-Kyoto rats. *J Hypertens* 17:983–991, 1999.
33. Fang Z and Wyss JM. Sympathetic nervous system overactivity contributes to NaCl-sensitive hypertension in estrogen depleted female spontaneously hypertensive rats. *Soc Neurosci Abstr* 25:550, 1999.
34. Ferguson AV and Latchford KJ. Local circuitry regulates the excitability of rat neurohypophysial neurones. *Exp Physiol* 85:153S–161S, 2000.
35. Ferrario CM and Averill DB. Do primary dysfunctions in neural control of arterial pressure contribute to hypertension? *Hypertension* 18(Suppl I):I-38, 1991.
36. Fisk GD and Wyss JM. Pressor and depressor sites are intermingled in the cingulate cortex of the rat. *Brain Res* 754:204–212, 1997.
37. Fisk GD and Wyss JM. Descending projections of infralimbic cortex that mediate stimulation-evoked changes in arterial pressure. *Brain Res* 859:83–95, 2000.
38. Folkow B. Physiological aspects of primary hypertension. *Physiol Rev* 62:347–504, 1982.
39. Gardiner SM and Bennett T. The contribution of the autonomic nervous system, the renin-angiotensin system and vasopressin to the maintenance of arterial blood pressure in adrenalectomized Wistar rats. *Clin Sci (Colch)* 71:357–365, 1986.
40. Gelband CH, Reaves PY, Evans J, Wang H, Katovich MJ, and Raizada MK. Angiotensin II type 1 receptor antisense gene therapy prevents altered renal vascular calcium homeostasis in hypertension. *Hypertension* 33:360–365, 1999.
41. Gerhard M, Walsh BW, Tawakol A, Haley EA, Creager SJ, Seely EW, Ganz P, and Creager MA. Estradiol therapy combined with progesterone and endothelium-dependent vasodilation in postmenopausal women. *Circulation* 98:1158–1163, 1998.
42. Grassi G and Esler M. The sympathetic nervous system in renovascular hypertension: lead actor or 'bit' player? *J Hypertens* 20:1071–1073, 2002.
43. Grassi G, Seravalle G, Cattaneo BM, Bolla GB, Lanfranchi A, Colombo M, Giannattasio C, Brunani A, Cavagnini F, and Mancia G. Sympathetic activation in obese normotensive subjects. *Hypertension* 25:560–563, 1995.
44. Grassi G, Seravalle G, Turri C, Bolla G, and Mancia G. Short-versus long-term effects of different dihydropyridines on sympathetic and baroreflex function in hypertension. *Hypertension* 41:558–562, 2003.
45. Green PS, Gridley KE, and Simpkins JW. Nuclear estrogen receptor–independent neuroprotection by estratrienes: a novel interaction with glutathione. *Neuroscience* 84:7–10, 1998.
46. Groppelli A, Giorgi DM, Omboni S, Parati G, and Mancia G. Persistent blood pressure increase induced by heavy smoking. *J Hypertens* 10:495–499, 1992.
47. Guyenet PG. Is the hypotensive effect of clonidine and related drugs due to imidazolinebinding sites? *Am J Physiol* 273:R1580–R1584, 1997.

48. Guyenet PG, Haselton JR, and Sun MK. Sympathoexcitatory neurons of the rostroventrolateral medulla and the origin of the sympathetic vasomotor tone. *Prog Brain Res* 81:105–116, 1989.
49. Hoang D, Macarthur H, Gardner A, and Westfall TC. Endothelin-induced modulation of neuropeptide Y and norepinephrine release from the rat mesenteric bed. *Am J Physiol Heart Circ Physiol* 283:H1523–H1530, 2002.
50. Huang BS and Leenen FH. Brain "ouabain" mediates the sympathoexcitatory and hypertensive effects of high sodium intake in Dahl salt-sensitive rats. *Circ Res* 74:586–595, 1994.
51. Hudson PM, Semenenko FM, and Lumb BM. Inhibitory effects evoked from the rostral ventrolateral medulla are selective for the nociceptive responses of spinal dorsal horn neurons. *Neuroscience* 99:541–547, 2000.
52. Ito S, Hiratsuka M, Komatsu K, Tsukamoto K, Kanmatsuse K, and Sved AF. Ventrolateral medulla AT1 receptors support arterial pressure in Dahl salt-sensitive rats. *Hypertension* 41:744–750, 2003.
53. Ito S and Sved AF. Blockade of angiotensin receptors in rat rostral ventrolateral medulla removes excitatory vasomotor tone. *Am J Physiol* 270:R1317–R1323, 1996.
54. Ito S and Sved AF. Influence of GABA in the nucleus of the solitary tract on blood pressure in baroreceptor-denervated rats. *Am J Physiol* 273:R1657–R1662, 2001.
55. Jamerson KA, Julius S, and Gudbrandsson T. Reflex sympathetic activation induces acute insulin resistance in the human forearm. *Hypertension* 21:618–623, 1993.
56. Janssen BJ, Lukoshkova EV, and Head GA. Sympathetic modulation of renal blood flow by rilmenidine and captopril: central vs. peripheral effects. *Am J Physiol (Renal Physiol)* 282:F113–F123, 2002.
57. Jin H, Yang RH, Chen YF, and Oparil S. Atrial natriuretic factor prevents NaCl-sensitive hypertension in spontaneously hypertensive rats. *Hypertension (Dallas)* 15:170–176, 1990.
58. Johnson AK, Cunningham JT, and Thunhorst RL. Integrative role of the lamina terminalis in the regulation of cardiovascular and body fluid homeostasis. *Clin Exp Pharmacol Physiol* 23:183–191, 1996.
59. Johnson AK and Gross PM. Sensory circumventricular organs and brain homeostatic pathways. *FASEB J* 7:678–686, 1993.
60. Johnson AK and Loewy AD. Circumventricular organs and their role in visceral functions. In: Loewy AD and Spyer KM, eds. *Central Regulation of Autonomic Functions*. New York: Oxford University Press, 1990, pp 247–267.
61. Kawasaki H, Nuki C, Saito A, and Takasaki K. Adrenergic modulation of calcitonin gene-related peptide (CGRP)-containing nerve-mediated vasodilation in the rat mesenteric resistance vessel. *Brain Res* 506:287–290, 1990.
62. Kawasaki H, Nuki C, Saito A, and Takasaki K. Role of calcitonin gene-related peptide-containing nerves in the vascular adrenergic neurotransmission. *J Pharmacol Exp Ther* 252:403–409, 1990.
63. Kawasaki H, Saito A, and Takasaki K. Age-related decrease of calcitonin gene-related peptide-containing vasodilator innervation in the mesenteric resistance vessel of the spontaneously hypertensive rat. *Circ Res* 67:733–743, 1990.
64. Kawasaki H, Saito A, and Takasaki K. Changes in calcitonin gene-related

peptide (CGRP)-containing vasodilator nerve activity in hypertension. *Brain Res* 518:303–307, 1990.
65. Kopp UC, Smith LA, and Dibona GF. Facilitatory role of efferent renal nerve activity on renal sensory receptors. *Am J Physiol* 253:F767–F777, 1987.
66. Kotchen JM, McKean HE, and Kotchen TA. Blood pressure trends with aging. *Hypertension* 4:128–134, 1982.
67. Kovács KJ and Sawchenko PE. Mediation of osmoregulatory influences on neuroendocrine corticotropin-releasing factor expression by the ventral lamina terminalis. *Proc Natl Acad Sci USA* 90:7681–7685, 1993.
68. Krukoff TL, MacTavish D, and Jhamandas JH. Effects of restraint stress and spontaneous hypertension on neuropeptide Y neurones in the brainstem and arcuate nucleus. *J Neuroendocrinol* 11:715–723, 1999.
69. Krukoff TL, MacTavish D, and Jhamandas JH. Hypertensive rats exhibit heightened expression of corticotropin-releasing factor in activated central neurons in response to restraint stress. *Brain Res Mol Brain Res* 65:70–79, 1999.
70. Kubo T. Cholinergic mechanism and blood pressure regulation in the central nervous system. *Brain Res Bull* 46:475–481, 1998.
71. Kubo T, Ishizuka T, Fukumori R, Asari T, and Hagiwara Y. Enhanced release of acetylcholine in the rostral ventrolateral medulla of spontaneously hypertensive rats. *Brain Res* 686:1–9, 1995.
72. Kumagai Y, Shiga T, Sunaga K, Cornelissen G, Ebihara A, and Halberg F. Usefulness of circadian amplitude of blood pressure in predicting hypertensive cardiac involvement. *Chronobiologia* 19:43–58, 1992.
73. Lewandowski J, Pruszczyk P, Elaffi M, Chodakowska J, Wocial B, Switalska H, Januszewicz W, and Zukowska-Grojec Z. Blood pressure, plasma NPY and catecholamines during physical exercise in relation to menstrual cycle, ovariectomy, and estrogen replacement. *Regul Peptides* 75/76:239–245, 1998.
74. Machado BH, Mauad H, Chianca Junior DA, Haibara AS, and Colombari E. Autonomic processing of the cardiovascular reflexes in the nucleus tractus solitarii. *Braz J Med Biol Res* 30:533–543, 1997.
75. Mancia G, Grassi G, Parati G, and Zanchetti A. The sympathetic nervous system in human hypertension. *Acta Physiol Scand Suppl* 640:117–121, 1997.
76. Martens JR, Reaves PY, Lu D, Katovich MJ, Berecek KH, Bishop SP, Raizada MK, and Gelband CH. Prevention of renovascular and cardiac pathophysiological changes in hypertension by angiotensi II type 1 receptor antisense gene therapy. *Proc Natl Acad Sci USA* 95:2664–2669, 1998.
77. Mauad H and Machado BH. Involvement of the ipsilateral rostral ventrolateral medulla in the pressor response to L-glutamate microinjection into the nucleus tractus solitarii of awake rats. *J Auton Nerv Syst* 74:43–48, 1998.
78. M'hamed SB, Sequeira H, Poulain P, Bennis M, and Roy JC. Sensorimotor cortex projections to the ventrolateral and the dorsomedial medulla oblongata in the rat. *Neurosci Lett* 164:195–198, 1993.
79. Morris ST and Reid JL. Monoxidine: a review. *J Hum Hypertens* 11:629–635, 1997.
80. Msghina M, Gonon F, and Stjarne L. Paired pulse analysis of ATP and noradrenaline release from sympathetic nerves of rat tail artery and mouse vas deferens: effects of K^+ channel blockers. *Br J Pharmacol* 125:1669–1676, 1998.
81. Msghina M, Gonon F, and Stjarne L. Facilitation and depression of ATP and noradrenaline release from sympathetic nerves of rat tail artery. *J Physiol* 515(Pt 2):523–531, 1999.

82. Myers J and Morgan T. The effect of sodium intake on the blood pressure related to age and sex. *Clin Exp Hypertheory Pract* 5:118, 1983.
83. Nishimura Y, Usui H, Suzuki A, Kajimoto N, and Yamanishi Y. Relaxant response of isolated basilar arteries to calcitonin gene–related peptide in stroke-prone spontaneously hypertensive rats. *Jpn J Pharmacol* 59:333–338, 1992.
84. Oberhauser V, Vonend O, and Rump LC. Neuropeptide Y and ATP interact to control renovascular resistance in the rat. *J Am Soc Nephrol* 10:1179–1185, 1999.
85. Oparil S, Chen Y-F, Berecek H, Calhoun DA, and Wyss JM. The role of the central nervous system in hypertension. In: Laragh JH and Brenner BM, eds. *Hypertension: Pathophysiology, Diagnosis and Management*. New York: Raven Press, 1995, pp 713–740.
86. Oppenheimer SM, Kedem G, and Martin WM. Left-insular cortex lesions perturb cardiac autonomic tone in humans. *Clin Auton Res* 6:131–140, 1996.
87. Osborn JW and Provo BJ. Salt-dependent hypertension in the sinoaortic denervated rat. *Hypertension* 19:658–662, 1992.
88. Palatini P, Penzo M, Racioppa A, Zugno E, Guzzardi G, Anaclerio M, and Pessina AC. Clinical relevance of nightime blood pressure and of daytime blood pressure variability. *Arch Intern Med* 152:1855–1860, 1992.
89. Peng N, Chambless BD, Oparil S, and Wyss JM. Alpha2A-adrenergic receptors mediate sympathoinhibitory responses to atrial natriuretic peptide in the mouse anterior hypothalamic nucleus. *Hypertension* 41:571–575, 2003.
90. Peng N, Chambless BD, and Wyss JM. Alpha-2 adrenergic receptor knockout mice do not respond to anterior hypothalamic nucleus microinjections of atrial natriuretic peptide. *Hypertension* 32:32, 1998.
91. Peng N, Clark JT, Wei CC, and Wyss JM. Estrogen depletion increases blood pressure and hypothalamic norepinephrine in middle-aged spontaneously hypertensive rats. *Hypertension*, 41:1160–1167, 2003.
92. Peng N, Wei CC, Oparil S, and Wyss JM. The organum vasculosum of the lamina terminalis regulates noradrenaline release in the anterior hypothalamic nucleus. *Neuroscience* 99:149–156, 2000.
93. Phillips MI. Antisense inhibition and adeno-associated viral vector delivery for reducing hypertension. *Hypertension* 29:177–187, 1997.
94. Phillips MI, Mohuczy-Dominiak D, Coffey M, Gali SM, Kimura B, Wu P, and Zelles T. Prolonged reduction of high blood pressure with an in vivo, nonpathogenic, adeno-associated viral vector delivery of AT1-R mRNA antisense. *Hypertension* 29:374–380, 1997.
95. Powis JE, Bains JS, and Ferguson AV. Leptin depolarizes rat hypothalamic paraventricular nucleus neurons. *Am J Physiol* 274:R1468–R1472, 1998.
96. Prichard BN and Graham BR. The use of monoxidine in the treatment of hypertension. *J Hypertens* 15:S47–S55, 1997.
97. Profant J and Dimsdale JE. Race and diurnal blood pressure patterns. *Hypertension* 33:1099–1104, 1999.
98. Raizada MK, Francis SC, Wang H, Gelband CH, Reaves PY, and Katovich MJ. Targeting of the renin-angiotensin system by antisense gene therapy: a possible strategy for the long-term control of hypertension. *J Hypertens* 18: 353–362, 2000.
99. Reis DJ. The nucleus tractus solitarius and experimental neurogenic hypertension: evidence for a central neural imbalance hypothesis of hypertensive disease. *Adv Biochem Psychopharmacol* 28:409–420, 1981.

100. Reis DJ. Neurons and receptors in the rostroventrolateral medulla mediating the antihypertensive actions of drugs acting at imidazoline receptors. *J Cardiovasc Pharmacol* 27(Suppl 3):S11–S18, 1996.
101. Rettig R, Ganten D, Lang RE, and Unger T. Brain angiotensin II: localization and possible functions. *Adv Biochem Psychopharmacol* 43:129–136, 1987.
102. Rettig R, Ganten D, Lang RE, and Unger T. The renin-angiotensin system in the central control of blood pressure. *Eur Heart J* 8(Suppl B):129–132, 1987.
103. Richard D and Bourque CW. Atrial natriuretic peptide modulates synaptic transmission from osmoreceptor afferents to the supraoptic nucleus. *J Neurosci* 16:7526–7532, 1996.
104. Sacks FM, Svetkey LP, Vollmer WM, Appel LJ, Bray GA, Harsha D, Obarzanek E, Conlin PR, Miller ER, III, Simons-Morton DG, Karanja N, and Lin PH. Effects on blood pressure of reduced dietary sodium and the Dietary Approaches to Stop Hypertension (DASH) diet. DASH-Sodium Collaborative Research Group. *N Engl J Med* 344:3–10, 2001.
105. Saigusa T, Iriki M, and Arita J. Brain angiotensin II tonically modulates sympathetic baroreflex in rabbit ventrolateral medulla. *Am J Physiol* 271:H1015–H1021, 1996.
106. Saleh TM and Connel BJ. Centrally mediated effect of 17beta-estradiol on parasympathetic tone in male rats. *Am J Physiol* 276:R474–R481, 1999.
107. Shek EW, Brands MW, and Hall JE. Chronic leptin infusion increases arterial pressure. *Hypertension* 31:409–414, 1998.
108. Steckelings U, Lebrun C, Qadri F, Veltmar A, and Unger T. Role of brain angiotensin in cardiovascular regulation. *J Cardiovasc Pharmacol* 19(Suppl 6):S72–S79, 1992.
109. Sturrock ND, Pound N, Peck GM, Soar CM, and Jeffcoate WJ. An assessment of blood pressure measurement in a diabetic clinic using random-zero, semi-automated, and 24-hour monitoring. *Diabet Med* 14:370–375, 1997.
110. Supowit SC, Hallman DM, Zhao H, and Dipette DJ. Alpha 2-adrenergic receptor activation inhibits calcitonin gene-related peptide expression in cultured dorsal root ganglia neurons. *Brain Res* 782:184–193, 1998.
111. Sutterer JR, Perry J, and DeVito W. Two-way shuttle box and lever-press avoidance in the spontaneously hypertensive and normotensive rat. *J Comp Physiol Psychol* 94:155–163, 1980.
112. Suzuki M, Guilleminault C, Otsuka K, and Shiomi T. Blood pressure "dipping" and "non-dipping" in obstructive sleep apnea syndrome patients. *Sleep* 19:382–387, 1996.
113. Sved AF, Ito S, and Yajima Y. Role of excitatory amino acid inputs to the rostral ventrolateral medulla in cardiovascular regulation. *Clin Exp Pharmacol Physiol* 29:503–506, 2002.
114. Todorov LD, Bjur RA, and Westfall DP. Inhibitory and facilitatory effects of purines on transmitter release from sympathetic nerves. *J Pharmacol Exp Ther* 268:985–989, 1994.
115. Todorov LD, Bjur RA, and Westfall DP. Temporal dissociation of the release of the sympathetic co-transmitters ATP and noradrenaline. *Clin Exp Pharmacol Physiol* 21:931–932, 1994.
116. Todorov LD, Mihaylova-Todorova S, Craviso GL, Bjur RA, and Westfall DP. Evidence for the differential release of the cotransmitters ATP and noradrenaline from sympathetic nerves of the guinea-pig vas deferens. *J Physiol* 496(Pt 3):731–748, 1996.

117. Toth MJ, Sites CK, and Poehlman ET. Hormonal and physiological correlates of energy expenditure and substrate oxidation in middle-aged, premenopausal women. *J Clin Endocrinol Metab* 84:2771–2775, 1999.
118. Toth MJ, Tchernof A, Sites CK, and Poehlman ET. Effect of menopausal status on body composition and abdominal fat distribution. *Int J Obes Relat Metab Disord* 24:226–231, 2000.
119. Toth MJ, Tchernof A, Sites CK, and Poehlman ET. Menopause-related changes in body fat distribution. *Ann NY Acad Sci* 904:502–506, 2000.
120. Vatta M, Rodriguez-Fermepin M, Bianciotti L, Perazzo J, Monserrat A, and Fernandez B. Atrial natriuretic factor enhances norepinephrine uptake in circumventricular organs, locus coeruleus and nucleus tractus solitarii of the rat. *Neurosci Lett* 197:29–32, 1995.
121. Vatta MS, Presas MF, Bianciotti LG, Rodriguez-Fermepin M, Ambros R, and Fernandez BE. B and C types natriuretic peptides modify norepinephrine uptake and release in the rat adrenal medulla. *Peptides* 18:1483–1489, 1997.
122. Verberne AJ and Owens NC. Cortical modulation of the cardiovascular system. *Progr Neurobiol* 54:149–168, 1998.
123. Verdecchia P and Porcellati C. The day–night changes in ambulatory blood pressure: another risk indicator in hypertension. *Giornale Ital Cardiol* 22:879–886, 1992.
124. Verdecchia P, Schillaci G, Boldrina F, Guerrieri M, and Porcellati C. Sex, hypertrophy and diurnal blood pressure variation in essential hypertension. *J Hypertens* 10:683–692, 1992.
125. Wang H and Leenen FH. Brain sodium channels mediate increases in brain "ouabain" and blood pressure in Dahl S rats. *Hypertension* 40:96–100, 2002.
126. Wang H, Reaves PY, Gardon ML, Keene K, Goldberg DS, Gelband CH, Katovich MJ, and Raizada MK. Angiotensin I-converting enzyme antisense gene therapy causes permanent antihypertensive effects in the SHR. *Hypertension* 35:202–208, 2000.
127. Westfall DP, Todorov LD, Mihaylova-Todorova ST, and Bjur RA. Differences between the regulation of noradrenaline and ATP release. *J Auton Pharmacol* 16:393–395, 1996.
128. Westfall TC, Han SP, Chen XL, del Valle K, Curfman M, Ciarleglio A, and Naes L. Presynaptic peptide receptors and hypertension. *Ann NY Acad Sci* 604:372–388, 1990.
129. Westfall TC, Han SP, Knuepfer M, Martin J, Chen XL, del Valle K, Ciarleglio A, and Naes L. Neuropeptides in hypertension: role of neuropeptide Y and calcitonin gene related peptide. *Br J Clin Pharmacol* 30(Suppl 1):75S–82S, 1990.
130. Westfall TC, McCullough LA, Vickery L, Naes L, Yang CL, Han SP, Egan T, Chen X, and MacArthur H. Effects of neuropeptide Y at sympathetic neuroeffector junctions. *Adv Pharmacol* 42:106–110, 1998.
131. Wieldbo B, Sernia C, Gyurko R, and Phillips MI. Antisense inhibition of hypertension in the spontaneously hypertensive rat. *Hypertension* 25:314–319, 1995.
132. Wilson PWF and Kannel WB. Hypertension, other risk factors, and the risk of cardiovascular disease. In: *Hypertension: Pathophysiology, Diagnosis, and Management*, 2nd ed., Vol 1. New York: Raven Press, 1995, pp 99–114.
133. Wyss JM and Carlson SH. The role of the central nervous system in hypertension. *Curr Hypertens Rep* 3:246–253, 1999.
134. Wyss JM, Oparil S, and Sripairojthikoon W. Neuronal control of the kidney: contribution to hypertension. *Can J Physiol Pharmacol* 70:759–770, 1992.

135. Wyss JM and Roysommuti S. The role of the nervous system in dietary NaCl-sensitive hypertension: peripheral and central mechanisms. *Thai J Physiol* 24:155–168, 1997.
136. Zhang Z and Oppenheimer SM. Characterization, distribution and lateralization of baroreceptor-related neurons in the rat insular cortex. *Brain Res* 760:243–250, 1997.
137. Zhang ZH, Dougherty PM, and Oppenheimer SM. Characterization of baroreceptor-related neurons in the monkey insular cortex. *Brain Res* 796:303–306, 1998.

14

Psychological Aspects of Heart Disease

CHRISTINE GAGNON, SRIKANTH RAMACHANDRUNI,
EDITH E. BRAGDON, AND DAVID S. SHEPS

Coronary artery disease (CAD) is the leading cause of death in the United States and other developed countries. Along with a number of other factors thought to contribute to the high prevalence of CAD in developed societies (longer life expectancy, obesity, sedentary lifestyles), various psychological and social factors seem to influence cardiac function in ways that promote heart disease. Several such psychological, social, and behavioral factors will be discussed in this chapter, including type A behavior pattern, hostility, anger, depression, vital exhaustion, anxiety, mental stress, low social support, and lifestyle factors such as diet and exercise.

TYPE A BEHAVIOR PATTERN, HOSTILITY, AND ANGER

Type A Behavior Pattern

Type A behavior pattern (TABP) is characterized by a tendency toward competitiveness, hostility, and exaggerated commitment to work. It has been proposed as an independent risk factor for coronary atherosclerosis and CAD.[132,148] Individuals with a healthy pattern of behavior, referred to as type B personality, are considered to be more resilient to CAD and are often used as a control group when studying TABP. People exhibiting TABP are reportedly at significantly greater risk of developing CAD than are those with type B personality, an association that is independent of other risk factors.[132] Another study indicated that TABP is associated with greater severity of disease in patients with angiographically confirmed CAD, but only in those under 45 years of age.[167] In contrast, TABP was unrelated to disease severity in a study of angiography patients.[38] Eaker and colleagues found that among individuals followed in the Framingham Study, TABP was linked to a greater than twofold increase in risk of angina pectoris.[39] Siegel et al. observed, however, that type A CAD patients were more likely than those with type B pattern to experience silent myocardial ischemia with exercise, but that silent ischemia patients with TABP were *less* likely to have a history of typical angina.[143] While the predictive value of TABP for incidence or severity of CAD is ambiguous, the finding that global TABP (i.e., the presence of the total group of behaviors comprising TABP) is unrelated to adverse cardiac outcomes (myocardial infarction [MI] or cardiac death) is consistent across numerous studies.[26,139,141,143] In fact, Ragland and Brand unexpectedly observed a *lower* mortality rate in type A than in type B patients who survived a MI by at least 24 hours.[127]

A number of investigators have found it more fruitful to focus on "toxic" components of the TABP. For example, one set of findings suggested that the most potent feature of the TABP for prospectively predicting cardiac disease is a constellation of traits consisting of aggravation, irritation, anger, and impatience (AIAI). Higher levels of AIAI were observed in patients with multivessel CAD than in those with single-vessel disease.[82] The "toxic components" that have received the most attention in the literature are hostility and anger (Table 14–1).

Hostility

Hostility incorporates the traits anger, cynicism, and mistrust; high anger-in denotes an exaggerated level of unexpressed angry emotion. Dembroski et al. have reported that of all components of the TABP scored for using the Structured Interview technique of type A assessment, only Potential for Hostility[36] or Potential for Hostility combined with Anger-In (i.e., suppressed anger[37]) were significantly associated with extent of CAD. In fact, several investigators have identified hostility as a stronger determinant than TABP of coronary attack among patients with ischemic heart disease.[10,11,42,64,65,79,88,97,107,109,139] It has also been shown that the hostility confers a twofold accelerated risk for carotid atherosclerosis and also increased risk for restenosis after percutaneous transluminal coronary angioplasty (PTCA).[70]

A number of physiological and behavioral factors may link hostility with increased cardiac risk. High hostility is associated with higher body mass index, more physical activity at work, and poorer pulmonary function. It is also associated with a higher concentration of unhealthy lifestyle behaviors, including smoking, poor diet, obesity, and alcoholism.[164] Hostile subjects manifest higher heart rate and blood pressure responses to

TABLE 14–1 Selected Studies Pertaining to Hostility and Anger and Coronary Artery Disease

Study	Risk Factor	End Points	Findings
Barefoot et al.[10,a]	Hostility	CD, ACD	Predicted both CD and ACD ($P < 0.005$)
Barefoot et al.[11,a]	Hostility	MI, ACD	RR (CI) = 1.6 (1.1–2.3) for MI
De Leon et al.[35,b]	Trait anger, PRI	Multivessel disease, recurrent event(s) after PTCA	RR (CI) = 1.80 (1.18–2.76) trait anger for multivessel disease; 2.1 (1.1–4.1) PRI for recurrent event after PTCA
Dembroski et al.[36,b]	Potential for hostility	CD, MI	RR = 1.7 ($P = 0.005$) (adjusted for traditional risk factors)
Everson et al.[42,a]	Cynical hostility	CD, MI, ACD	ACD: RR (CI) = 2.30 (1.47–1.39) CD: 2.18 (1.01–4.70)
Kawachi et al.[79,a]	Chronic anger	CD, MI, angina	RR (CI) = 2.66 (1.26–5.61)
Leon et al.[97,a]	Hostility	CD	No relationship
McCranie et al.[109,a]	Hostility	CD	No relationship
Shekelle et al.[141,a]	Hostility	CD, MI, ACD	Predicted ACD significantly ($P = 0.02$); predicted CD marginally ($P < 0.09$)

ACD, all-cause death; CD, cardiac death; CI, 95% confidence interval; MI, myocardial infarction; PRI, psychological risk index, which comprises trait anger and vital exhaustion; PTCA, percutaneous transluminal coronary angioplasty; RR, relative risk.
aStudies in subjects initially without heart disease.
bStudies in heart disease patients.

physiological stimuli, such as mental tasks,[152] as well as higher ambulatory blood pressure levels during daily life activity.[149] Also, evidence suggests that hostile individuals are more likely to exhibit hypercortisolemia and high levels of circulating catecholamines,[126,150] as well as diminished mononuclear leukocyte β-adrenergic receptor function.[151] Preliminary data suggest that hostile individuals may also manifest diminished vagal modulation of heart function[146] and increased platelet reactivity.[51,105]

Anger

Anger has received less attention as a potential risk factor for CAD than hostility and is often researched in combination with hostility, of which it is actually a component.[78] An angry temperament appears to have a stronger relation to CAD than reactive anger.[165] Anger, but not other mood states (anxiety, worry, sadness, happiness, challenge, feeling in control, or interest), was shown to trigger arrhythmias in patients with implantable cardioverter defibrillators.[94] Furthermore, a community-based sample of anger-prone normotensives was found to have higher mortality and morbidity risks for CAD than normotensives with low anger.[166] Risk for a MI appears to be increased within 1 to 2 hours following an anger episode.[112]

The literature includes some evidence to support both expressed and repressed anger as risk factors for CAD. Suppression, or "anger-in," and low "anger-out" were both found to be predictive of subsequent incidents of ischemic heart disease.[52] Conflict between cognition and behavioral expression of anger during stressful situations has been reported to result in greater flight-or-fight response in healthy males than when there is consistency between cognition and behavior.[166] There is also evidence favoring a larger role for expressed than for repressed anger in CAD.[144]

Increased serum lipids are associated with high trait anger and may constitute a pathophysiological mechanism linking anger and CAD.[166]

Depression and Vital Exhaustion

Depression

Depression is probably the most widely researched negative mood associated with risk for CAD. Major depressive disorder is characterized by the presence of at least five of the following: depressed mood, decreased interest or pleasure in previously enjoyable activities, significant change in weight or appetite, sleep disturbance, loss of energy, impaired cognitive abilities, feelings of guilt or worthlessness, motor problems, and morbid or suicidal thoughts.[2]

While some studies have failed to find a positive relationship between depression and cardiac events,[133] many more findings have substantiated the role of depression in developing CAD. The association between cardiovascular disease and affective disorder is supported by the observations that (1) there is a high rate of depression in the post-MI period, (2) depression adversely affects the prognosis of cardiac disease, and (3) affected patients have a higher-than-expected rate of sudden cardiac death.[131,133]

Patients with a lifetime history of MI have significantly more spells of depression[162] and depressed patients after an MI are more likely to be anxious or stressed than their counterparts without depression. Point prevalence rates of major depression in patients with coronary disease range from 17% to 23%,[61] and patients with CAD are three times more likely to be depressed than is the general population.[3]

Risk ratio for mortality in depressed patients with documented CAD has been reported to range between 1.25 and 5.0.[3,12] In patients hospitalized following an MI, major depression is an independent risk factor for mortality, increasing the risk by fourfold at 6 months,[47] and by eightfold at 18 months.[48] The risk is greatest among patients with ≥10 premature ventricular contractions (PVCs) per hour. These findings remained significant when adjusted for relevant covariates, including left ventricular dysfunction, tobacco use, or history of MI.[48] Frasure-Smith et al. found that, of post-MI patients receiving routine care after hospital discharge, those with higher levels of stress (indicated by the Stress Score on the General Health Questionnaire) had a threefold increase in risk of cardiac mortality over 5 years and an approximately 1.5-fold increase in risk of reinfarction over the same period. Major depressive disorder was the best predictor of adverse outcomes, followed by disease severity and left ventricular ejection fraction.[43]

Mortality risk appears to increase along with the severity of depression, and individuals with depressive symptomatology not meeting full diagnostic criteria are also at elevated risk for coronary events, with the relationship to CAD becoming stronger as the number of depressive symptoms increases.[3,122]

A number of mechanisms may link depression with poor cardiac outcomes. A higher prevalence of ventricular tachycardia was noted among the depressed patients, which may explain these patients' increased risk (by 30-fold) for cardiac mortality. Furthermore, ventricular tachycardia occurs with greater frequency in individuals with both depression and stable CAD.[22] Depressed patients also have significantly greater levels of catecholamines and higher blood pressure, heart rate, cardiac rhythm, and myocardial oxygen demand.[89] Impaired baroreflex sensitivity has also been documented in CAD patients with depression.[159] Patients with CAD and depression demonstrate less heart rate variability than those with low scores, a finding that suggests decreased levels of parasympathetic activation;[25,91,147] this may adversely alter their risk of death. Carney et al. found that cognitive behavioral therapy focused on the treatment of depression in CAD patients yielded increased heart rate variability and decreased heart rate, thus possibly reducing the risk of mortality.[23] Major depression may also be associated with increased platelet aggregability.[96,99] It still remains to be seen if treatment of depression in patients with heart disease will successfully decrease the adverse prognosis.

TABLE 14–2 Selected Studies Pertaining to Depression and Coronary Artery Disease

Study	Risk Factor	End Points	Findings
Anda et al.[3,a]	Depression, hopelessness	CD	Depressed affect: RR (CI) = 1.5 (1.0–2.3) Moderate hopelessness: 1.6 (1.0–2.5) Severe hopelessness: 2.1 (1.1–3.9)
Barefoot and Schroll[12,a]	Depression	CD, ACD	CD: $P = 0.002$ All death: $P = 0.001$
Carney et al.[24,b]	Depression	Death, MI, PTCA, CABG	RR = 2.5 (CI not reported)
Frasure-Smith et al.[47,b]	Depression	Fatal and nonfatal MI, unstable angina	Depression: RR (CI) = 3.6 (1.3–10.1) Depressive symptoms: 7.8 (2.4–25.3)
Frasure-Smith at al.[45,b]	Depressive symptoms	CD	RR (CI) = 3.05 (1.29–7.17)δ
Williams et al.[166,a]	Trait anger	CD, acute and silent MI, revascularization	RR (CI) = 1.54 (1.10–2.16) for combined end points; 1.75 (1.17–2.64) for acute MI and CD only

CABG, coronary artery bypass graft; CI, confidence interval; MI, myocardial infarction; PTCA, percutaneous transluminal coronary angioplasty; RR, relative risk.
[a]Studies in subjects initially without heart disease.
[b]Studies in heart disease patients.

Table 14–2 summarizes findings from selected studies that have related depression to established heart disease.

Vital Exhaustion

Chronic vital exhaustion is a psychological state consisting of fatigue, irritability, depleted energy levels, and demoralization.[5,6,8] It is a precursor to first MIs and is also associated with other cardiac events.[7,87]

There is, however, some controversy regarding the contribution of vital exhaustion in CAD. Some investigators argue that vital exhaustion and depression are not separate and distinct entities because of the strong relationships they found between measures of these constructs.[168] However, the two constructs exhibit differing relationships with other behavioral risk factors, which suggests that each is a unique entity. More specifically, stronger associations have been shown between depression and alcohol, drug use, hostility, cognitive dysfunctions, and congenital disorders, whereas vital exhaustion has been more strongly linked to cardiovascular complaints and treatment.[87] Additionally, vital exhaustion appears to be more strongly related to short-term risk, whereas depression has a greater relationship with long-term risk of CAD.[12] In a prospective observational study, frequent sense of exhaustion appeared to be independently associated with increased risk of CAD mortality in men.[30]

An imbalance between blood coagulation and fibrinolysis has been suggested as a possible mediator of vital exhaustion and subsequent MI.[86] Dysregulation of the hypothalamic–pituitary–adrenocortical (HPA) axis has also been proposed as a possible mechanism linking vital exhaustion with heart disease outcomes.[6,119] In a two-stage theoretical model of MI pathogenesis proposed by Goodkin and Appels, vital exhaustion constitutes a relatively brief second stage following a long period of hostility, occupational overexertion, and life stressors. The second stage is associated with subsequent immunosuppression and possible autoimmune reactions; of particular interest is the promotion of cytokine production in the brain, which may exacerbate the sense of exhaustion by overstimulating the HPA axis.[56]

ANXIETY

Anxiety is associated with a higher risk of CAD. High blood pressure,[163] smoking, and alcohol use exacerbate the influence of anxiety on progression of atherosclerosis. Anxiety is exceptionally common in patients with acute coronary syndrome, with an incidence approaching 50% among patients in the cardiac care unit.[27,115] The Normative Aging Study documented a three- to sixfold increased risk for MI and sudden cardiac death among highly anxious patients.[93] Frasure-Smith et al. found that following an MI, anxiety was associated with a 2.5-fold increase in risk for ischemic complications.[49] Similarly, a substudy from the Global Utilization of Streptokinase and Tissue Plasminogen Activator for Occluded Coronary Arteries (GUSTO) trial suggested that patients with acute MI and a high level of in-hospital anxiety had an almost fivefold increase in risk for recurrent ischemia, reinfarction, or death, compared with patients with MI without high levels of anxiety.[115] In fact, this study suggested that early in-hospital anxiety following MI was one of the strongest predictors for in-hospital complications.

Within the spectrum of anxiety disorders, phobic anxiety, generalized anxiety, panic disorder, and worry are predictors of MI and/or cardiac death,[60,77,80,93,161] although a few studies did not confirm this association.[108,154,155] Men with "phobic anxiety," a construct that appears to overlap substantially with panic disorder, also have higher rates of sudden cardiac death and CAD than control populations.[57,80] Men with panic disorder also exhibited excess mortality due to circulatory system disease.[31]

Patients with both generalized anxiety disorder and major depressive disorder have increased serum cholesterol, triglyceride, and LDL-C and reduced HDL-C levels, compared to patients with either disorder by itself, and thus may have a greater risk of mortality from CAD than patients with just one of these disorders.[138] Reduced heart rate variability[81,124] and reduction in vagal control of the heart[156,160] are associated with anxious symptomatology; reduction in the vagal control of heart rate and reduced heart rate variability are associated with increased cardiac mortality and morbidity, and predict fatal outcomes after MI.[15,69,84,95,113,171,172]

Paterniti et al. suggest that chronically high levels of anxiety may contribute to accelerating the evolution of carotid atherosclerosis.[121] This group followed 726 initially disease-free adults for 4 years and found that sustained anxiety was associated with a higher increase in common carotid intima–media thickness in both sexes and higher plaque occurrence in men than in individuals without sustained anxiety. Anxious symptomatology is also associated with sympathetic nervous system hyperactivation, which has been shown to damage the endothelium and to induce exaggerated heart rate and blood pressure responses to behavioral stimuli—both effects that may enhance the progression of atherosclerosis.[1,13,71,118,123]

An interesting side note on the implications of anxiety in diagnosing CAD is that among women with chest pain symptoms, a history of anxiety disorders is associated with a lower probability of significant angiographic CAD. Knowledge of anxiety disorder history may assist in the clinical evaluation of women with chest pain.[134]

Table 14–3 summarizes findings from studies that have related anxiety to development of established heart disease and established ischemic heart disease, respectively.

STRESS

Stress results when there is a discrepancy between the physical and/or psychological demands and the resources available for meeting those demands. The specific physical and/or psychological demands are called *stressors*. In general, the body's physiological reaction to stress includes increases in heart rate, blood pressure, respiration, muscle tension, and perspiration. Additionally, there is an increase in the levels of hormones, including corticosteroids and catecholamines, secreted by the adrenal glands.[59,125] Although stress can be uncomfortable, a certain amount of

TABLE 14–3 Selected Studies Pertaining to Anxiety Disorders and Coronary Artery Disease

Study	Risk Factor	End Points	Results
Coryell et al.[32]	Panic disorder	ACD	RR = 2.0 (CI not reported)
Haines et al.[60]	Phobic anxiety	ACD, MI	ACD: RR (CI) = 3.8 (1.6–8.6)
			MI: 1.3 (0.6–2.5)
Kawachi et al.[77]	Phobic anxiety	MI, sudden death	MI: RR (CI) = 0.9 (0.5–1.8)
			Sudden death: 4.5 (0.9–21.6)
Kawachi et al.[80]	Anxiety	CD, MI	CD: RR (CI) = 1.9 (0.7–5.4)
			MI: 2.4 (1.4–4.1)
Kubzansky et al.[93]	Worry	MI	RR (CI) = 2.4 (1.4–4.1)
Weissman et al.[161]	Panic disorder	MI, sudden death	MI: RR (CI) = 4.5 (1.7–12.3)
			Sudden death: 6.1 (2.4–15.7)

ACD, all-cause death; CD, cardiac death; CI, 95% confidence interval; MI, myocardial infarction; RR, relative risk. All studies were in subjects initially without CAD.

stress can be healthy, which is termed *eustress*.[111] Both too much and too little stress are believed to negatively affect quality of functioning.

It is well recognized that stress can be harmful to the cardiovascular system. Chronic elevations of catecholamines and corticosteroids damage arteries, contributing to the development of atherosclerosis, hypertension, and arteriosclerosis. Both prospective and retrospective studies have found the occurrence of major life events to precipitate MI.[72] Sudden death occurs when an individual who already has a cardiac vulnerability experiences an extreme stressor, such as the death of a loved one. The combination of the preexisting vulnerability and the major stressor are believed to result in cardiac arrhythmias leading to death.[116]

In a series of reports, Frasier-Smith and colleagues have described studies addressing the impact of high levels of psychological stress symptoms in the hospital after an acute MI.[43,44,46,50] One such study followed 461 men over 5 years who took part in a trial of psychological stress monitoring and intervention after an MI-related hospitalization. In patients receiving routine care after discharge, high stress was associated with a close to threefold increase in risk of cardiac mortality over 5 years and an approximately 1.5-fold increase in risk of reinfarction over the same period. In contrast, highly stressed patients who took part in the 1-year program of stress monitoring and intervention did not experience any significant long-term increase in risk.[43] In a similar study, for patients with non–Q-wave MIs receiving usual care, high stress in the hospital was associated with increased risk of cardiac mortality. In comparison, control patients with Q-wave MIs had no stress-related increase in risk, as in the patients with non–Q-wave MIs in the treatment group.[44]

Chronic Environmental Stress

The literature reflects a growing awareness of the importance of work-related stress as a serious CAD risk factor. For example, in a study of both male and female penitentiary staff personnel, individuals who subdued both their emotions and actions in anger-producing circumstances displayed ECG signs of CAD.[63] A number of fundamental factors tie shift work to CAD, including increased risk-related behaviors such as smoking and the disruption of circadian rhythm.[85,153]

Two theoretical models have been proposed to characterize the relationship between work-related stressor(s) and CAD. The first is the "job strain" model advanced by Karasek.[73] This model asserts that jobs in which high work demands are coupled with low decision latitude augment individuals' risk for CAD.[18,73] Elevated blood pressure has also been linked to job strain, especially in men. Several studies have appeared to document such a link,[73–75] although others[17,67] have failed to support this model. It is of interest that hypertension, one of the primary risk factors for CAD, has also been associated with job strain, especially in men.[135]

A more recently developed model, the effort-reward imbalance model, suggests that high-cost/low-gain occupational situations are stressful and may be associated with CAD.[145] Findings by Lynch et al. and by Bosma et al. provide some corroboration for this theory. Lynch and colleagues reported a significantly greater 4-year increase in plaque height and intima-media thickness in men with high-demand, low-income jobs than that in those with low-demand, high-income jobs.[103] Bosma and colleagues similarly reported an increase in new CAD for individuals (male and female), followed over approximately 5 years, whose jobs were characterized by high personal effort requirements and inadequate opportunity for rewards such as promotions.[67]

Acute Stress

The circadian variation in frequency of sudden cardiac death and myocardial ischemia is characterized by a morning peak. A meta-analysis of 66,635 patients with an acute MI and 19,390 patients with sudden death showed an excess of MIs (relative risk 1.38) and sudden deaths (relative risk 1.29) between the hours of 6 AM and noon, compared to the rest of the day.[28] These events were triggered by external factors, involving the activation of sympathetic nervous system. This finding is further supported by a study that reported absence of circadian variation in a sample of 1225 diabetic patients, particularly those with evidence of cardiac autonomic neuropathy and those taking β-blockers or aspirin.[9] Data from the Multicenter Investigation of the Limitation of Infarct size (MILIS) reported that 48% of 849 patients with an acute MI described one or more possible triggers, the most common one being emotional upset (14%).[157] Similarly, stressful life events occurred among 40 of 100 sudden-death victims on the day preceding death.[117]

An increase in cardiovascular events has also been associated with disasters. During the 5 days after the 1981 Athens earthquake, the incidence of cardiac deaths rose from the normal average of 2.6 deaths per day to an average of 5.4, with a peak of 8 deaths per day.[158] A sharp increase in early-morning cardiovascular mortality (relative risk [RR] = 2.4) was observed after the 1994 Los Angeles earthquake, compared to that of the week before the disaster.[98] This was not observed after the San Franscisco earthquake of 1989, which occurred in the afternoon. This suggests that MI is more likely to be precipitated by extreme life stress superimposed on a second trigger linked to circadian pattern, such as abrupt awakening in the morning.[19] A few other studies also support the above observations. A sudden increase in ischemic deaths was noted during the first week after blizzards in Massachusetts from 1974 to 1978.[54] In the 1991 Gulf War, incidence of acute infarction rose sharply in the first week after the missile attacks on Israel.[110] After the earthquake in Hanshin-Awaji, Japan, a similar observation was made.[76]

A model of the relationships between factors linking acute stress and cardiac pathology and death is depicted in Figure 14–1. Clinically, the effect of acute or subacute stress on established ischemic heart disease, including elevation of risk for recurrent ischemia, has been well demonstrated. Stress has been shown to provoke myocardial ischemia via numerous mechanisms in patients with CAD. Vasomotor abnormalities of atherosclerotic epicardial coronary arteries and the cardiac microcirculation have been noted in patients with CAD subjected to mental stress. Patients with CAD often exhibit an exaggerated systemic response to stress, characterized by an abnormally increased production of catecholamines, which can result in increased myocardial oxygen demand due to elevations in heart rate, blood pressure, and the rate of ventricular contraction. This increases vulnerability to ventricular tachycardia or ventricular fibrillation. Finally, abnormalities of thrombosis and hemostasis, including increases in platelet aggregability, and alterations in the fibrinolytic system (possibly as a consequence of elevated plasminogen activator inhibitor 1 levels) have been noted in patients subjected to chronic stress.[34,89,99,104,128,173]

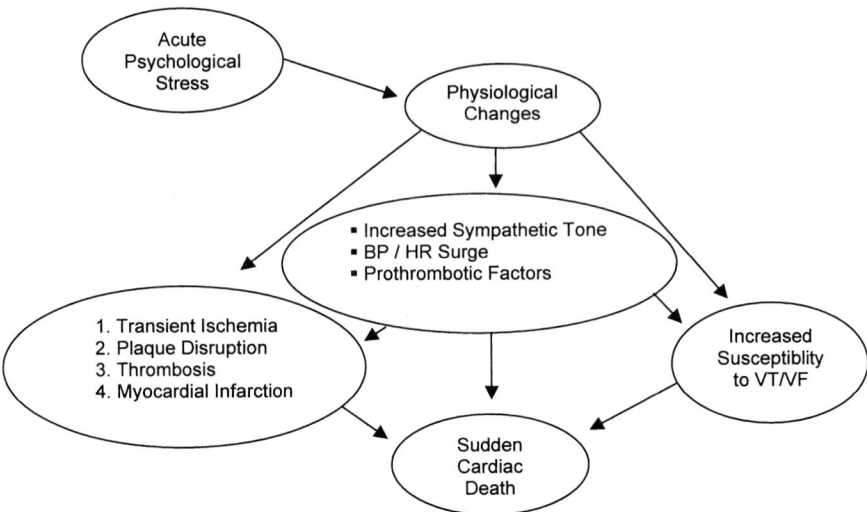

FIGURE 14–1 Model of the factors linking emotional stress with cardiac pathology and death. BP, blood pressure; HR, heart rate; VF, ventricular fibrillation; VT, ventricular tachycardia.

SOCIAL SUPPORT

Animal research has served as one important source of information pertaining to the cardiovascular benefits of social support. Experiments have shown social isolation to increase the coronary atherosclerosis in zoo mammals and birds,[129] swine,[130] and cynomolgus monkeys.[142]

In humans, a series of several prospective community-based studies have demonstrated an inverse correlation between the level of social support and CAD mortality and morbidity. Operational definitions of social support in these studies have variously used structural, functional, or subjective criteria. The earliest studies in particular were focused on social network, recording such measures as participation in group activities, family affiliations, and marital status. These studies measured both emotional support from very close persons ("attachment") and the support provided by the extended network ("social integration"). Later research often took account of subjects' own perceptions concerning the amount and adequacy of available emotional support. Some of these studies evaluated the access to guidance and perceived availability of needed assistance (i.e., tangible support).

Patients with small social networks have an elevated risk of mortality.[20,41,58,90,120] Participation in a relatively small network has been found, on average, to be associated with a two- to threefold increase in the incidence of CAD over time. Similarly, low levels of perceived emotional support confer an even greater increased risk for future cardiac events. In a 1-year longitudinal study of post-MI patients, insufficiency of tangible support with respect to health problems was an important prognostic factor for both decline in physical function and risk for death.[169]

Higher all-cause mortality risk has been found among men with low availability of emotional support and low adequacy of social participation and among men living alone.[62,68] Socially isolated men also demonstrate an increased risk of fatal CAD. Eng et al. observed that for older men, a greater number of close friends and higher religious-service attendance over time were both significantly predictive of decreased mortality.[40] Seeman et al. analyzed data from the Alameda County Study pertaining to the implications of different types of social ties for 17-year survival. Their results revealed that the strongest predictor of low mortality risk was married status for individuals under 60 years of age at baseline, but for persons aged 60 and over it was the number of close ties with friends and relatives.[137]

Social support has been implicated as a significant factor in recovery from MI and coronary artery bypass surgery.[4,83,100,114] Lack of social ties appears to be related to higher mortality, whereas emotional social support has been shown to be related to better chance of recovery from coronary events.[83] Social support may be especially important for maintaining compliance with rehabilitation programs for patients with CAD.[4] Among elderly patients hospitalized with clinical heart failure, the absence of emotional support, measured before admission, is a strong, independent predictor of the occurrence of fatal and nonfatal cardiovascular events in the year after admission.[92]

That social support interacts with other emotional factors has been shown in a few studies. For example, low emotional support accompanied by expressed anger has been shown to increase the risk of CAD progression, independent of medication or other risk factors. Persons with TABP who reported low levels of social support had more severe CAD than type A persons with high levels of social support; this relationship was not present for type B persons.[16]

The underlying pathophysiological mechanisms by which social support mitigates cardiovascular risk may involve alteration of high-risk behaviors. Emotional support may be associated with greater patient adherence to medical therapy and lifestyle modifications. However, it is relevant to note that the association between emotional support and cardiovascular outcomes does not appear to be mediated by smoking, obesity, or physical activity. Emotional support may also mitigate potentially damaging effects of negative emotional interactions on neuroendocrine and physiological regulatory systems, in part by dampening physiological responsivity to psychological challenges.[29,53,136] For example, in a laboratory experiment designed by Gerin et al., subjects played low- and high-stress versions of a videogame, both alone and together with a partner (social support). Participants exhibited lower diastolic blood pressure levels and rated the stressfulness of the game lower in the "together" condition than in the "alone" condition; furthermore, support moderated cardiovascular reactivity (change from baseline) when engaged in the high-stress, but not the low-stress, version of the game.[53]

LIFESTYLE CONTRIBUTIONS TO HEART DISEASE

Despite a significant decrease in the death rate due to cardiovascular illnesses during the last 3–4 decades, atherosclerotic CAD continues to be the leading cause of death and disability in the United States. But there is compelling evidence from random clinical trials in patients with CAD that risk factor alteration is helpful in diminishing cardiovascular mortality.[174] The two main lifestyle factors that are key for preventing these incapacitating conditions are diet and exercise. Both under- and overnutrition lead to diseases. The recommended diet patterns for avoiding hypertension and its related diseases such as stroke and dementia are low-sodium and high-potassium intakes, as well as the consumption of fruits and vegetables, and of the optimal quantity and types of fats, cholesterol, vegetable oils, and fish.[170] With respect to exercise, regardless of widespread knowledge of the benefits of including moderate to vigorous physical activity in one's daily life, more than 60% of the population is insufficiently active. Therefore, long-term remedies for CAD start with such basic lifestyle measures as weight reduction and control, including reduction of total fat calories to <30% of total calories, modification of fat intake to increased monounsaturated vegetable fat, increased intake of dietary fibers, increased physical activity, and controlled stress relaxation.[55] Research indicates that regular physical activity and healthy nutrition are effective in primary and secondary prevention of CAD. A percentage increase in physical activity with associated weight loss has a deep influence on peripheral lipoprotein metabolism and has shown to improve the atherogenic lipoprotein profile. Because a person's risk factors track down from childhood, it is imperative to prevent risk factors as early as possible.[14]

Numerous research studies suggest that dietary and lifestyle patterns in childhood influence CAD risk in adulthood. Harmful lifestyle and dietary habits such as smoking, high habitual dietary intake of total fat and saturated fat, low exercise level, and excessive alcohol consumption often characterize families collectively. These habits in turn are directly related to high levels of serum cholesterol, obesity, and hypertension in children, and with premature death from CAD. Long-term intervention involving reduction of dietary fat and work-related stress, increased exercise, and elimination of smoking have all been shown to significantly reduce coronary risk factors.[33]

Saturated fat consumed in high amounts is considered one of the main culprits of CAD. Hyperlipidemia is frequently left untreated in women. Initially, hormone replacement therapy (HRT) was considered first-line treatment for the management of hypercholesterolemia to prevent CAD in women. Recent research suggests, however, that HRT may not be effective for secondary prevention of coronary events, despite its beneficial effects on lipids.[102] According to a recent clinical trial, women with elevated cholesterol levels benefit from the lipid-lowering effects of statins for both high-risk primary and secondary prevention of CAD;[66] the revised National Cholesterol Education Program (NCEP) guidelines recommend statins as first-line therapy for women with hyperlipidemia. These recommendations are strongly supported by the American Heart Association and the American College of Cardiology.

The elderly percentage of the population is higher now than ever before. The average life span for a man of 45 years is now 77.3 years and 82.8 years for a woman. This increase in life expectancy is directly attributed to a decrease in CAD: over the past three decades, cardiovascular mortality has been decreasing at the rate of 3% per year. This corresponds to a decrease in both out-of-hospital (community) and hospital deaths and a decrease in nonfatal MI. In addition to advances in technology, a primary explanation behind this trend seems to be the adoption of healthier lifestyles, which appear to account for approximately half of the decline in CAD. Behavioral changes leading to reductions in blood pressure to within the normal range seem to be a particularly important contributor. However, the rate of decline in CAD differs by region and is influenced by socioeconomic factors.[101,106]

A common misconception among both health professionals and the public—namely a belief that heart disease primarily affects men—may constitute an impediment to the adoption of healthy life habits by women. Despite the overall trend toward healthier lifestyle choices, high-risk lifestyles have been reported to account for as much as 80% of women's coronary events,[101] yet many elderly women underestimate their risk for heart attack. This may partially explain the failure of some to make changes in their dietary habits, activity levels, and tobacco that could decrease their risk. In addition, many physicians do not treat cardiovascular risk factors aggressively in middle-aged and older women, despite data from primary and secondary prevention trials supporting the usefulness of interventions.[21]

REFERENCES

1. Ablad B, Bjorkman JA, Gustafsson D, Hansson G, Ostlund-Lindqvist and Pettersson K. The role of sympathetic activation in atherogenesis: effects of beta-blockade. *Am Heart J* 116:322–327, 1988.
2. American Psychiatric Association. *Diagnostic and Statistical Manual of Mental Disorders, Fourth Edition*. Arlington, VA: American Psychiatric Press. 1994.
3. Anda R, Williamson D, Jones D, Macera C, Eaker E, Glassman A, and Marks J. Depressed affect, hopelessness, and the risk of ischemic heart disease in a cohort of U.S. adults. *Epidemiology* 4:285–294, 1993.
4. Anderson D, Deshaies G, and Jobin J. Social support, social networks and coronary artery disease rehabilitation: a review. *Can J Cardiol* 12:739–744, 1996.
5. Appels A. Mental precursors of myocardial infarction. *Br J Psychiatry* 156:465–471, 1990.
6. Appels A. Exhausted subjects, exhausted systems. *Acta Physiol Scand* 640(Suppl):153–154, 1997A.
7. Appels A, Bar F, Lasker J, Flamm U, and Kop W. The effect of a psychological intervention program on the risk of a new coronary event after angioplasty: a feasibility study. *J Psychosom Res* 43:209–217, 1997.
8. Appels A and Mulder P. Fatigue and heart disease. The association between 'vital exhaustion' and past, present and future coronary heart disease. *J Psychosom Res* 33:727–738, 1989.
9. Aronson D, Weinrauch LA, D'Elia JA, Tofler GH, and Burger AJ. Circadian patterns of heart rate variability, fibrinolytic activity, and hemostatic factors in type I diabetes mellitus with autonomic neuropathy. *Am J Cardiol* 84:449–453, 1999.
10. Barefoot J, Dahlstrom WG, and Williams RB. Hostility, CHD incidence, and total mortality: a 25-year follow-up study of 255 physicians. *Psychosom Med* 45:59–63, 1983.
11. Barefoot JC, Larsen S, Lieth L, and Chroll M. Hostility, incidence of acute myocardial infarction, and mortality in a sample of older men and women. *Am J Epidemiol* 142:477–484, 1995.
12. Barefoot JC and Schroll M. Symptoms of depression, acute myocardial infarction and total mortality in a community sample. *Circulation* 93:1976–1980, 1996.
13. Barnett PA, Spence JD, Manuck SB, and Jennings JR. Psychological stress and the progression of carotid artery disease. *J Hypertens* 15:49–55, 1997.
14. Berg A, Halle M, Bauer S, Korsten-Reck U, and Keul J. Physical activity and eating behavior: strategies for improving the serum lipid profile of children and adolescents [in German]. *Wien Med Wochenschr* 144:138–144, 1994.
15. Bigger JT, Fleiss JL, Steinman RC, Rolnitzky LM, Kleiger RE, and Rottman JN. Frequency domain measures of heart period variability and mortality after myocardial infarction. *Circulation* 85:164–171, 1992.

16. Blumenthal JA, Burg MM, Barefoot J, Williams RB, Haney T, and Zimet G. Social support, type A behavior, and coronary artery disease. *Psychosom Med* 49:331–340, 1987.
17. Bosma H, Peter R, Siegrist J, and Marmot M. Two alternative job stress models and the risk of coronary heart disease. *Am J Public Health* 88:68–74, 1998.
18. Bosma H, Stansfeld SA, and Marmot MG. Job control, personal characteristics, and heart disease. *J Occup Health Psychol* 3:402–409, 1998.
19. Brown DL. Disparate effects of the 1989 Loma Prieta and 1994 Northridge earthquakes on hospital admissions for acute myocardial infarction: importance of superimposed triggers. *Am Heart J* 137:830–836, 1999.
20. Brummett, BH, Barefoot JC, Siegler IC, Clapp-Channing NE, Lytle BL, Bosworth HB, Williams RB, Jr, and Mark DB. Characteristics of socially isolated patients with coronary artery disease who are at elevated risk for mortality. *Psychosom Med* 63:267–272, 2001.
21. Carlsson CM and Stein JH. Cardiovascular disease and the aging woman: overcoming barriers to lifestyle changes. *Curr Womens Health Rep* 2:366–372, 2002.
22. Carney RM, Freedland KE, Rich MW, Smith LJ, and Jaffe AS. Ventricular tachycardia and psychiatric depression in patients with coronary artery disease. *Am J Med* 95:23–28, 1993.
23. Carney RM, Freedland KE, Stein PK, Skala JA, Hoffman P, and Jaffe AS. Change in heart rate and heart rate variability during treatment for depression in patients with coronary heart disease. *Psychosom Med* 62:639–647, 2000.
24. Carney RM, Rich MW, Freedland KE, Saini J, teVelde A, Simeone C, and Clark K. Major depressive disorder predicts cardiac events in patients with coronary artery disease. *Psychosom Med* 50:627–633, 1988.
25. Carney RM, Saunders RD, Freedland KE, Stein P, Rich MW, and Jaffe AS. Association of depression with reduced heart rate variability in coronary artery disease. *Am J Cardiol* 76:562–564, 1995.
26. Case RB, Heller SS, Case NB, and Moss AJ. The Multicenter Post Infarction Research Group: type A behavior and survival after acute myocardial infarction. *N Engl J Med* 312:737–741, 1985.
27. Cassem NH and Hackett TP. Psychiatric consultation in a coronary care unit. *Ann Intern Med* 75:9–14, 1971.
28. Cohen MC, Rohtla KM, Lavery CE, Muller JE, and Mittleman MA. Meta-analysis of the morning excess of acute myocardial infarction and sudden cardiac death. *Am J Cardiol* 79:1512–1516, 1997.
29. Cohen S. Psychosocial models of the role of social support in the etiology of physical disease. *Health Psychol* 7:269–297, 1988.
30. Cole SR, Kawachi I, Sesso HD, Paffenbarger RS and Lee IM. Sense of exhaustion and coronary heart disease among college alumni. *Am J Cardiol* 84:1401–1405, 1999.
31. Coryell W, Noyes R, and Clancy J. Excess mortality in panic disorder: a comparison with primary unipolar depression. *Arch Gen Psychiatry* 39:701–703, 1982.
32. Coryell W, Noyes R, and House JD. Mortality among outpatients with anxiety disorders. *Am J Psychiatry* 143:508–510, 1986.
33. Cunnane SC. Childhood origins of lifestyle-related risk factors for coronary heart disease in adulthood. *Nutrition Health* 9:107–115, 1993.

34. Dakak N, Quyyumi A, Eisenhofer G, Goldstein DS, and Cannon RO. Sympathetically mediated effects of mental stress on the cardiac microcirculation of patients with coronary artery disease. *Am J Cardiol* 76:125–130, 1995.
35. De Leon CF, Kop WJ, de Swart HB, Bar FW, and Appels PWM. Psychosocial characteristics and recurrent events after percutaneous transluminal coronary angioplasty. *Am J Cardiol* 77:252–255, 1996.
36. Dembroski TM, MacDougall JM, Costa PT, and Grandits GA. Components of hostility as predictors of sudden death and myocardial infarction in the Multiple Risk Factor Intervention Trial. *Psychosom Med* 51:514–522, 1989.
37. Dembroski TM, MacDougall JM, Williams RB, Haney TL, and Blumenthal JA. Components of type A, hostility, and anger-in: relationship to angiographic findings. *Psychosom Med* 47:219–233, 1985.
38. Dimsdale JE, Hackett TP, Hutter AM, Jr, Block PC, Canzano DM, and White PJ. Type A behavior and angiographic findings. *J Psychosom Res* 23:273–276, 1979.
39. Eaker ED, Abbott RD, and Kannel WB. Frequency of uncomplicated angina pectoris in type A compared with type B persons (the Framingham Study). *Am J Cardiol* 63:1042–1045, 1989.
40. Eng PM, Rimm EB, Fitzmaurice G, and Kawachi I. Social ties and change in social ties in relation to subsequent total and cause-specific mortality and coronary heart disease incidence in men. *Am J Epidemiol* 155:700–709, 2002.
41. Eriksen W. The role of social support in the pathogenesis of coronary heart disease. A literature review. *Fam Pract* 11:201–209, 1994.
42. Everson SA, Kauhanen J, Kaplan GA, Goldberg DE, Julkunen J, Tuomilehto J, and Salonen JT. Hostility, and increased risk of mortality, and acute myocardial infarction: the mediating role of behavioral risk factors. *Am J Epidemiol* 146:142–152, 1997.
43. Frasure-Smith N. In-hospital symptoms of psychological stress as predictors of long-term outcome after acute myocardial infarction in men. *Am J Cardiol* 67:121–127, 1991.
44. Frasure-Smith N, Lesperance F, and Juneau M. Differential long-term impact of in-hospital symptoms of psychological stress after non–Q-wave acute myocardial infarction. *Am J Cardiol* 69:1128–1134, 1992.
45. Frasure-Smith N, Lesperance F, Juneau M, Talajic M, and Bourassa MG. Gender, depression, and one-year prognosis after myocardial infarction. *Psychosom Med* 61:26–37, 1999.
46. Frasure-Smith N, Lesperance F, Prince R, Verrier P, Garber RA, Juneau M, Wolfson C, and Bourassa MG. Randomised trial of home-based psychosocial nursing intervention for patients recovering from myocardial infarction. *Lancet* 350:473–479, 1997.
47. Frasure-Smith N, Lesperance F, and Talajic M. Depression following myocardial infarction: impact on 6-month survival. *JAMA* 270:1819–1825, 1993.
48. Frasure-Smith N, Lesperance F, and Talajic M. Depression and 18-month prognosis after myocardial infarction. *Circulation* 91:999–1005, 1995.
49. Frasure-Smith N, Lesperance F, and Talajic M. The impact of negative emotions on prognosis following myocardial infarction: is it more than depression? *Health Psychol* 14:388–398, 1995.
50. Frasure-Smith N and Prince R. Long-term follow-up of the Ischemic Heart Disease Life Stress Monitoring Program. *Psychosom Med* 51:485–513, 1989.

51. Fukudo S, Lane JD, Anderson NB, Kuhn CM, Schanberg SM, McCown N, Muranaka M, Suzuki J, and Williams RB Jr. Accentuated vagal antagonism of beta adrenergic effects on ventricular repolarization: evidence of weaker antagonism in hostile type A men. *Circulation* 85:2045–2053, 1992.
52. Gallacher JE, Yarnell JW, Sweetnam PM, Elwood PC, and Stansfeld SA. Anger and incident heart disease in the caerphilly study. *Psychosom Med* 61:446–453, 1999.
53. Gerin W, Milner D, Chawla S, and Pickering TG. Social support as a moderator of cardiovascular reactivity in women: a test of the direct effects and buffering hypotheses. *Psychosom Med* 57:16–22, 1995.
54. Glass RI and Zack MM, Jr. Increase in deaths from ischemic heart diseases after blizzards. *Lancet* 1:485–487, 1979.
55. Gleichmann U, Gleichmann S, Mannebach H, and Baller D. Changes in life style as a causal therapeutic approach in coronary heart disease [in German]. *Z Kardiol* 87(Suppl 2):125–135, 1998.
56. Goodkin K and Appels A. Behavioral–neuroendocrine–immunologic interactions in myocardial infarction. *Med Hypotheses* 48:209–214, 1997.
57. Gorman JM and Sloan RP. Heart rate variability in depressive and anxiety disorders. *Am Heart J* 140(Suppl 4):77–83, 2000.
58. Greenwood DC, Muir KR, Packham CJ, and Madeley RJ. Coronary heart disease: a review of the role of psychosocial stress and social support. *J Public Health Med* 18:221–231, 1996.
59. Grignani G, Pacchiarini L, Zucchella M, Tacconi F, Canevari A, Soffiantino F, and Tavazzi L. Effect of mental stress on platelet function in normal subjects and in patients with coronary artery disease. *Haemostasis* 22:138–146, 1992.
60. Haines AP, Imeson JD, and Meade TW. Phobic anxiety and ischaemic heart disease. *BMJ* 295:297–299, 1987.
61. Hance M, Carney RM, Freedland KE, and Skala J. Depression in patients with coronary heart disease. A 12-month follow-up. *Gen Hosp Psychiatry* 18:61–65, 1996.
62. Hansen BS, Isacsson SO, Janzon L, and Lindell SE. Social network and social support influence mortality in elderly men: the prospective population study of men born in 1914, Malmo, Sweden. *Am J Epidemiol* 130:100–111, 1989.
63. Harenstam AB and Theorell TP. Work conditions and urinary excretion of catecholamines—a study of prison staff in Sweden. *Scand J Work Environ Health* 14:257–264, 1988.
64. Hearn MD, Murray DM, and Luepker RV. Hostility, coronary heart disease, and total mortality: a 33-year follow-up study of university students. *J Behav Med* 12:105–121, 1989.
65. Hecker MH, Chesney MA, Blacks GW, and Frautschi N. Coronary-prone behaviors in the Western Collaborative Group Study. *Psychosom Med* 50:153–164, 1988.
66. Herrington DM, Vittinghoff E, Lin F, Fong J, Harris F, Hunninghake D, Bittner V, Schrott HG, Blumenthal RS, Levy R, and HERS Study Group. Statin therapy, cardiovascular events, and total mortality in the Heart and Estrogen/Progestin Replacement Study (HERS). *Circulation* 105:2962–2967, 2002.
67. Hlatky MA, Lam LC, Lee KL, Clap-Channing NE, Williams RB, Pryor DB,

Califf RM, and Mark DB. Job strain and the prevalence and outcome of coronary artery disease. *Circulation* 92:327–333, 1995.
68. House JS, Robbins C, and Metzner HL. The association of social relationships and activities with mortality: prospective evidence from the Tecumseh community health study. *Am J Epidemiol* 116:123–140, 1982.
69. Huikuri HV, Linnaluoto MK, Seppanen T, Airaksinen KE, Kessler KM, Takkunen JT, and Myerburg RJ. Circadian rhythm of heart rate variability in survivors of cardiac arrest. *Am J Cardiol* 70:610–615, 1992.
70. Julkunen J, Salonen R, Kaplan GA, Chesney MA, and Salonen JT. Hostility and the progression of carotid atherosclerosis. *Psychosom Med* 56:519–525, 1994.
71. Kamarck TW, Everson SA, Kaplan GA, Manuck SB, Jennings JR, Salonen R, and Salonen JT. Exaggerated blood pressure responses during mental stress are associated with enhanced carotid atherosclerosis in middle-aged Finnish men: findings from the Kuopio Ischemic Heart Disease Study. *Circulation* 96:3842–3848, 1997.
72. Kaprio J, Koskenvuo M, and Rita H. Mortality after bereavement: a prospective study of 95,647 persons. *Am J Public Health* 77:283–287, 1987.
73. Karasek RA, Baker D, Marxer F, Ahlbom A, and Theorell T. Job decision latitude, job demands, and cardiovascular disease: a prospective study of Swedish men. *Am J Public Health* 71:694–705, 1981.
74. Karasek RA, Theorell TG, Schwartz J, Pieper C, and Alfredsson L. Job, psychological factors and coronary heart disease. Swedish prospective findings and US prevalence findings using a new occupational inference method. *Adv Cardiol* 29:62–67, 1983.
75. Karasek RA, Theorell T, Schwartz JE, Schnall PL, Pieper CF, and Michela JL. Job characteristics in relation to the prevalence of myocardial infarction in the US Health Examination Survey (HES) and The Health and Nutrition Examination Survey (HANES). *Am J Public Health* 78:910–918, 1988.
76. Kario K, Matsuo T, Kobayashi H, Yamamoto K, and Shimada K. Earthquake-induced potentiation of acute risk factors in hypertensive elderly patients: possible triggering of cardiovascular events after a major eathquake. *J Am Coll Cardiol* 29:926–933, 1997.
77. Kawachi I, Colditz GA, Ascherio A, Rimm EB, Giovannucci E, Stampfer MJ, and Willett WC. Prospective study of phobic anxiety and risk of coronary heart disease in men. *Circulation* 89:1992–1997, 1994.
78. Kawachi I, Sparrow D, Kubzansky LD, Spiro A 3rd, Vokonas PS, and Weiss ST. Prospective study of a self-report type A scale and risk of coronary heart disease: test of the MMPI-2 type A scale. *Circulation* 98:405–412, 1998.
79. Kawachi I, Sparrow D, Spiro A III, Vokonas P, and Weiss SC. A prospective study of anger and coronary heart disease: the Normative Aging Study. *Circulation* 94:2090–2095, 1996.
80. Kawachi I, Sparrow D, Vokonas PS, and Weiss ST. Symptoms of anxiety and risk of coronary heart disease. The Normative Aging Study. *Circulation* 90:2225–2229, 1994.
81. Kawachi I, Sparrow D, Vokonas PS, and Weiss ST. Decreased heart rate variability in men with phobic anxiety (data from the Normative Aging Study). *Am J Cardiol* 75:882–885, 1995.
82. Ketterer MW. The Ketterer Stress Symptom Frequency checklist: anger and

the severity of coronary artery disease. *Henry Ford Hosp Med J* 38:207–212, 1990.
83. King KB. Psychologic and social aspects of cardiovascular disease. *Ann Behav Med* 9:264–270, 1997.
84. Kleiger RE, Miller JP, Bigger JT, Moss AJ, and the Multicenter Postinfarction Research Group. Decreased heart rate variability and its association with increased mortality after acute myocardial infarction. *Am J Cardiol* 59:256–262, 1987.
85. Knutsson A. Shift work and coronary heart disease. *Scand J Soc Med* 44(Suppl):1–36, 1989.
86. Kop WJ, Hamulyak K, Pernot C, and Appels A. Relationship of blood coagulation and fibrinolysis to vital exhaustion. *Psychosom Med* 60:352–358, 1998.
87. Kopp MS, Falger PR, Appels A, and Szedmak S. Depressive symptomatology and vital exhaustion are differentially related to behavioral risk factors for coronary artery disease. *Psychosom Med* 60:752–758, 1998.
88. Koskenvuo M, Kaprio J, Rose RJ, Kesaniemi A, Sarna S, Heikkila K, and Langinvainio H. Hostility as a risk factor for mortality and ischemic heart disease in men. *Psychosom Med* 50:330–340, 1988.
89. Krantz D, Helmers K, Bairey CN, Nebel L, Hedges S, and Rozanski A. Cardiovascular reactivity and mental stress–induced myocardial ischemia in patients with coronary artery disease. *Psychosom Med* 53:1–12, 1991.
90. Kristenson M, Kucinskiene Z, Bergdahl B, Calkauskas H, Urmonas V, and Orth-Gomer K. Increased psychosocial strain in Lithuanian versus Swedish men: the LiVicordia study. *Psychosom Med* 60:277–282, 1998.
91. Krittayaphong R, Cascio WE, Light KC, Sheffield D, Golden RN, Finkel JB, Glekas G, Koch GG, and Sheps DS. Heart rate variability in patients with coronary artery disease: differences in patients with higher and lower depression scores. *Psychosom Med* 59:231–235, 1997.
92. Krumholz HM, Butler J, Miller J, Vaccarino V, Williams CS, Mendes de Leon CF, Seeman TE, Kasl SV, and Berkman LF. Prognostic importance of emotional support for elderly patients hospitalized with heart failure. *Circulation* 97:958–964, 1998.
93. Kubzansky LD, Kawachi I, Spiro A III, Weiss ST, Vokonas PS, and Sparrow D. Is worrying bad for your heart?: a prospective study of worry and coronary heart disease in the Normative Aging Study. *Circulation* 95:818–824, 1997.
94. Lampert R, Joska T, Burg MM, Batsford WP, McPherson CA, and Jain D. Emotional and physical precipitants of ventricular arrhythmia. *Circulation* 106:1800–1805, 2002.
95. La Rovere MT, Specchia G, Mortara A, and Schwartz PJ. Baroflex sensitivity, clinical correlates, and cardiovascular mortality among patients with a first myocardial infarction: a prospective study. *Circulation* 78:816–824, 1988.
96. Lederbogen F, Gilles M, Maras A, Hamann B, Colla M, and Heuser I. Increased platelet aggregability in major depression. *Psychiatry Res* 102:255–261, 2001.
97. Leon GR, Finn SE, Murray D, and Bailey JM. The inability to predict cardiovascular disease from hostility scores of MMPI items related to type A behavior. *J Consult Clin Psychol* 56:597–600, 1988.
98. Leor J, Poole WK, and Kloner RA. Sudden cardiac death triggered by an earthquake. *N Engl J Med* 334:413–419, 1996.

99. Levine SP, Towell BL, Saurez AM, Khierriem LK, Harris MM, and George JN. Platelet activation and secretion associated with emotional stress. *Circulation* 71:1129–1134, 1985.
100. Lindsay GM, Hanlon P, Smith LN, and Wheatley DJ. Assessment of changes in general health status using the short-form 36 questionnaire 1 year following coronary artery bypass grafting. *Eur J Cardiothorac Surg* 18:557–564, 2000.
101. Lloyd BL. Declining cardiovascular disease incidence and environmental components. *Aust N Z J Med* 24:124–132, 1994.
102. Lutfiyya MN and Henley E. HRT and vitamins C and E do not improve coronary disease in women. *J Fam Pract* 52:112–114, 2003.
103. Lynch J, Krause N, Kaplan GA, Salonen R, and Salonen JT. Work place demands, economic reward, and progression of carotid atherosclerosis. *Circulation* 96:302–307, 1997.
104. Manuck S, Olsson G, Hjemdahl P, and Rehnqvist N. Does cardiovascular reactivity to mental stress have prognostic value in postinfarction patients? A pilot study. *Psychosom Med* 54:102–108, 1992
105. Markovitz JH, Matthews KA, Kiss J, and Smitherman TC. Effects of hostility on platelet reactivity to psychological stress in coronary heart disease patients and in healthy controls. *Psychosom Med* 58:143–149, 1996.
106. Marmot MG and Syme SL. Acculturation and coronary heart disease in Japanese Americans. *Am J Epidemiol* 104:225–247, 1976.
107. Maruta T, Hamburgen ME, Jennings CA, Offord KP, Colligan RC, Frye RL, and Malinchoc M. Keeping hostility in perspective: coronary heart disease and the hostility scale on the Minnesota Multiphasic Personality Inventory. *Mayo Clin Proc* 68:109–114, 1993.
108. Matthews KA, Owens JF, Kuller LH, Sutton-Tyrrell K, and Jansen-McWilliams L. Are hostility and anxiety associated with carotid atherosclerosis in healthy postmenopausal women? *Psychosom Med* 60:633–638, 1998.
109. McCranie EW, Watkins LO, Brandsma JM, and Sisson BD. Hostility, coronary heart disease (CHD) incidence, and total mortality: lack of association in a 25-year follow-up study of 478 physicians. *J Behav Med* 9:119–125, 1986.
110. Meisel SR, Kutz I, Dayan KI, Pauzner H, Chetboun I, Arbel Y, and David D. Effect of Iraqi missile war on incidence of acute myocardial infarction and sudden death in Israeli civilians. *Lancet* 338:660–661, 1991.
111. Milsum JH. A model of the eustress system for health/illness. *Behav Sci* 30:179–186, 1985.
112. Mittleman MA, Maclure M, Sherwood JB, Mulry RP, Tofler GH, Jacobs SC, Friedman R, Benson H, and Muller JE. Triggering of acute myocardial infarction onset by episodes of anger. Determinants of Myocardial Infarction Onset Study Investigators. *Circulation* 92:1720–1725, 1995.
113. Molgaard H, Sorensen KE, and Bjerregaard P. Attenuated 24-h heart rate variability in apparently healthy subjects, subsequently suffering sudden cardiac death. *Clin Auton Res* 1:233–223, 1991.
114. Moser DK. Social support and cardiac recovery. *J Cardiovasc Nurs* 9:27–36, 1994.
115. Moser DK and Dracup K. Is anxiety early after myocardial infarction associated with subsequent ischemic and arrhythmic events? *Psychosom Med* 58:395–401, 1996.

116. Muller JE, Abela GS, Nesto RW, and Tofler GH. Triggers, acute risk factors and vulnerable plaques: the lexicon of a new frontier. *J Am Coll Cardiol* 23:809–813, 1994.
117. Myers A and Dewar HA. Circumstances attending sudden deaths from coronary artery disease with coroner's necropsies. *Br Heart J* 37:1133–1143, 1975.
118. Nesse RM, Cameron OG, Curtis GC, McCann DS, and Huber-Smith MJ. Adrenergic function in patients with panic anxiety. *Arch Gen Psychiatry* 41:771–776, 1984.
119. Nicolson NA and van Diest R. Salivary cortisol patterns in vital exhaustion. *J Psychosom Res* 49:335–342, 2000.
120. Orth-Gomer K, Rosengren A, and Wilhelmsen L. Lack of social support and incidence of coronary heart disease in middle-aged Swedish men. *Psychosom Med* 55:37–43, 1993.
121. Paterniti S, Zureik M, Ducimetiere P, Touboul PJ, Feve JM, and Alperovitch A. Sustained anxiety and 4-year progression of carotid atherosclerosis. *Arterioscler Thromb Vasc Biol* 21:136–141, 2001.
122. Penninx BWJH, Beekman ATF, Honig A, Deeg DJH, Schoevers RA, van Eijk JTM, and van Tilburg W. Depression and cardiac mortality: results from a community-based longitudinal study. *Arch Gen Psychiatry* 58:221–227, 2000.
123. Petterson K, Bejne B, Bjork H, Stawn WB, and Bondjers G. Experimental sympathetic activation causes endothelial injury in the rabbit thoracic aorta via beta 1-adrenoceptor activation. *Circ Res* 67:1027–1034, 1990.
124. Piccirillo G, Elvira S, Bucca C, Viola E, Cacciafesta M, and Marigliano V. Abnormal passive head-up tilt test in subjects with symptoms of anxiety power spectral analysis study of heart rate and blood pressure. *Int J Cardiol* 60:121–131, 1997.
125. Pickering TG. Mental stress as a causal factor in the development of hypertension and cardiovascular disease. *Curr Hypertens Rep* 3:249–254, 2001.
126. Pope ML, Smith TW. Cortisol excretion in high and low cynically hostile men. *Psychosom Med* 53:386–392, 1991.
127. Ragland DR and Brand RJ. Type A behavior and mortality from coronary heart disease. *N Engl J Med* 318:65–69, 1988.
128. Raikkonen K, Lassila R, Keltikanga-Jarvinen L, and Hautanen A. Association of chronic stress with plasminogen activator inhibitor-1 in healthy middle-aged men. *Arterioscler Thromb Vasc Biol* 16:363–367, 1996.
129. Ratcliffe HL and Cronin NT. Changing frequency of atherosclerosis in mammals and birds at the Philadelphia Zoological Garden. *Circulation* 18:41–52, 1958.
130. Ratcliffe HL, Lughibuhl H, Schnarr WR, and Chacko K. Coronary atherosclerosis in swine: evidence of a relation to behavior. *J Comp Physiol Psychol* 68:385–392, 1969.
131. Roose SP and Dalack GW. Treating the depressed patient with cardiovascular problems. *J Clin Psychiatry* 53(Suppl):25–31, 1992.
132. Rosenman RH, Brand RJ, Jenkins CD, Friedman M, Straus R, and Wurm M. Coronary heart disease in the Western Collaborative Group Study: final follow-up experience of 8 1/2 years. *JAMA* 233:872–877, 1975.
133. Ruberman W, Weinblatt E, Goldberg JD, and Chaudhary BS. Psychosocial influences on mortality after myocardial infarction. *N Engl J Med* 311:552–559, 1984.

134. Rutledge T, Reis SE, Olson M, Owens J, Kelsey SF, Pepine CJ, Reichek N, Rogers WJ, Merz CN, Sopko G, Cornell CE, Sharaf B, and Matthews KA. History of anxiety disorders is associated with a decreased likelihood of angiographic coronary artery disease in women with chest pain: the WISE study. *J Am Coll Cardiol* 37:780–785, 2001.
135. Schnall PL, Pieper C, Schwartz JE, Karase RA, Schlussel Y, Devereux RB, Ganau A, Alderman M, Warren K, and Pickering TG. The relationship between 'job strain,' workplace diastolic blood pressure and left ventricular mass index. *JAMA* 273:1929–1935, 1990.
136. Seeman TE, Berkman LF, Blazer DG, and Rowe JW. Social ties and support and neuroendocrine function. *Ann Behav Med* 16:95–106, 1994.
137. Seeman TE, Kaplan GA, Knudsen L, Cohen R, and Guralnik J. Social network ties and mortality among the elderly in the Alameda County Study. *Am J Epidemiol* 126:714–723, 1987.
138. Sevincok L, Buyukozturk A, and Dereboy F. Serum lipid concentrations in patients with comorbid generalized anxiety disorder and major depressive disorder. *Can J Psychiatry* 46:68–71, 2001.
139. Shekelle RB, Gale M, and Norusis M. Type A score (Jenkins Activity Survey), and risk of recurrent coronary heart disease in the aspirin myocardial infarction study. *Am J Cardiol* 56:221–225, 1985.
140. Shekelle RB, Gale M, Ostfeld AM, and Paul O. Hostility, risk of coronary heart disease, and mortality. *Psychosom Med* 45:109–114, 1983.
141. Shekelle RB, Hulley SB, Neaton JD, Billings JH, Borhani NO, Gerace TA, Jacobs DR, Lasser NL, Mittlemark MB, and Stamler J. The MRFIT Behavior Pattern Study, II: type A behavior and incidence of coronary heart disease. *Am J Epidemiol* 122:559–570, 1985.
142. Shively CA, Clarkson TB, and Kaplan JR. Social deprivation and coronary artery atherosclerosis in female cynomolgus monkeys. *Atherosclerosis* 77:69–76, 1989.
143. Siegel WC, Mark DB, Hlatky MA, Harrell FE, Jr, Pryor DB, Barefoot JC, and Williams RB, Jr. Clinical correlates and prognostic significance of type A behavior and silent myocardial ischemia on the treadmill. *Am J Cardiol* 64:1280–1283, 1989.
144. Siegman AW. Cardiovascular consequences of expressing, experiencing, and repressing anger. *J Behav Med* 16:539–569, 1993.
145. Siegrist J, Peter R, Junge A, Cremer P, and Seidel D. Low status control, high effort at work and ischemic heart disease: prospective evidence from blue-collar men. *Soc Sci Med* 31:1127–1134, 1990
146. Sloan RP, Shapiro PA, Bigger T, Jr, Bagiella E, Steinman RC, and Gorman JM. Cardiac autonomic control and hostility in healthy subjects. *Am J Cardiol* 74:298–300, 1994.
147. Stein PK, Carney RM, Freedland KE, Skala JA, Jaffe AS, Kleiger RE, and Rottman JN. Severe depression is associated with markedly reduced heart rate variability in patients with stable coronary heart disease. *J Psychosom Res* 48:493–500, 2000.
148. Stevens JH, Turner CW, Rhodewalt F, and Talbot S. The type A behavior pattern and carotid artery atherosclerosis. *Psychosom Med* 46:105–113, 1984.
149. Suarez EC and Blumenthal JA. Ambulatory blood pressure responses during daily life in high and low hostile patients with a recent myocardial infarction. *J Cardiopulm Rehabil* 11:169–175, 1991.

150. Suarez EC, Kuhn CM, Schanberg SM, Williams RB, Jr, and Zimmermann EA. Neuroendocrine, cardiovascular, and emotional responses of hostile men: the role of interpersonal challenge. *Psychosom Med* 60:78–88, 1998.
151. Suarez EC, Shiller AD, Kuhn CM, Schanberg S, Williams RB, Jr, and Zimmermann EA. The relationship between hostility and beta-adrenergic receptor physiology in healthy young males. *Psychosom Med* 59:481–487, 1997.
152. Sul J and Wan CK. The relationship between trait hostility and cardiovascular reactivity: a quantitative analysis. *Psychophysiology* 30:615–626, 1993.
153. Tenkanen L, Sjoblom T, and Harma M. Joint effect of shift work and adverse lifestyle factors on the risk of coronary heart disease. *Scand J Work Environ Health* 4:351–357, 1998.
154. Tennant CC and Langeluddecke PM. Psychological correlates of coronary heart disease. *Psychol Med* 15:581–588, 1985.
155. Tennant CC, Langeluddecke PM, Fulcher G, and Wilby J. Anger and other psychological factors in coronary atherosclerosis. *Psychol Med* 17:425–431, 1987.
156. Thayer JF, Friedman BH, and Borkovec TD. Autonomic characteristics of generalized anxiety disorder and worry. *Biol Psychiatry* 39:255–266, 1996.
157. Tofler GH, Stone PH, Maclure M, Edelman E, Davis VG, Robertson T, Antman EM, and Muller JE. Analysis of possible triggers of acute myocardial infarction (the MILIS Study). *Am J Cardiol* 66:22–27, 1990.
158. Trichopoulos D, Katsouyanni K, Zavitsanos X, Zavitsanos X, Tzonou A, and Dalla-Vorgia P. Psychological stress and fatal heart attack: the Athens (1981) earthquake natural experiment. *Lancet* 1:441–444, 1983.
159. Watkins LL and Grossman P. Association of depressive symptoms with reduced baroreflex cardiac control in coronary artery disease. *Am Heart J* 137:453–457, 1999.
160. Watkins LL, Grossman P, Krishnan R, and Sherwood A. Anxiety and vagal control of heart rate. *Psychosom Med* 60:498–502, 1998.
161. Weissman MM, Markowitz JS, Ouellette R, Greenwald S, and Kahn JP. Panic disorders and cardiovascular/cerebrovascular problems: results from a community survey. *Am J Psychiatry* 147:1504–1508, 1990.
162. Wells K, Rogers W, Burnam M, and Camp P. Course of depression in patients with hypertension, myocardial infarction or insulin dependent diabetes. *Am J Psychiatry* 150:632–638, 1993.
163. Whitehead WE, Blackwell B, De Silva H, and Robinson A. Anxiety and anger in hypertension. *J Psychosom Res* 21:383–389, 1997.
164. Whiteman MC, Fowkes FG, Deary IJ, and Lee AJ. Hostility, cigarette smoking and alcohol consumption in the general population. *Soc Sci Med* 44:1089–1096, 1997.
165. Williams JE, Nieto FJ, Sanford CP, and Tyroler HA. Effects of an angry temperament on coronary heart disease risk: the Atherosclerosis Risk in Communities Study. *Am J Epidemiol* 154:230–235, 2001.
166. Williams JE, Paton CC, Siegler IC, Eigenbrodt ML, Nieto FJ, and Tyroler HA. Anger proneness predicts coronary heart disease risk: prospective analysis from the Atherosclerosis Risk in Communities (ARIC) Study. *Circulation* 101:2034–2039, 2000.
167. Williams RB, Jr, Barefoot JC, Haney TL, Harrell FE, Jr, Blumenthal JA, Pryor DB, and Peterson B. Type A behavior and angiographically documented coronary atherosclerosis in a sample of 2,289 patients. *Psychosom Med* 50:139–152, 1988.

168. Wojciechowski FL, Strik JJ, Falger P, Lousberg R, and Honig A. The relationship between depressive and vital exhaustion symptomatology postmyocardial infarction. *Acta Psychiatr Scand* 102:359–365, 2000.
169. Woloshin S, Schwartz LM, Tosteson ANA, Chang CH, Wright B, Plohman J, and Fisher ES. Perceived adequacy of tangible social support and health outcomes in patients with coronary artery disease. *J Gen Intern Med* 12:613–618, 1997.
170. Woo J. Relationships among diet, physical activity and other lifestyle factors and debilitating diseases in the elderly. *Eur J Clin Nutr* 54(Suppl 3):S143–S147, 2000.
171. Yeragani VK, Balon R, Pohl R, Ramesh C, Glitz D, Weinberg P, and Merlos B. Decreased R-R variance in panic disorder patients. *Acta Psychiatr Scand* 81:554–559, 1990.
172. Yeragani VK, Pohl R, Berger R, Balon R, Ramesh C, Glitz D, Srinivasan K, and Weinberg P. Decreased heart rate variability in panic disorder patients: a study of power-spectral analysis of heart rate. *Psychiatry Res* 46:89–103, 1993.
173. Yeung A, Vekshtein V, Krantz D, Vita JA, Ryan TJ, Jr, Ganz P, and Selwyn AP. The effect of atherosclerosis on the vasomotor response of coronary arteries to mental stress. *N Engl J Med* 325:1551–1556, 1991.
174. Zafari AM and Wenger NK. Secondary prevention of coronary heart disease. *Arch Phys Med Rehabil* 79:1006–1017, 1998.

15
Epilogue: Relevance of the Cardiac Neuronal Hierarchy in Heart Disease

JEFFREY L. ARDELL, LOUIS J. DELL'ITALIA,
AND J. ANDREW ARMOUR

The overriding hypothesis of this book is that autonomic neuronal markers for the progression of cardiac disease and the risk of sudden cardiac death are complex, manifest early in the disease process, and are underappreciated given our current indirect methods of neurocardiac assessment. Furthermore, the genesis of autonomic dysfunction may depend on inherent rather than acquired factors that are subtle and presumably involve multiple facets of the cardiac neuronal hierarchy. Evidence based on data derived from single cells studied in vitro (Chapter 1), neuron–myocyte interactive cocultures (Chapter 2), whole animals (Chapters 3–12), and patients (Chapters 10–14) centers around the concept of the synergistic, multilevel neural interactions involved in cardiac control. Specifically, these studies have resulted in the evolving hypothesis that the cardiac chemical/mechanical milieu is transduced and reflexly modulated not only by the central nervous system but also by intrathoracic components of the cardiac neuronal hierarchy, including those of the paravertebral chain and those intrinsic to the heart.

Previously, cardiac function was considered to be controlled solely by the central nervous system and involve cardiac parasympathetic and sympathetic efferent postganglionic neurons acting in a reciprocal manner. Among the most exciting emerging developments in the field of neurocardiology is the idea that the cardiac nervous system comprises multiple nested intrathoracic (Chapters 1–4) and central (Chapters 5–7) feedback loops that interact to dynamically modulate cardiac efferent neurons coordinating regional cardiac function through all stages of life (Chapters 8 and 9). Moreover, various interactive way stations within the central nervous system and peripheral aspects of the cardiac nervous system are under longer-term control mediated by neurohumoral agents, both organ-specific and vascular delivered. Recently, it has become evident that the progression of cardiac disease is a translational process that involves reorganization or remodeling of neurohumoral systems, myocytes, and structural elements of the heart. To date, we have only scratched the surface in understanding the dynamics of these processes.

Interactions that occur among the varied peripheral and central neuronal cell stations within the cardiac neuronal hierarchy normally act to stabilize cardiac output in the presence of progressive pathology. The ultimate prognosis of the patient may well depend on how effectively cardiac afferent neurons transduce alterations in the cardiac chemical/mechanical milieu to the entire cardiac neuronal hierarchy and, as such, manifest either appropriate or inadequate reflex control of cardiac efferent neurons. That parts of the cardiac nervous system become remodeled in the maintainence of cardiac output during the evolution of various cardiac pathologies (Chapters 10–13), including when individuals are placed at risk by psychological and sociological factors (Chapter 14), may elicit varied and at times unexpected alterations in the function of its different cell populations. This neural remodeling in turn exerts a major functional impact on the course of cardiac disease.

The cardiac neuronal hierarchy comprises spatially distributed populations of neurons that display either tightly coupled or stochastic behavior, predicated on the capacity of its different populations to transduce cardiac mechanical as opposed to multimodal (mechanical and chemical) stimuli. That the cardiac milieu is transduced at the level of the heart independent of the influence of more centrally located neurons requires a thorough reassessment of how the cardiac nervous system should be approached. By taking into consideration how the entire cardiac neuronal hierarchy normally responds (in conjunction with circulating hormones) to altered cardiovascular status, one may be able to ascertain how its various neuronal substations adapt (remodel) during the evolution of specific cardiac pathologies.

In this volume, we have approached the issue of remodeling of the cardiac nervous system with the following definition in mind: *cardiac neuronal remodeling is represented as any alteration (acute or chronic) of the system's capacity to transduce the cardiac milieu or process descending inputs from higher center neurons to cardiac motor neurons*. Data presented in this book indicate that higher center neurons can exert profound and long-lasting stabilizing influences on any imbalance that might occur within the intrinsic cardiac nervous system secondary to inputs arising from the ischemic heart[5] (Chapter 5). Perhaps it is those individuals in whom a relative balance within this neuronal hierarchy is maintained during myocardial ischemic episodes who are thereby rendered relatively "resistant" to ischemia-induced cardiac arrhythmias, whereas those who can't are susceptible to arrhythmia formation.[12]

Remodeling of the cardiac nervous system directly affects any reorganization of cardiac myocyte function and the cardiac extracellular matrix that occurs during the evolution of specific cardiac diseases (Chapter 12). The remarkable effects of β-adrenoceptor blockade in clinical trials and in animal models of heart failure underscore the interplay between sympathetic neuronal outflow and cardiac disease. The central role of a hyperactive sympathetic nervous system in such a disease state is even more impressive because it is not intuitively obvious how blocking a pathway that increases contractility and has little or no effect on normal systemic arterial afterload could be of therapeutic benefit to heart failure patients. Recent evidence indicates that β-adrenergic receptor blockade may exert important clinical benefits by mitigating adverse remodeling of the cardiac nervous system in heart failure[14] (Chapter 12). Understanding the dynamic interplay between neurohumoral and myocyte factors indeed shapes our understanding of the genesis of symptoms arising from the diseased heart (Chapter 10), the pathogenesis of hypertension (Chapter 13), and the relevance of the psychological aspects of heart disease (Chapter 14).

Specifically, therapeutic targets for most cardiac pathologies have recently focused on the adrenergic and renin-angiotensin systems and their cross-regulation (Chapters 10–14). Many clinical and basic studies have demonstrated that modulation of the cardiac nervous system affects myocardial reactive inflammatory species, oxidative states, and extracellular matrix homeostasis (Chapter 12). Moreover, the concept of a cardiac neuronal hierarchy provides multiple and previously unrecognized targets for therapeutic development. Selective cardiothoracic surgical interventions[1] and radiofrequency catheter ablation procedures[11,16] can modify the transduction of the cardiac mechanical/chemical milieu by the cardiac neuronal hierarchy, including its target organ component.[13] Remodeling of the cardiac nervous system becomes manifest even after minor insults to the ventricular myocardium.[2] Such remodeling can involve both short-term[1,4] and long-term[10,13] alterations in the system's capacity to transduce the cardiac milieu to various cardiac efferent neurons. Remodeling can even be manifested at the histological level, as reflected by pathological changes that human intrinsic cardiac neurons undergo in the presence of compromised regional coronary arterial blood supply.[6]

The novel understanding of cardiac control presented in this volume suggests some promising guidelines. One representative treatment modality that is currently under intensive investigation is the application of electrical stimuli to the dorsal aspect of the thoracic spinal cord to manage symptoms associated with myocardial ischemia[9] (Chapter 5). Another is biventricular pacing in heart failure.[3,8] Both therapies may act in part by restraining the capacity of intrathoracic efferent neurons to respond excessively and reflexly to regional ventricular ischemia or mechanical overload. A balance is thereby reimposed on the cardiac neuronal hierarchy. This provocative concept can only be placed in proper context by expanding our current knowledge of the transduction of cardiac sensory information by neurons located throughout the cardiac neuronal hierarchy in such states.

Recent evidence points to the fact that neurohumoral derangement arising in response to cardiac stressors can initiate cardiac pathology. For example, exacerbated autonomic disturbance can contribute to the initiation of fatal ventricular arrhythmias (Chapter 11) and to adverse myocardial structural remodeling (Chapter 12). Thus, various cardiac pathological syndromes may be associated with adverse remodeling of the cardiac neuronal hierarchy that can cause or exacerbate morbidity or mortality.[2,7] An understanding of the varied neurohumoral responses elicited during the evolution of specific cardiac pathologies may be critical to determining why some patients experience sudden death while others sustain life in the presence of severely compromised cardiac function.[5]

The challenge before us is to determine how the cardiac neuronal hierarchy functions in an integrated manner in the normal state and to explore its varied interrelationships for neurotransmitter release in disease states. It is likewise critical to determine how various hormonal systems (e.g., renin-angiotensin system, circulating catecholamines), both target organ–specific and vascular-dependent, influence neuronal elements throughout the cardiac nervous system in normal and diseased hearts. In order to accomplish all of this, the function of the entire cardiac neuronal hierarchy must be analyzed as a whole, as any breakdown in communication among its peripheral and central neuronal populations can jeopardize cardiac regulation. Use of therapeutic strategies to restore balance to the neuronal hierarchy should result in significant improvements in the prognosis of some patients. The main purpose of this volume is to stimulate interest in the task of understanding how the functional interconnectivity of the cardiac nervous system can be reshaped during the development of cardiac pathology. The cardiac nervous system has now moved to the forefront as a research focus for understanding the development of heart disease and a basis for future treatment modalities.

REFERENCES

1. Arora RC, Ardell JL, and Armour JA. Cardiac denervation and cardiac function. *Curr Interv Cardiol Rep* 2:188–195, 2000.
2. Cao J-M, Chen LS, KenKnight BH, Ohara T, Lee M-H, Tsai J, Lai WW, Karagueuzian HS, Wolf PL, Fishbein MC, and Chen P-S. Nerve sprouting and sudden cardiac death. *Circ Res* 86:816–821, 2000.
3. El-Sherif N and Samet P. *Cardiac Pacing and Electrophysiology*. Philidelphia: W.B. Saunders Co., 1991.
4. Farrell DM, Wei CC, Tallaj J, Ardell JL, Armour JA, Hageman GR, Bradley WE, and Dell'Italia LJ. Angiotensin II modulates catecholamine release into interstitial fluid of canine ventricle in vivo. *Am J Physiol (Heart Circ Physiol)* 281:H813–H822, 2001.
5. Foreman RD, Linderoth B, Ardell JL, Barron KW, Chandler MJ, Hull SS, TerHorst GJ, DeJongste MJL, and Armour JA. Modulation of intrinsic cardiac neurons by spinal cord stimulation: implications for therapeutic use in angina pectoris. *Cardiovasc Res* 47:367–375, 2000.
6. Hopkins DA, MacDonald S, Murphy DA, and Armour JA. Pathology of intrinsic cardiac neurons from ischemic human hearts. *Anat Rec* 259:424–436, 2000.
7. Lathrop DA and Spooner PM. On the neural connection. *J Cardiovasc Electrophysiol* 12:841–844, 2001.
8. Leclercq C and Kass DA. Retiming the failing heart: principals and current clinical status of cardiac resynchronization. *Am J Cardiol* 39:194–201, 2002.
9. Linderoth B and Foreman RD. Physiology of spinal cord stimulation. *Neuromodulation* 2:105–164, 1999.
10. Murphy DA, Thompson GW, Ardell JL, McCraty R, Stevenson R, Sangalang VE, Cardinal R, Wilkinson M, Craig S, Smith FM, Kingma JG, and Armour JA. The heart reinnervates after transplant. *Ann Thorac Surg* 69:1769–1781, 2000.
11. Schauerte P, Scherlag BJ, Patterson E, Scherlag MA, Matsudaria K, Nakagawa H, Lazzara R, and Jackman WM. Focal atrial fibrillation: experimental evidence for a pathophysiologic role of the autonomic nervous system. *J Cardiovasc Electrophysiol* 12:592–599, 2001.
12. Schwartz PJ, La Rovere MT, and Vanoli E. Autonomic nervous system and sudden cardiac death. Experimental basis and clinical observations for postmyocardial infarction risk stratification. *Circulation* 85:I77–I91, 1992.
13. Smith FM, McGuirt AS, Hoover DB, Armour JA, and Ardell JL. Chronic decentralization of the heart differentially remodels canine intrinsic cardiac neuron muscarinic receptors. *Am J Physiol (Heart Circ Physiol)* 281:H1919–H1930, 2001.
14. Tallaj J, Wei CC, Hankes GH, Holland M, Rynders P, Dillon AR, Ardell JL, Armour JA, Lucchesi PA, and Dell'Italia LJ. β1-adrenergic receptor blockade

attenuates angiotensin II–mediated catecholamine release into the cardiac interstitium in mitral regurgitation. *Circulation* 225–230, 2003.
15. Task Force of the European Society of Cardiology and the North American Society of Pacing and Electrophysiology. Heart rate variability: standards of measurement, physiological interpretation and clinical use. *Circulation* 93: 1043–1065, 1996.
16. Tsai CF, Chen SA, Tai CT, Chiou CW, Prakash VS, Yu WC, Hsieh MH, Ding YA, and Chang MS. Bezold-Jarisch-like reflex during radiofrequency ablation of the pulmonary vein tissue in patients with focal atrial fibrillation. *J Cardiovasc Electrophysiol* 10:27–35, 1999.

Index

Accentuated antagonism, 200
Acetylcholine. *See also* Cardiac neurons, ligated ion channels; Nicotinic Cholinergic Receptors; Muscarinic Cholinergic receptors
  effect on
    autonomic ganglia, 125
    chronotropic function, 321
    inotropic function, 321
    intrinsic cardiac neurons, 6, 132, 320, 321
    myocytes, 125
    sympathetic efferent neurons, 321, 371
Acetylcholinesterase, cardiac distribution, 259
Adenosine
  antiadrenergic effects of, 274, 275, 278–280
    aging, effects on, 280
    decreased adenylyl cyclase activity, 278
    decreased β_1 coupling, 278
    decreased norepinephrine release by, 174, 279
  cardiac afferent neurons
    activation of, 87, 93, 97, 279
    algesic actions on, 174, 310
    analgesic actions on, 310
  cardiac interstitial levels of, 301
  cardioprotection and, 173, 287
  clearance of, 301
  cardiac electrophysiological effects, 260
    ontogeny of, 260
  fibroblasts
    lung, release of, 283
      aging, effects on, 283
    skin, release of, 283
      aging, effects on, 283
  intravenous infusion and
    pain perception, 301, 302, 304
  interstitial (cardiac) levels of, 279, 282
    aging, effects on, 279, 282, 285
    juvenile to old age, 285
  intrinsic cardiac neurons, stabilization by, 279
  ischemic preconditioning and, 173, 288
  K^+ ion channel (myocyte), effects on, 260
    ontogeny of, 260
  modulation of neurotransmitter release by, 174, 275, 279
    interactions with nicotinic receptors, 301, 304
  myocardial uptake, effects of aging on, 282
  preconditioning, cardiac, induced by, 173
  psychophysical effects of, 302
  release during myocardial ischemia, 110, 300, 301
  transport (cardiac), effects of aging on, 282
  vasomotor effects of, 174, 301
Adenosine A_1 receptor
  affinity (cardiac), effects of aging on, 282
  distribution (cardiac) of, 280–282
    aging, effects on, 280
    atrial, effects of aging, 281
    species specific differences in, 281, 282
    ventricular, effects of aging, 282
  G_i coupling, 275
    aging, effects on, 282

Adenosine receptor antagonists
    caffeine, effects on neuromodulation
        by, 173
Adenosine triphosphate (ATP)
    co-localization with NE in sympathetic
        nerves, 40
    distribution in intrinsic cardiac nervous
        system, 10
    effects on. *See also* Cardiac neurons,
            ligand gated ion channels;
            Cardiac neurons, voltage
            gated ion channels
        cardiac function, 40. *See also* Cardiac
            neurons, ligated ion channels;
            Cardiac neurons, voltage
            gated ion channels
        intrinsic cardiac afferent neurons,
            97
        intrinsic cardiac neurons, 40
        sympathetic efferents, 40. *See also*
            Cardiac neurons, ligated ion
            channels; Cardiac neurons,
            voltage gated ion channels
        vagal efferents, 40
Adenylate cyclase. *See also* cAMP
    adenosine/adrenergic interactions, 275,
        286
        juvenile to aged adults, 286
    adenosine inhibition of, 276, 286
        juvenile to aged adults, 286
    aging, effects on cardiac, 277
    beta adrenergic stimulation of, 276
    congestive heart failure and receptor
        modulation of, 344
    inhibitory guanine nucleotide (G_i)
        modulation of, 125
    muscarinic inhibition of, 125
    stimulatory guanine nucleotide (G_s)
        modulation of, 125
Adrenalectomy
    effects on
        cardiac catecholamine content, 130
        plasma catecholamine levels, 130
        sympathetic modulation of cardiac
            function, 130
    epinephrine replacement therapy
        restoration of sympathetic function
            by, 130

Adrenegic innervation, cardiac
    ontogeny of, 254, 259
        atrial/ventricular asymmetry in, 255
        tyrosine hydroxylase positive
            neurons, 259
Adrenergic receptors. *See also* Alpha
        adrenergic receptors; Beta
        adrenergic receptors
    activation of nodose afferent by, 87
    effect on intrinsic cardiac neurons, 132
Afferents, Cardiovascular
    adenosine and activation of, 279, 301, 309
    algesic actions of, 310
    analgesic actions of, 310
    age effects on, 308
    baroreceptor, low-pressure, 370
        central projections of, 370
        neuroanatomy of, 81
            atrial, 81
        ontogeny of, 253
        response characteristics of, 370, 378
    baroreceptor, high-pressure, 370. *See
            also* Baroreflex; Nucleus
            tractus solitarius
        central projections of, 121, 191, 222, 370
        inflammatory agents and effects on,
            194
        morphology of
            type A afferents, 81–83, 190
            type C afferents, 81, 83, 190
        ontogeny of, 253
        response characteristics of, 85, 91,
            370, 378
            type A afferents, 102, 190, 206
            type C afferents, 102, 190, 206
        remodeling associated with
            aging, 191
            capsaicin lesions of C-type fibers, 207
            cardiovascular pathology, 191
            development, 191
        sensory terminals, neuromodulator
            effects of
            ATP, 193
            calcitonin gene-related peptide, 192
            GABA, 193
            glutamate, 193
            histamine, 193
            norepinephrine, 194
            serotonin, 193
            substance P, 192
            VR1 receptors, 192
        stretch-activated ion channels in, 191
        voltage-gated ion channels in, 191
            type A afferents, 191
            type C afferents, 191, 192
    cardiopulmonary
        ontogeny of, 254
        reflex response to activation of, 254
            ontogeny of, 254
    chemoreceptor, 120, 370
        ontogeny of, 253

Index

reflex cardiovascular response to activation of, 370
reflex respiratory response to activation of, 370
response characteristics of, 120, 370
dorsal root ganglia afferents. See Dorsal root ganglia afferents
effects on
  hypothalamus, 369
  salt balance, 369
  water balance, 369
efferent functions of afferent nerves, 373
hypertension, effects on, 371
intrathoracic afferent neurons. See Cardiac neurons, extrinsic, afferents; Cardiac neurons, intrinsic, afferents
mechanoreceptor, 120, 258
  ontogeny of, 258
  response characteristics of, 120
memory function of, 120
myocardial ischemia and activation of, 279
nociceptors, cardiac
  response characteristics of, 107, 158
  projections of, 158
  spinothalamic projects modified by, 159
nodose afferent neurons. See Nodose ganglia afferents
ontogeny of, 101
opioid receptor mediated modulation of, 309
organization of, 369
osmoreceptor, 370
  response characteristics of, 370, 378
  reflex cardiovascular response to activation of, 370
pulmonary artery afferents, neuroanatomy of, 81
reflex mechanisms dependent upon, 369, 374, 378. See also Cardiac Neuronal Hierarchy
remodeling in cardiac pathology
  atrial arrhythmias, 111
  atrial fibrillation, 111
  ventricular arrhythmias, 111
renal, 369
sensory mechanisms of, 80, 84, 120, 369
  chemoreceptors, 120
  mechanosensors, 120
sensory transduction, fast-responding
  cardiac reflexes dependent on input from, 99, 102
    coordination of cardiac electrical function by, 104

coordination of cardiac mechanical function by, 104
decentralization, effects on, 99
limited memory function of, 99
mechanosensors and, 98
receptive fields for, 98
sensory transduction, mathematical models
  FitzHugh-Nagumo model, 106
    input- output functions of, 106
    noise, effects on, 106
    slow-responding inputs, effects on, 106
    time-scale effects on, 106
  Wilson and Cowan model, 107
    hysteretic function in, 107
      input filter, 107, 108
      memory, 107, 108
      state dependence, 107, 108
    input-output function in, 108
      descending modulation of, 108
      peripheral, 108
    noise reduction in, 108
sensory transduction, slow-responding
  cardiac reflexes dependent on input from, 100, 102
  long-term reflex modulation of cardiac output by, 104, 105
  memory function of, 100
  modality specificity, multimodal, 99
  neuromodulation of, 100
  noise in input function, 106
    amplifying effects of, 105
    aperiodic signals and, 105
    fast signals and 105
    minimizing adaptation, by, 105
  patterning of activity by, 99
  spatiotemporal transduction characteristics of, 105, 106
  threshold adaptation in, 100, 106
sympathetic, 159, 369
vagal, 165–169
  as immunological sensors, 168. See also Lipopolysaccharide, endotoxin
vena caval, neuroanatomy of, 81
ventricular, neuroanatomy of, 81
Aggravation, irritation, anger, impatience (AIAI)
  characteristics of, 394
Aging, effects on
  adenosine-adrenergic interactions, 284–287
    clinical implications of, 287

Aging, effects on (*Continued*)
  adrenergic-induced protein
      phosphorylation, cardiac, 277
  adrenergic modulation of cardiac
      contractile function
    models of, 273
    sex differences in, 273
  β-receptor kinase (βARK1), 277
  baroreflex, 272
  calcium influx into sympathetic nerve
      terminals, 275
  cardiac innervation, 272
  cardiac end-organ receptor
      mechanisms, 272
  cardiac neurons, ion channels of
    voltage-gated, 17–41
    ligand-gated, 42–47
  cholinergic-adrenergic interactions, 278
  GRK5, 277
  stroke tolerance, 236
  sympathetic nervous system, 272, 274, 275
    α_2 prejunctional receptors, 275
    β_2 prejunctional receptors, 275
    norepinephrine release, 275
    norepinephrine reuptake, 275
Aldosterone
  effects on myocardial remodeling, 341
Alpha adrenergic blockade
  as treatment for hypertension, 383
Alpha adrenergic receptors
  central α_2 receptors
    as treatment for hypertension, 383
    effects on parabrachial neural
        activity, 223
  distribution of, in heart, 274
    aging, effects on, 274
  effect on afferent release of CGRP, 373
  hypothalamic actions of, 373
  modulation of acetylcholine release
      from vagus, 5
  modulation of cardiac function
    sinoatrial node, 274
      aging, effects on, 274
    vasomotor tone, 274
      aging, effects on, 274
    ventricular contractility, 274
      aging, effects on, 274
  relative potency of agonists, 343
  signal transduction systems of
    α_1 receptors, 273
Amino acids
  effect on intrinsic cardiac neurons
    aspartate, 11

  gamma aminobutyric acid (GABA), 12
  glutamate, 11
Amygdala
  afferent projections from, 222
    infralimbic cortex, 229
    insular cortex, 229
    nucleus of solitary tract, 229
    parabrachial nucleus, 222
  autonomic-emotional interactions
      within, 228, 229, 235
    hypothalamic interactions and, 228
    lesion, effects on, 228
  central nucleus of, 228
  efferent neuronal projections to, 226
    dorsal motor nucleus, 228
    hypothalamus, 228
    infralimbic cortex, 229
    insular cortex, 229
    nucleus of solitary tract, 228
    parabrachial nucleus, 228
    thalamus, medial dorsal n., 229
  electrical stimulation, effects on
    blood pressure
      anesthetized, 228
      awake, 228
      sleep, 228
    heart rate
      anesthetized, 228
      awake, 228
  efferent projections to
    Diencephalon, 375
    Pons/Medulla, 375
  modulation of
    blood pressure, 228, 378
    cardiac electrical stability (VF
        potential), 228
    sympathetic nervous system, 375
  stroke, effects on neurotransmitters in, 235
Anger
  cardiac effects associated with
    ECG abnormalities, 233
    ventricular arrhythmias, 233
    ventricular fibrillation, 233
  coronary artery disease and, 394
  characteristics of in relation to cardiac
      disease, 232, 396
  sympathoexcitation and, 233
Angina pectoris. *See also* Silent Ischemia;
    Syndrome X
  adenosine and
    myocardial ischemia, 300
    interactions with nicotine in, 305

Index

interactions with substance P in, 305
adenosine/β endorphin interactions in, 309
afferent sensory transduction in, 155
  neurotransmitters in, 158
  response characteristics of, 158
  sympathetic afferents mediating, 158
antinociception, definition of, 158
autonomic aspects of, 139, 155
basis of, 155, 298, 311
anger as risk factor for, 394
behavior, Type A and, 394
chronic refractory, 139, 153
  definition of, 156
  incidence of, 156
  lifestyle effects of, 153
chronic stable, 156
emotional aspects of, 155
exercise induced angina, 155, 302, 305, 308
  bamiphylline (A_1) blockade of, 305
  theophylline blockade of, 305
hostility as risk factor for, 395
ischemic heart disease and perception of, 139, 304
localization of
  central substernal, 299
  diffuse, 300
  radiating, 299
  referred, 159, 160, 162
  versus cardiac outcome, 299
opioid receptor mediated effects on, 309
oxygen supply/demand in, 139, 155, 298, 300
physical deconditioning resulting from, 306
physical training and effects on
  adenosine-provoked chest pain, 307
  exercise capacity, 306
  pain perception, 306
  ST segment depression, 307
quality of pain
  aching, 299
  burning-pricking, 299
  multimodal, 155, 300
  pressing-throbbing, 299
  dyspnoea-suffocation, 155, 299
  anxiety, 299
silent ischemia in patients with, 303
spinal cord processing of nociceptive inputs, 158
  thoracic, 158
sympathectomy, effects on, 162
symptoms, cardiac, in, 298

syndrome X and, 303, 304
therapeutic approaches for treatment of. *See also individual treatments*
  angiotensin converting enzyme inhibitors, 156
  angiotensin II receptor blockade, 332
  beta adrenergic receptor blockade, 156, 332
  calcium channel blockers, 156
  electrical neuromodulation. *See also* SCS and TENS
    spinal cord stimulation (SCS), 139, 153, 156, 170, 332, 333
    Transcutaneous electrical nerve stimulation (TENS), 156
  revascularization, coronary artery
    angioplasty, 156
    bypass, 139, 156
vagal afferent neuronal modulation of, 162
Angiotensin 1–7
modulation of sympathetic nerves, 372
Angiotensin II
activation of
  nodose afferents by, 87
  sympathetic nerves by, 35, 139, 319, 349
control of cardiac function
  chronotropic response, 319
  inotropic response, 331
effects on
  area postrema, 375, 376
  baroreflex, 372
  cardiac neuronal hierarchy, 35, 319, 375
  intrinsic cardiac neuronal activity, 35, 319
  ontogeny of, 260
  neuronal norepinephrine release by, 331, 372, 375, 359
  paraventricular nucleus, 377
  subfornical organ (SFO), 375
  sympathetic nervous system, 35, 128, 129, 352, 375
interactions with
  inflammatory cytokines, 352
  reactive oxygen species, 352
myocardial remodeling modulated by, 139, 341, 352
production of, 358
receptor systems mediating cardiac effects,
  direct myocyte effects, 319
  neural dependent, 35, 129, 139, 319

Angiotensin III
  modulation of sympathetic nerves, 372
Angiotensin Converting Enzyme (ACE)
  antisense gene therapy targeting, 383
  effects on intrinsic cardiac nervous system, 335
  β adrenergic blockade and activity of, 352
  production of angiotensin II by, 359
  as treatment for
    angina pectoris, 156
    hypertension, 383
Angiotensin converting enzyme inhibitors
  effects on sympathetic neurons, 349
Angiotensinogen
  antisense gene therapy targeting, 383
  sympathetic stimulation and increases in, 349
Anterior hypothalmic nucleus. See also Hypothalamus
  modulation of
    blood pressure by, 380
    catecholamine release by, 379
    sympathetic nerve activity by, 375, 380
Anxiety. See also Panic disorder
  cardiac effects of, 399
  characteristics of in relation to cardiac disease, 232
  pain perception during, 308
Apoptosis, myocyte
  β adrenergic receptors and, 348
  β_2 adrenergic receptors and mitigation of, 348
  Ca^{++} overload and, 348
Arachidonic acid, activation of nodose afferents by, 87
Area Postrema (AP)
  angiotensin II, effects on, 375, 376
  arginine vasopressin, effects on, 375, 376
  modulation of sympathetic nervous system by, 375
  ontogeny of coordinated activity within, 253
  paraventricular nucleus modulation of, 376
  as plasma peptide sensor, 376
Arginine Vasopressin (AVP)
  modulation of area postrema by, 375, 376
  modulation of sympathetic nervous system by, 375
Arrhythmias, cardiac. See also Atrial arrhythmias; Atrial Fibrillation; Ventricular arrhythmias; Ventricular Fibrillation
  anger as risk factor for, 396
  bradykinin facilitation of, 358
  congestive heart failure and, 341, 342
  therapeutic options for treatment of
    AT1 receptor blockade, 351
    AT1a receptor knockout, 351
AT1 receptor
  antisense gene therapy targeting, 383
  interdependent interactions with β_1 adrenergic receptor, 351
  intrinsic cardiac neuronal distribution of, 319, 349
  myocyte distribution of, 319, 349
  sympathetic nerve distribution of, 139, 349
AT1 receptor blockade
  mitigation of angiotensin II induced
    myocyte necrosis, 350
    coronary vascular damage, 350
  effects on
    intrinsic cardiac nervous system, 335
  as treatment for hypertension, 383
AT2 receptor
  inhibitory effects of, 359
Atherosclerosis
  anger as risk factor for, 232
  anxiety as risk factor for, 232, 399
  psychological stress as risk factor for, 232, 401
  social isolation as risk factor for, 404
Atherosclerosis, carotid
  hostility and risk of, 394
Atrial afferent neurons. See Afferent neurons, cardiovascular
Atrial arrhythmias
  autonomic imbalance and potential for, 134, 137
  focal neural activation and, 134
  nerve network filter characteristics and, 134
  myocyte electrical remodeling and potential for, 137
Atrial conduction
  ontogeny of, 256
Atrial contractile function
  ontogeny of, 257
  regulation of. See Parasympathetic nervous system; Sympathetic nervous system
Atrial electrical activity. See also Atrial repolarization; Effective refractory period

Index

intrinsic cardiac neuronal modulation of
  in canines, 324
  in humans, 325
  maze surgical procedure and effects on, 328
  parasympathetic modulation of, 324, 328
  regional difference in, 324
  right vs. left vagal effects on, 324
  unipolar electrograms, extracellular, as index of, 322
Atrial fibrillation. *See also* Maze procedure
  remodeling of cardiac nervous system in, 111
  treatment of
    surgical, 327, 328
    Maze procedure, 328
Atrial Natriuretic Peptide (ANP)
  central nervous system effects modulating
    sympathetic tone by, 372
  modulation of neuronal norepinephrine release by, 372, 375
  sympathoinhibitory effects of, 372
Atrial repolarization
  intrinsic cardiac neural effects on, 322
  parasympathetic effects on, 322
  unipolar extracellular electrograms as index of, 322
Atrial septal defects
  adenylate cyclase activity in, 262
  β adrenergic receptor downregulation in, 262
  cardiac blood shunts resulting from, 262
  depletion on myocyte contractile elements in, 262
  intrinsic cardiac nervous system, changes in, 262
  neural/myocyte connections in, 262
  perineural fibrosis in, 262
  volume overload in, 262
Atrio-ventricular block
  induced by parasympathetic nerve stimulation, 134
  ontogeny of, 254
Atrio-ventricular conduction
  intrinsic vs. extrinsic control of, 134, 254
  ontogeny of, 254
  parasympathetic influences on, 134
Atrio-ventricular node
  adenosine and modulation of, 279
  autonomic innervation of, 134
    remodeling in sinus node disease, 134
  innervation of, 254

intrinsic cardiac, 134
sympathetic, 254
  ontogeny of, 254
parasympathetic, 134
  ontogeny of, 256
reflex control of
  ontogeny of, 254
Atropine. *See* Muscarinic cholinergic blockade
Autoimmune reactions in cardiac disease, 399
Autonomic nervous system. *See also*
  Afferents, cardiovascular
  Cardiac neuronal hierarchy;
  Cardiac neurons, extrinsic;
  Cardiac neurons, intrinsic;
  Parasympathetic nervous system; Sympathetic nervous system
  neuropathy and effects on cardiac control, 403
  peripheral afferent/efferent interactions, 373

Baroreceptors, arterial. *See* Afferents, Cardiovascular
Baroreceptors, low-pressure. *See* Afferents, Cardiovascular
Baroreflex. *See also* Caudoventrolateral nucleus; Nucleus Ambiguus; Nucleus tractus solitarius; Parasympathetic nervous system; Rostroventrolateral nucleus; Sympathetic nervous system
  afferent neurons. *See* Afferents, Cardiovascular
  aging, effects on reflex control of, 272
    heart rate, 272
    muscarinic receptor function, cardiac, 278
    parasympathetic efferents, 272
    sympathetic efferents, 272
  anatomical organization of, 188, 189
  angiotensin II effects on, 372, 374
  area postrema, neurohumoral interactions and, 376
  brainstem neural interactions mediating, 85, 121, 221. *See also*
    Medulla oblongata; Nucleus Tractus Solitarius; Nucleus Ambiguus
  cortical modulation of, 227, 231, 377
  depression and effects on sensitivity, 397

Baroreflex (*Continued*)
   effect of myocardial infarction on sensitivity of, 187
   efferent neurons. *See also* Sympathetic Nervous System; Parasympathetic Nervous System
      parasympathetic efferent neurons, 85, 101, 188, 200, 206
      sympathetic efferent neurons, 85, 101, 188, 200, 206, 375
   estrogen effects on, 381
   GABA mediated effects on, 196, 376
   gain as risk factor for
      myocardial infarction, 142
      sudden cardiac death, 142
   gain, modulation by
      infralimbic cortex, 227
      insular cortex, 231
      ion channels, afferent, 192
      supramedullary inputs, 189
   glutamate effects on, 195
   inspiratory-related inhibition of, 203
   maladaption of, 368
      afferent ion channels in cardiac disease, 192
   obesity, effects on, 371
   ontogeny of,
      afferent input, 253
      central processing, 253
         area postrema, 253
         nucleus tractus solitarius, 253
      gain, 253, 254
      heart control, 253
   resetting, 368
Behavior, Type A. *See also* AIAI
   cardiovascular response to stress, 234
   characteristics of, 393
   coronary artery disease in, 394
   toxic components of, 394
Behavior, Type B
   cardiovascular response to stress, 234
   characteristics of, 394
Beta adrenergic agonists. *See* Epinephrine; Norepinephrine
Beta adrenergic antagonists
   effects on
      leukocytes, oxidative capacity of, 358
      reactive inflammatory species, 357
      ventricular contractile function, 356
   mitigation of angiotensin II induced
      coronary vascular damage, 350
      hypertension, 350
      myocyte fibrosis, 350
   as treatment for
      angina pectoris, 156
      cardiomyopathy, 355
      congestive heart failure by, 139, 355, 421
      hypertension, 383
Beta adrenergic receptor
   adenosine, antiadrenergic effects of, 274, 280
   aging, effects on, 274, 280, 284–287
   affinity, cardiac, effects of aging on, 277
   β_1 receptor mediated effects, 347
   β_1 adrenergic receptor overexpression and cardiomyopathy, 348
   β_1 downregulation with chronic angiotensin II exposure, 350
   β_1 interdependent interactions with AT1 receptor, 351
   β_2 receptor mediated effects, 348
      pre-synaptic modulation of catecholamine release, 130
   β_2 adrenergic receptor overexpression and
      cardiac effects of, 348
      non-pathological consequences of, 348
   β_2 polymorphism and effects on cardiac pathology
      Gln27, effects of, 349
      Gly16, effects of, 349
      Ile164, effects of, 349
      Thr164, effects of, 349
   changes in congestive heart failure, 344, 347
   control of cardiac function
      atrial contractility, 278
         adenosine antagonism of, 278
      heart rate, 273
         aging and effects on, 273
      ventricular contractility, 276
         adenosine antagonism of, 278, 285
           juvenile to aged adults, 285
         aging and effects on, 273, 284, 285
           juvenile to aged adults, 285
   coupling to adenylate cyclase, 125, 273, 276, 348
   distribution of β_1 and β_2 receptors in heart, 348
      effects of aging on, 277
   distribution of β_2 receptors on sympathetic neurons, 130, 348
   effect on
      Ca^{++} permeability and handling, 276, 348
         adenosine antagonism of, 278
      intrinsic cardiac nervous system, 335

intrathoracic sympathetic neurons, 130, 348
matrix metalloproteinases in CHF, 352
neurohumoral remodeling in CHF, 352
guanine nucleotide inhibitory proteins (G_i)
  role of, 348
guanine nucleotide stimulatory proteins
  (G_s), role of, 125, 273, 276, 348
relative potencies of agonists, 343
reverse remodeling in CHF for
  extracellular matrix, cardiac, 352
  left ventricular chamber function, 353
  myocyte contractile function, 353
signal transduction mechanisms for
  β_1 receptors, 276
  congestive heart failure, 344, 348
Birth
  cardiovascular stress of, 258
Biventricular pacing
  effects on cardiac nervous system, 422
Blood. *See also* Coagulation
Blood pressure
  age-related changes in, 379
  circadian rhythm of, 379
  control, long-term, 369
  control, short-term, 369
  depression and effects on, 397
  hostility and effects on, 394
  stress and effect on, 400
Body mass index
  hostility and relationship to, 394
Bradykinin
  afferent activation and pain perception, 161
  chemical stimulation of
    cardiac afferents by, 161, 163
    intrinsic cardiac afferents by, 97
    intrinsic cardiac neurons by, 36, 319
    nodose afferents by, 87
  effects on (via BK_2 receptor)
    arrhythmias, 358
    sympathetic release of norepinephrine, 358
    ventriclar fibrillation, 358
  modulation of myocardial remodeling by, 341
  myocardial ischemia and release of, 110, 359
Bundle of His, 256
  ontogeny of, 256

Calcitonin gene-related peptide (CGRP)
  α_2 adrenergic modulation of neural release by, 373
  effect on
    intrinsic cardiac neurons, 132, 319
    mast cells, 193
    nodose afferent neurons, 87
    NTS neurons, 198
    parabrachial neurons, 223
    sympathetic neurons, 375
    vasomotor tone, 193, 334, 373
  released from cardiac afferent neurons, 193, 373
  spinal cord stimulation and peripheral release of, 173, 334
Calcium channel current, L-type
  beta adrenergic modulation of, 273
Calcium channel antagonists, as treatment for
  angina pectoris, 156
  hypertension, 383
cAMP. *See also* Adenylate cyclase
  adenosine A_1 receptor inhibition of, 276
  adrenergic beta receptor stimulation of, 276
  inhibitory guanine nucleotide (G_i) modulation of, 125
  modulation of cardiac contractility by, 276
  modulation of neuronal excitability by, 29
  muscarinic inhibition of, 125
  protein kinase A (PKA) activation by, 276
  protein phosphorylation modulated by, 276
  receptor systems modulating levels of, 276
  stimulatory guanine nucleotide (G_s) modulation of, 125, 276
Capsaicin
  activation of cardiac afferent neurons by, 161
  depletion of cardiac substance P by, 9
Cardiac Neuronal Hierarchy. *See also* Afferents, cardiovascular; Baroreflex; Spinal cord, segmental interactions; Parasympathetic nervous system; Spinal cord stimulation; Sympathetic nervous system
  anatomical organization of, 315, 369, 419
  central nervous system components, 123, 154, 174, 221, 222, 226, 229

Cardiac Neuronal Hierarchy (*Continued*)
    peripheral components, 6, 7, 123, 154, 174, 221
    autonomic dysfunction in, 109, 176, 263, 349, 357, 358, 419, 422
    activity patterns within, 420
    central nervous system organization of, 174, 220
        ascending projections for visceral sensory inputs, 222
        descending projections for, 226
        medullary interactions for, 159, 187, 208
        spinal cord interactions for, 153, 159, 174
            intersegmental, 154
            spinothalamic projections, 159
    control of cardiac function by, 103, 221, 420
        short-term (seconds), 103
        long-term (minutes to hours to days), 103
    coordination of activity within
        afferent dependent mechanism, 79, 80, 97, 101, 112, 126, 127, 134
            fast-responding inputs and, 106, 112
            slow-responding inputs and, 106, 112
        descending projections and, 126
        local circuit neurons and, 126, 127, 134
    hysteretic behavior of
        filter characteristics of, 107
        in adverse neurohumoral remodeling, 109
        local circuit neuronal mediation of, 107
        memory function of, 107
    neural interactions within, 123, 154, 177, 220, 419
    neurohumoral interactions within, 118, 123, 141, 349, 357, 358, 420
    ontogeny of, 71, 253, 254
        central reflex mechanisms, 254
        efferent output, 71, 254
        peripheral reflex mechanisms, 259
    peripheral neural interactions
        feedback loops and, 1, 103, 133, 141
        intrathoracic, 118, 123, 133, 141
        intrinsic cardiac, 1, 118, 123, 125, 133
        network filter characteristics, 133
    radiofrequency catheter ablation effects on, 421
    feedback loops within
        central nervous system, 79, 97, 123
        intrathoracic nervous system, 6, 79, 97, 112, 123
    remodeling during cardiac pathology, 107, 111, 137, 141, 176, 220, 307, 349–359, 420
    remodeling during CNS pathology, 235–237
    remodeling during cardiac stress, 107
    sudden infant death syndrome and dysfunction of, 263
    syndrome X and supersensitivity of, 307
Cardiac neurons, discharge characteristics
    current injections, effects on, 15
    functional classification of
        accommodating, 15
        phasic, 15
        tonic, 15
    muscarine-sensitive K^+ current and, 15
    in vivo versus *in vitro* models, 15
    spontaneous activity *in vivo*, 16
Cardiac neurons, extrinsic (intrathoracic, extracardiac) ganglia. *See also* Cardiac neuronal hierarchy; Parasympathetic nervous system; Sympathetic nervous system
    afferent neurons
        hypoxia and activation of, 97
        intrathoracic feedback reflex loops and, 79, 121
        morphology of, Aδ fibers, 84
        response characteristics of, 91, 92
            chemoreceptors, 93
            mechanoreceptors, 92
        modality specificity of, 121
            chemosensitive, 84, 93
            mechanosensitive, 84, 89
        sensory neurites, distribution of, 79, 80, 89, 121
        soma locations of
            mediastinal ganglia, 84
            middle cervical ganglia, 84
            stellate ganglia, 84
        transduction of
            adenosine, 93
            peptides, 93
            purines, 95
    anatomical organization of, 350
    angiotensin II- AT1 receptor mediated effects on
        ventricular contractility, 350
        heart rate, 350

cholinergic receptor mechanisms
within, 65, 67, 132
control of. *See also* Parasympathetic
nervous system; Sympathetic
nervous system
atrial contractility, 122
atrioventricular node, 122
sinoatrial node, 122
ventricular contractility, 122
coordination of activity within, 131
afferent dependent mechanism, 85, 99
convergence of input and, 131
filter characteristics and, 131, 132
decentralization, effects on, 131
efferent neurons, sympathetic postganglionic, 122
mediastinal ganglia, 122
middle cervical ganglia, 122
stellate ganglion, 122
local circuit neurons
definition of, 122
function of, 124
generation of basal nerve activity, 122
interganglionic neural interactions, 122
intraganglionic neural interactions, 122
peripheral integration/reflexes, 122
neuronal subtypes within
afferents (see above)
efferents, sympathetic (see above)
local circuit neurons (see above)
reflex mechanisms within, 80, 124
Cardiac neurons, in cell culture with
cardiomyocytes
adrenergic receptors
β agonist rate effects in, 64, 305
sole cardiomyocyte culture, 63
autonomic neuron-cardiomyocyte
co-culture, 63
β blockade, rate effects, 64
basal conditions, 63
isoproterenol stress, 63
tetrodotoxin (TTX), rate effects, 64
basal conditions, 63
isoproterenol stress, 63
angiotensin II- AT1 receptor mediated
effects on
agonist challenge, rate effects in
sole cardiomyocyte culture, 68
autonomic neuron-cardiomyocyte
co-culture, 68, 350
β adrenergic blockade and blunting
of rate effects to, 68

receptor blockade, rate effects on,
sole cardiomyocyte culture, 68
autonomic neuron-cardiomyocyte
co-culture, 68
basal myocyte function in nerve-
myocyte co-cultures
contractile, 62
electrical, 62
coordination of activity in, 74
muscarinic receptors, 67
agonist challenge, rate effects in
sole cardiomyocyte culture, 67
autonomic neuron-cardiomyocyte
co-culture, 67
receptor blockade, rate effects in
sole cardiomyocyte culture, 66
autonomic neuron-cardiomyocyte
co-culture, 66
myocyte morphology
sole myocyte culture, 62
with autonomic neuron co-culture, 62
neurochemical profile in
acetylcholinesterase, 72
bradykinin, 72
calcitonin gene-related peptide, 72
choline acetyltransferase, 72
NADPH, 72
neuropeptide Y, 72
oxytocin, 72
Protein gene product 9.5, 72
tryosine hydroxylase, 72
vasoactive intestinal peptide, 72
nicotinic receptors, 65
nicotine challenge, rate effects in, 66
sole cardiomyocyte culture, 65
autonomic neuron-cardiomyocyte
co-culture, 65
receptor blockade, rate effects in, 66
sole cardiomyocyte culture, 65
autonomic neuron-cardiomyocyte
co-culture, 65
nitric oxide (NO)
β-adernoreceptor attenuation of rate
effects to NO stress, 69
intrinsic cardiac neuronal production
of, 69
NO donor challenge, rate effects in
sole cardiomyocyte culture, 69
autonomic neuron-cardiomyocyte
co-culture, 69
ontogeny, effects on autonomic neuron-
cardiomyocyte co-cultures
postsynaptic effects, neonate
mediated, 70

Cardiac neurons, in cell culture with
    cardiomyocytes (*Continued*)
  presynaptic effects, adult mediated, 70
  purinergic agonists
    ATP and P_2 mediated rate increase in, 69
    adenosine and P_1 mediated rate increase in, 69
  technique for
    cardiomyocyte-intrinsic cardiac neuron co-culture, 62
    cardiomyocyte-stellate neuron co-culture, 62
Cardiac neurons, intrinsic
  acetylcholine, effects on
    autonomic ganglia, 125
    myocytes, 125
    neurotransmitter release, 125
  activity, spontaneous
    cardiac related, 6, 131
    respiratory related, 6, 131
  adenosine and modulation of, 279, 301
  adenosine triphosphate (ATP)
    chronotropic response to, 10, 69
    histochemical location of, 10
    modulation of
      neuronal activity, 11, 40, 69
      norepinephrine release, 10, 40
      vagal afferents by, 10, 40
    myocardial ischemia and release of, 11
  afferent neurons
    intrinsic cardiac feedback reflex loops and, 79, 80, 121
    modality specificity of, 121
      chemosensory, 83
      mechanosensory, 83, 97
      multimodal, 83, 97
    neurotransmitters contained in
      calcitonin gene-related peptide, 5
      substance P, 5
    morphology of, 84, 97
    projections
      higher centers of cardiac neuronal hierarchy, 84
      intrinsic cardiac nervous system, 5, 84
    sensory neurites, distribution of, 80, 84, 97, 121
    transduction of
      adenosine, 97
      ATP, 97
      bradykinin, 97

      catecholamines, 97
      nitric oxide, 97
      substance P, 97
    amino acids
      effects on neuronal activity
        aspartate, 11
        GABA, 12
        glutamate, 11
      glutamate receptors distribution
        cardiac, 12
        neuronal, 12
    anatomy of
      canine, 316, 318
      feline, 321
      guinea pig, immunoreactive neurochemical profile, 73
      human, 317, 318, 325
      porcine, 317
    angiotensin II- AT1 receptor mediated effects on
      catecholamine spillover into coronary sinus, 350
      heart rate, 319, 350
      ontogeny of, 260
      neural activity within, 35, 36, 132, 260
      sympathetic release of
        epinephrine, 346, 350
        norepinephrine, 331, 346, 350
      ventricular contractility, 319, 331, 350
    AT1 receptors on, 349
    autonomic nerve interactions within, 5, 125
    bradykinin—BK_2 receptor mediated effects on
      neuronal activity within, 36, 319
      regional cardiac function, 319
      sympathetic neuronal release of norepinephrine, 358
    calcitonin gene-related peptide (CGRP)
      distribution in, 9
      effects on neuronal activity in, 132, 319
    catecholamines
      effects on neuronal activity in, 5, 6, 9, 132
        α mediated effects, 8, 65
        β mediated effects, 8, 65
      decentralization, effects on, 8
      reuptake mechanism in, 8
      synthesis within, enzymes for, 8
        dopamine β-hydroxylase, 8
        L-amino acid decarboxylase, 8
    chemical stimulation of
      chronotropic response, 319, 321

dromotropic response, 319, 321
inotropic response, 321, 330
cholinergic synaptic mechanisms
    within, 6
  muscarinic, 67, 132, 319
  nicotinic, 65, 132, 319, 321
C-type natriuetic peptide (CNP) effects on
  neuronal activity in, 319
  regional cardiac function, 319
coordination of activity in, 315
  afferent dependent mechanisms, 9, 85, 126, 127
  descending input and, 9
  local circuit neurons and, 127
  synaptic-mediated, 4
  nonsynaptic-mediated, 4
decentralized from CNS, effects on, 6, 131, 319, 321
  effects on neuronal activity in, 6
  effects on neurochemical coding in, 8
efferent distribution from, 316, 321
  atrial, 322–324, 329
  ventricular, 326, 327
efferent neurons, parasympathetic postganglionic, 79, 319, 321, 326, 330
  ontogeny of, 71, 259
efferent neurons, parasympathetic preganglionic, input to, 5, 125. See also Nucleus ambiguus
efferent neurons, sympathetic postganglionic, 79, 122, 319, 321, 326
  catecholamine uptake by, 130
electrical stimulation, 316
  chrontropic effects of, 318
  dromotropic effects of, 318, 322, 324
  inotropic, ventricular, effects of, 330
  neuronal electrophysiology, effects on, 5
electrophysiological properties. See Cardiac neurons, discharge characteristics; Cardiac neurons, passive membrane properties ; Cardiac neurons, ligand-gated ion channels; Cardiac neurons, voltage-gated ion channels
endothelin, effects on neuronal activity in, 132
enkephalin (D-Ala^2 D-Leu^5) effects on neuronal activity in, 37, 319
extracellular activity recorded from, 319

extrapericardial input to, 131, 141
  parasympathetic, 123, 316, 328–330
  sympathetic, 123, 318
final common pathway for cardiac control, 3, 330
ganglionated plexi
  anatomical organization of, 317
  defined, 317
  functional organization of, 3, 316
heterogeneous activation and induction of
  cardiac arrhythmias, 137
  ventricular fibrillation, 137
histamine, 260
  cardiac distribution of, 10
  H_1 versus H_2 receptor mediated effects, 260
  neural activity in response to, 10, 260
  mast cells as source for, 10
  ontogeny of, 260
ion channels, ligand-gated. See Cardiac neuron, ligand-gated ion channels
ion channels, voltage-gated. See Cardiac neuron, voltage-gated ion channels
ischemic heart disease, effects on, 137, 262
local circuit neurons (LCNs), 79
  definition of, 122
  function of, 124
    generation of basal nerve activity, 122
    interganglionic neural interactions, 5, 122, 125
    intraganglionic neural interactions, 5, 122, 125
    peripheral integration/reflexes, 122
  hysteretic information processing by, 107
  filter characteristics of, 107
  memory function of, 107
low pass filter characteristics of, 131, 132
modulation of regional cardiac function
  atrial conduction, 322, 323
  atrial contractility, 319, 321
  atrial electrical activity, 324, 329
  atrioventricular node, 316
  sinoatrial node, 316, 319, 329
  ventricular conduction, 326
  ventricular electrical activity, 326
  ventricular contractile function, 258
  ontogeny of, 258

Cardiac neurons, intrinsic (*Continued*)
  morphology of neurons in,
    bipolar, 3, 72
    multipolar, 3, 72
    unipolar, 3, 72
  myocardial ischemia, activation of, 279
  neurochemical coding for
    ATP, 6
    catecholamines, 6
    dynorphin B, 8
    histamine, 6
    nitric oxide, 6
    neuropeptide Y, 8
    serotonin, 6
    somatostatin, 8
    substance P, 8
    vasoactive intestinal peptide, 8
  neuronal subtypes within
    afferents. *See* Cardiac neurons, intrinsic, efferent neurons
    efferents, parasympathetic. *See* Cardiac neurons, intrinsic, efferent neurons, parasympathetic postganglionic
    efferents, sympathetic. *See* Cardiac neurons, intrinsic, efferent neurons, sympathetic postganglionic
    local circuit neurons. *See* Cardiac neurons, intrinsic, local circuit neurons
  neurokinin, effects on neuronal activity in, 132
  neuropeptide Y
    effects on neuronal activity in, 38, 132
    localization within, 125, 259
    ontogeny of, 259
    vasomotor effect, 10
  nicotine effects on
    intrinsic cardiac nervous system parasympathetic efferent neurons, 321
    sympathetic efferent neurons, 321
  nitric oxide
    effects on
      neural activity in, 6, 11, 69, 260
      ontogeny of, 260
      presynaptic terminals, vagal efferent neurons, 11
    immunoreactivity for, 11
  noncholinergic synaptic mechanisms within, 68, 132
  norepinephrine neuronal release by, 125
  oxytocin effects on
    neuronal activity in, 319

    regional cardiac function, 319
  pituitary adenylate cyclase-activating polypeptide (PACAP)
    effects on neuronal activity in, 39
  purinergic agonists, effects on, 132, 137
  reflex mechanism in, cardio-cardiac
    characteristics of, 80, 124
      focused, 103
      limited memory, 104
      minimal computation, 103
      rapid, 103
    coordination of regional cardiac function by, 104
      electrical function, 104
      mechanical function, 104
  receptor mechanisms associated with. *See individual* putative neurotransmitters
  serotonin
    effects on activity in, 6
    distribution in, 10
  small intensely fluorescent (SIF) cells in, 5, 8, 122
  somatostatin effects on, 36, 260
    ontogeny of, 260
  substance P
    effects on
      neuronal activity in, 132, 319
        neuromediator effects, 10, 40
        neuromodulator effects, 10, 40
      regional cardiac function, 319
    fiber distribution to
      intrinsic cardiac nervous system, 9
      myocytes, 9
  sympathetic/parasympathetic interactions within, 125
    chorotropic control and, 125
  sympathetic preganglionic projections to, 5, 7. *See also* Sympathetic nervous system
  synaptic transmission. *See also* Cardiac neurons, ligand-gated ion channels; Cardiac neurons, voltage-gated ion channels
    cholinesterase inhibition and, 47
    nicotinic acetylcholine receptor channels and fast excitatory post-synaptic potentials (EPSPs), 48
    muscarinic receptor channels and
      M_1 mediated slow EPSPs, 48
      M_2 (or M_3) mediated slow inhibitory post-synaptic potentials

Index

post-synaptic summation and
    convergence of input, 47
vasoactive intestinal peptide (VIP)
    effects on
        neuronal activity in, 36, 125, 132, 319
        ontogeny of, 260
        regional cardiac function, 319
veratridine, effects on activity of, 19
Cardiac neurons, ligand-gated ion
    channels
    ATP P2X purinoceptor channels, 46
        characteristics of
            current-voltage relationship, 46
            ion selectivity, 46
            rapid depolarization, 46
            rectification, 46
            reversal potential, 46
        decentralization and expression of, 47
        cardiac disease and expression of, 47
    nicotinic acetylcholine receptor
        channels, 41
        blockade of, 41
        channel subtypes of, 42, 44
            α subunits and, 43, 44
            β subunits and, 43, 44
        characteristics of
            cation selectivity, 41
            current-voltage relationship, 41
            latency, 41
            retification, 41
            reversal potential, 41
        excitatory potentials, rapid, and, 41
        neuropeptide modulation, 44
            pituitary adenylate cyclase-
                activating polypeptide
                (PACAP) and potentiation of, 44
            substance P inhibition of, 35
            vasoactive intestinal polypeptide
                (VIP) and
                potentiation of, 44
        synaptic neurotransmission and, 43
Cardiac neurons, passive membrane
    properties
    input resistance, determination of, 13, 14
    ion channel rectification, 14
    leaky conductance in, 14
    membrane time constant, 13
    ontogeny of, 14
    resting membrane potential, 12, 13, 14
Cardiac neurons, voltage-gated ion
    channels
    Ca^{++} channels, 20
        adrenergic modulation, α-receptor
            mediated attenuation of, 34

antagonists for, 21
characteristics of
    activation, 20
    conductance, 20
    inactivation, voltage dependence
        of, 20
    recovery, rate of, 20
    threshold, 20
    ion selectivity of, 20
modulation of
    intracellular Ca^{++} dependent
        processes, 20
    neuronal excitability, 20
neurochemical modulation of, 21, 36, 37
ontogeny, 21, 23
subtypes of, 21
K^+ channel, ATP-sensitive, 26
characteristics of
    ATP concentration threshold, 26
    conductance, 26
function, transduce changes in cell
    metabolism to
    changes in membrane potential, 26
hypoxia and activation of, 27
myocardial ischemia and activation
    of, 27
ontogeny of, 26
resting membrane potential and, 27
K^+ channels, Ca^{++} dependent, 25
characteristics of
    conductance, 25
    voltage sensitivity, 25
function, hyperpolarize cell after
    action potentials that raise
    intracellular Ca^{++} levels, 25
resting membrane potential and, 25
K^+ channel, delayed outward
    rectifying, 23
characteristics of
    activation, 23
    deactivation, 23
    rectification, outward, 23
    threshold, 24
function, rapid termination of action
    potential, 23
K^+ channel, inward rectifying, 26
characteristics of
    gating, 26
    inward rectification, 26
ontogeny of, 26
K^+ channel, muscarine-sensitive, 27
    acetylcholine modulation of, 27
characteristics of
    activation of, voltage dependence, 27

Cardiac neurons, voltage-gated ion
　　channels (*Continued*)
　　deactivation of
　　　time dependence, 27
　　　voltage dependence, 27
　　　threshold, 27
　　function of, 27
　　　modulation of neuronal
　　　　excitability, 27
　　　resting membrane potential and, 27
　　ontogeny of, 30–34
　　receptor subtypes, mediated
　　　responses of
　　　　M_1 receptors, 30
　　　　M_2 receptors, 33
　　　　M_3 receptors, 33
　　　　M_4 receptors, 33
　K^+ channel, transient outward, 24
　　characteristics of
　　　activation, 24
　　　inactivation
　　　　time dependence, 24
　　　　voltage dependence, 24
　　　ontogeny, 24
　　　recovery of, 24
　　　threshold, 24
　　function, reduce excitatory effects of
　　　depolarizing
　　　stimuli in time-dependent manner,
　　　　24
　Na^+ channels, 17
　　action potential dependence on, 17
　　characteristics of
　　　conductance, 17
　　　inactivation of, voltage
　　　　dependence, 19
　　　recovery of, 19
　　ciguatoxin, effects on, 19
　　tetrodotoxin (TTX), effects on, 17
　　veratridine, effects on, 19
　nonselective cation channels,
　　　hyperpolarization-activated
　　characteristics of
　　　conductance, 29
　　　rectification, 28
　　　time dependence, 28
　　　voltage dependence, 28
　　modulation of neuronal excitability
　　　by, 29
　　neurotransmitter modulation and
　　　regulation
　　　of synaptic efficacy by, 29
　peptide modulation of, 35, 36
　　angiotensin II and modulation of
　　　Ca^{++} channels, 35, 36

　　bradykinin, 36
　　met-enkephalin and modulation of
　　　Ca^{++} channels, 36, 37
　　ontogeny of, 37
　　neuropeptide Y and modulation of
　　　Ca^{++} channels, 36, 38
　　somatostatin and modulation of
　　　Ca^{++} channels, 36
　　substance P and modulation of
　　　nicotinic acetylcholine receptors
　　　(nAChR), 36, 39
　　nonselective cation conductance, 40
　　pituitary adenylate cyclase-activated
　　　peptide (PACAP) and
　　　modulation of nAChR, 36, 39
　　ontogeny of, 39
　　vasoactive intestinal peptide and
　　　modulation of nAChR, 36
　purinergic modulation of, 40
　　receptors subtypes associated with,
　　　40
　　$P2Y_2$ receptors mediated modulation
　　　of
　　　Ca^{++} dependent K^+ channels, 40
Cardiac Nervous System. *See* Cardiac
　　Neuronal Hierarchy
Cardiac preconditioning
　adenosine induced, 173
　opioid induced, 173
Cardiomyopathy, idiopathic dilated
　β adrenergic receptor blockade, effects
　　on
　　α-myosin heavy-chain mRNA, 355
　　β-myosin heavy-chain mRNA, 355
　　β adrenergic receptors, 355
　　LV chamber function, 356
　　myocyte calcium handling, 355
　　sarcoplasmic reticulum Ca^{++} ATPase
　　　mRNA, 355
Cardiomyopathy, ischemic
　β adrenergic receptor blockade, effects
　　on
　　myocyte Ca^{++} transients, 355
　　sarcoplasmic reticulum Ca^{++}
　　　ATPase, 355
Cardiomyopathy, non-ischemic
　β adrenergic receptor blockade, effects on
　　myocyte Ca^{++} transients, 355
　　sarcoplasmic reticulum Ca^{++}
　　　ATPase, 355
Cardiovascular afferents. *See* Afferents,
　　cardiovascular; Parasym-
　　pathetic Nervous System;
　　Sympathetic Nervous System;
　　Baroreflex

Carotid atherosclerosis. *See*
    Atherosclerosis, carotid
Cardiovascular stressors
    anger, 395
    hostility, 394
    mental tasks, 395
Catecholamines. *See also* Alpha adrenergic
        receptors; Beta adrenergic
        receptors; Epinephrine;
        Norepinephrine
    activation of cardiac afferent neurons
        by, 97
    depression and effects on, 397
    effect on intrinsic cardiac neurons, 6
    hostility and circulating levels of, 395
    modulation of sensory afferent
        sensitivity by, 100
    psychological stress and release of, 400,
        403
    vascular spillover of, 371
Caudoventrolateral medulla (CVLM)
    afferent projection from
        nucleus tractus solitarius, 188
    baroreflex and modulation of activity
        in, 188, 375
    GABA as putative neurotransmitter, 374
    modulation of sympathetic nervous
        system by, 188, 375
    suppression of rostroventrolateral
        nucleus, 374
Central nervous system. *See specific regions*
    and nuclei
c-fos, as marker for neuronal activity, 161
CGRP. *See* Calcitonin gene-related
        peptide
Chemoreceptors. *See* Afferent neurons,
        Cardiovascular
Chemoreflex
    afferent neuronal inputs for
        ontogeny of, 253
    central processing of
        ontogeny of, 253
            area postrema, 253
            nucleus tractus solitarius, 253
    inspiratory-related inhibition of, 203
Cholecystokinin
    effects on parabrachial neurons, 223
Cholesterol
    effects of anxiety on, 400
    effects of depression on, 400
Choline acetyltransferase
    distribution within heart, 6, 73
Cholinergic innervation, cardiac. *See also*
        Cardiac neurons, intrinsic;
        Parasympathetic nervous system

atrial-ventricular asymmetry
    ontogeny of, 255
    acetylcholinesterase positive neurons,
        259
    ontogeny of, 259
    ontogeny of, 254, 255, 259
Cholinergic receptors. *See* Muscarinic
        cholinergic receptors;
        Nicotinic cholinergic receptors
Chymase
    cardiac production of angiotensin II by,
        359
Circumventricular organs
    hypothalamic projects from, 377
Circadian rhythm
    in blood pressure, 379
    in hypertension, 379
    in NaCl homeostasis, 379
    stroke, effects on, 230
    ventral basal thalamus, role in, 224
CNP (type C natriuretic peptide)
    central nervous system mediated effects
        on sympathetic tone, 372
    effects on intrinsic cardiac neuronal
        activity, 319
    modulation of neuronal norepinephrine
        release by, 372
    sympathoinhibitory effects of, 372
Coagulation, blood
    exhaustion and impact on, 399
Colchicine, axoplasmic transport inhibitor,
    effect on intrinsic cardiac NPY
        expression, 8
Cognitive behavior therapy in cardiac
        disease,
    impact on cardiac control, 397
    impact on mortality, 397
Conditioned heart rate response
    intralimbic modulation of, 227
Congestive heart failure. *See also*
        Ventricular remodeling;
        Remodeling; Norepinephrine;
        Epinephrine; Apoptosis,
        Myocyte; Necrosis, Myocyte;
        Cardiomyopathy; Heart failure
    adrenergic receptor signal transduction
        in, 344
    afferent transduction mechanisms in,
        111
    angiotensin II—sympathetic
        interactions in, 138, 352
    adverse cardiac effects of, 139
    beta adrenergic receptor
        β_1 mediated adverse cardiac effects
            of, 347

Congestive heart failure (*Continued*)
  β_1 downregulation in, 344
  β_2 desensitization in, 349
  β_2 polymorphism and effects on progression of, 349
  β_2 mediated effects on
    calcium transients, 348
    cardiac contractility, 348
  β_1/β_2 shifts during progression of, 348
  LV pressure/volume loops, effects on, 355
  signal transduction and, 347
  cardiac catecholamine content, 344, 345
  cardiac effects of stellate stimulation in, 345
  clinical measures of, left ventricular
    shape, 355
    ejection fraction, 355
    mass, 355
    volume, 355
  inotropic responses in, 345
  LV pressure/volume loops in, 355
  MMP/TIMP interactions in, 342, 352
  models of
    angiotensin II infusion, 352
    mitrial regurgitation, volume overload, 352
    pacing-induced, 352
  nerve growth factor (NGF)
    decreased cardiac content in, 351
    decreased transcardiac gradient in, 351
  neurohumoral interactions in, 138, 352
  norepinephrine
    cardiac content in, 343
    kinetics during progressive of heart failure, 343–345
    turnover and, 347
    reuptake and, 347
  ouabain effects on, 373
  oxidative stress and, 342, 357
  remodeling of
    extracellular matrix, 342
    left ventricular wall structure, 340
    myocytes, 340
    neurohumoral systems, 111, 340, 351
  tyrosine hydroxylase activity and, 347
  stages of, 340–344
  social support and impact on, 405
  sympathetic overdrive associated with, 138, 340, 342, 347, 357
  therapeutic approaches for treatment of, 139, 342
    AT1 blockade versus ACE inhibitors, 351
    β_1 versus nonselective β adrenergic blockade, 139, 349, 352, 354–357
  ventricular fibrillation threshold in, 340
Contractility, Cardiac. *See* sympathetic nervous System; Parasympathetic nervous system
Coronary angioplasty, percutaneous transluminal treatment for
  chronic stable angina, 156
  coronary artery disease, 156
Coronary artery disease (CAD)
  adenosine
    exercise induced release of, 308
    intracoronary infusion and pain perception in, 302
    intravenous infusion and pain perception in, 302
  age effects on, 393
  anger as risk factor for, 395
  anxiety as risk factor for, 399
  behavior, type A and, 393
  blood flow control in, 153
  depression as risk factor for, 396
  exercise induced angina and, 155, 308. *See also* Angina pectoris
    characteristics of, 155
    perceived location of, 155
  exhaustion as risk factor for, 399
  hostility as risk factor for, 394
  hypercholesterolemia in, 407
  hyperlididemia in, 407
  lifestyle factors and impact on, 406
  models of, chronic ameroid constrictor, 333
  psychological aspects of, Chapter 14
  stress as risk factor for, 233, 400
  sympathetic activity in response to stress, 332
  social support and recovery from, 404
  spinal cord stimulation, effects on
    cardiac supply/demand, 332
    coronary blood flow redistribution, 333
    ST segment displacement during angiotensin II
    activation of cardiac nervous system, 333
    ST segment depression during exercise, 333
    ST segment depression during cardiac pace, 333

therapeutic approaches for treatment
    of. *See also individual therapies*
  angiotensin II receptor blockade, 332,
      335
  angiotensin converting enzyme
      inhibitors, 335
  beta adrenergic receptor blockade,
      332, 335
  intrinsic cardiac nervous system as
      target for, 335
  spinal cord stimulation, 332, 333, 335
Coronary atherosclerosis
  behavior, type A and, 393
Coronary blood flow
  autoregulation, 155, 300
  spinal cord modulation of, 333
  stress and effects on, 403
Coronary artery bypass surgery,
      treatment for
  chronic stable angina, 156
  coronary artery disease, 156
Coronary syndrome, acute
  anxiety as risk factor in, 399
Corticosteroids
  effects of stress on release of, 400
Corticotrophin-releasing factor
  paraventricular release of during stress,
      379
CVLM. *See* Caudoventrolateral medulla
Cytokines, inflammatory. *See*
      Inflammatory cytokines

Depression
  characteristics of in relation to cardiac
      disease, 396
Diabetes, Type 2
  blood pressure regulation in, 371
  sympathetic nerve activity in, 371
Diencephalon. *See also* Hypothalamus;
      Organum vasculosum of
      lamina terminalis; Subfornical
      organ
  modulation by descending inputs, 375
  modulation of sympathetic activity by,
      375
Diet. *See* Lifestyle
Digitalis glycosides inhibition of Na^+-K^+
      ATPase activity by, 373
DiI as neuronal tract tracer, 204
Dorsal motor nucleus of the vagus
  parasympathetic preganglionic neurons
      location of, 369
  vagal efferent neuronal projections
      from, 2

Dorsal root ganglia afferent neurons
  afferent projections of, spinal cord, 79,
      80, 83
    Aδ fibers, 83
    C fibers, 83
  modality specificity of, 121
    chemosensitive, 83, 89
    mechanosensitive, 83
    multimodal, 83, 87
    myocardial ischemia, activation of,
        109
  sensory neurite distribution of, 79, 80,
      87, 121
  reflex responses to activation of
    cardiovascular, 121, 137
    somatic, 121
  response characteristics of, 87
    activity domains of, 89
    fast-responding
      mechanosensitive, 88
      memory, limited, 88
    slow-responding
      chemosensitive, 89
      memory function of, 89
  transduction of
    purines, 89, 110
    substance P, 89, 110
Dynorphin
  distribution to intrinsic cardiac nervous
      system, 8
  hypothalamic actions of, 230

Effective refractory period. *See also* Atrial
      repolariation; Ventricular
      repolarization
  atrial heterogeneity in, 322
  determination of, 322
  right vs. left parasympathetic influences
      on, 322
Effort-reward imbalance. *See also* Stress,
      mental
  defination and effect on cardiac
      pathology, 402
Endothelin effect on intrinsic cardiac
      neurons, 132
Enkephalin (D-Ala^2 D-Leu^5) effects on
      intrinsic cardiac neurons, 37, 319
Enkephalin, Met
  cardiac distribution of, 37
  modulation of
    cardiac neurons by, 37. *See also*
        Cardiac neurons, Voltage-
        gated ion channels
    vagal efferents by, 37

Epinephrine. *See also* Adenylate cyclase;
    Beta adrenergic receptor;
    cAMP
  $\beta 1$ vs. $\beta 2$ receptor mediated effects of,
      130
    $\beta 1$ mediated
      chronotropic effects, 130
      inotropic effects, 130
    $\beta 2$ mediated presynaptic effects on
        sympathetic
        catecholamine release, 130
  cardiac content, 129, 343
  compartmentalization of, 343
    cardiac interstitial fluid versus
        plasma levels, 345
  congestive heart failure, effects on
      neural release of, 354
  infusion and pain perception during,
      306
  interstitial fluid levels (cardiac) in
      response to
    angiotensin II, 129, 345, 346, 354
    spinal cord stimulation, 173
    stellate stimulation, 129, 130, 345,346
  kinetics of
    extraction from blood, 343
    neuronal release, 129, 139, 342, 343
    neuronal reuptake, 343
    spillover, 129
    synthesis of, 343
  kinetics in cardiac pathologies of
    congestive heart failure, 139
    mitrial regurgitation, 353
  plasma levels of, 129, 274
    effects on aging on, 274
  selectivity for adrenergic receptor
      subtypes, 343
Estrogen
  antihypertensive effects of, 381
  interactions with
    catecholamines release, 381
    nitric oxide release, 381
  replacement therapy, BP effects of, 382
Eustress, defination of, 401
Exercise. *See also* Lifestyle factors
  behavioral stressors impacting on, 394
  catecholamine release and, 273
  inotropic effects of, 273
Exhaustion, vital
  characteristics of, 398
  as precursor for cardiac pathology, 398
Extracellular matrix, cardiac
  matrix metalloproteinases (MMP's)
      and, 342, 352

  mitigation of collagen degradation by
      β-adrenergic blockade, 352
  reactive inflammatory species and
      modulation of, 357
  remodeling in
    congestive heart failure, 341, 342
    mitrial regurgitation, 352
  plasticity in, 342
  tissue inhibitors of metalloproteinases
      (TIMP's), 342

Fibrillation, atrial. *See* Atrial fibrillation
Fibrillation, ventricular. *See* Ventricular
    fibrillation
Fibrinolysis, exhaustion and effects on,
    399
Fight-or-flight, 396
FK506 binding protein
  sympathetic overdrive and depletion
      of, 356
FKBP12.6 binding protein
  sympathetic overdrive and depletion
      of, 356
  β adernergic blockade and retention of
      in CHF, 356
Forebrain. *See also* Insular cortex;
    Infralimbic cortex
  anesthesia, cardiovascular effects of,
      230
  cardiovascular control, lateralization of,
      230, 231
  stroke, insular, effects on
    cardiovascular system, 230
    circadian rhythms, 230

GABA (γ-aminobutyric acid)
  CVLM modulation of RVLM by, 374
  effects on
    parabrachial neurons, 223
    hypothalamic neurons, 230
    nucleus tractus solitarius, 196, 197
    nucleus ambiguus neurons, 202
Galinin, modulation of norepinephrine
    release, 372
Ganglia, intrathoracic. *See also* Cardiac
    neurons, intrinsic; Cardiac
    neurons, extrinsic
  activity within, spontaneous, 255
    ontogeny of, 255
  modulation of cardiac function,
    chronotropic function, 255
      ontogeny of, 255
    inotropic function, 255
      ontogeny of, 255

Index

Gap junctions, cardiac, ontogeny of, 257
Gate control theory of pain. *See* Pain, neuromodulation
Glutamate
  cervical cord neurons, excitatory effects of, 163
  hypothalamic actions of, 230
  nucleus ambiguus neurons, neuromodulation of, 202
  nucleus tractus solitarius, excitatory effects of, 196
G proteins
  Gs
    adenylate cyclase activation and, 125, 273, 276, 348
    aging, effects on, 277
    β_1 adrenergic receptors and stimulation of, 125, 276
    norepinephrine β_1 receptor mediated myocyte
      toxicity and, 348
  Gi
    A_1 adenosine receptors and stimulation of, 276, 278, 279
    adenylate cyclase inhibition and, 125
    aging, effects on, 277
    β_2 receptors and stimulation of, 348
    M_2 receptors and stimulation of, 125
Growth factors
  myocardial remodeling and, 341

Heart failure. *See also* Congestive heart failure
  cardiac neurons, changes in, 262
  cardiac reflex control, blunting in, 111
  congenital cardiac malformations and, 262
    atrial septal defects and, 262
    ventricular septal defects and, 262
    genetic defects and, 262
  parasympathetic activity, remodeling in, 200
  sensory transduction mechanisms in, 111
Heart rate. *See also* Heart Rate Variability; Sympathetic nervous system; Parasypathetic nervous system
  baroreflex modulation of, 253
    ontogeny of, 253
  beta-adrenergic modulation of, 372
  chemoreflex modulation of, 253
    ontogeny of, 253
  depression and effects on, 397
  conditional response of, 227
    intralimbic modulation of, 227
  hostility and effects on, 394
  neural control of, 255
    ontogeny of, 255
  neural control following sinoatrial node parasympathectomy, 125
  parasympathetic efferent neuronal control of, 263
    ontogeny of, 263
  stress and effects on, 400, 403
  sympathetic efferent neuronal control of, 263
    ontogeny of, 263
Heart Rate Variability (HRV)
  adrenergic blockade, effects on, 261
    ontogeny of, 261
  anxiety and effects on, 400
  as index of cardiac electrical instability, 264
  as risk factor for
    myocardial infarction, 142
    sudden cardiac death, 142
  baroreflex and modulation of, 261
    ontogeny of, 261
  cardiac transplant, effect on, 262
  cholinergic blockade, effects on, 261
    ontogeny of, 261
  cognitive behavior therapy and, 397
  depression and effects on, 397
  high frequency component in, 261
    ontogeny of, 261
  low frequency component in, 261
    ontogeny of, 261
  respiratory inputs, effects on, 261
    ontogeny of, 261
  stroke, effects on, 236
  sudden infant death syndrome and, 263
  sympathetic modulation of, 263
  premature birth and, 261
Hippocampus, GABA receptor mechanisms within, 197
Hostility
  characteristics of, 394
  coronary artery disease and 394
Hypothalamic-pituitary-adrenocortical (HPA) axis
  link to progression of cardiac disease, 399
Histamine
  activation of nodose afferents by, 87
  cardiac effects of, 10, 260
    ontogeny of, 260
HDL-C
  effects of depression on, 400
  effects of anxiety on, 400

Hormone Replacement Therapy (HRT)
  as treatment for coronary artery
    disease, 407
Hydrogen peroxide, activation of nodose
  afferents by, 87
Hydroxyl radical, activation of nodose
  afferents by, 87
Hypercortisolemia, hostility and relation
  to, 305
Hyperlipidemia, sex related differences,
  407
Hypertension
  age related effects in, 381
  animal models of
    chronic angiotensin II infusion, 350,
      371
    DOCA-NaCl treatment, 371
    high renin, 376
    kidney clamp, 371
    salt-sensitive, 376, 379, 380
    Spontaneously hypertensive rat
      (SHR), 371, 376, 379, 380
  anger as risk factor for, 232
  anxiety as risk factor for, 232
  area postrema modulation of, 376
  arterial baroreflexes in, 368
  catecholamines, circulating in, 371
  central processing of Na^+ inputs to, 380
  circadian rhythms in, 368, 379
  CNS α_2-adrenergic receptor modulation
    of, 373
  CNS imidazoline-receptor modulation
    of, 373
  estrogen effects in, 381
  heart rate in, 371
  hypothalamic neural mechanisms in, 376
  neural mechanisms, 369, 380
  neurohumoral remodeling in, 380
  maintenance phase of, 371
  menopause and, 381
  microneurography in, 371
  NTS modulation of, 376
  neurotransmitter imbalance and
    induction of, 376
  obesity as factor in, 371, 382
  onset phase of, 371
  oubain effects on, 373
  parasympathetic efferent activity,
    remodeling in, 200
  psychological stress as risk factor for,
    232, 233, 400
  renal mechanisms, 369, 371
  RVLM modulation of, 374
  salt-sensitive individuals and, 378
  sex related differences in, 381
  smoking as factor in, 371
  target-organ damage in, 380
  Type 2 diabetes as factor in, 371
Hypothalamus. *See also* Diencephalon and
    individual nuclei including
    Anterior hypothalmic nucleus;
    Lateral hypothalamic area;
    Posterior hypothalamic
    nucleus
  anatomical organization of, 376
  anterior hypothalamic nuclei
    modulation of blood pressure by, 377
    projections from, 377
  ANP/norepinephine mediated
    interactions within, 379
  AV3V modulation of blood pressure,
    377
  cardiovascular afferent input to, 378
  corticotrophin-releasing factor released
    from, 379
  cortical projections into, 378
  estrogen effects on, 382
  lateral hypothalamus
    afferent input from
      infralimbic cortex, 230
      insular cortex, 230
    efferent projections to
      spinal cord, intermediolateral cell
        column, 230
      ventral lateral medulla, 230
    functional organization of, 229
    neurotransmitter mechanisms in
      dynorphin, 230
      GABA, 230
      glutamate-NMDA, 230
      neuropeptide Y, 230
  medial n., spinothalamic afferent
    projections to, 159
  median preoptic nucleus modulation of
    blood pressure, 377
  modulation of sympathetic nervous
    system by, 376
  Na^+/K^+ ATPase activity and
    sympathetic tone, 373
  neural interactions within, 379
  parabrachial nucleus input to, 222
  paraventricular nucleus (PVN)
    magnocellular neurons, 376
    modulation of blood pressure by, 376
    parvocellular neurons, 376
    projections to
      area postrema, 376
      NTS, 376
      RVLM, 376
    release of AVP from, 376

Index

plasma Na$^+$ modulation of, 378
preoptic nuclei
  modulation of
    blood pressure by, 377
    sympathetic nervous system by, 377
  plasma volume, 377
  water balance and, 377
spinal cord projections from, 376
sympathoexcitation and
  lateral hypothalamic area, 376
  posterior hypothalamic area, 376
sympathoinhibition and
  anterior hypothalamic nuclei, 377
  preoptic area, 377
supraoptic nucleus, release of AVP from, 376
vasomotor effects from stimulating on colonic circulation, 252
ventral posterior lateral (VPL) n. spinothalamic projections to, 159

Ibotenic acid (excitotoxin)
  effects on spinal cord neurons, 168
Idiopathic dilated cardiomyopathy
  norepinephrine kinetics in, 343
IL-1β
  β adrenergic receptor blockade, effects on production of, 357
  heart failure and induction of, 357
  myocardial infarction and production of, 357
IL-6
  β adrenergic receptor blockade, effects on production of, 357
  heart failure and induction of, 357
  myocardial infarction and production of, 357
Immunosuppression in cardiac disease, 399
Imidazoline receptors
  central effects as antihypertensive therapy, 383
  cardiovascular response to activation of, 373
  CNS distribution of, 373
  relationship to α_2-adrenergic receptors, 373
Inflammatory cytokines
  cardiac remodeling in heart failure and, 354
  cardiac contractile dysfunction induced by, 357
    β adrenergic signal transduction and, 357

myocyte Ca^{++} handing and, 357
nitric oxide production and, 357
peroxynitrite formation and, 357
extracellular matrix alterations and, 357
fetal gene program induction and, 357
lipopolysaccharide (LPS) induced release of, 168. *See also* Lipopolysaccharide, endotoxin
myocyte growth and, 357
myocyte apoptosis and, 357
remodeling of neuronal ion channels by, 192
vagal afferent neuronal activation and antinociceptive effects during inflammation, 169
hypothalamic-pituitary-adrenal axis, 169
hypothalamic expression of interleukin IL-1β, 169
Infralimbic cortex, modulation of blood pressure by, 378
Innervation density, methods for evaluating cardiac, 254
Intermediolateral nucleus of spinal cord. *See also* Sympathetic nervous system, preganglionics
parabrachial nucleus modulation of, 223
paraventricular nucleus modulation of, 376
Infralimbic cortex
  ablation, effects on
    baroreflex gain, 227
    conditioned heart rate response, 227
  afferent input from, 222
    amygdala, 227
    entorhinal cortex, 227
    hippocampus, 227
    insular cortex, 227
    nucleus tractus solitarius, 227
    parabrachial nucleus, 227
  efferent projections to, 226
    amygdala, central nucleus, 228
    hypothalamus
      anterior, 228
      lateral, 228
    insular cortex, 228
    nucleus of solitary tract, 228
    parabrachial nucleus, 228
    spinal cord, IML cell column, 228
    thalamus, ventral basal, 228
  stimulation, effects on
    blood pressure, 227
    heart rate, 227
    sympathetic nervous system, 230

Infralimbic cortex (*Continued*)
  sympathoinhibition mediated by modulation
    of ventrolateral medulla, 227
  sympathetic-parasympathetic interactions, 232
Inositol triphosphate, alpha adrenergic modulation of, 273
Insular cortex
  ablation, effects on
    blood pressure, 235
    catecholamines, circulating, 235
    sudden cardiac death, 235
    sympathetic nervous system, 226, 235
  afferent inputs to
    baroreceptor sensitive, 231
    parabrachial nucleus, 225
    ventral basal thalamus, 226
  anesthesia, effects on
    cardiovascular control mechanisms, 231
    sympathetic neuromodulation by, 231
  cortical interactions with infralimbic cortex, 227
  electrical stimulation, effects on
    arrhythmias, 227, 235
    blood pressure, 226, 227, 230, 235
    catecholamines, circulating, 226
    gastrointestinal system, 226
    heart rate, 226, 227, 230, 235
    respiration, 226
    sudden cardiac death, 235
  electrocardiogram changes during stimulation of, 227
  functional organization of, 225
  heart rate/blood pressure phase relationships and, 377
  lateralization of CV responses from, 231, 377
    parasympathetic modulation, left side, 231
    sympathetic modulation, right side, 231
  lesions, effects on
    cardiovascular response to stress, 231
    catecholamines, circulating levels of, 231
    sympathetic tone, 231
  modulation of
    baroreflex gain by, 231
    blood pressure by, 377
    parasympathetic nervous system by, 231, 377
    sympathetic nervous system by, 230, 231, 377
    sympathetic-parasympathetic interactions, 232
  viscerotopic map of
    gustatory inputs, 225
    visceral inputs, 225
Intrinsic Cardiac Nervous (ICN) system. *See* Cardiac neurons, intrinsic
Intrathoracic Cardiac Nervous system. *See* Afferents, cardiovascular; Cardiac neuronal hierarchy, cardiac neurons, extrinsic; Cardiac Neurons, intrinsic; Parasympathetic nervous system; Sympathetic nervous system
Ischemic heart disease
  adenosine (iv) and pain perception in, 304
  pain
    intensity in, 304
    threshold in, 304
Isoproterenol, myocyte toxic effects during high level exposure to, 348
Ischemic preconditioning
  cardioprotection from, 288
    aging, effects on, 288
  infarct reduction by, 288
    aging, effects on, 288
  stunning and, 288

Job strain. *See also* Stress, mental
  definition and relation to coronary artery disease, 402

Kallikrein-kinin system, 358
  interactions with renin-angiotensin system, 358, 359
  modulation of catecholamine release by, 358, 359

Lateral hypothalamic area
  cortical projections into, 378
  modulation of sympathetic nervous system by, 375, 376
Lateral Parabrachial Nucleus
  modulation of RVLM, 374
  modulation of sympathetic nervous sytem by, 375
Left ventricle dysfunction
  models of
    angiotension II infusion, 352

Index

mitrial regurgitation, 352
  pacing-induced, 352
  neurohumoral remodeling and relation to, 344, 352
  remodeling in progressive congestive heart failure, 341
  role of excessive sympathetic activation in, 340, 352
Leptin, modulation of paraventricular nucleus activity by, 377
Leukocyte, hostility and β-adrenergic receptor function in, 395
Lifestyle factors in cardiac disease
  age dependent effectiveness, 406
  angina and, 153
  as risk factors, 406
  impact of diet, 406
  impact of exercise, 406
LDL-C
  effects of anxiety on, 400
  effects of depression on, 400
Lipopolysaccharide (LPS) endotoxin
  acute inflammatory reactions induced by, 168
  inflammatory cytokines released following infusion of
    interleukins, IL-1, IL-6, IL-1β, 168
    tumor necrosis factor-α (TNF-α), 168
  systemic response to
    altered pain sensitivity, 169
    glucocorticoid release, 169
    hyperthermia, 169
    liver acute-phase protein release, 169

Matrix, extracellular collagen, 420
  neurohumoral factors influencing, 422
  remodeling during cardiac pathology, 420
Matrix metalloproteinases (MMP's). *See also* Extracellular matrix; TIMP's
  activation during congestive heart failure, 352
  β adrenergic blockade, effects on, 352
  degradation of collagen and, 342
  modulation of activity by
    angiotensin II, 354
    inflammatory cytokines, 354
    norepinephrine, 354
    reactive oxygen species, 354
Maze procedure. *See also* Atrial Fibrillation
  atrial electrical activity
    parasympathetic effects following, 328
  heterogeneity in following, 328
  atrial wavelet formation and, 328
  canine model of, 328
  chronotropic incompetence following, 328
  rationale underlying, 328
Medulla oblongata. *See also individual* brainstem nuclei including RVLM, CVLM,
  NTS, and Area Postrema
  generation of basal autonomic nerve activity by, 375
  integrative capabilities of, 375
  modulation by descending inputs, 375, 378
Mental stress. *See* Stress, mental
Microdialysis, cardiac. *See also* Norepinephrine; Epinephrine
  Angiotensin II sympathetic stimulation and cardiac interstitial levels of
    epinephrine, 129
    norepinephrine, 129
  stellate stimulation and cardiac interstitial fluid (ISF) levels of
    epinephrine, 129, 345, 346
    norepinephrine, 129, 345, 346
  myocardial ischemia and cardiac ISF levels of
    norepinephrine, 345
Middle cervical ganglion. *See also* Cardiac neurons, extrinsic; Sympathetic nervous system
  afferent, modality specificity of
    chemosensory, 83
    mechanosensory, 83
    multimodal, 83
  cholinergic receptor mechanisms in, 132
  neuronal sub-types in
    afferent, 121
    local circuit neurons, 122
    sympathetic postganglionic soma, 122
  control of cardiac function by, 122
  reflex mechanisms in, 124
Muscarinic cholinergic receptors. *See also* Cardiac neurons, voltage gated ion channels
  aging, effects on cardiac, 278
  cAMP dependent effects mediated by, 125
  cardiac distribution of, 278
  effect on intrathoracic sympathetic neurons, 5, 132

Muscarinic cholinergic receptors (*Continued*)
  effect on intrinsic cardiac neurons, 27, 30–34, 132
  G_i protein effects mediated by, 125
  inhibition of norepinephrine release by, 5
  signal transduction by, 125
Myocardial infarction
  alterations in
    baroreflex sensitivity, 137
    cardiac autonomic activity, 167, 200
    heart rate variability, 167
  anger as risk factor for, 232–234, 395
  angina pectoris, history of proceeding, 303
  anxiety as risk factor for, 232, 399
  anxiety and impact on recovery from, 399
  β adrenergic receptor blockade, cardiac remodeling and, 357
  baroreflex sensitivity as risk factor for, 142
  cardiovascular reaction to stress following, 234
  depression following, 396
  circadian variation, 402
  electrocardiogram QRS changes in, 298
  heart rate variability as risk factor for, 142
  inflammatory cytokines, production of, 357
  neurohumoral remodeling of cardiac nervous system, 137
    ventricular fibrillation resistant, 137
    ventricular fibrillation susceptible, 137
      depressed baroreflex sensitivity and, 137
      reduced heart rate variability and, 137
  parasympathetic tone as factor in recovery from, 137, 167, 200
  psychological stress as risk factor for, 232, 401
  recurrent ischemia following acute, 399
  reinfarction following, 399, 401
  reinnervation following, 136
  remodeling of
    cardiac nervous system, 135–138
    myocyte electrical activity, 136
    neurochemical profile of cardiac innervation, 136
      calcitonin gene-related peptide, 136
      vasoactive intestinal peptide, 136
    sympathetic innervation, 136, 142
  silent ischemia, history of preceding, 303
  social support and recovery from, 405
  sympathetic activation and risk for, 142
  therapeutic approaches for treatment of β adrenergic blockade, 357
Myocardial ischemia.
  adenosine receptor blockade
    effects on sensory transduction of, 111
  adenosine release during, 288, 300, 301
    aging, effects on, 288
    cardioprotective effects of, 288
  adenosine triphosphate release during, 11
  afferent nerves activated by, 109–111, 158
    adenosine transduction in, 111
    sympathetic, 158
    vagal, 158
  anger as risk factor for, 232
  anxiety as risk factor for, 232
  arrhythmias, reperfusion, 351
  ATP release during, 300, 301
  behavioral stress as risk factor for, 232
  bradykinin
    facilitation of catecholamine release by, 359
    intracardiac release during, 359
  creatine phosphate in, 300, 301
  effect on
    intrinsic cardiac neurons during, 174
    intrinsic cardiac neuronal ultrastructure, 262
    myocyte excitation-contraction coupling, 153
    parasympathetic efferent nerves during, 137
    heart rate, 137
    vasomotor activity, 153
  electrocardiogram changes in, QRS complex, 298
  neuromodulation and attenuation of, 170
    cardiac metabolism, 173
    coronary blood flow, 173
  oxygen supply/demand in, 153, 173, 300
  release of
    acetylcholine, 298
    adenosine, 155, 298
    bradykinin, 155, 298
    lactate, 155
    norephinephrine, 345
    potassium, 155
    prostaglandins, 155

serotonin, 298
substance P, 298
remodeling of
cardiac nervous system, 135, 137
myocyte electrical function, 137
spinal cord stimulation, stabilizing
effects on
cardiac nervous system during, 174.
See also Cardiac neurons,
intrinsic; Spinal cord
stimulation
Myocardial oxygen demand, depression
and effects on, 397
Myocardial supply/demand
blood flow autoregulation in, 155
coronary artery disease, 155
normal hearts, 155
cardiorespiratory threshold in, 155
coronary artery disease and imbalances
in, 139, 155
excitation-contraction (EC) coupling,
effects on, 155
exercise and, 155
lactate production and, 155
Myocyte
action potential, generation of, 256
ontogeny of, 256
apoptosis. *See* Apoptosis, myocyte
calcium hemeostasis in, 341, 348
ontogeny of, 256, 257, 258
contractile function of, 258
ontogeny of, 258
cell cultures
neonatal versus adult derived cells, 70
co-cultures with autonomic neurons,
62–75
contractile proteins within, 258
ontogeny of, 258
excitation-contraction coupling in, 256
ontogeny of, 256, 257
extrinsic control of. *See* Cardiac
Neuronal Hierarchy; Cardiac
neurons, extrinsic; Cardiac
neurons, intrinsic;
Parasympathetic nervous
system; Sympathetic nervous
system
gap junctions between, 256
ontogeny of, 256, 257
growth of, 341
intrinsic control mechanisms of, 61
mechanosensitive ion channels within,
258
ontogeny of, 258
necrosis. *See* Necrosis, myocyte

ontogeny of receptor systems for
angiotensin II, 260
histamine, 260
remodeling during cardiac pathology,
341, 353, 420
reverse remodeling of, 353
sarcoplasmic reticulum, 256
ontogeny of, 256

NaCl
circadian rhythm of, 379
effects on organum vasculosum of
lamina terminalis, 375
modulation of sympathetic nervous
system by, 375
Necrosis, myocyte
beta adrenergic receptors and, 348
Ca^{++} overload and, 348
Nerve growth factor (NGF)
cardiac content of, 351
intracardiac changes in congestive heart
failure, 351
transcardiac gradient of, 351
Neural disorders, hypersensitive
Syndrome X. *See* Syndrome X
Neuroendocrine function, psychological
factors and, 405
Neurokinin, effects on intrinsic cardiac
neurons, 132
Neuronal transplant. *See* Transplant,
neuronal
Neuropeptide Y (NPY)
interactions with
adrenergic receptor system, 372
adenosine triphosphate (ATP)
receptor system, 372
parasympathetic efferents,
neurotransmitter release, 38
cardiac innervation and, 8, 259
ontogeny of, 259
co-localization with norepinephrine in
sympathetic nerves, 372
intrinsic cardiac neurons, effects on, 38,
132. *See also* Cardiac neurons,
voltage-gated ion channels
hypothalamic actions of, 230
modulation of sympathetic nervous
system by, 375
Neurotensin, effects on parabrachial
neurons, 223
Neuropeptides. *See individual
neurochemicals*
Nicotinic cholinergic blockade
effect on intrinsic cardiac neurons, 319,
321

Nicotinic cholinergic receptors
  cardiac nervous system and modulation of
    chronotropic function, 321
    inotropic fucntion, 321
  effect on (neural)
    intrinsic cardiac neurons, 132, 319, 320 321. See also Cardiac neurons, ligand-gated ion channels; Cardiac neurons, voltage- gated ion channels
    nucleus ambiguus neurons, 205
    sympathetic neurons, 321, 371
Nitric oxide (NO/EDRF)
  activation of
    intrinsic cardiac afferents by, 87
    nodose afferents by, 87
  distribution in intrinsic cardiac nervous system, 11
  modulation intrinsic cardiac neurons by, 260
  ontogeny of, 260
  and β adrenergic response, 357
Nitrergic innervation, cardiac, ontogeny of, 260
Nociceptin, modulation of nucleus ambiguus neurons by, 202
Nodose ganglion afferent neurons. See also Nucleus tractus solitarius
  afferent projections of, 79, 80, 85, 188, 191
    Aδ fibers, 83
    C fibers, 83
  ion channel mechanisms in
    Na$^+$ channels
    Ca^{++}-activated K$^+$ channels
  memory function of, 120
  modality specificity of
    chemosensory, 83, 85, 86, 120
    mechanosensory, 83, 86, 120
    multimodal, 83, 120
  myocardial ischemia, activation of, 109
  reflex response to activation of, 137
  response characteristics of
    chemoreceptors
      slow-responding, 87
      memory function of, 87
    mechanoreceptors
      fast-responding, 86
      limited memory, 86
  sensory neurite distribution of, 79, 80, 120
  sensory transduction of,
    adenosine, 83, 87, 110
    angiotensin II, 87

  arachidonic acid, 87
  bradykinin, 83, 87
  calcitonin gene-related peptide, 87
  catecholamines, 87
  histamine, 87
  hydrogen peroxide, 87
  hydroxyl radicals, 87
  nitric oxide donors, 87
  oxygen free radicals, 87
  pH, 87
  substance P, 83, 87, 110
  vasoactive intestinal peptide, 87
Norepinephrine. See also Adenylate cyclase; Alpha adrenergic receptor; Beta adrenergic receptor; cAMP
  adenosine and sympathetic neuronal release of, 279
  agonist selectivity for adrenergic receptor subtypes, 343
  alpha-adrenergic effects
    presynaptic neural actions, 173, 275, 372
    vasomotor actions, 372
  angiotensin II effects on sympathetic release of, 129, 139, 353, 372
  anti-arrhythmic effects of, 173
  atrial natriuretic peptide (ANP) effects on release of, 372
  beta-adrenergic effects
    β_1 vs. β_2 receptor mediated effects of, 343, 348
    cardiac effects, 372
    β_2 neural effects on release of, 275, 348
    vasomotor effects, 372
  bradykinin effects on release of, 359
  cardiac content, 343
    aging, effects on, 274
    in congestive heart failure, 344, 345
  cardiac preconditioning in response to, 173
  compartmentalization of, 342
    cardiac interstitial versus plasma levels, 345
  congestive heart failure, effects on release of, 353
  effects on
    afferent sensitivity, 100
    intrinsic cardiac neurons, 132
  estrogen effects on release of, 381
  excessive release and cardiac end-organ effects in
    myocyte toxicity, 139, 340
    myocardial fibrosis, 340

Index

ventricular fibrillation threshold, 340
ventricular wall stress, 139, 340
hypothalamic modulation of release, 379
interstitial fluid levels (cardiac) in response to
  angiotensin II, 129, 345, 346, 353
  spinal cord stimulation, 173
  stellate stimulation, 129, 345,346
kinetics, 344
  synthesis, 345, 347
  neuronal release, 129, 343, 344
    aging and, 272, 274, 275
  neuronal clearance (uptake 1), 343–345
    aging and, 272, 275
  uptake by non-neuronal tissue (uptake 2), 343
  spillover, 129, 343–345
kinetics in cardiac pathologies of
  congestive heart failure, 139, 345
  idiopathic dilated cardiomyopathy, 343
  mitrial regurgitation, 353
  valvular heart disease, 343
modulation of cardiac
  conductile tissue by, 340
  contractile function by, 340
  pacemakers by, 340
myocardial remodeling and, 139, 341
myocyte toxicity and
  Ca^{++} influx, 348
  Ca^{++} overload, 348
myocyte viability and, 347
plasma levels of, 129, 274
  aging, effects on, 274
sympathetic stimulation-induced release of, 129, 274
  aging, effects on, 274, 346
Type C natriuretic peptide (CNP) effects
  on release of, 372
tyrosine hydroxylase and synthesis of, 347
NTS. *See* Nucleus tractus solitarius
Nucleus ambiguus
  acetylcholine as neurotransmitter
    for cardiopulmonary neural interactions, 205
    nicotinic receptor effects, 204
      pre-synaptic, 204
      post-synaptic, 204
    interactions with
      GABAergic responses, 204
      glycinergic responses, 204

  non-NMDA receptors, 204
  afferent input from
    nucleus of tractus solitarius, 121, 188, 202
    superior larnygeal neurons, 204
    cardiorespiratory interactions and, 201, 203, 205
  efferent neuronal projections to
    intrinsic cardiac nervous system, 2, 188
  GABA as neurotransmitter, 202
    for cardiopulmonary neural interactions, 205
    nociceptin, interactions with, 202
    shaping of neuronal activity by, 202
    μ-opioids, interactions with, 202
  glutamate as neurotransmitter, 202
    for fast excitatory neurotransmission, 205
    non-NMDA receptor effects, 202
    NMDA receptors effects, 202
  neural activity
    basal, generation of, 201
    effects of anesthesia on, 201
    synaptic mediated, 201
  parasympathetic preganglionic neurons
    location of, 121, 188, 369
  respiratory sinus arrhythmia,
    generation of, 203
    GABAergic inputs and modulation of, 203
Nucleus tractus solitarius (NTS)
  afferent neurotransmission involving
    glutamate, 195
    non-NMDA receptors (primary), 195, 196
    NMDA receptors, 195, 196
  afferent projections to
    aortic depressor nerve, 121, 375
    carotid sinus nerve, 121, 188, 375
    vagal, 121, 188, 375
  baroreflex. *See* Baroreflex
  feedback inhibition within, GABA mediated, 197
    $GABA_A$-mediated, post-synaptic effects, 196
    $GABA_B$-mediated, pre-synaptic effects, 196
  functional organization of, 194
  glutamate mediated excitation of
    non-NMDA receptors (fast neurotransmission), 199
    NMDA receptors, 199
  hypertension, role in, 376
  lesions, effects on blood pressure, 374

Nucleus tractus solitarius (NTS) (*Continued*)
  modulation of sympathetic nervous system by, 375
  Na^+ sensitive inputs to, 378
  neuromodulation of activity by
    biogenic amines, 197
    peptides, 197
      calcitonin gene-related peptide, 198, 199
      substance P, 198
  osmolality sensitive inputs to, 378
  ontogeny of coordinated activity with, 253
  paraventricular nucleus modulation of, 376
  projections from, 375
  efferent neuronal projections to
    caudoventrolateral nucleus, 188, 375
    nucleus ambiguus, 188
    parabrachial nucleus, 221
    rostroventrolateral nucleus, 221
  sensory (afferent neuron) inputs
    cardiovascular, 189, 221
    gastrointestinal, 189, 221
    respiratory, 189, 221
  vicerotropic organization of afferent inputs to, 188

Opioids
  cardioprotective effects of, 173, 334
  modulation of nucleus ambiguus neurons by, 202
  spinal cord stimulation and release of, 334
Organum vasculosum of lamina terminalis (OVLT)
  drinking behavior modulated by, 378
  modulation of
    ANP release by, 379
    blood pressure by, 379, 380
    hypothalamus by, 375, 378
    sympathetic nervous system by, 375, 380
  plasma Na^+ modulation of activity in, 378, 379
  plasma osmolarity modulation of activity in, 378, 379
  projections to anterior hypothalamic nucleus, 379
Osmoreceptors. *See* Afferents, Cardiovascular
Orthostatic intolerance
  aging, effects on induction of, 272

  baroreflex function in, 272
  characteristics of, 272
  end-organ receptor mechanisms in, 272
  sympathetic nervous system and, 272
Ouabain. *See* Digitalis glycosides
Oxidative stress, congestive heart failure and, 342
Oxygen free radicals, nodose afferent activation by, 87
Oxytocin effects on intrinsic cardiac neuronal activity, 319

Pacemaker, cardiac. *See* Sinoatrial node
Pain, ischemic
  adenosine and perception of peripheral, 305
  theophylline blockade of, 305
Pain, neuromodulation of. *See also* Angina pectoris; Spinal cord stimulation; Transcutaneous electrical nerve stimulation
  gate control theory, 157, 169, 172
  vagal afferents, antinociceptive effects on
    cardiac pain, 166
    tail-flick response, 166
Pain, neuropathic
  sensitization of
    central neurons in, 172
    peripheral neurons in, 172
  spinal cord stimulation. *See also* Spinal Cord Stimulation
    GABA release in spinal cord by, 172
    neuronal inhibition in spinal cord by, 172
Pain, referred, neural substrate for, 159. *See also* Angina pectoris
Panic disorder as predictor of cardiac disease and mortality, 400
Parabrachial Nucleus
  efferent projections to
    amygdala (central nucleus), 222
    dorsal motor nucleus, 223
    hypothalamus
      paraventricular nucleus, 222
      supraoptic nucleus, 222
    intermediolateral nucleus of spinal cord, 223
    intralimbic cortex, 222
    nucleus ambiguus, 223
    thalamus, ventral basal, 222
  electrical stimulation, effects on blood pressure, 223
  functional organization of, 221, 223
  integrative function of, 223

Index 455

neuropeptides modulating activity within,
  calcitonin gene-related peptide, 223
  cholecystokinin, 223
  neurotensin, 223
  somotostatin, 223
  substance P, 223
neurotransmitter mechanisms within
  α_2 adrenergic receptors, 223
  GABAa receptors, 223
  NMDA receptors, 223
nucleus of solitary tract, input to
  cardiovascular related, 221
  gustatory related, 222
Parasympathetic nervous system. *See also* Baroreflex; Cardiac neurons, intrinsic; Dorsal motor nucleus; Muscarinic cholinergic receptor; Nucleus ambiguus; Nucleus tractus solitarius; Nicotinic cholinergic receptor; Spinal cord, sacral
  aging, effects on
    antiadrenergic action, 278
    muscarinic receptor activity, 278
  anatomical organization of, 2, 122, 369
  antiadrenergic effects of, 278
  anxiety and effects on activity of, 400
  baroreflex control of. *See* Baroreflex
  cardiac innervation, 122, 255
    ontogeny of, 255
  coordination of activity in, 200
    cardiac periodicity in, 206
    respiratory periodicity in, 203
  depression and effects on activity, 397
  effect on
    atrial electrical function, 2, 122, 324, 328
    cardiac conduction, 2, 122, 316, 322
    cardiac contractility, 2, 80, 122, 369
      ontogeny of, 255
    cardiac pacemakers, 2, 80, 122, 316, 369, 395
      ontogeny of, 255
  exercise training, effects on, 200
  ganglia, intracardiac, 317–321. *See also* Cardiac neurons, intrinsic
  interactions with sympathetic nerves, 125, 200, 419
    ontogeny of, 255
    pre-junctional interactions, 125
    post-junctional interactions, 125
  maze surgical procedure and effects on, 328
  parabrachial nucleus, effects on, 223

postganglionic projections from, 2, 122, 324, 328, 369. *See also* Cardiac neurons, intrinsic
preganglionic projections from, 2, 122, 328, 329, 369
  asymmetry in, 2
  divergence of inputs to intrinsic cardiac nervous system, 2
  remodeling in progressive cardiovascular disease
    heart failure, 200
    hypertension, 200
Paraventricular Hypothalamic Nucleus (PVN). *See also* Hypothalamus; Paraventricular nucleus (PVN)
  modulation of RVLM, 374
  neurohumoral modulation of, 377
Paravertebral sympathetic ganglia, organization of, 368. *See also* Sympathetic nervous system
Peptides. *See individual neurochemicals*
Peptidergic innervation, cardiac
  ontogeny of, 254
    atrial versus ventricular tissues, 255
    intrinsic cardiac nerves containing neuropeptide Y, 73, 259
    somatostatin, 259, 260
    vasoactive intestinal peptide, 73, 259, 260
Periaqueductal gray
  brainstem projections, 374
  cortical modulation of, 378
  modulation of RVLM, 374
Percutaneous transluminal coronary angioplasty (PTCA)
  hostility and need for, 394
  restenosis following, 394
Petrosal ganglia, afferent projections of, 191
Pituitary adenylate cyclase-activating polypeptide (PACAP)
  cardiac distribution of, 39
  co-localization with parasympathetic neurons, 39
  ontogeny of, 39
  PAC_1 receptors mediated effects on intracardiac neurons. *See also* Cardiac neurons, voltage-gated ion channels
    depolarization of, 39
    modulation of excitability, 39
    inhibition of current I_A, 39
Plasma volume
  neurohumoral modulation of, 369
  renal regulation of, 369

Platelet reactivity
  depression and relation to, 397
  hostility and relation to, 395
  psychological stress and effects on, 403
Pons/midbrain. See also Lateral Parabrachial N.; Periaqueductal Gray
  modulation by descending inputs, 375
  modulation of sympathetic activity by, 375
Posterior hypothalamic nucleus
  modulation of
    blood pressure by, 380
    sympathetic activity by, 375, 376, 380
Power spectral analysis. See Heart rate variability
Preconditioning, Cardiac. See Cardiac preconditioning
Prefrontal cortex, modulation of blood pressure by, 378
Premature Ventricular Contractions (PVC)
  intrinsic cardiac neronal stimulation and induction of, 264
  post-MI depression and relation to, 397
Prevertebral sympathetic ganglia, organization of, 369. See also Sympathetic nervous system
Protein kinase C (PKC), adrenergic receptor modulation of, 273
Pseudorabies virus as transneuronal marker, 204
Psychological aspects of heart disease. See Anger; Anxiety; Behavior; Depression; Exhaustion; Hostility; Stress (mental); Social support; Lifestyle
Pulsus alternans, afferent transduction of, 92
Purinergic innervation, cardiac, ontogeny of, 259
Purinergic receptors. See also Adenosine; Adenosine triphosphate
  afferent activation and pain perception, 302
  cardiomyocyte effects of, 301
  effects on
    dorsal root afferents, 89, 95
    intrathoracic afferents, 95
    intrinsic cardiac neurons, 132
    parasympathetic efferent neurons,
      A1 inhibition of, 302
      A2 excitation of, 302

    sympathetic efferent neurons
      A1 inhibition of, 302
    vasomotor actions of
      A_1 versus A_2 receptor mediated, 302

Radiofrequency catheter ablation, effects on cardiac nervous system, 421
Reactive inflammatory species (RIS)
  myocardial remodeling and, 341, 354, 357
  reactive inflammatory species (RIS), 357
  β adrenergic receptor blockade and, 357
  reactive oxygen species (ROS), 357
  iNOS expression in CHF, 357
  nitric oxide (NO) and β adrenergic response, 357
Remodeling in progressive cardiac disease. See also Ventricular remodeling
  β-adenoreceptor blockade effects on, 352, 411
  cardiac matrix, extracellular, 421
    in congestive heart failure, 341
    mitral regurgitation, 352
  chamber, left ventricular in
    mitral regurgitation, 352
    pacing induced heart failure, 352
  electrical remodeling, myocyte, 118, 136, 141, 421
  ion channels, in response to
    axotomy, 192
    growth factors, 192
    increased activity, 192
    inflammatory agents, 192
  neurohumoral, cardiac nervous system, in, 106, 118, 128, 174, 421
    atrial arrhythmias, 111
    atrial fibrillation, 111
    cardiac neuronal ablation, 47, 110, 134
    coronary artery disease, 187
    chronic angiotensin II infusion, 350, 352
    congestive heart failure, 111, 128, 342, 344, 345, 351
    chronic myocardial ischemia, 47, 107, 110, 310
    development, 191
    hypertension, 379
    mitrial regurgitation, 352
    myocardial infarction, 136, 200, 352
    myocardial ischemia, 136
    pacing induced heart failure, 352
    post-cardiac surgery, 47, 110
    silent ischemia, 310

sinus node disease, 134
sudden infant death syndrome, 263
syndrome x, 307
ventricular arrhythmias, 111
Remodeling, neural
 in aging, 191, 272
 following
  nerve damage, 47, 131, 134, 206, 207
   capsaicin induced, 207
  stimulation, 192, 198
Respiratory sinus arrhythmia,
 afferent modulation of, 203
 cardiovascular disease, effects on, 202
 central neuronal generation of, 203
 characteristics of, 202
Reverse remodeling in cardiac pathology
 β-adenoreceptor blockade effects on
  extracellular matrix, 352
  LV chamber function, 353, 355, 356
  myocytes, 352
Renin
 increased activity in congestive heart
   failure
  cardiac mechanisms, 352
  renal mechanisms, 352
Renin-angiotensin system, 358
 interactions with kallikrein-kinin
   system, 358, 359
 modulation of catecholamine release
   by, 358, 359
Rostroventrolateral Medulla (RVLM)
 acetylcholine effects on, 374
 AMPA receptors and, 374
 AT1-angiotensin II receptors and
   modulation of, 374
 Baroreflex. See Baroreflex
 bulbospinal projections to IML, 188
 caudoventrolateral medulla (CVLM),
   interactions with, 374
 descending projections to, 374
 excitatory inputs to, 374
 GABA effects on, 374
 glutamate effects on, 230, 374
  AMPA receptors, 230
  Kainate receptors, 230
 inhibitory inputs to, 374
 modulation of
  blood pressure by, 380
  sympathetic tone by, 188, 374, 375,
    380
 muscarinic receptors within, 374
 pacemaker activity within, 374
 paraventricular nucleus modulation of,
   376

peptides as putative neurotransmitters,
   374
RVLM. See Rostroventrolateral Medulla
Ryanodine receptor (RyR2)
 β adrenergic blockade and maintenance
   of, 356
 congestive heart failure and, 356
 sympathetic overdrive and expression
   of, 355

Salt. See NaCl
Serotonin, distribution to cardiac nervous
   system, 10
Sex-related differences in
 adrenergic modulation of cardiac
   contractile function, 273
  aging, effects on, 273
 catecholamine release from sympathetic
   nerves, 274
  aging, effects on, 274
Silent ischemia
 frequency of, 303
 symptoms in, 303
Sinoatrial node
 adenosine and
  modulation of, 279
  pacemaker shifts induced by, 279
 intrinsic cardiac neuronal modulation of,
  posterior atrial ganglionated plexus,
    134
  right atrial ganglionated plexus, 134
 pacemaker activity in, 256
  ontogeny of, 256
 parasympathetic influences on, 133,
   134. See also Parasympathetic
   nervous system
 reflex control of, 98
 sympathetic, parasympathetic
   interactions, 126, 200
 sympathetic influences on, 126, 254. See
   also Sympathetic nervous
   system
  ontogeny of, 254
Social Support
 definition and factors involved in, 404
 impact on recovery from cardiac
   disease, 404
Somatostatin
 cardiac innervation and, 8, 259
  ontogeny of, 259
 effect on
  intrinsic cardiac neurons, 260
   ontogeny of, 260
  parabrachial neurons, 223

Spinal cord
  intermediolateral cell column, convergence of input at, 375
  parasympathetic preganglionics, 368
    sacral spinal cord organization of, 369
  sympathetic preganglionics, 368
Spinal cord, segmental interactions
  cervical (C1–C2) modulation of upper thoracic cord
    inhibition of, 153, 162, 163
    propriospinal projections mediating, 163, 164, 165
    supraspinal modulation of, 163
    vagal afferent modulation of, 153, 162,165
  cervical (C1–C2) modulation of lumbosacral cord,
    propriospinal projections mediating, 165
  cervical (C3 and below), vagal afferent modulation of, 166
  thoracic
    cardiac afferent input to, 158–161
      lamina activate by cardiac afferent inputs, 161
    efferent projections from, spinothalamic tract, 159
    inhibition, descending of, 160, 162
    vagal afferent suppression of, 167
      C1–C2 as relay for, 168
  vagal afferent modulation of
    cervical neurons, 153
      direct projection to, 168
      nucleus tractus solitarius as relay for, 168
      subcoeruleus/parabrachial pathway in, 168
    thoracic neurons, 167
Spinal Cord Stimulation (SCS)
  angina, treatment of, 139, 156, 162, 171, 332, 422
  caffeine, attenuation of neuromodulation effects by, 174
  cervical versus thoracic stimulation, effects of, 171
  effects on
    angina warning system, 156
    autonomic reflex function, 169
    cardiac electrophysiology, ST segment, 139
    cardiac interstitial catecholamines, 173
    cardiac nervous system, 333, 335, 422
      in basal conditions, 140, 174, 333
      during transient myocardial ischemia, 140, 174, 333
    cardiac metabolism, 173
    cardiac supply/demand, 173, 332, 333
    coronary blood flow redistribution, 169, 172, 173, 333
    exercise tolerance, 140
    intrinsic cardiac neurons, stabilization of
      local circuit neurons, 141
      neuronal activity in
        basal conditions, 140, 174
        during myocardial ischemia, 140, 174
    ischemic pain, 170
    skin temperature, 169
    spinal cord inhibitory neuronal networks, 172
    sympathetic nerve activity, 172, 173
  efferent projections mediating peripheral effects, 140
  ischemia, protection from tissue damage by
    calcitonin gene-related peptide (CGRP), 173
    heat shock proteins, 173
  neural memory of, 171
  neurogenic pain, effects on, 332
  neuropathetic pain, effects on, 169
  peripheral neurotransmitter release of
    calcitonin gene-related peptide, 141, 334
    endorphins, 141
    opioids, 334
    substance P, 141
  technique for, 139, 170, 171
Statins, as treatment for hyperlipidemia, 407
Stellate ganglion. *See also* Cardiac neurons, extrinsic; Sympathetic nervous system
  afferent neurons, modality specificity of
    chemosensory, 83
    mechanosensory, 83
    multimodal, 83
  cholinergic receptor mechanisms in, 132
  control of cardiac function by, 122
  neuronal sub-types in
    afferent, 121
    local circuit neurons, 122
    sympathetic postganglionic soma, 122

Index

reflex mechanisms in, 124
Stress, behavioral
  effects on
    cardiac function, 232
    cardiac pathology, 232
    ventricular fibrillation, 232
Stress, mental
  angina associated with, 155
  effects on cardiac function and
      pathology, 234, 400
  coronary artery stenosis, 155, 233
  myocardial infarction, 233
  hypertension, associated with, 233
  intervention therapy and cardiac effects
      of, 401
  psychological definition of, 400
  reactors versus non-reactors
    blood pressure response in, 235
    characteristics of, 235
    heart rate response in, 235
    lateralization of CV control in, 235
    sympathetic neuromodulation in, 235
  work related and impact on cardiac
      pathology, 402
Stroke
  aging, effects on cardiovascular deficits
      following, 236
  insular strokes, effects on
    blood pressure, 232, 236
    catecholamines, circulating, 232, 236
    heart rate variability, 236
    modulation of sympathetic tone, 232,
        236, 377
    neurotransmitter profile in amygdala,
        235
    heart rate/blood pressure phase
        relationships, 377
    mortality, 232, 236
  cardiac dysfunction associated with,
      220, 236
Subfornical organ (SFO)
  angiotensin II modulation of, 378
  modulation of hypothalamus by, 375,
      378
  modulation of sympathetic nervous
      system by, 375
Substance P
  distribution in intrinsic cardiac nervous
      system, 8, 9, 40
  effects on
    cardiac function, 40
    dorsal root afferent neurons, 89
    intrinsic cardiac neurons, 40, 97, 132,
        319. *See also* Cardiac neurons,
        voltage-gated ion channels

nodose ganglion afferent neurons, 87
    NTS neurons, 198
    parabrachial neurons, 223
    parasympathetic nervous system, 40
    sympathetic nervous system, 40
  extrasynaptic effects of, 198
  myocardial ischemia and release of, 110
  release from cardiac afferents, 193
    effects on mast cells, 193
    effects on vasomotor tone, 193
  synaptic effects of, 198
Sudden cardiac death
  anger as risk factor for, 232, 234
  anxiety as risk factor for, 232, 399
  autonomic dysfunction in cardiac
      nervous system and, 137, 142,
      200, 422
  baroreflex gain as marker of, 142
  heart rate variability as marker of,
      142
  circadian variation, 402
  congestive heart failure and, 341
  handedness as risk factor for, 232
  heterogeneous sympathetic innervation
      and risk of, 352
  myocyte electrical remodeling and
      potential for, 137
  neurological pathology as factor in, 235
  parasympathetic tone as factor in, 200
  post MI-depression as risk factor for,
      396
  psychological stress and impact on, 232,
      235, 401
  seizures, limbic, and, 232 , 234
  stroke and neural substrate for, 236
Sudden Infant Death Syndrome (SIDS)
  autonomic dysfunction and, 203, 263
  cardiopulmonary control dysfunction
      and, 203
  heart rate variability and potential for,
      263
  maternal smoking and risk for, 203
  postnatal nicotine exposure and risk
      for, 203
Sympathetic nervous system. *See also*
      Cardiac nerve, extrinsic;
      Cardiac nerves, intrinsic
  adrenalectomy, effects on, 130. *See also*
      Adrenalectomy
  adenosine receptor mediated effects on,
      301, 305
  anatomical organization, 1, 121, 368
  angiotensin II receptor mediated effects
      on, 128, 129, 349, 372
  angiotensin II production by, 129

Sympathetic nervous system (*Continued*)
  anxiety and effects of activity of, 400
  area postrema modulation of, 376
  atrial natriuretic peptide (ANP) receptor mediated effects on, 372
  bradykinin receptor mediated effects on, 359
  cardiac innervation density
    ontogeny of, 254, 255
    reduction with chronic NE, 351
  cardiac periodicity in activity, ontogeny of, 253
  catecholamines
    circulating as index of, 130, 370
    release by
      angiotensin II-AT1 receptor nerve stimulation, 129
      stellate electrical stimulation, 129, 130
  central nervous system modulation of, 222, 223, 226, 229. *See also* Amygdala; Baroreflex; Parabrachial nucleus; Insular Cortex; Infralimbic cortex; Hypothalamus; Nucleus tractus solitarius; Rostroventrolateral medulla; Thalamus, ventral basal
  cholinergic synaptic mechanisms in, 301
  circadian variation in activity of, 402
  congestive heart failure and, Chapter 12
  cortical modulation of, 377
  diabetes, Type 2, effects on, 371
  effect on
    cardiac conduction, 1, 122
    cardiac contractility, 1, 80, 122, 344, 369
    cardiac pacemakers, 1, 80, 122, 369
    peripheral vascular resistance, 369
  epinephrine, pre-junctional effects on norepinephrine release, 130
  estrogen effects on, 381, 382
  galanin receptor mediated effects on, 372
  ganglia, intracardiac. *See* Cardiac neurons, intrinsic; Cardiac neurons, extrinsic
  hypothalamic modulation of, 375–379
  interaction with parasympathetic efferents, 125, 200, 419
    ontogeny of, 255
    pre-junctional interactions, 125
    post-junctional interactions, 125
  microneurography as index of, 343, 371
  myocardial infarction, remodeling of, 352
  neuropeptide Y (NPY)
    interaction with adrenergic systems, 125, 372
    release from, 372
  hyper-activity in hypertension, 371
  intersegmental coordination, ontogeny of, 253
  obesity, effects on, 371
  paravertebral ganglia, 368
  prevertebral ganglia, 369
  psychological stress and effects of activity on, 403
  renal sympathetic innervation, 371
  respiratory modulation of activity, ontogeny of, 253
  stimulation and release of angiotensin II by, 349
  type C natriuretic peptide (CNP) mediated effects on, 372
Synaptic transmission. *See specific receptor types*
Syndrome X
  adenosine (iv) and pain perception in, 304
  adenosine-induced analgesia in, 309
  anxiety and pain perception in, 308
  cardiac neuronal hierarchy and, 307
  epinephrine (iv) and pain perception in, 306
  exercise induced
    angina in, 306, 309
    ST depression in, 306
  microvascular angina pectoris, 306
  neural remodeling in, 307
  pain
    perception and, 304
    threshold in, 304
  sympathetic tone and, 306

Thalamus, ventral basal
  afferent input from
    parabrachial nucleus, 222
    spinal cord, 224
  circadian rhythm and, 224
  efferent projections to
    infralimbic cortex, 224
    insular cortex, 222
  modality specificity within, 224
  neurotransmitter mechanisms within
    muscarinic receptors
      M_2 inhibitory effects, 224
      M_3/M_5 excitatory effects, 224
    non-NMDA, excitatory effects, 224

visceral inputs to, 222
  baroreceptor related, 223
  chemoreceptor related, 223
  gustatory related, 223
  pulmonary related, 223
Telencephalon, modulation of sympathetic activity by, 375. *See also* Amygdala
Tissue inhibitors of metalloproteinases (TIMP's), inhibition of MMP activation by, 342. *See also* Extracellular matrix, Matrix metalloproteinases
TNF-α
  β adrenergic receptor blockade, effects on production of, 357
  heart failure and induction of, 357
  myocardial infarction and production of, 357
Transcutaneous electrical nerve stimulation (TENS)
  algesic effects of, 308
  caffeine effects of response to, 308
  effects on
    angina pectoris, 156
    angina warning system, 156
    coronary blood flow, 173
Transgenic mice
  AT1a receptor knockout and reduced arrhythmia formation on myocardial reperfusion, 351
  β_2 adrenergic receptor overexpression and
    cardiac effects of, 348
    non-pathological consequences of, 348
  β_1 adrenergic receptor overexpression and cardiomyopathy, 348
  BK$_2$ receptor knockout and reduced norepinephrine release from sympathetics, 359
Transplant, neuronal, induction of hypertension by, 376
Type A behavior, see Behavior, Type A
Type B behavior, see Behavior, Type B
Tyrosine hydroxylase
  congestive heart failure and effects on, 344, 347
  synthesis of norepinephrine and, 347

Vagus nerve. *See* Afferent neurons, cardiovascular; Parasympathetic nervous system

Valsalva maneuver
  ontogeny of cardiovascular response to, 252, 254
Valvular heart disease, norepinephrine kinetics in, 343
Vasoactive Intestinal Peptide
  cardiac innervation and, 8, 259
  ontogeny of, 259
  effect on
    intrinsic cardiac neurons, 36, 125, 132, 319
    ontogeny of, 260
  nodose afferents, 87
Vasomotor control
  adenosine and, 301
  effects of stress on, 403
  estrogen effects on, 382
Vasopressin. *See* Arginine Vasopressin
Ventricular arrhythmia
  anger as risk factor for, 232
  autonomic imbalance and potential for, 131, 134
    focal neural activation and, 134
    myocardial ischemia and, 137
    nerve network filter characteristics and, 134
  anxiety as risk factor for, 232
  bradykinin facilitation of, 358
  epileptic seizures and, 232
  infralimbic stimulation and induction of, 232
  insular cortex stimulation and induction of, 227, 232
  myocyte electrical remodeling and potential for, 137
  psychological stress as risk factor for, 232
  remodeling of cardiac nervous system in, 111
  stress induced
    central nervous system and, 134
    intrathoracic nervous system and, 134
  stroke and neural substrate for, 236
  sudden infant death and, 264
  sympathetic-parasympathetic interactions mediating, 264
Ventricular conductile system, 256
  ontogeny of, 256, 257
  sudden infant death and degeneration within, 264
Ventricular contractile function
  afterload effects on, 257
  ontogeny of, 257, 258
  Ca^{++} handling and modulation of, 257

Ventricular contractile function (*Continued*)
  ontogeny of, 258
  congenital cardiac malformations and, 262
  echocardiographic evaluation of in infants, 257
  intrinsic cardiac neuronal modulation of, 258
    ontogeny of, 258
  neurochemical profile for innervation
    neuropeptide Y, 9
    somatostatin, 9
    tryosine hydroxylase, 9
    vasoactive intestinal peptide, 9
  preload effects on, 257
    ontogeny of, 257, 258
  pressure volume loops and evaluation of, 257
    ontogeny of, 257
  reflex control of, 99. *See also* Parasympathetic nervous system; Sympathetic nervous system
  stretch, response in, 258
    ontogeny of, 258
Ventricular dysfunction
  angiotensin II-sympathetic interactions and induction of, 139
  intrinsic cardiac nervous system imbalance in, 140
    descending inputs stabilizing, 140
  congestive heart failure and, 139, 340
  excessive sympathetic stimulation and, 340
Ventricular electrical activity. *See also* Effective refractory period
  activation-recovery intervals
    intrinsic cardiac neuronal modulation of, 326, 331
    regional difference in, 326
  angiotensin II effects on, 331
  evaluation of using
    activation-recovery interval, 326
    QRST area, 326
    unipolar electrograms, extracellular, as index of, 326
Ventricular fibrillation. *See also* Ventricular arrhythmia
  anger as risk factor for, 233
  autonomic dysfunction and
    induction of, 109, 137, 142, 176, 340, 422
    preceding, 109
  baroreflex sensitivity and risk of, 137
  bradykinin facilitation of, 358
  congestive heart failure and, 340
  heart rate variability and risk of, 137
  heterogeneous sympathetic innervation and risk of, 352
  induced by
    amygdala stimulation, 228
    intrinsic cardiac neuronal stimulation, 264
  myocardial infarction and induction of, 352
  myocardial ischemia and induction of, 228
    amygdala modulation of, 228
  myocyte electrical remodeling and potential for, 137
  parasympathetic activity and reduced risk of, 142
  psychological stress as risk factor for, 232, 403
  public access defibrillators (PAD) and, 142
  resistant animals, 137, 420
  stress induced, 233
  susceptible animals, 137, 420
  sympathetic activity and risk of, 109, 340
Ventricular function curves
  β adrenergic blockade, effects on 356
  congestive heart failure, effects on 356
Ventricular remodeling in cardiac pathology
  chamber diameter and, 341, 355
  extracellular matrix and, 341, 352, 354
  growth factors in, 341
  hemodynamic factors in, 341
  LV chamber stiffness, 356
  LV isovolumetic relaxation in, 356
  LV systolic elastance, 356
  LV wall thickness/diameter ratio in, 341
  myocardial wall stress and, 341, 352
  myocytes and, 341
  neurohumoral factors
    aldosterone, 341
    angiotensin, 341, 352
    bradykinin, 341
    norepinephrine, 341, 352
  reactive inflammatory species in, 341, 354
  stages of, 341
  therapeutic approaches targeting
    cardiac nervous system, 341, 355

Index   463

noradrenergic system, 341, 353, 355
renin-angiotensin system, 341
wall thickening and, 341
Ventricular repolarization. *See also*
        Effective refractory period;
        Ventricular Electrical
        Activity
    activation-recovery interval as index of,
        326
    QRST area as index of, 326
    sympathetic effect on, 331
Ventricular septal defects
    cardiac blood shunts resulting from,
        262
    depletion of myocyte contractile
        elements in, 262

intrinsic cardiac nervous system,
        changes in, 262
    neural/myocyte connections in, 262
    perineural fibrosis in, 262
    volume overload in, 262
Ventricular tachycardia. *See also*
        Ventricular arrhythmias
    depression as risk factor for, 397
    heterogeneous sympathetic innervation
        and risk of, 352
    induced by intrinsic cardiac neuronal
        stimulation, 264
    psychological stress as risk factor for, 403
Visceral afferent neurons. *See* Afferent
        neurons, cardiovascular
Vital exhaustion. *See* Exhaustion, vital